McGraw-Hill's

EMT-Paramedic

Peter A. DiPrima, Jr., EMT-P
Program Coordinator for Basic, Advanced Cardiac,
and Pediatric Life Support
Emergency Training Institute
New York-Presbyterian Hospital
Weill Cornell Medical Center
New York City
Lead Paramedic/Certified Instructor Coordinator
Holbrook Fire District
Holbrook, New York

George P. Benedetto, Jr., DHA(c), MPA, EMT-P
Trauma Coordinator
Department of Surgery
New York Hospital Queens
Flushing, New York
EMS Emergency Care Instructor and Educator
New York-Presbyterian Hospital
The University Hospital of Columbia and Cornell
New York, New York

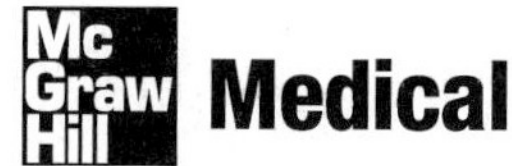

New York Chicago San Francisco Lisbon London Madrid Mexico City Milan New Delhi
San Juan Seoul Singapore Sydney Toronto

McGraw-Hill's EMT-Paramedic

1 2 3 4 5 6 7 8 9 0 QDP/QDP 0 9 8

ISBN 978-0-07-149680-3
MHID 0-07-149680-7

NOTICE

Medicine is an ever-changing science. As new research and clinical experience broaden our knowledge, changes in treatment and drug therapy are required. The authors and the publisher of this work have checked with sources believed to be reliable in their efforts to provide information that is complete and generally in accord with the standards accepted at the time of publication. However, in view of the possibility of human error or changes in medical sciences, neither the authors nor the publisher nor any other party who has been involved in the preparation or publication of this work warrants that the information contained herein is in every respect accurate or complete, and they disclaim all responsibility for any errors or omissions or for the results obtained from use of the information contained in this work. Readers are encouraged to confirm the information contained herein with other sources. For example and in particular, readers are advised to check the product information sheet included in the package of each drug they plan to administer to be certain that the information contained in this work is accurate and that changes have not been made in the recommended dose or in the contraindications for administration. This recommendation is of particular importance in connection with new or infrequently used drugs.

The book was set in Minion by International Typesetting and Composition.
The editors were Catherine A. Johnson and Kim J. Davis.
The production supervisor was Sherri Souffrance.
Project management was provided by Arushi Chawla, International Typesetting and Composition.
The designer was Eve Siegel; the cover designer was Handel Low.
The cover photo was provided by RF-Veer.
The index was prepared by Susan Hunter.
Quebecor World/Dubuque was the printer and binder.

This book is printed on acid-free paper.

Library of Congress Cataloging-in-Publication Data

DiPrima, Peter A.
McGraw-Hill's EMT-Paramedic / Peter A. DiPrima Jr., George Benedetto Jr.
p. ; cm.
Includes bibliographical references.
ISBN 978-0-07-149680-3 (pbk. : alk. paper) 1. Medical emergencies—Examinations, questions, etc. 2. Emergency medical technicians—Examinations, questions, etc. I. Benedetto, George. II. Title.
[DNLM: 1. Emergency Medical Services—United States—Examination Questions. 2. Emergencies—United States—Examination Questions. 3. Emergency Medical Technicians—United States—Examination Questions. 4. Emergency Treatment—United States—Examination Questions. WB 18.2 D596e 2008]
RC86.9.D57 2008
616.02'5076—dc22

2007036799

To my wife, Sue, and our children, Gabrielle and Jack, thank you for being there, with love.

PAD

To my daughter, Alessandra (Ale), you are the center of my universe and the reason I exist. To my brothers and sisters, Nancy, George-Anne (Jan), Michael, Christopher, James, RoseMarie, and Paul, thank you for your loving support and encouragement; and to Angela, Anna, Christopher, and Peter, you four have made my life and career come full circle. I love and cherish you all so very much. To Nayna Shah and Kenneth M. Rifkind, MD, FACS, my teachers, mentors, and friends for life. Thank you.

GPB

CONTENTS

PREFACE

The concept of the team approach is important in responding to emergencies in the prehospital environment. Each health-care professional must not only perform the duties of his or her own role but must understand the roles of other involved professionals.

Nurses, physicians, emergency medical technicians, first responders, police officers, and firefighters, must work together in a coordinated and efficient manner to achieve optimal results for patient survival.

This review book is divided into seven sections that correspond with the Paramedic National Curriculum. Each chapter provides a scenario to further assist the student in understanding emergency medicine as it relates to real-life situations, and, at the end of each chapter, questions are provided to complete the learning process of each subject.

The review book also provides the theory adapted by the American Heart Association 2005 Guidelines for Cardiopulmonary Resuscitation and Emergency Cardiovascular Care, the National Incident Management System, and updated hazardous materials information for the first responder.

The practice exam questions and answers included in this book are also available online to help you prepare for exam day. Visit www.mcgrawhillemt.com to take the test and assess your results.

We hope you enjoy utilizing this book as an adjunct learning tool. Be safe!

Peter A. DiPrima, Jr., EMT-P
George P. Benedetto, Jr., EMT-P

EXAM PREPARATION TIPS

Start studying now! Give yourself ample time to prepare by arranging your notes and making sure you have covered all the required course material. Organize all information that was given during your course—this includes textbooks, lecture notes, handouts, and the like.

ANATOMY OF A MULTIPLE-CHOICE QUESTION

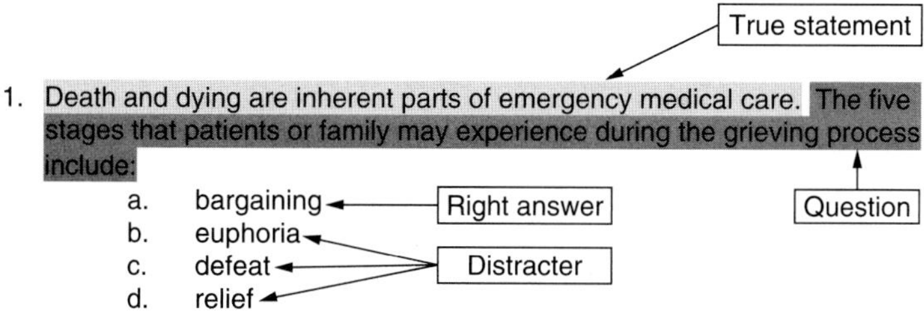

THE DO'S AND DON'TS OF ANSWERING MULTIPLE-CHOICE QUESTIONS

Do's

- If the question is "theoretical," carefully read and understand the stem of the question before looking at the alternatives. Circle or underline key words in the stem. Use your knowledge of headings to think about where in your text, lecture notes, etc. that question is drawn from. Recall a few relevant points about the information. This does not have to take much time but this recall is an essential step!
- Predict an answer, if possible.
- Uncover all of the alternatives and check the format of the question. Are one of the alternatives correct or can several or all of the alternatives be correct?
- Read each alternative carefully for understanding. Pay careful attention to qualifying words. Keeping the stem of the question in mind, respond to each alternative with a yes, no, or maybe/not sure.
- If you know the answer, carefully mark the correct answer on your answer sheet.
- If you do not know the answer, re-check the stem of the question. Narrow your choices, by eliminating any alternative that you know is incorrect. If two options still look equally tempting, compare each to the stem of the question, making sure that the one you eventually choose answers what is asked.
- If you are still not sure, make an educated guess.
- If you were unable to make a choice and need to spend more time with the question, or you answered the question but are not at all sure that you made the correct choice, put a big question mark beside that question, and move on to the next. Avoid

getting bogged down on one question part of the way through the exam. It is much better to move on and finish all of those questions that you can answer and then to come back later to process the problematic questions. If necessary, when looking over the questions again, change an answer ONLY if you can logically justify the change.

Don'ts

- Don't select an alternative just because you remember learning the information in the course; it may be a "true" statement in its own right, but you have to make sure that it is the "correct" answer to the question.
- Don't pick an answer just because it seems to make sense.
- Don't dismiss an alternative answer because it seems too obvious and simple.
- Don't be wowed by fancy terms in the question.
- Don't pick "c" every time you are unsure of the answer.
- Don't pick your answer based on a pattern of responses.

PHYSICAL PREPARATION

It is crucial to know the material to pass the exam, but it is equally important to be prepared physically as well. Physical preparation includes staying healthy, getting adequate sleep, eating balanced meals, and exercising regularly. Reward yourself after a successful study session.

Finally, keep anxiety in check! Stretch, breathe deeply, breathe often, take frequent short breaks, and stay positive.

Section 1

Preparatory

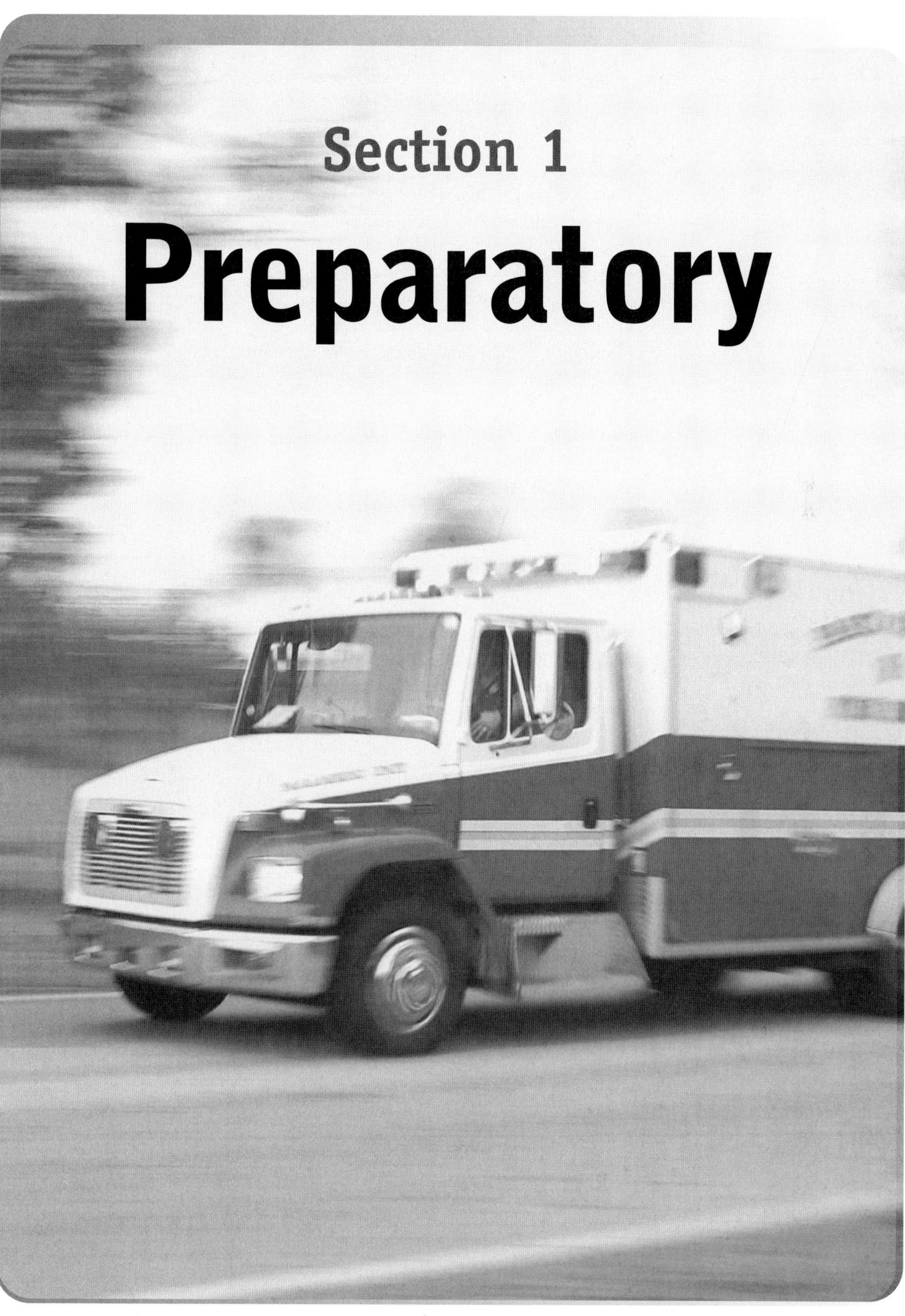

Chapter 1
EMS Systems/Roles and Responsibilities

WHAT IS AN EMS SYSTEM?

An emergency medical services (EMS) system is a network of coordinated medical services that provides support and medical care to a given community.

National Highway Traffic Safety Administration (NHTSA) Technical Assistance Program Assessment Standards for EMS include:

- Integration of health services
- EMS research
- Legislation and regulation
- System finance
- Human resources
- Medical direction
- Education systems
- Public education
- Prevention
- Public access
- Communication systems
- Clinical care
- Information systems
- Evaluation

WHO ARE THE KEY PLAYERS IN AN EMS SYSTEM?

- EMS personnel:
  - First responders
  - Basic life support (BLS) responders
  - Advanced responders
- EMS physicians
- EMS dispatchers
- Public safety organizations
- Specialized resources
- Medical educators
- Citizens
- Regulatory agencies
- EMS system leaders
- Receiving facilities

- Receiving physicians
- Health-care staff
- Researchers
- Community leaders

EMS CREDENTIALING

- **Certification**—Agency or association grants recognition.
- **Licensure**—Governmental agency's competency standards are met.
- **National Registry**—National organization grants standardized recognition.
- **Reciprocity**—Agency grants certification/licensure to person with equivalent certification/licensure from another agency.

NATIONAL EMS CERTIFICATION LEVELS

Basic Life Support (BLS)	**Advanced Life Support (ALS)**
• First responder	• EMT-Intermediate
• EMT-Basic	• Paramedic

MEDICAL DIRECTION

- Required for ALS providers and many BLS providers.
- EMS providers are the designated agent of the system's medical director.
- An EMS system's medical director grants authority to practice within a specific EMS system.

MEDICAL CONTROL/DIRECTION

- **On-Line** (occurs at the time of need)
  - Direct orders from a qualified physician
- **Off-Line** (established prior to the time of need)
  - In form of policies, standing orders, protocols, etc.

THE PARAMEDIC: PREHOSPITAL HEALTH-CARE WORKER

Innovative roles for the modern paramedic:

- Primary care
  - Transport to nonemergency facilities
  - Treatment without transport
- Public health and preparation
  - Community injury and illness prevention
  - Community training and education
  - Follow-up care
- Research and education

Responsibilities of a modern paramedic:

- Emergency responder
- Field triage specialist
- Diagnostician (limited)
- Emergency health-care provider
- Transporter

- Record keeper
- Data manager
- Primary care provider
- EMS profession advocate
- Patient advocate
- Emergency planner
- EMS/Public educator
- Community servant
- Clinical researcher
- Lifelong student

CHAPTER QUESTIONS

1. The National Highway Act charged the ______________ with developing an EMS system and upgrading prehospital emergency care.
   a. Department of Transportation
   b. American Red Cross
   c. Department of Health and Human Services
   d. State EMS agencies
2. The National Highway Traffic Safety Administration provides a set of recommended standards for EMS systems called the *Technical Assistance Program Assessment Standards.* These 10 standards include:
   a. personnel scheduling
   b. vehicle maintenance
   c. system access
   d. medical direction
3. Of the four levels of prehospital emergency medical training, the level of training that allows for cardiac pacing, decompressing the chest cavity, and cricothyroidotomy is the:
   a. First responder level
   b. EMT-Basic level
   c. EMT-Intermediate level
   d. EMT-Paramedic level

Suggested Readings

Ambulance service in New York City. Report by the Committee on Public Health; the New York Academy of Medicine. *Bull N Y Acad Med.* 1967;43(4):336–45.

Delbridge TR, Anderson PB, Aufderheide TP. EMS Agenda for the Future Implementation Guide. http://www.nhtsa.dot.gov/people/injury/ems/agenda/index.html 1998. Accessed January 2, 2007.

Lew BJ. A successful prehospital quality assurance program in compliance with New York State regulations. *J Emerg Nurs.* 1992 Oct;18(5):390–6.

Spaite D, Benoit R, Brown D, et al. Uniform prehospital data elements and definitions: a report from the uniform prehospital emergency medical services data conference. *Ann Emerg Med.* 1995 Apr; 25(4):525–34.

US Department of Transportation, National Highway Traffic Safety Administration. *EMT-Paramedic: National Standard Curriculum.* Washington, DC: US Department of Transportation, National Highway Traffic Safety Administration; 1998.

Chapter 2

The Well-Being of the Paramedic

Ms. Ronner, a 92-year-old woman living alone, summons her neighbor to help her because she is unable to get up from bed. Her neighbor calls emergency medical services (EMS) and states to the call receiving operator that her neighbor is having chest pain and cannot move. An advanced life support ambulance is dispatched. On the patient's refrigerator is a copy of a hospital discharge summary from 2 months ago, at which time she was admitted for a myocardial infarction. Her medical history is notable for a myocardial infarction 4 years ago, emphysema, a stroke 2 years ago, hypertension, and multiple infarct dementia. She presents alert, pale, and diaphoretic with mild dyspnea. You and your partner start taking vital signs and putting her on high concentration oxygen. She states that under no circumstances does she want to be revived if her heart stops. As the ECG machine is being connected, she says, "My heart stopped when I had my heart attack, and they brought me back, but I was on a breathing machine for 6 weeks. I'd rather die than go through that again. I've lived a good life, but it's getting hard for me to live at home, and I don't want to live in a nursing home!" She says that she has discussed this with her private physician, but the paperwork is currently unavailable, and the physician cannot be reached. She has no available relatives. The patient states she is not afraid to die: "I am comfortable with death!"

What stage of the grieving process is this?

Physical, mental, and emotional well-being affects work performance and judgement. The need to be physically, mentally, and emotionally ready is vital to performing as a paramedic.

WELLNESS AND PERSONAL INJURY PREVENTION

Physical Well-being

Physical fitness reduces the risk of some injuries, but DOES NOT provide injury immunity.

Physical Fitness

Some EMS systems may provide exercise facilities and dedicate work-time to fitness. This works best if stretching occurs before strenuous activity.

Nutrition

Good nutritional habits are difficult, but are not impossible to maintain in EMS. Preplanning and discipline are the answer to eating healthy.

Habits and Addictions

Tobacco Smoking

- Cigarette smoking and other tobacco use imposes a huge and growing global public health burden. Tobacco use is currently estimated to kill nearly 5 million people worldwide each year, accounting for 1 of every 5 deaths among males over age 30 and 1 in 20 deaths among females over age 30.
- Second-hand smoke endangers EMS partners.
- Smoke odor can cause a negative impact for a sensitive patient.

Drugs and Alcohol

- Health-care providers are not immune to substance abuse.
- Substance abuse can often be a career-ending choice.
- Personal issues typically involved.

Personal Safety

- The frequency of EMS vehicle collisions is steadily increasing.
- Emergency vehicle operations pose the greatest risk of death to an EMS provider.
- EMS systems should provide an emergency vehicle operations course that teaches EMS personnel to drive defensively.
- Aggressive emergency driving seldom saves much time.
- *Due regard* for the safety of others; defined as how reasonably a careful person performing under similar circumstances would act.

Emergency Vehicle Driving Considerations

- What are the road conditions?
- When responding, choosing the best travel route, best approach, and best parking place ensures safe driving.

The ultimate responsibility for SAFE vehicle operation is YOURS!

LIFTING AND MOVING

- Being physically fit reduces the risk of injury.
- Proper body mechanics are also critical, but are not always possible in the daily operation of a paramedic and will not prevent a cumulative injury.
- To prevent injury, reduce the load (force).

Tools for Assistance

- Sharing the load among multiple personnel

Aggravating Factors

- Sporadic lifting
- Constant sitting in the vehicle
- Burst of exertion without warm-up
- Feeling of invincibility
- Lifestyle
- Stress
- Poor physical fitness and conditioning

Lifting and Moving Tips

- Evaluate situation if time permits
- Plan ahead and know your limits
- Get help or use an assist device
- Use team leader and communicate with team
- Have good footing and balance
- Exhale during exertion
- Keep close to your body and below shoulder
- Use leg muscles and avoid twisting
- Change positions and stretch

HAZARDOUS ENVIRONMENTS

Physical or Chemical Hazards That Can Injure Paramedics During Their Course of Work

- Noise
- Radiation
- Chemical substances
- Confined space
- Machinery and electricity

Risk Reduction for Physical and Chemical Hazards

- Annual audiograms and hearing protection
- Awareness training and procedures
- Confined space training
- Hazardous material (Haz-mat) training
- Electrical lockout
- Know specific hazards in your response area

HOSTILE ENVIRONMENTS

- Incidents on the roadway.
- Industrial response.
- Assault and domestic violence.
- Congregating intoxicated persons.
- Anticipate potential hazards during response.
- Request specialized resources.
- Stage if necessary.
- The unknown may be greatest risk!

PERSONAL HEALTH AND SAFETY—INFECTION CONTROL AND DISEASE TRANSMISSION

Disease Transmission

EMS providers must anticipate potential disease transmission via splash, spray, person-to-person contact, and airborne particles with each patient they come in contact with. Gloves, barrier gowns, masks, goggles, and face shields help protect from contact with patients' potentially infectious fluids while respirators help protect from airborne particles.

Diseases of Greatest Concern to EMS Health-Care Providers

- Human immunodeficiency virus (HIV)/Acquired immune deficiency syndrome (AIDS)
- Hepatitis B and hepatitis C
- Influenza
- Tuberculosis
- Meningitis
- Staphylococcus (VRSA/MRSA)

Infection Control Methods

The New *Hand Hygiene Guidelines* for Healthcare Settings published by the Centers for Disease Control and Prevention (CDC) on October 25, 2002, offer some major changes. The following are the key new CDC hand hygiene changes that are listed as "strongly recommended" and "required for implementation" as recommended by federal and/or state regulation:

- Wash hands with non-antimicrobial soap and water when not contaminated. Note that antimicrobial soap is not the same as antibacterial soap. Antibacterial soaps are not recommended for routine hand-washing procedures. Antibacterial soaps kill off the resident bacteria that are on your skin to protect you from pathogens. Antimicrobials only reduce the number of organisms present and remove transient flora, not your normal flora.
- If hands are not visibly soiled, use an alcohol-based waterless antiseptic agent for routine decontamination.
- To improve hand hygiene in high workload areas with a high intensity of patient care, make an alcohol-based waterless antiseptic available at the entrance to the patient room or at the bedside. Provide hand hygiene products that have a low irritancy potential or provide hand lotions or creams to minimize irritant contact dermatitis.
- Do not wear artificial fingernails or extenders when providing patient care.
- Keep nails natural and one-quarter inch long.

POSTEXPOSURE FOLLOW-UP

- Washing and first aid
- Medical attention and consultation as appropriate
- Prophylactic medications
- Baseline testing
- Follow-up and testing

DEATH AND DYING

"... The survival rate of patients who fail to respond to effective ALS care in the field has never been improved by high-speed, potentially dangerous transportation to an Emergency Department." "... High speed transport of pulseless patients persists to a large extent because EMS personnel are uncomfortable with having to stop efforts in a victim's home and, in effect, making such a public acknowledgment of failure."

The grieving process has five- distinct or predictable stages. They are:

- **Denial** ("Not me.") Defense mechanism creating a buffer between shock of dying and dealing with the illness/injury.

- **Anger** ("Why me.") Paramedics may be the target of the anger. Don't take anger or insults personally, be tolerant and do not become defensive. Employ good listening and communication skills. Be empathetic.
- **Bargaining** ("OK, but first let me . . .") Agreement that, in the patient's mind, will postpone the death for a short time.
- **Depression** ("OK, but I haven't . . .") Characterized by sadness and despair. The patient is usually silent and retreats into his own world.
- **Acceptance** ("OK, I am not afraid.") Does not mean the patient will be happy about dying. The family will usually require more support during this stage than the patient.

Dealing with the needs of a dying patient and/or the family members includes performing the following:

- Respect; keeping an open line of communication, and allowing the patient and family a means for privacy.
- Treat them with dignity by allowing them to feel in control.
- Family members may express rage, anger, and despair.
- Listen empathetically.
- Do not offer false reassurance.
- Use a gentle tone of voice.
- Let the patient know that everything that can be done to help will be done.
- Use a reassuring touch, if appropriate.
- Comfort the family.
- Be respectful of religious beliefs, and, when possible, honor requests of the family while adhering to regional or state protocols.

STRESS

In addition to responding to day-to-day assignments, paramedics may encounter stressful situations while performing their duties. Examples of situations that may produce a stress response include:

- Mass casualty situations (i.e., Oklahoma City bombing, September 11th, Hurricane Katrina)
- Infant and child trauma (i.e., child struck by a car)
- Amputations
- Infant/child/elder/spouse abuse
- Death/injury of coworker or other public safety personnel

The paramedic will experience personal stress as well as encounter patients and bystanders in severe distress. Therefore, understanding how to manage stress and stressful situations is paramount. ***Remember, what constitutes an emergency to others may not necessarily be an emergency to you. Be respectful!***

Understanding the warning signs of stress:

- Irritability to coworkers, family, friends
- Inability to concentrate
- Difficulty sleeping/nightmares
- Anxiety
- Indecisiveness
- Guilt
- Loss of appetite

- Loss of interest in sexual activities
- Isolation
- Loss of interest in work

Keeping Stress Under Control

Reducing stress by making lifestyle changes is helpful to avoid "burnout." Lifestyle changes include:

- Changing your diet
- Reducing sugar, caffeine, and alcohol intake
- Avoiding fatty foods
- Increasing carbohydrates
- Exercising regularly
- Practicing relaxation techniques, meditation, and visual imagery
- Balancing work, recreation, family, health

The following work-environment changes can also reduce stress.

- Request work shifts allowing for more time to relax with family and friends.
- Request a rotation of duty assignment to a less busy area.

Seek/refer professional help. (Employee assistance program [EAP])

CRITICAL INCIDENT RESPONSE

Critical incident stress debriefing (CISD) or Critical incident stress management (CISM) is a team of peer counselors and mental-health professionals who help emergency care workers deal with critical incident stress.

A meeting is held within 24 to 72 hours of a major incident.

- Open discussion of feelings, fears, and reactions.
- Not an investigation or interrogation.
- All information is confidential.
- CISD leaders and mental-health personnel evaluate the information and offer suggestions on overcoming the stress.

CISD/CISM is designed to accelerate the normal recovery process after experiencing a critical incident.

- Works well because feelings are ventilated quickly.
- Debriefing environment is nonthreatening.
- The paramedic should review how to access their local CISD system.

Comprehensive CISM includes:

- Preincident stress education
- On-scene peer support
- One-on-one support
- Disaster support services
- Defusing
- CISD
- Follow-up services
- Spouse/family support
- Community outreach programs
- Other health and welfare programs such as wellness programs (employee assistance program)

CHAPTER QUESTIONS

1. To avoid infectious diseases, the paramedic should wear protective clothing such as:
   a. leather gloves
   b. latex gloves
   c. a helmet
   d. turnout gear
2. Professional attributes are important to maximize effectiveness as a paramedic. Meeting the physical demands of the job includes:
   a. leadership ability
   b. good moral character
   c. good eyesight and color vision
   d. being able to make appropriate decisions quickly
3. Death and dying are inherent parts of emergency medical care. The five stages of grief include which of the following:
   a. bargaining
   b. euphoria
   c. defeat
   d. relief

4 The refusal of the patient to accept the possibility of death occurs during the __________ stage.
   a. anger
   b. denial
   c. bargaining
   d. relief

5. A state of exhaustion and irritability that can markedly decrease one's effectiveness in delivering emergency medical care is referred to as:
   a. eustress
   b. stress
   c. anguish
   d. burnout

Suggested Readings

Guidelines for Cardiopulmonary Resuscitation and Emergency Cardiovascular Care. American Heart Association. August 22, 2000.

The *New Hand Hygiene Guidelines for Healthcare Settings*. The Centers for Disease Control and Prevention (CDC) on October 25, 2002. Healthcare Infection Control Practices Advisory Committee and the HICPAC/SHEA/APIC/IDSA Hand Hygiene Task Force. MMWR 2002;51(No. RR-16). January 5, 2007.

US Department of Transportation, National Highway Traffic Safety Administration. *EMT-Paramedic: National Standard Curriculum*. Washington, DC: US Department of Transportation, National Highway Traffic Safety Administration; 1998.

Chapter 3

Illness and Injury Prevention

According to the National Institute for Occupational Safety and Health (NIOSH), acute trauma at work remains a leading cause of death and disability among U.S. workers. *Trauma* is defined as an injury or wound to a living body caused by the application of external force or violence. Acute trauma can occur with the sudden, one-time application of force or violence that causes immediate damage to a living body.

During the period from 1980 through 1995, at least 93,338 workers in the United States died as a result of trauma suffered on the job, for an average of about 16 deaths per day (NIOSH). The Bureau of Labor Statistics ([BLS] Department of Labor) Census of Fatal Occupational Injuries (CFOI) has identified 5915 workplace deaths from acute traumatic injury in 2000. BLS also estimates that 5.7 million injuries to workers occurred in 1997 alone; while NIOSH estimates that about 3.6 million occupational injuries were serious enough to be treated in hospital emergency rooms in 1998.

- Injury surpassed stroke as third leading cause of death.
- Estimated lifetime cost of injuries >$114 billion.

Effects of early release from hospital on EMS services across the United States:

- Increased access to EMS services for supportive care and intervention

COMMON DEFINITIONS

- *Injury* is defined as intentional or unintentional damage to a person.
- *Injury risk* is defined as real or potential hazardous situations that put individuals at risk for sustaining an injury.
- *Injury surveillance* is defined as ongoing systematic collection, analysis, and interpretation of injury data essential to the planning, implementation, and evaluation of public health practice, closely integrated with the timely dissemination of these data to those who need to know.

The final link in the surveillance chain is the application of this data to prevention and control.

- *Primary injury prevention* is defined as keeping an injury from ever occurring.
- *Secondary and tertiary prevention* is defined as care and rehabilitation activities (respectively) that are preventing further problems from an event that has already occurred.
- *Teachable moment* is defined as the time after an injury has occurred when the patient and observers remain acutely aware of what has happened and may be more receptive to teaching about how the event or illness could be prevented.
- *Years of productive life* are defined as the calculation by subtracting age of death from 65.
- *Epidemiology* is defined as the study of factors that influence the occurrences of injury, illness, and health-related events.

? CHAPTER QUESTIONS

Match the following terms with their definitions.

1. Primary injury prevention
2. Secondary and tertiary prevention
3. Teachable moment
4. Years of productive life
   a. Defined as the calculation by subtracting age of death from 65.
   b. Defined as keeping an injury from ever occurring.
   c. Defined as the time after an injury has occurred when the patient and observers remain acutely aware of what has happened and may be more receptive to teaching about how the event or illness could be prevented.
   d. Defined as care and rehabilitation activities (respectively) that are preventing further problems from an event that has already occurred.

Suggested Readings

Centers for Disease Control and Prevention (CDC). [1988] Guidelines for Evaluating Surveillance Systems. *MMWR* 37 (S-5):1–18. October 12, 2007.

National Safety Council. *Injury Facts.* Itasca, Il: National Safety Council 2002.

Research Needs and Priorities: A Report by the NORA Traumatic Injury Team, DHHS (NIOSH) Publication No. 98-134. www.cdc.gov/niosh/injury/NIOSH. Accessed October 12, 2007.

Safety and Health Topic: Traumatic Occupational Injuries: Traumatic Occupational Injury.

http://origin.cdc.gov/niosh/injury/. Accessed February 12, 2007.

US Department of Transportation, National Highway Traffic Safety Administration. *EMT-Paramedic: National Standard Curriculum.* Washington, DC: US Department of Transportation, National Highway Traffic Safety Administration; 1998.

Chapter 4
Medical/Legal Issues

Overall outcomes of cardiopulmonary resuscitation (CPR) are less favorable in elderly people than in younger people, although the most important determinant of outcome appears to be the burden of associated illnesses rather than aging per se. For individuals with metastatic cancer, sepsis, and multiorgan failure, survival rates after CPR are close to zero. Rates of survival to hospital discharge after cardiac arrest are best for people who arrest in public places, whereas most studies have found that nursing home residents with serious chronic illnesses and functional disability rarely survive until hospital discharge.

You and your partner respond to an area nursing home for an unconscious patient. Upon arrival, the nursing staff greets you in the lobby and states Ms. Roberts was in the cafeteria and just collapsed. As you enter the room, the patient is found in the rear of the cafeteria, supine, and what appears to be unconscious and cyanotic. As you establish unresponsiveness, your partner states that Ms. Roberts has no pulse. The nurse states the patient has no advanced directives that she knows of. She also gives a list of medications and past medical history. Your partner states, "Let's call medical control for a pronouncement time! She is 92 and has an extensive medical history." You ask your partner, "Does she have a valid do not resuscitate order (DNR) in her paperwork." Your partner replies, "No." You begin CPR and your partner looks at you in amazement and says, "What are you doing?"

With the scenario above, do you have a moral, legal, or ethical responsibility to provide basic and advanced care?

MEDICAL/LEGAL ASPECTS OF PREHOSPITAL CARE

Legal, Ethical, Moral Responsibilities

What are the differences?

- Legal responsibilities; established by the law-making bodies of government.
- Ethical standards are principles of conduct identified by members of a group or profession.
- Morality is defined as an individual's assessment of right and wrong.

Categories of Law

- Criminal Law—Law that deals with crimes and their punishments.
- Civil Law—Law concerned with noncriminal matters.
- Tort Law—Legislation governing wrongful acts, other than breaches of contract by one person against another or his or her property, for which civil action can be brought. Tort law and Contract law define civil liability exposures. The four areas of torts are negligence, intentional interference, absolute liability, and strict liability.

Common Terminology

- Appeal—The transfer of a case from a lower to a higher court for a new hearing
- Plaintiff—The party that institutes a suit in a court

- Defendant—The party against which an action is brought
- Deposition—Testimony under oath, especially a statement by a witness that is written down or recorded for use in court at a later date
- Documentation—The act or an instance of the supplying of documents or supporting references or records
- Interrogation—The process of formally and systematically questioning a suspect in order to elicit incriminating responses

Laws Affecting EMS

- Scope of practice—This term is used by licensing boards for various medical-related fields that define the procedures, actions, and processes that are permitted for the licensed individual. The scope of practice is limited to that which the individual has received education and clinical experience, and in which he/she has demonstrated competency. Each state has specific regulation based on entry education and additional training and practice.
- Specific state motor vehicle laws.
- Infectious disease exposure.
- Assault against public safety officer.
- Obstruction of duty.
- Good Samaritan Law—This principle of Tort law provides that a person who sees another individual in imminent and serious danger or peril cannot be charged with negligence if that first person attempts to aid or rescue the injured party, provided the attempt is not made recklessly.
- Ryan White CARE Act—The Ryan White CARE (Comprehensive AIDS Resource Emergency) Act was originally signed August 18, 1990, as a federal program designed to improve the quality and availability of care for persons with HIV/AIDS and their families. The act was amended and reauthorized in May 1996 with 4 years of funding at levels determined annually as part of the federal budget process. The program is administered by the Health Resources and Services Administration (HRSA) which is within the U.S. Department of Health and Human Services (DHHS).

Paramedics have a legal responsibility to report certain incidents, such as:

- Domestic violence
- Child and elder abuse
- Criminal acts
- GSW, stabbing, and assault victims
- Animal bites
- Communicable diseases
- Out-of-hospital deaths
- Possession of controlled substances

Accountability and Malpractice Issues

- *Standard of Care*—The expected care, skill, and judgement demonstrated under similar circumstances by a similarly trained, reasonable paramedic.
- *Negligence*—Deviation from accepted or expected standards of care expected to protect from unreasonable risk of harm.
  - Elements required to prove negligence
    - — Duty to act
    - — Breach of duty
    - — Actual damage or harm
    - — Proximate cause

- *Borrowed servant doctrine*—The borrowed servant doctrine is based on the idea that an employee can be "borrowed" by someone other than the employer. The person who "borrows" the employee becomes liable for the employee's actions.
- Patients' civil rights.
- Liability when off duty.

CIVIL CASES

- Proof of guilt required by a "preponderance of evidence"
- Burden of proof shifts to the defendant
- Simple versus gross negligence

SPECIFIC PARAMEDIC-PATIENT ISSUES

- Issues surrounding consent
- Refusals
- Restraint
- Abandonment
- Transfer of patient care
- Advance directives and end-of-life decisions
- Out-of-hospital death
- Confidentiality and privacy

CONSENT

To obtain proper consent, the patient must have the legal and mental capacity. Does the patient understand the consequences of his or her actions?

Types of Consent

- Informed—Consent by a patient to a medical procedure after achieving an understanding of the relevant medical facts and the risks involved.
- Expressed—Expressed consent is a more formal type of permission founded on words, either oral or written, and it applies to more invasive procedures. The so-called written informed consent is an expressed consent in written form which includes the signature of (at least) both the health-care professional and the patient (or the patient's legal guardian). The written informed consent is particularly beneficial to the health-care provider if questions concerning treatment should develop.
- Implied Consent—When a patient is unable to give expressed consent, the law assumes that the patient would desire to have life-saving treatments rendered.
- Involuntary—Court ordered.

Specific Consent Issues

Emancipated Minor—An emancipated minor is a child who has been granted the status of adulthood by a court order or other formal arrangement. Emancipated minor status is not automatically bestowed on those who have simply moved away from their parents' home. The majority of emancipated minor cases involve working teenagers who have demonstrated an ability to support themselves financially. A professional actress or musician over the age of 14 is more likely to be considered an emancipated minor than a runaway working for minimum wage.

There are three ways for a teenager to earn emancipated minor status.

- The first method is to demonstrate to a court that he or she is financially independent and the parents or legal guardians have no objections to his or her living arrangements.

A petition is usually filed in a family courtroom, and the judge can either approve or disallow the emancipated minor's petition. This is to prevent disgruntled teenagers from arbitrarily leaving home and declaring themselves to be emancipated. Becoming an emancipated minor through financial independence is not considered a "divorce" from parents, but rather a means for successful teens to protect their assets.

- Another recognized way to earn emancipated minor status is to become legally married. This option does not supersede other laws governing the age of consent, however. A 12-year-old girl seeking emancipated minor status cannot become legally married until she has reached her state's minimal age of consent.
- The third means of becoming an emancipated minor is to enlist in any of the U.S. armed forces.

REFUSAL

- Establishing capacity—Does the patient understand the nature of his or her medical condition and the potential consequences of refusing treatment and/or transport?
- Assessment of decision-making capacity—The patient should have absence of deficits in:
  - Cognition
  - Judgement
  - Understanding
  - Choice
  - Expression of choice
  - Stability

RESTRAINT

- False imprisonment is restraint without proper justification or authority.
- Intentional and unjustifiable detention of an individual without his consent

ASSAULT AND BATTERY

- Assault—Unlawfully placing an individual in apprehension of immediate body harm without consent
- Battery—Unlawfully touching an individual without consent

PATIENT CONFIDENTIALITY AND PRIVACY

You have treated and transported a 50-year-old local politician who was originally diagnosed in the emergency room with Pneumocystis carinii pneumonia (PCP). At the station, you discuss this case including the name of the patient. Since PCP is associated with HIV/AIDS, your coworker suspects this man is infected. Your coworker discusses this case with a friend who then discusses this matter with other people who know this patient.

What are the possible consequences of your discussing this pertinent patient information?

- Defamation—Communication of false information, knowing the information to be false or with reckless disregard of whether it is true or false
- Slander—Malicious, false, and injurious statement spoken about a person
- Libel—Published false statement damaging a person's character

INTERACTION WITH LAW ENFORCEMENT

Crime Scenes

- Request law enforcement if they are not already on-scene
- Await law enforcement arrival if possible
- Minimize areas of travel and contact with scene
- Document any alterations to the scene created by EMS personnel
- Minimize personnel within scene if possible
- Document pertinent observations

Evidence Preservation

- Avoid cutting through penetrations in the clothing
- Save everything—clothing of assault victim, items found on person, and the like
- Prevent sexual assault victim from washing
- Follow sound chain of evidence procedures

VEHICLE OPERATION ISSUES

It is 3:00 am. While responding to a motor vehicle collision (MVC), you fail to proceed through an intersection with "due regard." The traffic signal is red. You attempt to stop but are unable to do so. Witnesses state your emergency lights were on but do not recall hearing your siren. The driver of the car you struck is injured.
What is due regard?

MEDICAL CONTROL ISSUES

- Failure to follow medical control direction
- Following obviously harmful direction
- Implementing therapies without prior authorization
- Following direction of an unauthorized person
- Medical control directs EMS to an inappropriate hospital
- The paramedic exceeds the scope of his training or medical authorization

HOSPITAL SELECTION ISSUES

- Was the paramedic and medical control decision appropriate?
- Was the closest and appropriate facility chosen?
- Did the paramedic follow the written policies or guidelines?

DISPATCH ISSUES

- Untimely dispatch
- Failure to provide responding units with adequate directions (incorrect address)
- Dispatch of inadequate level of care
- Failure to provide prearrival instructions
- Inadequate recordkeeping

CHAPTER QUESTIONS

1. All of the following are components to establishing negligence, except:
   a. the EMT's action or lack of action caused additional injury to the patient
   b. the EMT violated the standard of care
   c. the EMT was on duty with a paying EMS service (not volunteer)
   d. the EMT has a duty to act
2. By law, the EMT is allowed to release confidential patient information without the patient's or guardian's permission in all of the following situations except:
   a. when the press requests identifying information about the patient
   b. a third-party billing form requires the information
   c. another health-care provider needs to know the information for continued care
   d. when the EMT is required by legal subpoena to provide information to the court
3. While providing patient care at a secured crime scene, the EMT should:
   a. not cut through holes in clothing possibly caused by bullets or stabbing(s)
   b. pick up any evidence found and deliver directly to a police officer
   c. cover the deceased patient with a sheet and remove the body to the ambulance
   d. use the telephone to call in a report to medical control
4. Most states require an EMT to report certain conditions or situations, including:
   a. use of patient restraints
   b. gunshot or stab wounds
   c. suspected child abuse
   d. all of the above

Suggested Readings

"Civil law." The American Heritage Dictionary of the English Language, Fourth Edition. Houghton Mifflin Company, 2004. http://www.answers.com/topic/civil-law. Accessed January 26, 2007.

Cohn BM, Azzara AJ. *Legal Aspects of Emergency Medical Services.* Philadelphia (PA): W. B. Saunders Company; 1998.

"Criminal law." The American Heritage Dictionary of the English Language, Fourth Edition. Houghton Mifflin Company, 2004. http://www.answers.com/topic/criminal-law. Accessed January 26, 2007.

The American Heritage Dictionary of the English Language, 4th ed. Houghton Mifflin Company, 2004. http://www.answers.com. Accessed January 26, 2007.

"Tort Law." Dictionary of Insurance Terms. Barron's Educational Series, Inc, 2000. 26 Jan. 2007. http://www.answers.com/topic/tort-law. Accessed January 26, 2007.

US Department of Transportation, National Highway Traffic Safety Administration. *EMT-Paramedic National Standard Curriculum.* Washington, DC: US Department of Transportation, National Highway Traffic Safety Administration; 1998.

Chapter 5
Ethics

ETHICS VERSUS MORALS

- Ethics—Refer to the rules or standards that govern the conduct of members of a particular group or profession. Ethics often help shape our legal views.
- Morals—Generally considered to be social, religious, or personal standards of right and wrong. Personal beliefs of right and wrong behavior often influence our ethics development.

ETHICAL CONSIDERATIONS IN PATIENT CARE

- **Beneficence**—The paramedic's responsibility to "do well" for the patient
- **Nonmalfeasance**—The paramedic's responsibility to not harm the patient
- **Autonomy**—Patient's right of self determination
- **Justice**—Treat all patients fairly

SPECIFIC ETHICAL ISSUES FACING PARAMEDICS

Resuscitation

- Is a valid do not resuscitate (DNR) present but patient is breathing and has a pulse?
- Family conflict in the presence of a DNR.
- Terminating resuscitation when efforts appear futile, or valid DNR now presented.

Ethical Issues in Health Care

- Is it in the patient's best interest?
- Determining what the patient wants, whether stated or written. In certain instances, input from family should also be considered.

The role of "good faith" in making ethical decisions includes providing patient benefit, avoiding harm, and recognizing patient autonomy.

Confidentiality

- Confidentiality is a fundamental right of all patients.
- Does this supersede ethical considerations?
- What if public health would benefit?

Consent

- Remember the patient has a right to make decisions regarding his or her own health care.

- Fundamental element of the patient-physician relationship.
- AMA code of medical ethics.

Ethics of Implied Consent

- Does the patient understand the issues at hand?
- Can the patient make an informed decision in his or her best interest?

APPLICATIONS OF ETHICAL PRINCIPLES TO PATIENT-CARE SITUATIONS

Care in Futile Situations

- Futile—With no practical effect or useful result.
- Who makes the decision?

Obligation to Provide Prehospital Care

- Good Samaritan
- Inability to pay
- Isn't in the "health plan"
- Patient "dumping"
- Economic triage

Advocacy refers to speaking on behalf of patients in order to protect their rights and help them obtain needed information and services.

Ethical Issues Involving the Physician Extender, Paramedic

The physician orders something which:

- The paramedic believes is contraindicated
- The paramedic believes is medically acceptable but not in the patient's best interests
- The paramedic believes is medically acceptable but morally wrong

CHAPTER QUESTIONS

1. The fundamental right of any patient is called confidentiality.
   a. True
   b. False
2. Morals refer to the rules or standards that govern the conduct of members of a particular group or profession. Ethics often help shape our legal views.
   a. True
   b. False
3. Ethics are generally considered to be social, religious, or personal standards of right and wrong. Personal beliefs of right and wrong behavior often influence our ethics development.
   a. True
   b. False

References

Code of Medical Ethics: Current Opinions with Annotations, Chicago, IL: American Medical Association; 2006–2007.

Iserson K, Saunders AB, Mathieu D. *Ethics in Emergency Medicine.* 2nd Ed. Tucson, AZ: Galen Press; 1995.

US Department of Transportation, National Highway Traffic Safety Administration. *EMT-Paramedic National Standard Curriculum.* Washington, DC: US Department of Transportation, National Highway Traffic Safety Administration; 1998.

Chapter 6
General Principles of Pathophysiology

To better understand pathophysiology, you need to understand basic anatomy and physiology. Below is a brief review of anatomy and physiology (A&P).

- Anatomy—Study of the structure of body parts
- Physiology—Study of the function of body parts

ORGANIZATION OF THE BODY

- Atoms—The atomic level consists of basic elements such as hydrogen and oxygen.
- Macromolecules (biomolecules)—Many atoms that join to form a structure.
- DNA—A long chain formed of carbon, hydrogen, and oxygen.
- Organelle—Tiny structure within a cell that carries out functions.
- Mitochondria—Produce energy for the cell.
- Cell—A basic unit in the living system that carries out many functions simultaneously to live and grow.
- Tissue—Similar cells working together to perform a function.
- Organ—Composed of several types of tissues and performs a specific function.
- Organ system—A system that performs a specific function.
- Organism—A complex being made of separate systems functioning as one human being.

CHEMISTRY OF LIFE

Atom—Smallest unit in our body

- Nucleus contains protons (+) and neutrons (no electric charge).
- Neutrons determine the atomic number. They are usually the same. When they are not the same, they can be radioactive (emit radiation).
- Orbit of the atom contains the electrons (−).
- The number of electrons = the number of protons.

Reactions Between Atoms

- A reaction is the gaining, losing, or sharing of electrons. When this happens, a chemical bond is formed. If this bond is magnetic (loss or gain of electrons) it is known as an *ionic bond.* An example of this is $Na^+ + Cl^- = NaCl$ (sodium chloride; salt).
- If atoms are sharing electrons, it is known as a *covalent bond.* An example of this is $2H^+ + O^{2-} = H_2O$ (water).

TYPES OF CHEMISTRY

- Inorganic—The branch of chemistry that deals with inorganic compounds
- Organic—The branch of chemistry that deals with carbon compounds

IMPORTANT INORGANIC MOLECULES

- Water can also form a hydrogen bond between molecules. This is weaker than the chemical bond caused by the slight charge of each atom. Electrons are shared, but are mostly around oxygen. Electrons are negative, so oxygen is slightly negative. Hydrogen has to be slightly positive. This bond is what makes water harder to boil or freeze.
- In our body, water easily absorbs or gives off heat.

ACIDS, BASES, AND PH

Molecules disassociate (or split up).

- Ions that give off molecules (charged molecules) in water:
  - If ions are H^+, it is an acid.
    - — Solution becomes acidic
    - — Lowers the pH
  - If ions are OH^- (hydroxide), it is a base.
    - — Solution becomes basic (alkaline)
    - — Raises the pH

pH is a measure of the acidity or alkalinity of a solution.

- pH ranges from 0–14.
- A pH of 7 is considered neutral (equal balance of H^+ and OH^-).
- All life needs a constant pH (blood pH is about 7.4).
- *Buffers* are solutions that can absorb the excess ions.

MOLECULES OF LIFE

Proteins

- Are mostly structural and are considered the building blocks of life.
- Can also be enzymes (catalysts that speed reactions).
- Made up of amino acids.
  - About 20 different amino acids
  - Only 8–10 essential amino acids
- Amino acids join together to form peptide bonds.
  - Amino acids are made up of the amino (+) part and the acid (–) part.
  - A long chain of amino acids is called a polypeptide.
- Proteins have three levels of structure.

Carbohydrates (Sugars)

- Sources of fuel.
- A single carbohydrate is a monosaccharide.
- Glucose is a six-carbon monosaccharide.
- Two carbohydrates bonded together are called a disaccharide.

- Maltose is two glucoses with a covalent bond.
- Polysaccharides contain many monosaccharides.
  - Found in plants and animals.
  - Glycogen, starch, cellulose.
- Glycogen.
  - Human storage form of glucose.
  - Stored in the blood and muscles.
  - Produced by the liver.
- Starch.
  - Plant storage form of glucose.
  - Cellulose (fiber).
  - Humans don't have the enzymes to break down cellulose.
  - Passes through system undigested.

Lipids

- Nonpolar (no charge) and do not dissolve in water
- Triglycerides (fats):
  - Contain one glycerol and three fatty acids.
  - Fatty acids are carbon chains with H^+ attached.
  - Saturated refers to the number of H^+ attached.
  - Found in meat, dairy products.
  - One double bond, monounsaturated.
  - Two or more double bonds, polyunsaturated.
    - Found in vegetable products

Phospholipids

Similar to triglycerides, but instead of fatty acid, they have phosphate and nitrogen.

Steroids (Sex Hormones)

Similar in structure to cholesterol.

Nucleic Acids

- Huge biomolecules with specific functions.
  - An example would be DNA (deoxyribonucleic acid), RNA (ribonucleic acid).
- Polymers of nucleotides.
  - Nucleotides are specific molecules.
  - Polymer = chain of a specific molecule.
- RNA is single stranded.
- DNA is double stranded.
  - Held together by hydrogen bonds.
  - Sequences of bases (adenine, guanine, thiamine, cytosine) determines genetic structure.
- ATP (energy source).
- Adenine + ribose (sugar) = adenosine.
- Also has three phosphates when one phosphate is broken off, energy is released.
- ATP = ADP + P + energy.

CELL STRUCTURE AND FUNCTION

Organelles

Cell (Plasma) Membrane

- "Gate" to the cell (regulates which substances enter and exit the cell).
- Made of a double layer of phospholipids.
- Protein molecules are embedded in the membrane.
- Some serve as receptors, others serve as transporters.

Cytoplasm

- Fluid of the cell that is inside the membrane and houses the organelles.
- Molecules and organelles move within it.

Nucleus

- "Control center" of the cell.
- It is the largest organelle in the cell.
- Enclosed by a nuclear envelope (permeable membrane).
- Contains a nucleolus.
- Contains RNA.
  - RNA calls for production of ribosomes.
  - Ribosomes leave the nucleus to remain in the cytoplasm.
  - May attach to the endoplasmic reticulum.
  - Contains fluid, called nucleoplasm.
  - Also contains chromatin.
- Condenses to chromosomes during cell division.
- Chromosomes contain the DNA.
  - DNA codes for specific protein production.
- Many proteins serve as enzymes.
  - Breaking down of molecules (catabolism).
  - Building complex molecules (anabolism).

Endoplasmic Reticulum (ER)

- Is called the "factory."
- Membranous canals beginning at the nuclear envelope.
- Ribosomes may attach; if so, is considered to be a rough ER.
  - Involved in protein synthesis
- If there are no ribosomes attached, it is called smooth ER.
  - Involved in production of lipids

Golgi Complex (Apparatus)

- "Shipping and receiving."
- Receives packages (vesicles) from the ER.
- ER breaks off to form vesicles.
  - Packages these for transport outside the cell
  - Also called vesicles
  - Also produces lysosomes
  - Remains in the cell

  - Breaks down large molecules
  - Can eat away on the cell itself

Mitochondria

- "Powerhouse of the cell"—produces ATP for use as energy
- Double membrane
  - Inner membrane contains cristae (folds).
  - These folds contain the ATP-producing molecules.
  - Burns glucose products to make ATP.
  - Uses oxygen during the process.
  - Gives off carbon dioxide, water.
- Glycolysis
  - Breaking down of glycogen
  - Breaking down of oxygen
  - Kreb's cycle

Centrioles

- Exact function is unknown.
- May help move material in cytoplasm.
- Are short cylinders at right angles.
- Contain small tubules called microtubules.

Cilia and Flagella

- If present, are on the outside of the cell
- Help in movement
- Whiplike—Move the cell in a fluid (sperm)
- Oarlike—Cell moves particles (upper respiratory tract)

Movement Into and Out of the Cell

Movement is accomplished by active or passive transport.

Passive Transport (Three Types)

1. Diffusion
   - Molecules move from higher to lower concentration.
   - Human examples:
     - Oxygen entering blood in lungs through alveoli (air sacks)
     - Waste leaving kidneys during dialysis
   - No energy is expended by the cell.
2. Osmosis
   - Special type of diffusion involving solutes.
   - Involves the movement of water to lower concentration of solutes.
   - Equal amounts of water on each side of the membrane—isotonic.
   - Higher concentration of water—hypotonic.
   - Lower concentration of water—hypertonic.
3. Filtration
   - Molecules move through membranes under pressure.
   - Smaller molecules pass through membrane.

Active Transport

- Carries molecules from lower to higher concentration.
- Requires receptor proteins and energy (ATP).
- Examples:
  - Thyroid gland (iodine)
  - Small intestines (glucose)
  - Kidneys (sodium)
- To work, requires a large amount of ATP.
- Typically, these types of cells have more mitochondria.

Phagocytosis/Pinocytosis

- Another way molecules enter cells.
- Molecule forms a vesicle within the cell membrane.
- If it is a large vesicle, it is called *phagocytosis* (cell eating).
- If it is a small vesicle, it is called *pinocytosis* (cell drinking).

TYPES OF CELLULAR INJURY

Hypoxic Injury

- Most common cause of cellular injury
- May result from:
  - Decreased amounts of oxygen in the air
  - Loss of hemoglobin or hemoglobin function
  - Decreased number of red blood cells
  - Disease in respiratory or cardiovascular system
  - Loss of cytochromes

Chemical Injury

- Chemical agents causing cellular injury
  - Poisons
  - Lead
  - Carbon monoxide
  - Ethanol
  - Pharmacological

Infectious Injury

- Virulence or pathogenicity of microorganisms depends on their ability to survive and reproduce in the human body, where they injure cells and tissues.
- Disease-producing potential depends upon its ability to:
  - Invade and destroy cells
  - Produce toxins
  - Produce hypersensitivity reactions

BACTERIA

- Survival and growth depend upon the effectiveness of the body's defense mechanisms and the bacteria's ability to resist the mechanisms.
- Coating protects the bacterium from ingestion and destruction by phagocytes.

- Not all virulent extracellular pathogens are encapsulated—mycobacterium tuberculosis can survive and be transported by phagocytes.
- Bacteria also produce substances such as enzymes or toxins which can injure or destroy cells.
- Toxins are produced by many microorganisms.
  - Exotoxins
  - Endotoxins
- Fever is caused by the release of endogenous pyrogens from macrophages, or circulating white blood cells that are attracted to the injury site.
- Inflammation is one of the body's responses to the presence of bacteria.
- Ability to produce hypersensitivity reactions is an important pathogenic mechanism of bacteria toxins.
- Bacteremia or septicemia is proliferation of microorganisms in the blood.

VIRUSES

- Viral diseases are among the most common afflictions seen in humans.
- Intracellular parasites take over the control of metabolic machinery of host cells for use to replicate the virus.
- Protein coat (capsid) encapsulating most viruses allows them to resist phagocytosis.
- Viral replication occurs within the host cell.
- Having no organelles, viruses are incapable of metabolism.
- Cause decreased synthesis of macromolecules vital to the host cell.
- Viruses do not produce exotoxins or endotoxins.
- There may be a symbiotic relationship between viruses and normal cells.
- Viruses result in a persistent unapparent infection.
- Viruses can evoke a strong immune response but can rapidly produce irreversible and lethal injury in highly susceptible cells (as in AIDS).
- Immunologic and inflammatory injury.
  - Cellular membranes are injured by direct contact with cellular and chemical components of the immune or inflammatory process as in phagocytes (lymphocytes and macrophages) and others such as histamine, antibodies, and lymphokines.
  - Membrane alterations are associated with rapid leakage of potassium out of the cell and an influx of water.
- Viruses contain injurious genetic factors.
- Viruses contain injurious nutritional imbalances.
- Viruses contain injurious physical agents.
- Viruses contain manifestations of cellular injury.
- Viruses contain cellular manifestations.
- Viruses contain systemic manifestations.
- Viruses contain cellular death/necrosis.

BODY TISSUES AND MEMBRANES

Tissues are composed of similar cells, performing similar functions.

Epithelial Tissue (Epithelium)

- Covers the body's surface
- Externally, provides protection from:
  - Drying

- Injury
- Bacterial invasion

- Internally, may be specialized for protection
  - Secretion of mucous (respiratory tracts)
  - Absorption of molecules (kidney)

Three Main Types of Epithelial Tissue

- Squamous—Flat cells, found lining lungs and blood vessels
- Cuboidal—Cube shaped cells that line the kidney tubules
- Columnar—Cells that resemble pillars or columns that line the digestive tract

Three Other Divisions of Epithelial Tissue

Simple

- Single layer of cells

Stratified

- Layers piled upon layers.
- Examples of stratified squamous epithelium: nose, mouth, esophagus, outer skin also, but reinforced with keratin for strength.

Pseudostratified

- Appears to be stratified
- Instead, each cell attaches to the baseline

Glandular

- Described as glandular if secretes a product.
- Glands may be a single cell (digestive tract) or can be composed of many cells.
  - If the cell secretes product into ducts (exocrine glands):
    - — Salivary and sweat glands
  - If the cell secretes into blood stream (endocrine glands):
    - — Pituitary and thyroid glands

Connective Tissue

- Binds structures together, provides support and protection.
- Fills spaces.
- Stores fat.
- Cells are widely separated by a *matrix.*

Loose Connective Tissue

- Commonly lies below the epithelium.
- Used to bind structures together.
- Composed of star-shaped cells that produce extracellular fibers called *fibroblasts.*
- Cellular area separated by jellylike fluid.
  - Fluid contains white and yellow fibers.
    - — White fibers

      Occur in bundles

Contain collagen

Provide strength and some flexibility

— Yellow fibers

Occur in networks (show difference between network and bundle)

Contain elastin, provides most of the elasticity

- Adipose tissue is a type of loose connective tissue.
  - Fibroblasts enlarge and store fat while the matrix reduces.

Fibrous Connective Tissue

- Composed of collagen (strength/flexibility).
- Fibers are in close proximity to one another.
- Found in tendons and ligaments.
  - Tendon, muscle to bone
  - Ligament, bone to bone
- No blood flows to this tissue.

Cartilage

- Cells are present in *lacunae* (small chambers).
- Cells are separated by a solid yet flexible matrix.

Three types of cartilage—based on fiber type

1. Hyaline Cartilage
   - Most common type, contains very fine fibers, and has a milk-glass appearance
   - Located in the nose, ends of bone, rings of trachea, fetal skeleton
2. Elastic Cartilage
   - Contains elastic and collagen fibers, and is, therefore, more flexible
   - Located in the outer ear
3. Fibrocartilage
   - Matrix composed of strong collagenous fibers.
   - Absorbs shock, reduces friction between joints, and is found in pads that absorb pressure.
     - Menisci (between the condyles/epicondyles of knee)
     - Intervertebral disks (between vertebral bodies)

Bone

- Most rigid of the connective tissues.
- Is made up of calcium salt deposits around protein fibers.
  - Calcium provides the rigidity.
- Proteins provide the elasticity and strength.
- Bones are classified into three types.
  - Long bones—structure and support
  - Short bones—facilitate movement
  - Flat bones—protection

For anatomical purposes

1. Compact bone
   - Osteocytes (cells) are in lacunae around Haversian canals. The canals supply blood to the cells.

2. Spongy bone
   - Exists on the ends of bone and is composed of bars and plates for reinforcement.
   - Spongy bone is not as dense as compact bone, but stronger.

Blood

- Also considered a connective tissue and is separated by plasma.
- Two types of blood cells.
  - Red blood cells (erythrocytes)
    - Contain the hemoglobin which carries oxygen
  - White blood cells (leukocytes)
    - Fight infection
- Also present in the plasma are platelets which are important in blood clotting.

Muscular Tissue

Muscular tissue is composed of fiber that contains *actin* and *myosin* microfilaments. Movement (muscular contraction) occurs when these two interact. Three types of muscular tissue exist: skeletal, smooth, and cardiac.

Skeletal (Striated)

- Attaches to the bones.
- Function is to move the skeleton.
- Fibers are cylindrical and run the length of the muscle.
- Skeletal muscles have many nuclei and have concentric bands that give a striated appearance.
- Skeletal muscle is under voluntary control.

Smooth

- Lacks dark bands, and has no striations.
- Smooth muscle is involuntary muscle (not under voluntary control, for most—biofeedback).
- Found in the intestines, stomach, and arteries.
- Muscles contract more slowly and can remain contracted for a longer period of time.

Cardiac

- Appears to combine both smooth and striated features.
- Fibers appear branched, so that the contractions occur in many directions.
- Is present in the heart, and is responsible for the heartbeat.
- Cardiac muscle is an involuntary muscle.

Nervous Tissue

- Found in the brain and spinal cord.
- Composed of neurons and neuroglial (glial) cells.
  - Neurons are composed of:
    - Dendrite—Conducts impulse (sends message)
    - Cell body—Contains nucleus
    - Axon—Conducts impulse away from the body
    - Nerve fibers—Are just long axons or dendrites

- ◦ Glial cells
  - — Support and protect the neurons.
  - — Those that encircle the fibers are called *Schwann cells.*
  - — The outer layer is called the *neurilemma.*
  - — Promotes growth in damaged cells.
  - — Inner fatty layer called *myelin.*
    Provides insulation
    There are "gaps" between these cells
  - — The nodes pass on the nervous impulse.

THE INTEGUMENTARY SYSTEM

Structure of the Skin

Skin has accessory organs such as epidermis, dermis, hair follicles, nerve endings, and glands.

Epidermis

- Outer and thinner region.
- Cells are squamous.
- Has several layers, therefore they are stratified.
- Bottom layer referred to as germinal layer (stratum germinativum).
- Called *basal cells*; they lie next to the dermis.
- Constant cell division pushes cells upward. As they move upward, the cells receive less oxygen and nutrients from blood.
- The cells die and fall off in about 2–4 weeks.
- As cells move upward, keratin (protein) enters and hardens the cell.
- There are more keratinized cells on certain parts of body, such as:
  - ◦ Palms, soles of feet
- Skin colorations result from certain proteins in the epidermis.
  - ◦ Melanin (produced by melanocytes)
    - — More production of melanin, darker color
  - ◦ Carotene
    - — Develops a yellowish color
- Absence of melanin production referred to as albinism.

Dermis

- The region of tissue below the epidermis. This region is thicker than the epidermis and is composed of connective tissue, not epithelial tissue like the epidermis.
  - ◦ Contains collagen and elastin fibers
    - — Collagen = flexibility and strength
    - — Elastin = elasticity
- Has projections into the epidermis (to anchor it).
- Causes spiraling patterns in the epidermis (fingerprints).
- Contains blood vessels (arteries and veins).
- Also contains nervous tissues.

Subcutaneous Region

- Lies below the dermis.
- This is where fat (stored energy) is stored in adipose tissue (which is loose connective tissue).

- Also provides protection to the body from shock.
- Especially noticeable near kidneys.

Accessory Structures of the Skin

Hair

- Found over most of the body
  - Can be fine (thin) or coarse (thick)
- Hair development
  - Epidermal cell grows from a hair follicle.
  - Cells die and move outward.
  - Become keratinized and harden.
- Parts of the hair
  - Hair follicle
  - Root (within the follicle)
  - Shaft (outside the follicle)
  - Sebaceous glands (secrete oils into the follicle)
  - Erector pili muscle (holds hair upright)
  - Interesting that if cold, these muscles contract
  - Causes a pocket of warm air to develop
- Life span is about 3–5 months

Nails

- Also grow from epithelial cells.
- As cells move out, they become more keratinized.
- Three portions to the nail.
  - Nail root (germinal area).
  - Pink region has vascular dermal tissue beneath.
  - Ends are keratinized cells without blood flow.

Glands

- All glands of the epidermal system are exocrine.
  - Secrete substances into ducts

Sebaceous glands

- Secrete sebum into the hair follicle.
- Lubricates and waterproofs the hair and skin.
- When these glands don't work, whiteheads/blackheads are formed.
  - Bacteria in the follicle produces the reddened pimple.
  - May become inflamed during adolescence.
  - Due to presence of certain hormones in high levels.

Sweat glands (sudoriferous glands)

- Present in large numbers all over the body
- Three types
  - Apocrine glands
    - — Excrete sweat into hair follicles
    - — Activate when under stress

- ◦ Eccrine glands
  - — Excrete directly onto the skin
  - — Activate to cool the body down
- ◦ Ceruminous glands (in the ear) excrete cerumen (ear wax)

Mammary glands

- Modified sweat glands
- Located within the breasts
- Produce milk after a child is born

Functions of the Skin

Protection

- From trauma.
- From bacterial infection.
- From growth of pathogenic organisms (organisms that kill).
- Sweat glands products are slightly acidic.
- Retains/repels water.
- Exposed cells are dead and keratinized.
- Waterproof.

Sensory Reception and Communication

- Receptors located in the dermal tissue for:
  - ◦ Heat, cold, pain, pressure sensation

Synthesis of Vitamin D

- Precursor molecules exposed to UV rays turn to Vitamin D.
- Vitamin D converts to hormone (calcitronin) in kidneys.
  - ◦ Regulates calcium and phosphorus in the body.
- Prevents rickets (bone-softening disease).

Regulation of Body Temperature

- The chemical reactions in our body produce heat.
  - ◦ Glucose to ATP
  - ◦ ATP to ADP
- To maintain warmth, blood flow through the dermis is increased. Increased blood flow warms epidermis.
- To reduce heat, sweat glands produce more sweat. Air evaporates sweat off the epidermis, thus cooling it.

Disorders of the Skin

- Many exist (acne, athlete's foot, eczema, psoriasis, dandruff, moles, warts)
- Most are not serious (life-threatening)

Cancer

- Malignant melanoma (most serious)
  - ◦ Resembles a mole (darkly pigmented spot)
  - ◦ Occurs in light skinned people from constant exposure to sun
  - ◦ Can lead to death

- Two types, both occur from UV rays:
  - Squamous cell carcinoma
    - Epithelium is affected
  - Basal-cell carcinoma
    - Dermis is affected
- Both can usually be treated surgically

THE SKELETAL SYSTEM

- Bones (206 in the adult body)
- Joints (there are many, but we are concerned with about 20)
- Cartilage (covers joints)
- Ligaments (connects bones)

Functions of the Skeletal System

- Support the body
- Protection for organs
- Produce red blood cells
- Storage for nutrients
- Provide sites for muscle attachments

Classification of Bones

- Long bones
  - Support
- Short bones
  - Facilitate movement
- Flat bones
  - Provide protection
  - Produce RBCs
- Irregular bones
  - Help make connections between typical bones

Anatomy of Long Bones

- Periosteum
  - Encloses the bone
  - Fibrous connective tissue that contains blood vessels
- Epiphysis
  - Expanded portion at the end
  - Made of spongy bone
  - Compact bone at the end
- Diaphysis
  - Between the epiphysis
  - Made of compact bone
- Medullary cavity
  - Cavity in center of the bone contains yellow marrow
- Articular cartilage
  - Connection between bones

Classification of Joints

- Synarthrodial—Immoveable (slight movements for shock absorption)
- Amphiarthrodial—Slight mobility (intervertebral)
  - Cartilage disk between bones
- Diarthrodial—Limited mobility (several types)

Structure of Diarthrodial Joints

- Joint cavity—Houses the synovial fluid (lubricates), provides space for movement
- Hyaline cartilage—Protects bones from abrasion, absorbs shock between bones
- Synovial membrane—Encapsulates the joint
  - Articular capsule—Surrounds the articulation (helps keep it together)
  - Ligaments—Connect the bones
  - Tendons—Attach muscle to the bone

Joints of the Skeletal System

- Ball and socket
- Condyloid (ellipsoidal)
- Gliding
- Hinge
- Pivot
- Saddle

Growth and Development

- Skeletal growth begins as cartilage in prenatal development.
- Osteoblasts begin to deposit calcium (ossification).
- First begins in the center of the long bones.
- Called primary ossification points.
- Ossification extends along the shaft.
- At birth, shaft is fully ossified.
- Postnatal bone growth occurs at secondary ossification points called *epiphyseal plates* or "growth plates."
- The epiphyseal plate has four layers
  - Zone of resting cells—Serves as reservoir for future growth
  - Proliferative zone—Cartilage cells increase in size
  - Hypertrophic zone—Cartilage cells arrange themselves in vertical columns
  - Calcified cartilage zone—Cartilage cells erode and bone is deposited by osteoblasts

Ossification of Short Bones

- Ossify from the center outward.
- At birth, about 400 ossification centers exist.
- After birth, another 400 more develop.
- After puberty, growth plates ossify and bone stops growing (evidence that excessive stress can cause premature ossification).
- Bone is constantly being broken down (osteoclasts).
- Rebuilt again by osteoblasts.
- Else, we could not recover from a broken bone.

Fractures

- Simple—Bone does not pierce the skin.
- Compound—Bone does pierce the skin.
- Incomplete—Bone broken, but not into two separate parts.
- Greenstick—Incomplete break, usually occurring in children (young bones).
- Impacted—Bone is wedged into bone, usually longitudinally..
- Comminuted—Broken into several pieces.
- Spiral—Resulting from torsion (twisting).

Surface Features of Bone

The adult human skeleton consists of 206 bones:

- 28 skull bones (8 cranial, 14 facial, and 6 ear bones).
- The horseshoe-shaped hyoid bone of the neck.
- 26 vertebrae (7 cervical or neck, 12 thorax, 5 lumbar or loins, the sacrum which is five fused vertebrae, and the coccyx, human vestigial tail, which is four fused vertebrae).
- 24 ribs plus the sternum or breastbone; the shoulder girdle (2 clavicles, the most frequently fractured bone in the body, and 2 scapulae).
- Pelvic girdle (2 fused bones).
- 30 bones in human arms and legs (a total of 120).
- There are also a few partial human bones, ranging from 8–18 in number.

Appendicular System—126

- Upper right and left extremities—32 each
  - Shoulder girdle to phalanges
- Lower right and left extremities—31 each
  - Pelvic girdle to phalanges

Skeletal Muscle Structure

- Tendons connect muscle to bone.
- Fascia connects the muscle to tendon.
  - Fascia is connective tissue, several layers thick.
  - Innermost layer called "epimysium."
- Fascicles exist within the epimysium.
  - The fascicles are separated by "perimysium."
- Muscle "fibers" within the fascicle are separated by *endomysium*
- Muscle fibers contain *myofibrils*
  - They run the length of the muscle fiber.
- Myofibrils contain protein filaments called *actin* and *myosin.*
  - Actin and myosin move in opposite directions to cause muscular contraction.
  - Muscles shorten no more than about 60% of resting length.

Parts of the Myofibrils

- Actin and myosin protein filaments make up much of the muscle fiber.
  - Actin is the thin, light filament.
  - Myosin is the thicker, darker filament.

- The arrangement of these fibers produces darker and lighter areas (striations).
  - The dark areas of myosin are called the "A bands."
  - The light areas of actin are called the "I bands."
- Actin filaments also occur inside the A bands during contraction; the actin filaments slide further into the A bands.
- The area in the middle of the A band that has no actin is called the "H zone."
  - Myosin filaments grow thicker here and are called the "M line."
  - During contraction, this area grows smaller due to the actin filaments.

What else would get smaller? (Answer: I bands)

- In the I band, the actin filaments are connected in a zigzag arrangement.
- This is referred to as the "Z line."
- The area from one Z line to the next is a "sarcomere."

Structure of Actin and Myosin

- Each of these are protein filaments.
  - Myosin is the most abundant.
    - — Accounts for about 2/3 of the muscle protein.
    - — Molecule composed of two twisted protein strands.
    - — Many of these molecules form a filament.
    - — Strands have globular parts.
    - — Called "cross bridges."
    - — Cross bridges project outward.
  - Actin accounts for about 1/4 of the muscle protein.
    - — Molecule is a globular structure composed of ADP molecules.
    - — These molecules serve as active sites for the cross bridges.
    - — Filament formed from double twisted strand (helix) of actin molecules.

Other Muscle Proteins

- Tropomyosin and troponin (each are associated with the actin filament)
- Tropomyosin
  - Rod-shaped; occupy the longitudinal grooves of the actin molecule.
- Troponin
  - Is a molecule on the tropomyosin and is called a tropomyosin/troponin complex.

HOW CONTRACTIONS OCCUR

Muscle at Rest

- Troponin/tropomyosin complex is exposed to the myosin.
- No linkage can be formed between the two molecules.

Contraction

- High concentration of calcium ions become present.
- Calcium ions bind to the troponin, moving the position of the complex. This exposes the active sites on the actin to the myosin cross bridges.
  - Linkages can be formed which cause the shortening.

Where Does the Calcium Come From?

The sarcoplasmic reticulum contains a high level of calcium ions.

- Stimulus (action potential) reaches the sarcoplasmic reticulum—the sarcoplasmic membrane becomes more permeable to calcium ions.

Where Does the Stimulus Come From?

- Stimulus, muscle impulse, action potential is all the same.

Muscle contraction needs stimulation from a specific neurotransmitter; that neurotransmitter is acetylcholine. Acetylcholine is produced in the cytoplasm of motor neurons and is shipped in vesicles to the motor nerve fiber. It remains in the distal end of the axon.

As the nerve impulse reaches the end of the axon, acetylcholine is released into gap between axon and motor nerve plate.

- Acetylcholine binds with receptor molecules in the sarcolemma.
    - This binding causes the muscle stimulus (action potential).
- Stimulus travels in all directions over the surface of the sarcolemma.
- Reaches deep into the muscle and finally to the sarcoplasmic reticulum.

Relaxation

- An active transport system (calcium pump) begins to work.
    - Rapidly moves the calcium ions back into the sarcoplasmic reticulum.
    - At this point, calcium is moving both into and out of the sarcoplasmic reticulum.

Also, *cholinesterase* begins the rapid decomposition of acetylcholine.

- With the acetylcholine gone, the sarcoplasmic membrane is no longer permeable to calcium.
- Linkages between actin and myosin break, troponin is exposed, and muscular contraction is inhibited.

Muscular Contraction Review

- Mentally, when you want to contract a muscle:
    - Nerve cell that controls muscle sends impulse toward that muscle.
    - When impulse reaches neuromuscular junction (synaptic gap), *acetylcholine* is released.
    - Acetylcholine binds with the receptor molecules in the cell.
    - Causes an action potential (AP) to be generated in the muscle.
    - AP reaches deep into muscle to the sarcoplasmic reticulum (SR).
    - AP causes SR to become more permeable to calcium (Ca).
    - Ca leaves the SR and binds with troponin (located on the tropomyosin).
    - Causes the tropomyosin-troponin complex to invert itself.
    - This exposes the active sites, which bind to the myosin cross bridges.
    - Presence of ATP causes bending at this connection, resulting in muscular contraction.

Breakdown of Contractions

When an action potential is created, a single signal is sent to the muscle to contract (shorten).

- Contraction ends and then relaxation (lengthening) occurs.
- This process can be divided into three periods:
    - Latency period
        - After the stimulus reaches the muscle and before contraction begins

  - Contractile period
    - From beginning to end of contraction
    - Beginning of shortening to beginning of lengthening
  - Relaxation period
    - Period where muscle fiber is lengthening

Typically, many stimuli are sent to contracting muscles to cause contractions.

- This can result in a condition of maximal contraction, called *tetanus.*
- With prolonged tetanus, muscular fatigue will occur.
- Muscular lengthening with continued stimulus—hold a 50-lb crate with elbows at 90°.
- Inability of muscle to rapidly relax—seen in hamstring tears (quad too strong for hams).

Recruitment

Neural stimulation causes electrical impulse to be sent to muscle.

- Causes shortening.
- Similarly, electric shock also causes muscular contraction.
- Electrical impulses are sent to the muscle from motor neurons.
- Connection occurs at the neuromuscular junction.
- A motor end plate is formed.
- Mitochondria and nuclei are abundant.
- This is called a *motor unit*—a single motor neuron and all the muscle fibers it innervates.

All or None Principle

- Motor units contract on an "all or none" principle.
- Not speaking of entire muscle, just the motor unit.
- The motor neuron receives electrical signals from brain. When the neuron reaches a threshold, an action potential is created.
- Larger motor units exist in the larger muscles.
- Provides greater contractile force faster.
- Results in smaller control of muscle contraction.
- Smaller motor units exist in the smaller muscles.
  - Gives us the fine motor control versus gross motor control.

Energy Sources for Contraction

- The energy used to contract comes from ATP (adenosine triphosphate).
  - This is supplied by mitochondria in the sarcoplasm.
- Globular portions of myosin contain an enzyme called ATPase.
  - The enzyme causes ATP to decompose to ADP + P + energy.
  - The energy causes the cross bridge to bend.
  - This causes the contraction.
  - Only a very small amount of ATP is present in the sarcoplasm.
  - Contractions from this ATP are very short.
  - ATP can be resynthesized from creatine phosphate (CP).
  - CP stores excess energy.
  - Given off by the mitochondria during the Krebs cycle.
  - Uses this energy to form a bond with the phosphate.
  - ADP has a greater polarity than CP.
  - It uses the energy and the phosphate to make more ATP.

CELLULAR METABOLISM

Metabolism

Anabolic Metabolism

- Smaller molecules used to build larger molecules.
- Process used is *dehydration synthesis*.
  - H^+ and OH^- are removed (H_2O).
- Monosaccharides (glucose) synthesize complex carbohydrates.
- Glycerol and fatty acids synthesize lipids.
- Amino acids synthesize proteins.
  - Peptide bonds occur (between C and N atoms)

Catabolic Metabolism

- Larger molecules are broken down to smaller molecules.
- Process used is *hydrolysis*.
- H_2O is added (as H^+ and OH^-).
- Opposite reactions occur as far as:
  - Complex carbohydrates
  - Lipids
  - Proteins

Enzymes

- Usually proteins, these speed up/assist reactions.
- May contain inactive part used for binding.
  - Called a cofactor
  - If organic, is a coenzyme
    - — Coenzymes are frequently vitamin molecules.

Energy for Metabolic Reactions

- Energy is stored in the bonds between atoms.
- When molecules are broken down, energy is given off.
- Some energy is captured chemically (ATP).
- ATP has high energy bonds.
- Some energy escapes (warms the body).

Production of Energy (Two Phases)

- Anaerobic metabolism
- Aerobic metabolism

Anaerobic Metabolism

- Glucose is broken down to pyruvic acid (pyruvate).
- 6-carbon glucose => two 3-carbon pyruvates.
- This is called glycolysis.
- This gives off energy for two ATP molecules.
  - Occurs very fast
  - Rapid form of energy

- Pyruvate is unstable, quickly converted to lactic acid (lactate).
- Lactate is later removed by oxygen.

Aerobic Metabolism

- Pyruvate breaks down to 2-carbon acetyl group.
  - Two pyruvates => three acetyls.
- Acetyl group combines with coenzyme A (acetyl CoA).
- Acetyl CoA acted on by oxygen.
  - Goes through a series of steps (citric acid cycle—Krebs cycle).
  - Gives off 36 ATP molecules.
  - By-products are CO_2 and H_2O.
- Requires oxygen.
- Produces ATP slowly.

Metabolic Pathways

A series of reactions to convert substance to ATP.

Carbohydrate Pathway (described above)

Lipid Pathway

- Fats must first undergo hydrolysis (addition of water).
- Are then converted to acetyl-CoA (through beta-oxidation).
- Others are converted first to ketone bodies, then to acetyl-CoA; is the efficient way of burning fuel.
- The body always uses the most efficient method.

Protein Pathways

- Proteins are converted to amino acids.
- Amino acids have aminos removed (deamination).
- Various pathways occur, depending upon the amino acid.
  - Some paths lead to acetyl-CoA.
  - Others lead to various steps in the Krebs cycle.
- By-product is urea (high in nitrogen) and is hard on the liver to deaminate proteins.

? QUESTIONS

1. Which of the following structures is NOT part of the respiratory system?
   a. The epiglottis
   b. The pharynx
   c. The esophagus
   d. The larynx
2. At the end of the bronchioles are thousands of tiny air sacs known as:
   a. alveoli
   b. bronchi
   c. pleurae
   d. capillaries

3. A thin layer of connective tissue covers the outer surface of the lungs. This is called the:
   a. inferior pleura
   b. parietal pleura
   c. interpleural space
   d. visceral pleura
4. The upper chambers of the heart are called the:
   a. myocardium
   b. aorta
   c. ventricles
   d. atria
5. To cause the heart to contract, an electrical impulse must travel through the following route:
   a. the SA node, the AV node, the Purkinje fibers, the bundle of His
   b. the SA node, the AV node, the bundle of His, and the Purkinje fibers
   c. the AV node, the SA node, the bundle of His, and the Purkinje fibers
   d. the AV node, the SA node, the Purkinje fibers, and the bundle of His

Suggested Readings

Seeley R, et al. *Anatomy and Physiology.* 6th ed. New York: McGraw-Hill; 2002.

US Department of Transportation, National Highway Traffic Safety Administration. *EMT-Paramedic: National Standard Curriculum.* Washington, DC: US Department of Transportation, National Highway Traffic Safety Administration; 1998.

Chapter 7
Pharmacology

Your patient is a 55-year-old male who presents to EMS sitting at the kitchen table in moderate respiratory distress. His elbows are on the table allowing him to be seated in a tripod position, and he appears to be really working at breathing. Although this problem came on gradually today, his family states that he has had lung disease for a long time. He is a lifetime smoker and is on home oxygen at 3 lpm via nasal cannula.

He takes the following medications:

- Atrovent MDI
- Theolair (theophylline)
- Proventil MDI
- Advair 250/50

He appears very thin and barrel chested with a pink complexion. You immediately notice pronounced accessory muscles in his neck and chest along with retractions. His breathing is labored, pursing his lips during exhalation. His vital signs are pulse 94 irregular, BP 140/80, respiratory rate of 40 labored, skin is warm and pink, diffuse wheezes, and his SpO_2 is 90%.

What would be the pharmacologic treatment of choice for this patient?

Pharmacology—The study of drugs and their actions on the body.

Chemical Name—A description of the drug's chemical composition and molecular structure.

Generic Name—Official name approved by the Food and Drug Administration (FDA)

Trade Name—The brand name registered to a specific manufacturer or owner.

Official Name—The name assigned by the U.S. Pharmacopeia (official volumes of drug standards).

WHAT IS A DRUG?

A drug is a chemical agent that is used in the diagnosis, treatment, or prevention of disease.

ORIGIN OF DRUGS

- Plants
  - Alkaloids
  - Glycosides
  - Gums
  - Oils

- Animals and humans
- Minerals or mineral products
- Chemical substances made in a laboratory

DRUG CLASSIFICATION

Drugs are classified by body system, class of agent, and mechanism of action.

Sources for Drug Information

- AMA drug evaluation
- Physician's Drug Reference (PDR)
- Hospital formulary
- Drug inserts

DRUG LEGISLATION IN THE UNITED STATES

- The purpose of legislation is to protect the public from adulterated or mislabeled drugs.
- History of particular drug legislation includes:
  - Pure Food and Drug Act, 1906
  - Harrison Narcotic Act, 1914
  - Federal Food, Drug, and Cosmetic Act, 1938

SCHEDULE OF CONTROLLED SUBSTANCES (TABLE 7-1)

Controlled Substance Act of 1970—Purpose was to schedule controlled substances based on potential for abuse. They are numbered from I to V.

INVESTIGATIONAL DRUGS

- Investigational drugs may take years to progress through the FDA testing sequence.
- Animal studies may be used to ascertain:
  - Toxicity
  - Therapeutic index
  - Modes of absorption, distribution, metabolism, and excretion
- Human studies may be used for investigational drugs as well.

TABLE 7-1: Schedule of Controlled Substances

Schedule	Abuse Potential	Medical Use	Examples
I	High	No accepted medical use	Heroin, mescaline, LSD
II	High	Accepted medical uses, may lead to severe medical and/or psychological dependence	Opium, morphine, codeine, oxycodone, methadone, cocaine, secobarbital
III	Less potential	Accepted medical uses, may lead to moderate to low physical dependence and/or high psychological dependence	Acetaminophen with codeine, aspirin with codeine
IV	Lower than schedule III	Accepted medical use, may lead to limited physical or psychological dependence	Phenobarbital, diazepam, lorazepam
V	Lower abuse than schedule IV	Accepted medical use, may lead to limited physical or psychological dependence	Medications containing limited quantities of certain opiates

SPECIAL CONSIDERATIONS IN DRUG THERAPY

Pregnant Patients

U.S. FDA Pregnancy Category Definitions

A—Controlled studies in women fail to demonstrate a risk to the fetus in the first trimester, and the possibility of fetal harm appears remote.

B—Animal studies do not indicate a risk to the fetus and there are no controlled human studies; animal studies do show an adverse effect on the fetus, but well-controlled studies in pregnant women have failed to demonstrate a risk to the fetus.

C—Studies have shown that the drug exerts animal teratogenic or embryocidal effects, but there are no controlled studies in women, nor are studies available in animals.

D—Positive evidence of human fetal risk exists, but benefits in certain situations (i.e., life-threatening situations or serious diseases for which safer drugs cannot be used or are ineffective) may make use of the drug acceptable despite its risks.

X—Studies in animals or humans have demonstrated fetal abnormalities or there is evidence of fetal risk based on human experience, or both, and the risk clearly outweighs any possible benefit.

DRUG ADMINISTRATION—PEDIATRIC PATIENTS

Based on the patient's weight and body surface area.

DRUG ADMINISTRATION—GERIATRIC PATIENTS

The physiological effects of aging can lead to altered pharmacodynamics and pharmacokinetics.

Management of Drug Administration

- Paramedics are responsible for the safe administration of any drug they administer.
- They must deliver the medication via the appropriate route, observe and document the effects of the drugs, and identify drug indications and contraindications.
- Paramedics must take a thorough patient history, including:
  - Prescribed medication name, strength, and daily dosage
  - Over-the-counter medications
  - Vitamins
  - Drug reactions
- Consult with medical control, when appropriate.

AUTONOMIC PHARMACOLOGY

The autonomic nervous system is composed of the sympathetic and parasympathetic divisions. It functions to stimulate smooth muscle, cardiac muscle, and exocrine glands. It also regulates:

- Heart rate and blood pressure
- Sweat, salivary, and gastric secretions
- Pupil diameter and eye accommodation

- Gastrointestinal motility
- Diameter of the bronchioles

DIVISIONS OF THE AUTONOMIC NERVOUS SYSTEM

Each parasympathetic and sympathetic nerve:

- Originates in the central nervous system (CNS).
- Has its activity controlled and integrated by the brain, and contains a preganglionic neuron, whose cell of origin lies within the CNS, and a postganglionic neuron, whose cell of origin lies within a ganglion outside the CNS.
- The pre- and postganglionic neurons synapse at a ganglion.

Parasympathetic Division (Feed and Breed)

- Most preganglionic fibers originate in the midbrain or medulla oblongata of the brain.
- Ganglia are found close to, or within, innervated organs.
- A few preganglionic nerves leave the CNS in the sacral portion of the spinal cord. These fibers also synapse with postganglionic nerves close to, or within, the innervated organs.
- The parasympathetic nervous system carries on many of the mundane day-to-day functions, such as, flow of saliva, peristalsis, constriction of pupils, and accommodation for near vision.

Sympathetic Division (Fight or Flight)

- Sympathetic preganglionic fibers begin in the intermediolateral columns of the spinal cord and extend from the first thoracic to the second or third lumbar segments.
- Once outside the spinal cord, preganglionic fibers synapse with postganglionic nerves at ganglia located in three areas of the body:
  - Paravertebral ganglia, which lie on each side of the vertebral column
  - Prevertebral ganglia (i.e., celiac, superior mesenteric, inferior mesenteric, and aorticorenal ganglia) in the abdominal cavity
  - Terminal ganglia near the urinary bladder and rectum
- Stimulation of the sympathetic nervous system prepares the body to meet stress in the following ways:
  - Increasing heart rate
  - Elevating cardiac output
  - Stimulating intermediary metabolism
  - Dilating bronchioles
  - Redistributing blood from the gastrointestinal (GI) tract to the skeletal muscles

NEUROTRANSMITTERS (CHEMICAL TRANSMISSION OF IMPULSES)

Ganglia

- **Acetylcholine** is the neurotransmitter at all autonomic ganglia. Released by preganglionic nerve endings, acetylcholine stimulates nicotinic receptors on the postganglionic neurons.

Parasympathetic Nerve Endings

- **Acetylcholine** is also the neurotransmitter at all parasympathetic nerve endings. Following its release, acetylcholine stimulates muscarinic receptors on the innervated tissue.

Sympathetic Nerve Endings

- **Norepinephrine** (noradrenaline) is the neurotransmitter released from most sympathetic postganglionic neurons. Once released, it stimulates alpha-1 receptors on blood vessels to cause vasoconstriction, or beta-1 receptors in the heart to increase both heart rate and force of contraction.
- **Acetylcholine** is the neurotransmitter released by a few sympathetic postganglionic nerves (such as, sympathetic innervation of the sweat glands), where it stimulates muscarinic receptors.

Adrenal Medulla

- **Epinephrine** (adrenaline) is an emergency hormone released by the adrenal medulla. It increases heart rate by stimulating cardiac beta-1 receptors and dilates the bronchioles by stimulating beta-2 receptors. Adrenaline redistributes blood in the body, shunting it from the peritoneal area to the skeletal muscles. It does this by stimulating alpha-1 receptors on visceral vessels and beta-2 receptors on vessels in skeletal muscle.

Synthesis and Inactivation of Neurotransmitters

- **Acetylcholine**—Synthesized within nerves from acetylcoenzyme A and choline by the enzyme choline acetylase; acetylcholine is stored in vesicles within the nerve until released. The enzyme acetylcholine esterase, also formed within the nerve, rapidly inactivates acetylcholine.

Why is it important to understand how a neurotransmitter is inactivated when treating a patient with organophosphate poisoning? ***Organophosphate poisoning inhibits the production of acetylcholine esterase which causes a large accumulation of acetylcholine. This is what causes the signs and symptoms of S.L.U.D.G.E.M. (Salivation, Urination, Defecation, GI Upset, Emesis, Muscle twitching).***

Norepinephrine and Epinephrine

- Epinephrine, norepinephrine, and dopamine are often called **catecholamines**.
- In the noradrenergic neurons, the end product is norepinephrine. In the adrenal medulla, the synthesis is carried one step further. An enzyme found in the adrenal medulla, phenylethanolamine-methyltransferase, converts norepinephrine to epinephrine. The human-adrenal medulla contains approximately four times as much epinephrine as norepinephrine. The absence of phenylethanolamine-*N*-methyltransferase in noradrenergic neurons accounts for the absence of significant amounts of epinephrine in noradrenergic neurons.
- The final step in the synthesis of norepinephrine, the conversion of dopamine to norepinephrine, takes place within intraneuronal storage vesicles. Norepinephrine is released from noradrenergic nerve endings by action potentials through exocytosis. The norepinephrine contents of entire vesicles are emptied into the synaptic region, where they may interact with adrenergic receptors.
- Norepinephrine is removed from the area of the synapse and receptors by:
  - Reuptake into the secreting neuron. Neuronal reuptake is the most important mechanism for terminating the action of released norepinephrine.
  - Following neuronal reuptake, norepinephrine is either stored in vesicles or inactivated by mitochondrial monoamine oxidase (MAO); diffused from the synapse into the circulation and ultimate enzymatic destruction in the liver by

MAO or catechol-*O*-methyltransferase (COMT); and catecholamine is actively transported into effector cells (extraneuronal uptake), followed by enzymatic inactivation by COMT.

AUTONOMIC RECEPTORS

Cholinergic Receptors

- Nicotinic receptors (so-called because the effects of nicotine in ganglia and on skeletal muscle mimic the actions of acetylcholine).
- Found in all autonomic ganglia. Nicotinic receptors are also found on skeletal muscle.
- However, nicotinic receptors in ganglia are not identical to those on skeletal muscle. Nicotinic receptors in ganglia can be blocked competitively by ganglionic blockers. Ganglionic blockers do not block nicotinic receptors on skeletal muscle; rather, these receptors are blocked by neuromuscular blockers.

Muscarinic Receptors

- Named because of the effects of muscarine on receptors innervated by parasympathetic postganglionic nerves and sympathetic cholinergic nerves mimic the actions of acetylcholine on these receptors.
- Found in smooth muscle, cardiac muscle, and exocrine glands innervated by parasympathetic nerves. They are involved in the constriction of bronchioles, slowing of heart rate, increase in GI motility, and secretion of salivary, gastric, and bronchiolar glands. They are also found in sweat glands innervated by the sympathetic nervous system. Muscarinic receptors are also located in the brain. Several subtypes of muscarinic receptors have been detected:
  - M1 receptors are found in various secretory glands.
  - M2 receptors predominate in the myocardium and also appear to be found in smooth muscle.
  - M3 and M4 receptors are located in smooth muscle and secretory glands.
  - All subtypes are found in the CNS.

Adrenergic Receptors

Alpha-1 postsynaptic receptors are found on smooth muscle innervated by sympathetic nerves. Important functions include vasoconstriction of precapillary resistance vessels (arterioles) and capacitance vessels (veins).

Alpha-2 presynaptic receptors are found on adrenergic nerve terminals. They are responsible for reducing the release of norepinephrine from sympathetic nerves.

Beta-1 postsynaptic receptors are found on postsynaptic effector cells, especially in the heart. They are responsible for the sympathetically mediated increase in heart rate and force of contraction. They are also found on fat cells where they are responsible for the sympathetically mediated increase in lipolysis. Beta-1 receptors also mediate the release of renin.

Beta-2 postsynaptic receptors are found on the bronchioles, where they mediate sympathetic bronchodilation. They are located on precapillary resistance vessels (arterioles) in skeletal muscle where they mediate vasodilation. Beta-2 receptors relax the bladder and decrease intestinal motility.

Biological Model Systems and Receptor Characterization

General properties of drugs:

- Drugs do not present any new functions on a tissue or organ in the body, they only modify existing functions.
- Drugs in general exert multiple actions rather than a single effect.

- Drug action results from a physiochemical interaction between the drug and a functionally important molecule in the body.
- Drugs that interact with a receptor to stimulate a response are known as agonists.
- Drugs that attach to a receptor but do not stimulate a response are called antagonists.
- Drugs that interact with a receptor to stimulate a response, but inhibit other responses, are called partial agonists.

Once administered, drugs go through four stages:

1. Absorption
2. Distribution
3. Metabolism
4. Excretion

Drug Forms

Liquid Forms

- Solutions
- Tinctures
- Suspensions
- Spirits
- Emulsions
- Elixirs
- Syrups

Solid Drug Forms

- Pills
- Powders
- Tablets
- Suppositories
- Capsules

Gas Forms

- Oxygen

Routes of Drug Administration

- The mode of drug administration affects the rate at which onset of action occurs and may affect the therapeutic response that results.
- The choice of the route of administration is crucial in determining the suitability of a drug.
- Drugs are given for either their local or systemic effects.
- The routes of drug administration are categorized as:
  - Inhalation route (nebulized medications)
  - Enteral (drugs administered along any portion of the gastrointestinal tract):
    - — Sublingual
    - — Buccal
    - — Oral
    - — Rectal
    - — Nasogastric
  - Parenteral (any medication route other than the alimentary canal):
    - — Subcutaneous

— Intramuscular
— Intravenous
— Intrathecal
— Pulmonary
— Intralingual
— Intradermal
— Transdermal
— Umbilical
— Intraosseous
— Nasal
— Endotracheal

Mechanisms of Drug Action

- To produce optimal desired or therapeutic effects, a drug must reach appropriate concentrations at its site of action.
- Molecules of the chemical compound must proceed from point of entry into the body to the tissues with which they react.
- The magnitude of the response depends on the dosage and the time course of the drug in the body.
- Concentration of the drug at its site of action is influenced by various processes, which are divided into three phases of drug activity.

Pharmaceutical

- Disintegration of dosage form
- Dissolution of drug

Pharmacokinetic—The body's reaction to drugs, including their absorption, distribution, metabolism, and elimination

Pharmacodynamics—The study of the effects of drugs on the body

- Drug-receptor interaction

Pharmacokinetics

Absorption

Mechanisms involved in absorption:

- Diffusion
- Osmosis
- Filtration

Variables that affect drug absorption:

- Nature of the absorbing surface
- Blood flow to the site of administration
- Solubility of the drug
- pH
- Drug concentration
- Dosage form
- Routes of drug administration
- Bioavailability

Distribution

When a drug is introduced into the body, where it ends up depends on a number of factors:

- Blood flow—Tissues with the highest blood flow receive the drug first.
- Protein binding—Drugs stuck to plasma proteins are crippled, they can only go where the proteins go.
- Lipid solubility and the degree of ionisation—This describes the ability of drugs to enter tissues (highly lipid soluble/unionised drugs can basically go anywhere).

Metabolism

- Is necessary to eliminate the drug.
- Many drugs are nonpolar and their theoretical half lives (t1/2) might be days to weeks unless they were metabolized.
- Having a drug accumulate in the body that long, without being eliminated, would be deadly!
- Sometimes metabolism yields a more active metabolite.

Excretion

Organs of excretion:

- Kidneys
- Intestine
- Lungs
- Sweat and salivary glands
- Mammary glands

Drug-Response Relationship

- Plasma level profile of a drug
- Biologic half-life
- Therapeutic threshold or minimum effective concentration
- Therapeutic index—Ratio of dose of drug that has a toxic effect to that which has a therapeutic effect
  - Minimum toxic dose/minimum therapeutic dose
  - Also termed "margin of safety"

Factors Altering Drug Responses

- Age
- Body mass
- Gender
- Environmental milieu
- Time of administration
- Pathologic state
- Genetic factors
- Psychological factors

Predictable Responses

- Desired action
- Side effects

Unpredictable Adverse Responses

- Drug allergy
- Anaphylactic reaction
- Delayed reaction ("serum sickness")
- Hypersensitivity
- Idiosyncrasy
- Tolerance
- Cross tolerance
- Tachyphylaxis
- Cumulative effect
- Drug dependence
- Drug interaction
- Drug antagonism
- Summation (addition or additive effect)
- Synergism
- Potentiation
- Interference

Drug Interactions

- Variables influencing drug interaction include:
    - Intestinal absorption
    - Competition for plasma protein binding
    - Drug metabolism or biotransformation
    - Action at the receptor site
    - Renal excretion
    - Alteration of electrolyte balance
- Drug-drug interactions
- Other drug interactions
    - Drug-induced malabsorption of foods and nutrients
    - Food-induced malabsorption of drugs
    - Alteration of enzymes
    - Alcohol consumption
    - Cigarette smoking
    - Food-initiated alteration of drug excretion
- Drug incompatibilities—occur when drugs are mixed

Drug Storage

- Certain precepts should guide the manner in which drugs are secured, stored, distributed, and accounted for.
- Refer to local protocol.
- Drug potency can be affected by:
    - Temperature
    - Light
    - Moisture
    - Shelf life
- Applies also to diluents.
- Security of controlled medications.

Components of a Drug Profile

- Drug names
- Classification
- Mechanisms of action
- Indications
- Pharmacokinetics
- Side/adverse effects
- Routes of administration
- How supplied
- Dosages
- Contraindications
- Considerations for pediatric patients, geriatric patients, pregnant patients, and other special patient groups

Commonly Administered Prehospital Medications (Listed in Alphabetical Order)

Activated Charcoal

INDICATIONS:	• Used to treat certain types of poisonings and overdoses
ADMINISTRATION:	• Administered PO
DOSAGE: ADULT: PEDIATRIC:	 • 50 g • 1 g/kg
THERAPEUTIC EFFECTS:	• Binds and absorbs various chemicals and poisonous compounds, thereby reducing their absorption into the body
CONTRAINDICATIONS:	• Caustic/Corrosive substances • Cyanide poisonings • Semiconscious or unconscious patients
SIDE EFFECTS:	• Abdominal cramping, constipation, dark stools, nausea, and vomiting
SPECIAL NOTES/RESTRICTIONS:	• Does not absorb all drugs or toxic substances (i.e., cyanide, lithium, iron, lead, arsenic, etc.) • Has no effect in methanol or organophosphate poisonings • Has little therapeutic value in caustic alkalis and acid poisonings • Should not be given with ice cream, milk, sherbet, or syrup of ipecac

Adenosine (Adenocard)

INDICATIONS:	• Paroxysmal supraventricular tachycardia • Supraventricular tachycardia • Wolf-Parkinson-White syndrome
ADMINISTRATION:	• Rapid intravenous (IV), rapid intraosseous (IO) followed by normal saline (NS) flush
DOSAGE:	
ADULT:	• Supraventricular tachycardia: initial 6 mg IV bolus over 1–2 seconds, increase to 12 mg every 1–2 min as needed for 2 doses, maximum single dose 12 mg
PEDIATRIC:	• Initial: 0.1 mg/kg intravenous pyelogram (IVP) (MAX: 6 mg) • Repeat: 0.2 mg/kg IVP (MAX: 12 mg)
THERAPEUTIC EFFECTS:	• Slows conduction time through atrioventricular (AV) node • Interrupts reentry pathways through AV node • Restores sinus rhythm in patients with supraventricular tachycardia (SVT)
CONTRAINDICATIONS:	• Hypersensitivity to adenosine • Second or third degree AV block • Sinus node dysfunction, such as sick sinus syndrome or symptomatic bradycardia • Atrial flutter/atrial fibrillation • Sick sinus syndrome • Ventricular tachycardia
SIDE EFFECTS:	• Transient AV block, asystole, and other dysrhythmias • Chest pressure • Dizziness • Flushing • Nausea • Shortness of breath
SPECIAL NOTES/RESTRICTIONS:	• Onset is generally within less than 1 minute • Adverse effects are usually short-lived and easily tolerated • Effects may be more pronounced in patients on dipyridamole • Effects may be attenuated in patients on theophylline preparations

Albuterol (Ventolin, Proventil)

INDICATIONS:	• Acute bronchospasm
ADMINISTRATION:	• Handheld nebulizer, nebulizer mask, endotracheal tube (ETT)
DOSAGE:	
ADULT:	• 2.5 mg/3 cc normal saline solution (NSS)
PEDIATRIC:	• 2.5 mg/3 cc NSS
THERAPEUTIC EFFECTS:	• Decreases bronchospasm via beta receptors • Improves pulmonary function
CONTRAINDICATIONS:	• Hypersensitivity to any of the contents of the solution • Tachydysrhythmias
SIDE EFFECTS:	• Cough • Dizziness or nervousness • Nausea • Tachycardia • Tremor
SPECIAL NOTES/RESTRICTIONS:	• May be put down the ETT in intubated asthmatics or COPD patients

Amiodarone (Cordarone)

INDICATIONS:	• Ventricular fibrillation, ventricular tachycardia, rapid atrial fibrillation, rapid atrial flutter, SVT
ADMINISTRATION:	• IVP or IV infusion
DOSAGE:	
ADULT:	• Pulseless ventricular fibrillation/ventricular tachycardia (VF/VT)—Initial: 300 mg IVP • Pulseless VF/VT—Repeat: 150 mg IVP • Rapid Atrial Fib/Flutter: 2.5—5 mg/kg slow IVP • Rapid A Fib/Flutter (alternative): 150 mg/100 cc D_5W over 10 minutes • SVT: 2.5—5 mg/kg IVP • SVT (alternative): 150 mg/100 cc D_5W over 10 minutes • Stable V Tach: 2.5—5 mg/kg slow IVP • Stable V Tach (alternative): 150 mg/100 cc D_5W over 10 minutes
PEDIATRIC:	• Pulseless VF/VT: 5 mg/kg IVP • Rapid A Fib/Flutter: 5 mg/kg IV over 20–60 minutes • SVT: 5 mg/kg IV over 20–60 minutes • Stable V Tach: 5 mg/kg IV over 10 minutes
THERAPEUTIC EFFECTS:	• Prolongs action potential and refractory period • Reduces ventricular dysrhythmias and raises fibrillatory threshold

CONTRAINDICATIONS:	• Cardiogenic shock • Hypersensitivity to amiodarone • Second or third degree AV block • Severe sinus bradycardia • Severe sinus node dysfunction
SIDE EFFECTS:	• Hypotension • Bradycardia, asystole, and pulseless electrical activity
SPECIAL NOTES/RESTRICTIONS:	• Serial use of calcium channel blockers, beta blockers, and other antiarrhythmics may cause additive hypotensive, bradycardic, and proarrhythmogenic effects • Draw up slowly to prevent bubbling

Aspirin

INDICATIONS:	• Myocardial infarction, chest pain
ADMINISTRATION:	• Chewed PO
DOSAGE: ADULT: PEDIATRIC:	 • 4 baby aspirin (81 mg each) • Not indicated
THERAPEUTIC EFFECTS:	• Inhibits platelet aggregation by blocking formation of thromboxane A2 • Reduces overall mortality of acute MI • Reduces nonfatal reinfarction
CONTRAINDICATIONS:	• Hypersensitivity to aspirin • Active bleeding condition or ulcer • Pregnancy
SIDE EFFECTS:	• Heartburn • Indigestion • Nausea
SPECIAL NOTES/RESTRICTIONS:	• Patients on Coumadin (warfarin) MAY take aspirin in the acute setting

Atropine (Atropine, Component of Mark I Auto-Injector)

INDICATIONS:	• Symptomatic bradycardia, asystole, pulseless electrical activity, nerve agent poisoning, organophosphate poisoning
ADMINISTRATION:	• IV, IO, endotracheal (ET), intramuscular (IM)
DOSAGE: ADULT:	 • Asystole: 1 mg IVP or 2 mg ETT q3–5min (up to 0.04 mg/kg) • Bradycardia: 0.5–1 mg IVP (up to 0.04 mg/kg)

	• Nerve agents: 2 mg IVP/IM q5min until relief of symptoms
PEDIATRIC:	• Bradycardia: 0.02 mg/kg IVP (min 0.1 mg, max 1 mg; up to 0.04 mg/kg) • Nerve agents: 2 mg IVP/IM q5min until relief of symptoms
THERAPEUTIC EFFECTS:	• Blocks acetylcholine receptor sites • Decreases vagal tone • Increases SA and AV nodal conduction • Dries secretions
CONTRAINDICATIONS:	• Tachycardia
SIDE EFFECTS:	• Blurred vision • Dry mouth • Headache • Pupillary dilatation • Tachycardia
SPECIAL NOTES/RESTRICTIONS:	• Organophosphate or nerve agent poisoning may require large doses • Consider atropine before epinephrine in pediatric bradycardia only if the bradycardia is suspected to be from increased vagal tone or primary AV block

Calcium Chloride

INDICATIONS:	• Hyperkalemic cardiac arrest, calcium channel blocker overdose, hypocalcemia
ADMINISTRATION:	• IV, IO
DOSAGE:	
ADULT:	• 1 g (10 cc of 10% solution) IVP
PEDIATRIC:	• 20 mg/kg (0.2 cc/kg of 10% solution) up to 500 mg IVP
THERAPEUTIC EFFECTS:	• Stabilizes cardiac tissue to effects of high potassium
CONTRAINDICATIONS:	• Digoxin toxicity • Hypercalcemia
SIDE EFFECTS:	• Arrhythmias • Bradycardia • Cardiac arrest • Hypotension
SPECIAL NOTES/RESTRICTIONS:	• Do not administer with sodium bicarbonate or it may crystallize in the intravenous line • Not to be routinely used during cardiac arrest

Cyanide Antidote Kit

Dextrose (D50, D25, D10)

INDICATIONS:	• Hypoglycemia
ADMINISTRATION:	• IV, IO
DOSAGE:	
ADULT:	• 25 g (50 cc D_{50}) IVP
PEDIATRIC:	• Newborn: 5 cc/kg D_{10} slowly (1 cc/kg D_{50} mixed with 4 cc/kg NS) • Less than 13 years: 2 cc/kg D_{25} (1 cc/kg D_{50} mixed with 1 cc/kg NS) • 13 or older: 1 cc/kg D_{50}
THERAPEUTIC EFFECTS:	• Immediate source of glucose
CONTRAINDICATIONS:	• CVA with normal serum glucose
SIDE EFFECTS:	• Local irritation
SPECIAL NOTES/RESTRICTIONS:	• Dilute dextrose before administration to pediatric patients • To make D_{25} from D_{50}: Dilute D_{50} 1:1 with sterile water or NS • To make D_{10} from D_{50}: Dilute D_{50} 1:4 with sterile water or NS • Can potentially precipitate acute neurologic symptoms in alcoholics • Causes local tissue necrosis if IV infiltrates

Diazepam (Valium)

INDICATIONS:	• Major motor seizures, status epilepticus, premedication for painful procedures, combative patients
ADMINISTRATION:	• IV, IO, PR, IM (if necessary)
DOSAGE:	
ADULT:	• Procedural sedation and pain management: 2–5 mg IV • Seizures: 5 mg IV over 2 minutes, 10 mg PR, or 2–5 mg IM • Eclamptic seizures: 2 mg IV q5min for effect or 10 mg PR • Nerve agents: 2–10 mg IV or 10 mg IM titrated to effect
PEDIATRIC:	• Procedural sedation and pain management: 0.1 mg/kg IV/IO • Seizures: 0.1 mg/kg IV over 2 minutes or 0.5 mg/kg PR • Nerve agents: 0.1 mg/kg IV/IM MAX DOSES: 5 mg in children and 10 mg in adolescents

THERAPEUTIC EFFECTS:	• Suppresses spread of seizure activity through the motor cortex • Skeletal muscle relaxant • Reduces anxiety and causes sedation
CONTRAINDICATIONS:	• Respiratory depression • Hypotension
SIDE EFFECTS:	• Hypotension • Respiratory depression • Use is cautioned in elderly patients
SPECIAL NOTES/RESTRICTIONS:	• Intramuscular administration leads to widely variable absorption and should be avoided if possible

Diphenhydramine (Benadryl)

INDICATIONS:	• Anaphylaxis, allergic reactions, dystonic reactions
ADMINISTRATION:	• IV, IM, IO
DOSAGE:	
ADULT:	• 25-mg IVP or 50-mg IM
PEDIATRIC:	• 1 mg/kg (0.02 cc/kg) IVP (MAX: 25 mg)
THERAPEUTIC EFFECTS:	• Inhibits histamine release and effects • Anticholinergic effects antagonize extrapyramidal symptoms
CONTRAINDICATIONS:	• Acute asthma exacerbation • Acute glaucoma • Pregnancy
SIDE EFFECTS:	• Blurred vision • Headache • Palpitations • Sedation

Dobutamine (Dobutrex)

INDICATIONS:	• Cardiogenic shock, septic shock
ADMINISTRATION:	• IV infusion, IO infusion
DOSAGE:	
ADULT:	• 5–20 mcg/kg/min infusion
PEDIATRIC:	• 5–20 mcg/kg/min infusion
THERAPEUTIC EFFECTS:	• Improves cardiac output with little systemic vasoconstriction • Increases cardiac contractility

CONTRAINDICATIONS:	• Idiopathic hypertrophic subaortic stenosis (IHSS) • Hypovolemia (uncorrected)
SIDE EFFECTS:	• Bronchospasm • Ectopy • Hypertension or hypotension • Palpitations • Tachycardia
SPECIAL NOTES/RESTRICTIONS:	• If systolic blood pressure is less than 70, dopamine should be used • 6 mg/kg in 100 cc D_5W at 1.0 cc/h equals 1 mcg/kg/min • Hypovolemia should be corrected with volume expansion fluids prior to the administration of dobutamine

Dopamine (Intropin)

INDICATIONS:	• Cardiogenic shock, neurogenic shock, sepsis, refractory hypotension, bradycardia
ADMINISTRATION:	• IV infusion, IO infusion
DOSAGE:	
ADULT:	• 5–20 mcg/kg/min infusion
PEDIATRIC:	• 5–20 mcg/kg/min infusion
THERAPEUTIC EFFECTS:	• Stimulates alpha, beta, and dopamine receptors, depending on dose • Increases cardiac output and systemic arterial pressure • Dilates vessels to brain, heart, and kidneys • Increases heart rate
CONTRAINDICATIONS:	• Uncorrected hypovolemic shock • Uncorrected tachydysrhythmias
SIDE EFFECTS:	• Angina • Ectopy • Headache • Tachydysrhythmias
SPECIAL NOTES/ RESTRICTIONS:	• Titrate to blood pressure • Use dobutamine in cardiogenic shock with systolic BP over 70 • 6 mg/kg in 100 cc D_5W at 1 cc/h equals 1 mcg/kg/min • Hypovolemia should be corrected with volume expansion fluids prior to the administration of dopamine

Epinephrine

INDICATIONS:	• Cardiac arrest, anaphylaxis, bronchospasm, shock
ADMINISTRATION:	• IV, IO, SC, ET, IV infusion, IO infusion, handheld nebulizer
DOSAGE:	
ADULT:	• Cardiac arrest: 1 mg IVP q3–5min or 2 mg ET q3–5min • Bradycardia: 0.5–1 mg IVP or 2–10 mcg/kg/min infusion • Septic or spinal shock: 1–4 mcg/min infusion • Allergic rxn: 0.1–0.3 mg 1:1000 SC or 0.1–0.5 mg 1:10000 slow IVP • Respiratory distress: 0.1–0.3 mg 1:1000 SC
PEDIATRIC:	• Cardiac arrest—INITIAL: 0.01 mg/kg IVP/IO or 0.1 mg/kg ET • Cardiac arrest —REPEAT: 0.1 mg/kg IVP, IO, or ET q3–5min • Bradycardia—INITIAL: 0.01 mg/kg IVP/IO or 0.1 mg/kg ET • Bradycardia—REPEAT: 0.1 mg/kg IVP, IO, or ET q3–5min • Septic or spinal shock: 0.1–1 mcg/kg/min infusion • Allergic rxn: 0.01 mg/kg (0.1 cc/kg) 1:1000 SC or 1:10000 slow IVP • Respiratory distress: 5 cc 1:1000 via handheld nebulizer
THERAPEUTIC EFFECTS:	• Stimulates alpha and beta adrenergic receptors • Increases heart rate, systemic blood pressure, and coronary blood flow
CONTRAINDICATIONS:	• Hypertension • Tachycardia
SIDE EFFECTS:	• Hypertension • Palpitations • Tachycardia • Tremors
SPECIAL NOTES/RESTRICTIONS:	• Pay special attention to using correct concentration (1:1000 or 1:10,000)

Furosemide (Lasix)

INDICATIONS:	• Pulmonary edema
ADMINISTRATION:	• IV
DOSAGE: ADULT: PEDIATRIC:	 • 40 mg IVP or double patient's prescribed dose up to 120 mg IVP • Not applicable
THERAPEUTIC EFFECTS:	• Loop diuretic which inhibits resorption of sodium and chloride • Mild vasodilator
CONTRAINDICATIONS:	• Hypokalemia • Hypovolemia • Pregnancy
SIDE EFFECTS:	• Dehydration • Dysrhythmias

Glucagon

INDICATIONS:	• Hypoglycemia, refractory allergic reaction, beta blocker overdose, GI smooth muscle relaxation
ADMINISTRATION:	• IV, IO, IM
DOSAGE: ADULT: PEDIATRIC:	 • Hypoglycemia: 1 mg IM • Refractory allergic reaction: 1–4 mg IV slow push • Hypoglycemia: 0.1 mg/kg IM (MAX: 1 mg) • GI smooth muscle relaxation: IV 0.25–2.0 mg
THERAPEUTIC EFFECTS:	• Promotes breakdown of hepatic glycogen to glucose • Bypasses blocked beta receptors to stimulate heart rate and contractility
CONTRAINDICATIONS:	• Insulinoma • Pheochromocytoma • Hypersensitivity to glucagon
SIDE EFFECTS:	• Nausea and vomiting • Urticaria
SPECIAL NOTES/RESTRICTIONS:	• Patients need carbohydrate replacement after administration to prevent secondary hypoglycemic events • May not be effective in patients with poor glycogen stores (cancer patients, chronic alcoholics, malnutrition)

Lidocaine

INDICATIONS:	Ventricular arrhythmias
ADMINISTRATION:	IV, IO, ET, IV infusion, IO infusion
DOSAGE:	
ADULT:	• 1 mg/kg IV or 2 mg/kg ET (repeated at 0.5 mg/kg to max of 3 mg/kg)
PEDIATRIC:	• 1 mg/kg IV/IO or 2 mg/kg ET (repeated at 0.5 mg/kg to max of 3 mg/kg)
THERAPEUTIC EFFECTS:	• Suppresses ventricular ectopy • Elevates threshold for ventricular fibrillation • Suppresses reentry arrhythmias
CONTRAINDICATIONS:	• Idioventricular rhythms • Second and third degree AV block • Allergy to local anesthetics • Sinus bradycardia
SIDE EFFECTS:	• Arrhythmias • Hypotension • Irritability • Muscle twitching • Seizures
SPECIAL NOTES/RESTRICTIONS:	• Successful use of lidocaine IVP should be followed by additional boluses • Boluses should be reduced in cases of shock, congestive heart failure (CHF), or elderly patients

Magnesium

INDICATIONS:	• Ventricular arrhythmias, preeclampsia, eclampsia, asthma, torsades de pointes
ADMINISTRATION:	• IV, IO
DOSAGE:	
ADULT:	• Cardiac arrest: 2 g IVP • Ventricular tachycardia: 1–2 g IV over 5–20 min • Asthma: 1–2 g IV over 5–20 min • Preeclampsia: 4 g IV over 20 minutes • Eclampsia: 1 g/min IVP until seizure stops (MAX: 4 g)
PEDIATRIC:	• Cardiac arrest: 20–50 mg/kg IVP/IO
THERAPEUTIC EFFECTS:	• Affects myocardial impulse formation and conduction time • Relaxes smooth muscle

ABSOLUTE CONTRAINDICATIONS:	• None
RELATIVE CONTRAINDICATIONS:	• Active labor • Heart block • Hypocalcemia • Renal failure
SIDE EFFECTS:	• Bradycardia • Hyporeflexia • Hypotension • Respiratory depression
SPECIAL NOTES/RESTRICTIONS:	• Dilute to at least 10 cc before administration • Preferred antidysrrhythmic for patients with torsades de pointes

Mark 1 Auto-Injector (Atropine/Pralidoxime)

INDICATIONS:	• Nerve agent poisoning
ADMINISTRATION:	• IM
DOSAGE:	
ADULT:	• Mild symptoms: 1 kit IM • Moderate symptoms: 1 kit IM q5min for 3 doses • Severe symptoms: 3 kits IM immediately
PEDIATRIC:	• Contact medical command
THERAPEUTIC EFFECTS:	• Blocks acetylcholine receptor sites • Dries secretions • Reactivates acetylcholinesterase enzymes
SIDE EFFECTS:	• Laryngospasm • Muscle rigidity • Blurred vision • Dry mouth • Headache • Pupillary dilatation • Tachycardia
SPECIAL NOTES/RESTRICTIONS:	• Contains 2-mg atropine and 600-mg pralidoxime

Morphine

INDICATIONS:	• Pain management, pulmonary edema, procedural sedation
ADMINISTRATION:	• IV, IO, IM

DOSAGE:	
ADULT:	• Chest pain or pulmonary edema: 2–4 mg IV • Pain: 2–5 mg IV, titrated to effect • Procedural sedation: 3–5 mg IV
PEDIATRIC:	• Pain: 1–3 mg IV/IO, titrated to effect • Procedural sedation: 1–3 mg IV/IO
THERAPEUTIC EFFECTS:	• Binds with opiate receptors to reduce pain • Peripheral vasodilatation
CONTRAINDICATIONS:	• Use of monoamine oxidase inhibitors (MAOIs) within past 14 days • Asthma • COPD • Head injury • Hypotension • Hypovolemia • Respiratory depression
SIDE EFFECTS:	• Bradycardia • Hypotension • Nausea and vomiting • Respiratory depression
SPECIAL NOTES/RESTRICTIONS:	• Naloxone and respiratory equipment should be immediately accessible

Naloxone (Narcan)

INDICATIONS:	• Opiate overdose
ADMINISTRATION:	• IV, IM, SC, ET, intranasal (IN)
DOSAGE:	
ADULT:	• 2 mg IV/IM/SC/ET/IN
PEDIATRIC:	• <5 years or <20 kg 0.1 mg/kg IV/IM/SC/ET • >5 years or >20 kg 2 mg IV/IM/SC/ET
THERAPEUTIC EFFECTS:	• Reverses effects of most narcotic agents
CONTRAINDICATIONS:	• Hypersensitivity to naloxone
SIDE EFFECTS:	• Acute narcotic withdrawal • Hypertension • Irritability • Nausea and vomiting • Tachycardia
SPECIAL NOTES/RESTRICTIONS:	• Does not reverse benzodiazepine overdoses • May precipitate acute withdrawal symptoms • Caution should be exercised when administering naloxone to patients addicted to narcotics

Nitroglycerin (Nitro-Bid, Nitrostat)

INDICATIONS:	• Angina pectoris, pulmonary edema, hypertension
ADMINISTRATION:	• SL
DOSAGE:	
ADULT:	• Angina: 1 metered dose SL q5min for 3 doses • Pulmonary edema—SBP > 160: 2 metered doses SL q3–5min • Pulmonary edema—SBP 100–160: 1 metered dose SL q3–5min
PEDIATRIC:	• Not indicated
THERAPEUTIC EFFECTS:	• Dilates coronary and systemic arteries
CONTRAINDICATIONS:	• Head trauma • Hypertrophic cardiomyopathy • Glaucoma • Hypotension • Use of Viagra (sildenafil) within preceding 48 hours
SIDE EFFECTS:	• Dizziness • Headache • Hypotension
SPECIAL NOTES/RESTRICTIONS:	• Contact medical command prior to administration if taking Viagra

Nitrous Oxide

INDICATIONS:	• Pain management
ADMINISTRATION:	• Inhalation
DOSAGE:	
ADULT:	• Self-administered by mask
PEDIATRIC:	• Self-administered by mask (must be old enough to self-administer)
THERAPEUTIC EFFECTS:	• Decreases sensitivity to pain
CONTRAINDICATIONS:	• Altered mental status • Decompression sickness • Suspected pneumothorax • Chronic lung disease • Head injury • Hypotension • Obvious intoxication • Suspected bowel obstruction
SIDE EFFECTS:	• Dizziness • Drowsiness • Nausea and vomiting
SPECIAL NOTES/RESTRICTIONS:	• Effects diminish 2–5 minutes after removing source

Pralidoxime (2-PAM, Protopam, Component of Mark I Auto-Injector)

INDICATIONS:	• Nerve agent poisoning
ADMINISTRATION:	• IV, IM
DOSAGE: ADULT: PEDIATRIC:	 • 600 mg IM or 1000 mg IV over 15–30 min • 20–50 mg/kg IV over 15–30 min
THERAPEUTIC EFFECTS:	• Reactivates acetylcholinesterase enzymes
SIDE EFFECTS:	• Laryngospasm • Muscle rigidity • Tachycardia

Sodium Bicarbonate

INDICATIONS:	• Cardiac arrest, tricyclic antidepressant, aspirin overdose, hyperkalemia, acidosis
ADMINISTRATION:	• IV, IO
DOSAGE: ADULT: PEDIATRIC:	 • 1 mEq/kg IV • 1 mEq/kg IV/IO
THERAPEUTIC EFFECTS:	• Buffers strong acids in the blood • Antagonizes sodium channel blockade in tricyclic antidepressant (TCA) overdoses • Prevents resorption of salicylates in renal tubules
CONTRAINDICATIONS:	• Hypokalemia • Pulmonary edema
SIDE EFFECTS:	• Dysrhythmias secondary to potassium effects • Metabolic alkalosis • Pulmonary edema
SPECIAL NOTES/RESTRICTIONS:	• Not to be used in place of proper ventilation to prevent acidosis • If less than 2 years old, must be diluted 1:1 with NS or D_5W • Use for cyanide poisoning only if antidotes not available or ineffective

Sodium Thiosulfate

INDICATIONS:	• Victims of cyanide poisoning in severe distress (shock)
ADMINISTRATION:	• IV
DOSAGE: ADULT: PEDIATRIC:	 • 12.5 g (50 cc) IV over 10 minutes (adults and children >25 kg) • 75 mg/kg (0.3 cc/kg) IV over 10 minutes (children <25 kg)
THERAPEUTIC EFFECTS:	• The role of sodium thiosulfate alone is an adjunct to the normal rhodanase metabolism of free cyanide
SIDE EFFECTS:	• No significant side effects
SPECIAL NOTES/RESTRICTIONS:	• Repeat at half dose if symptoms persist

Topical Benzocaine

INDICATIONS:	• Use of topical benzocaine is limited to assisting with the placement of an ETT
ADMINISTRATION:	• Topical
DOSAGE:	• Spray mucous membranes (nose or mouth) for 1 second • This may be repeated ONE time • Avoid sprays in excess of 2 seconds
THERAPEUTIC EFFECTS:	• Topical benzocaine is a local anesthetic chemically related to lidocaine used to facilitate the placement of an endotracheal intubation
ABSOLUTE CONTRAINDICATIONS:	• Known hypersensitivity to benzocaine or other local anesthetics
SIDE EFFECTS:	• Methemoglobinemia • Diminished gag reflex, edema of the airway mucosa, increased chance of aspiration
SPECIAL NOTES/RESTRICTIONS:	• Use cautiously around the eyes • Do not apply to large inflamed tissue areas • Due to retention of the medication, topical benzocaine should not be used underneath dentures or applied to a cotton ball applicator • The use of mouth sprays containing benzocaine may impair swallowing and increase the risk of aspiration

Vasopressin

INDICATIONS:	• Pulseless Arrest
MECHANISM OF ACTION:	• Increases cyclic adenosine monophosphate (cAMP) which increases water permeability at the renal tubule resulting in decreased urine volume and increased osmolality; causes peristalsis by directly stimulating the smooth muscle in the GI tract; direct vasoconstrictor without inotropic or chronotropic effects
DOSAGE:	• 40 Units/IV

Verapamil (Calan, Isoptin, Verelan, Covera)

INDICATIONS:	• Supraventricular tachydysrhythmias
ADMINISTRATION:	• IV, IO
DOSAGE:	
ADULT:	• 2.5–5 mg IV over 2 minutes
PEDIATRIC:	• Not indicated
THERAPEUTIC EFFECTS:	• Calcium channel blocker • Delays impulse propagation through AV node • Dilates coronary and systemic arterial systems
CONTRAINDICATIONS:	• Wolf-Parkinson-White (WPW) syndrome • AV block • Cardiogenic shock • Hypotension
SIDE EFFECTS:	• AV blockade • Bradycardia • Dizziness • Headache • Hypotension
SPECIAL NOTES/RESTRICTIONS:	• Do NOT use in WPW patients as it can cause cardiac arrest • Use caution if wide complex tachycardia

VAUGHN WILLIAMS' ANTIARRHYTHMIC DRUG CLASSIFICATION

- Class I: Agents that block sodium channels
- Class II: Agents that antagonize catecholamine effects
- Class III: Agents that prolong the action potential duration
- Class IV: Agents that block calcium channels

? CHAPTER QUESTIONS

1. The main source of drugs is:
   a. animals
   b. plants
   c. minerals
   d. all of the above
2. Which of the following is one of the "six" rights of medication administration?
   a. The right container
   b. The right doctor
   c. The right route
   d. The right pharmacy
3. An example of the enteral route of drug administration is:
   a. sublingual
   b. intravenous
   c. subcutaneous
   d. topical
4. Buccal administration of a drug is accomplished:
   a. by nasal spray
   b. through a newborn's umbilical vein or artery
   c. between the cheek and gum
   d. through an intraosseous needle
5. A liquid form of a drug prepared using an alcohol extraction process is called a/an:
   a. solution
   b. tincture
   c. emulsion
   d. spirit
6. The prototype opioid antagonist is:
   a. opium
   b. versed
   c. narcan
   d. ibuprophen
7. The central nervous system stimulants known as the methylxanthines include:
   a. ritalin
   b. dexedrine
   c. theophylline
   d. amphetamine sulfate

8. Benzodiazepines and barbiturates are the two main pharmacologic classes in the functional class of:
   a. antiseizure or antiepileptic drugs
   b. analgesics and antagonists
   c. antianxiety and sedative-hypnotic drugs
   d. anesthetics
9. Stimulation of the parasympathetic nervous system results in:
   a. papillary dilation
   b. secretion of the digestive glands
   c. increase in heart rate and cardiac contractile force
   d. bronchodilation

Questions 10 through 14: Match the term with the definition.

10. Atropine	a. Proventil
11. Terbutaline	b. Drug used to treat high cholesterol
12. Insulin	c. Antidote for organophosphate poisoning
13. Antihyperlipidemics	d. Secreted from the beta cells in the pancreas
14. Beta-2 Medication	e. Beta-2 medication used for asthma treatment

Suggested Readings

Circulation 2005 112 [Suppl I]: IV-78 - IV-83; published online before print November 28, 2005, doi:10.1161/CIRCULATIONAHA.105.166559

Halperin HR, Tsitlik JE, Gelfand M, et al. A preliminary study of cardiopulmonary resuscitation by circumferential compression of the chest with use of a pneumatic vest. *N Engl J Med.* 1993;329:762–8.

Paradis NA, Martin GB, Rivers EP, et al. Coronary perfusion pressure and the return of spontaneous circulation in human cardiopulmonary resuscitation. *JAMA.* 1990; 263:1106–13.

US Department of Transportation, National Highway Traffic Safety Administration. EMT-Paramedic: National Standard Curriculum. Washington, DC: US Department of Transportation, National Highway Traffic Safety Administration; 1998.

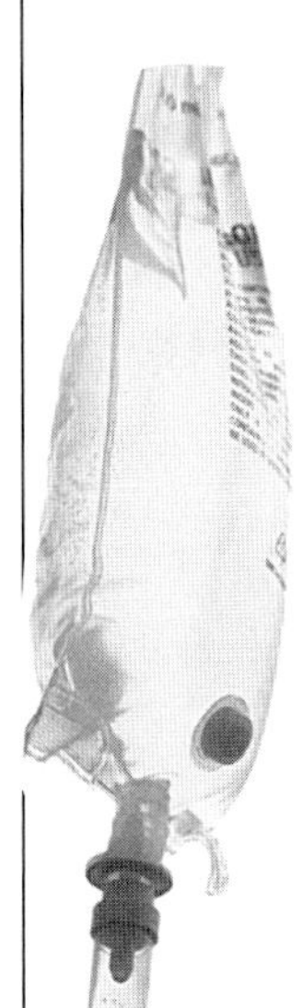

Chapter 8

Venous Access and Medication Administration

Your medical control physician orders an intravenous (IV) drip of lidocaine at 2 mg/min. You mix 2 g of lidocaine in 500 mL of normal saline. You are using a microdrip administration set.

How many drops per minute will your infusion be?

MATHEMATICAL EQUIVALENTS USED IN PHARMACOLOGY

- The metric system
- Conversions between household units and the metric system
- Fahrenheit scale for temperature reading
- Celsius (centigrade) scale for temperature reading
- Converting between Fahrenheit and Celsius temperatures

CALCULATING DRUG DOSAGES

Calculation methods

- Fraction method
- Ratio method
- Desired dose over available concentration method

LEGAL CONSIDERATIONS

Policies and procedures specify regulations of medication administration.

PRINCIPLES OF MEDICATION ADMINISTRATION

- Local drug distribution system—policies which establish stocking and supply of drugs
- Paramedic's responsibility associated with the drug order includes:
  - Verification of the drug order
  - The "six rights" of medication administration
    - — Right patient
    - — Right drug

- Right dose
- Right route
- Right time
- Right documentation

MEDICAL ASEPSIS

- Clean technique versus sterile technique
- Sterilization
- Antiseptics
- Disinfectants

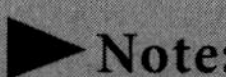
Note:

Universal precautions and body substance isolation (BSI) in medication administration should be used.

PHARMACOLOGY CALCULATIONS

Basic Units of the Metric System

- Meter (m)
- Gram (g, Gm)
- Liter (L, l)
- kilo (k) = 1000 × more
- hecto = 100 × more
- deca = 10 × more
- deci = 10 × less
- centi (c) = 100 × less
- milli (m) = 1000 × less
- micro (mc, μ) = 1,000,000 × less

Apothecary

- Weight
- 480 grains = 1 oz
- 12 oz = 1 lb
- (1.0 grain = 60 mg)
- Volume
- 1 dram = 60 grains (= 4 mL)
- (1 ounce = 30 mL)

Household

- Tablespoon (T, tbs)
- 1 T = 15 mL
- Teaspoon (t, tsp)
- 1 t = 5 mL
- Drop (gtt)
- 60 gtts = 1 tsp

Additional Measures

- International units (U)
- Percentage measures (%)
- g/100 mL
- Milliequivalent measures (mEq)
- Ratio measures (#:###)

Equivalencies

- 5280 feet = 1 mile
- 5280 feet/mile
- 1000 mg = 1 gram
- 1000 mg/g
- 60 mg = 1 gr
- 60 mg/gr
- 2.2 lb = 1 kg
- 2.2 lb/kg
- 1000 mL = 1 liter
- 1000 mL/L
- 60 drops = 1 mL
- 60 gtts/mL
- 100 mg = 1 mL
- 100 mg/mL

Math Review

- Numerator = top number
- Denominator = bottom number

Conversions

- 1 × 1000 = 1000
- 1 × 100 = 100
- 1 × 10 = 10
- 1 × 1 = 1
- 1/10 = 0.1
- 1/100 = 0.01
- 1/1000 = 0.001
- 1 kg = 1000 g
- 1 mg = 0.001 g
- 1000 mg = 1 g
- 0.001 mL = 1 l
- 1 l = 1000 mL
- 1 kg = 1000 g
- 1 g = 1000 mg

Multiplying Fractions

- Multiply the numerators
- Multiply the denominators
- Reduce the product to the lowest common denominator

Dividing Fractions

- Invert the divisor portion of the problem
- Multiply the two numerators
- Multiply the two denominators
- Reduce answer to lowest terms

Dimensional Analysis

- Identify desired units
- Identify relevant givens
- Identify necessary conversion factors
- Set up problem
- Cancel units
- Reduce fractions
- Solve remaining math

CHAPTER QUESTIONS

1. A patient is to be given 3 mg of Diazepam orally. Syrup available has stock strength 2 mg in 5 mL. What volume will you administer?
2. A patient is ordered 0.25 mg of Digoxin. 250 μg tablets are available. How many tablets will you give the patient?
3. A patient is ordered 120 mg of Propanolol three times a day. 40-mg tablets are available. How many tablets will be administered at each dose?
4. A patient is to receive 10 mL of Amoxicillin suspension. 100 mg in 5 mL suspension is available. How many milligrams of Amoxicillin will the patient receive?
5. A patient is ordered 100 mg of medication T by intramuscular (IM) injection. Available is 50 mg in 1 mL of liquid. What volume will you administer?
6. A patient is ordered 40 mg of Loxapine by IM injection. 50 mg in 1 mL ampules are available. What volume will you administer?
7. An adult is ordered 24 mg of medication P as premedication. On hand are ampules containing 20 mg/mL. What volume should be drawn up into the syringe?
8. A patient is to receive 1 L of normal saline over 6 hours. What will the flow rate be?
9. 300 mL of Dextrose is to be given over 4 hours. At what rate should it be delivered?
10. A child is to receive 350 mL of solution Z over 8 hours. What will the flow rate be?
11. A patient is given Dextrose 5% for 8 hours. The flow rate is set at 100 mL/h. How much will the patient receive in liters?
12. A young girl is given Dextrose solution 5%. The pump rate is set to 40 mL/h. How much will she receive after 12 hours?
13. A child is to receive 400 mL of Dextrose 5% over 8 hours. This is to be delivered using a microdrip administration set. Calculate the drip rate.
14. A patient is to receive 0.6 L of Dextrose 5% over 6 hours using a standard administration set for crystalloids (15 gtts/mL). Calculate the drip rate.
15. 600 mL of Nitro-Glycerin is to be given to a patient intravenously. How long will it take if the pump is set at 75 mL/h?
16. A female patient is to receive 500 mL of normal saline. The drip chamber is set to deliver 50 mL/h. How long will this take?
17. A patient is to receive 1 L of normal saline over 6 hours. The IV set delivers 20 drops/mL. What is the infusion rate?

18. A child is to receive 350 mL of normal saline solution over 8 hours using a microdrip set. Calculate the drip rate.
19. A patient is to receive 1 unit of blood (500 mL) over 6 hours.
    The IV set delivers 15 drops/mL. Calculate the drip rate.
20. A patient is ordered 100 mg of Loxapine by IM injection. 50 mg in 5 mL ampoules are available. How many ampoules will you administer?
21. The main source of drugs is:
    a. animals
    b. plants
    c. minerals
    d. all of the above
22. Which of the following is one of the "six" rights of medication administration?
    a. The right container
    b. The right doctor
    c. The right route
    d. The right pharmacy
23. An example of the enteral route of drug administration is:
    a. sublingual
    b. intravenous
    c. subcutaneous
    d. topical
24. Buccal administration of a drug is accomplished:
    a. by nasal spray
    b. through a newborns' umbilical vein or artery
    c. between the cheek and gum
    d. through an intraosseous needle
25. A liquid form of a drug prepared using an alcohol extraction process is called a/an:
    a. solution
    b. tincture
    c. emulsion
    d. spirit
26. Stimulation of the parasympathetic nervous system results in:
    a. papillary dilation
    b. secretion of the digestive glands
    c. increase in heart rate and cardiac contractile force
    d. bronchodilation
27. When administering medication by the IM route, insert the needle at a:
    a. 10°–15° angle
    b. 25° angle
    c. 45° angle
    d. 90° angle
28. In standard microdrip administrations sets, 1 mL of fluid is:
    a. 10 gtts
    b. 15 gtts
    c. 45 gtts
    d. 60 gtts

29. How many milligrams are in a gram?
    a. 10
    b. 100
    c. 1000
    d. 10,000
30. Your medical control physician orders an IV drip of Lidocaine at 2 mg/min. You mix 2 g of Lidocaine in 500 mL of normal saline. You are using a microdrip administration set. How many drops per minute will your infusion be?
    a. 15 gtts
    b. 30 gtts
    c. 45 gtts
    d. 60 gtts
31. A dopamine drip is ordered at 5 mcg/kg/min. You are to set up your IV drip by injecting 400 mg of dopamine into a 500 mL IV bag of normal saline. You are using a standard microdrip administration set. The patient weighs 176 lb. What is the patient's weight in kilograms?
    a. 100 kg
    b. 70 kg
    c. 50 kg
    d. 80 kg
32. What is the drip rate?
    a. 30 gtts/min
    b. 15 gtts/min
    c. 45 gtts/min
    d. 60 gtts/min

Suggested Reading

US Department of Transportation, National Highway Traffic Safety Administration. *EMT-Paramedic: National Standard Curriculum*. Washington, DC: US Department of Transportation, National Highway Traffic Safety Administration; 1998.

Chapter 9
Therapeutic Communications

PROCESS OF COMMUNICATION

Communication is the ability to share information with people, and to understand what information and feelings are being conveyed by others. Communication can take on many forms including gestures, facial expressions, signs, and vocalizations (including pitch and tone), in addition to speech and written communications.

Communication Processes

- Source
  - Common symbols
  - Clear format
  - Medium
    - Written
    - Verbal
    - Other symbols
- Encoding
  - The act of placing a message in an understandable format
  - Procedure of translating a message into a code that is understood by sender and receiver
- Message
  - Code and format intended to deliver idea
- Decoding
  - Act of interpreting symbols and format
  - The decoding process can have many flaws
    - Symbols or words sent in the message are not common to both parties
    - Interpretation of message is based on different understandings of symbols or format
- Receiver
  - Person intended to understand message
  - In order for a message to be successful, the source must try to encode in a way the receiver understands
- Feedback
  - The response to a message

HURDLES OF EFFECTIVE COMMUNICATION

There are a wide number of sources of noise or interference that can enter into the communication process. In a patient interview setting, it is even more common since interactions involve people who do not have experience with each other. The following suggests a number of sources of noise:

- Language—The choice of words or language in which a sender encodes a message will influence the quality of communication. Because language is a symbolic representation of a phenomenon, room for interpretation and distortion of the meaning exist.
- Defensiveness, distorted perceptions, guilt, project, transference, distortions from the past.
- Misreading of body language, tone, and other nonverbal forms of communication.
- Noisy transmission.
- Receiver distortion—Selective hearing, ignoring nonverbal cues.
- Power struggles.
- Self-fulfilling assumptions.
- Language—Different levels of meaning.
- Assumptions—That is, assuming others see the situation the same as you, or have the same feelings as you.
- Distrusted source, erroneous translation, value judgment, state of mind of two people.
- Perceptual biases—People attend to stimuli in the environment in very different ways. We each have shortcuts that we use to organize data. Invariably, these shortcuts introduce some biases into communication. Some of these shortcuts include stereotyping, projection, and self-fulfilling prophecies. Stereotyping is one of the most common. This is when we assume that the other person has certain characteristics based on the group to which they belong without validating that they in fact have these characteristics.
- Interpersonal relationships—How we perceive communication is affected by the past experience with the individual. Perception is also affected by the organizational relationship two people have. For example, communication from a superior may be perceived differently than that from a subordinate or peer.
- Cultural differences—Effective communication requires deciphering the basic values, motives, aspirations, and assumptions that operate across geographical lines. Given some dramatic differences across cultures in approaches to such areas as time, space, and privacy, the opportunities for miscommunication while we are in cross-cultural situations are plentiful.

READING NONVERBAL COMMUNICATION CUES

A large percentage of the meaning we derive from communication comes from the nonverbal cues that the other person gives. Often a person says one thing but communicates something totally different through vocal intonation and body language. Mixed signals force the receiver to choose between the verbal and nonverbal parts of the message. Most often, the receiver chooses the nonverbal aspects. Mixed messages create tension and distrust because the receiver senses that the communicator is hiding something or is being less than candid.

Nonverbal communication is made up of the following parts:

- Visual
- Tactile
- Vocal
- Use of time, space, and image

Visual

This is often called body language and includes facial expression, eye movement, posture, and gestures. The face is the biggest part of this. All of us *read* people's faces for ways to interpret what they say and feel. This fact becomes very apparent when we deal with someone with dark sunglasses. Of course we can easily misread these cues especially when communicating across cultures where gestures can mean something very different in another culture. For example, in American culture, agreement might be indicated by the head going up and down, whereas in India, a side-to-side head movement might mean the same thing. We also look to posture to provide cues about the communicator; posture can indicate self-confidence, aggressiveness, fear, guilt, or anxiety. Similarly, we look at gestures such as how we hold our hands, or a handshake. Many gestures are culture bound and susceptible to misinterpretation.

Tactile

This involves the use of touch to impart meaning as in a handshake, a pat on the back, an arm around the shoulder, a kiss, or a hug.

Vocal

The meaning of words can be altered significantly by changing the intonation of one's voice. Think of how many ways you can say "no." You could express mild doubt, terror, amazement, or anger, among other emotions. Vocal meanings vary across cultures. Intonation in one culture can mean support; in another culture it can mean anger.

Use of Time as Nonverbal Communication

Use of time can communicate how we view our own status and power in relation to others. Think about how a subordinate and his/her boss would view arriving at a place for an agreed-upon meeting.

Physical Space

For most of us, someone standing very close to us makes us uncomfortable. We feel our "space" has been invaded. People seek to extend their territory in many ways to attain power and intimacy. We tend to mark our territory either with permanent walls, or in a classroom with our coat, pen, paper, etc. We like to protect and control our territory. For Americans, the "intimate zone" is about 2 ft; this can vary from culture to culture. This zone is reserved for our closest friends. The "personal zone" from about 2–4 ft usually is reserved for family and friends. The "social zone" (4–12 ft) is where most business transactions take place. The "public zone" (over 12 ft) is used for lectures. At the risk of stereotyping, we will generalize and state that Americans and Northern Europeans typify the noncontact group with small amounts of touching and relatively large spaces between them during transactions. Arabs and Latinos normally stand closer together and do a lot of touching during communication. Similarly, we use *things* to communicate. This can involve expensive things, neat or messy things, photographs, plants, etc.

Image

We use clothing and other dimensions of physical appearance to communicate our values and expectations.

NONVERBAL COMMUNICATION

The use of gestures, movements, material things, time, and space can clarify or confuse the meaning of verbal communication.

A *majority* of the meaning we attribute to words comes not from the words themselves, but from nonverbal factors such as gestures, facial expressions, tone, body language, etc. Nonverbal cues can play five roles:

1. Repetition—They can repeat the message the person is making verbally.
2. Contradiction—They can contradict a message the individual is trying to convey.
3. Substitution—They can substitute for a verbal message. For example, a person's eyes can often convey a far more vivid message than words, and often do.

4. Complementing—They may add to or complement a verbal message. A boss who pats a person on the back in addition to giving praise can increase the impact of the message.
5. Accenting—Nonverbal communication may accept or underline a verbal message. Pounding the table, for example, can underline a message.

Skillful communicators understand the importance of nonverbal communication and use it to increase their effectiveness, as well as use it to understand more clearly what someone else is really saying.

A word of warning. Nonverbal cues can differ dramatically from culture to culture. An American hand gesture meaning "A-OK" would be viewed as obscene in some South American countries. Be careful.

DEVELOPING COMMUNICATION SKILLS

Listening Skills

There are a number of situations when you need to solicit good information from others; these situations include:

- Interviewing the patient
- Solving problems
- Seeking information from bystanders or family members

The skill of communication involves a number of specific strengths. The first involves listening skills.

- Listen openly and with empathy.
- Judge the content, not the messenger or delivery; comprehend before you judge.
- Use multiple techniques to fully comprehend (ask, repeat, rephrase, etc.).
- Active body state; fight distractions.
- Ask the other person for as much detail as he/she can provide; paraphrase what the other is saying to make sure you understand it and check for understanding.
- Respond in an interested way that shows you understand the problem and the patient's concern.
- Attend to nonverbal cues, body language, not just words; listen between the lines.
- State your position openly; be specific, not global.
- Communicate your feelings but don't act them out (i.e., tell a person that his behavior really upsets you; don't get angry).
- Be descriptive, not evaluative; describe objectively, your reactions, consequences.
- Be validating, not invalidating ("You wouldn't understand"); acknowledge other's uniqueness, importance.
- Be conjunctive, not disjunctive (not "I want to discuss this regardless of what you want to discuss").
- Don't totally control conversation; acknowledge what was said.
- Own up; use "I", not "They" . . . not "I've heard you are noncooperative."
- Don't react to emotional words, but interpret their purpose.
- Practice supportive listening, not one-way listening.
- Decide on specific follow-up actions and specific follow-up dates.

A major source of problems in communication is defensiveness. Effective communicators are aware that defensiveness is a typical response in a situation especially when negative information or criticism is involved. Be aware that defensiveness is common, particularly with subordinates when you are dealing with a problem. Try to make adjustments to compensate for the likely defensiveness. Realize that when people feel threatened they will try to protect themselves; this is natural. This defensiveness can take the form of aggression, anger, competitiveness, or avoidance among other responses. A skillful listener is aware of the potential for defensiveness and makes needed adjustments. He or she is aware that self-protection is necessary and avoids making the other person spend energy, defending the self.

In addition, a supportive and effective listener does the following:

- Stops talking; asks the other person for as much detail as he/she can provide; asks for other's views and suggestions.
- Looks at the person, listens openly and with empathy to the employee; is clear about his position; is patient.
- Listens and responds in an interested way that shows he understands the problem and the other's concern.
- Is validating, not invalidating ("You wouldn't understand"); acknowledges other's uniqueness, importance.
- Checks for understanding; paraphrases; asks questions for clarification.
- Doesn't control conversation; acknowledges what was said; let's the other finish before responding.
- Focuses on the problem, not the person; is descriptive and specific, not evaluative; focuses on content, not delivery or emotion.
- Attends to emotional as well as cognitive messages (i.e., anger); aware of nonverbal cues, body language, etc.; listens between the lines.
- Reacts to the message, not the person, delivery or emotion.
- Comprehends before judging; asks questions.
- Uses many techniques to fully comprehend.
- Stays in an active body state to aid listening.
- Fights distractions.
- (If in a work situation) Takes notes; decides on specific follow-up actions and specific follow-up dates.

? CHAPTER QUESTIONS

1. Nonverbal communication is made up of the following parts:
   a. visual
   b. tactile
   c. vocal
   d. use of time, space, and image
   e. none of the above
2. A *receiver* is a person intended to understand a message.
   a. True
   b. False

Suggested Reading

US Department of Transportation, National Highway Traffic Safety Administration. *EMT-Paramedic: National Standard Curriculum*. Washington, DC: US Department of Transportation, National Highway Traffic Safety Administration; 1998.

Chapter 10
Life-Span Development

PHYSIOLOGICAL (TABLE 10-1)

INFANCY (BIRTH TO 1 YEAR)

Weight

- ◦ Normally 3.0–3.5 kg at birth
- ◦ Normally drops 5–10% in the first week of life due to excretion of extracellular fluid
- ◦ Exceeds birth weight by second week
- ◦ Grows at approximately 30 gm/day during the first month
- ◦ Should double weight by 4–6 months
- ◦ Should triple weight at 9–12 months
- ◦ Infant's head equal to 25% of the total body weight

Cardiovascular System

- Circulation changes soon after birth
  - Closing of the ductus arteriosus
  - Closing of the ductus venosus
  - Closing of the foramen ovale
  - Immediate increase in systemic vascular resistance
  - Decrease in pulmonary vascular resistance
- Left ventricle strengthens throughout first year

Pulmonary System

- Airways shorter, narrower, less stable, more easily obstructed
- Infants primarily nose breathers until 4 weeks
- Lung tissue is fragile and prone to barotrauma
- Fewer alveoli with decreased collateral ventilation
- Accessory muscles immature, susceptible to early fatigue
- Chest wall less rigid
- Ribs positioned horizontally, causing diaphragmatic breathing
- Higher metabolic and oxygen consumption rates than adults
- Rapid respiratory rates lead to rapid heat and fluid loss

Renal System

- Kidneys unable to concentrate urine
- Specific gravity rarely exceeds 1.020

TABLE 10-1: Normal Vital Sign Ranges for All Age Groups

Age	Heart Rate	Respiratory Rate/Tidal Volume	Systolic Blood Pressure	Temperature
Infancy (birth to 1 year)	• First 30 minutes the heart rate is 100–160 bpm • Averaging out around 120 bpm	• Initially 40–60 • Dropping to 30–40 after the first few minutes of life • Slowing to 20–30 by 1 year of life • 6–8 mL/kg initially • Increasing to 10–15 mL/kg by 1 year old	Systolic blood pressure increases from 70 mmHg at birth to 90 mmHg at 1 year	98–100°F
Toddler (12–36 months) Preschool (3–5 years old)	• Toddlers: 80–130 bpm • Preschoolers: 80–120 bpm	• Toddlers: 20–30 bpm • Preschoolers: 20–30 bpm	• Toddlers: 70–100 mmHg • Preschoolers: 80–110 mmHg	96.8–99.6°F
School Age (6–12 years old)	70–110 bpm	20–30 bpm	80–120 mmHg	98.6°F
Adolescence (13–18 years old)	55–105 bpm	12–20 bpm	100–120 mmHg	98.6°F
Early adulthood (20–40 years old)	70 bpm	16–20 bpm	120 mmHg	98.6°F
Middle adulthood (40–60 years old)	70 bpm	16–20 bpm	120 mmHg	98.6°F
Late Adulthood (61 to older)	Depends on health status	Depends on health status	Depends on health status	98.6°F

Immune System

- Passive immunity retained through the first 6 months of life
- Based on maternal antibodies

Nervous System

- Movements
  - Strong, coordinated suck and gag
  - Well-flexed extremities
  - Extremities move equally when infant is stimulated
- Reflexes
  - Moro reflex
  - Palmar grasp

  - Sucking reflex
  - Rooting reflex
- Fontanelles
  - Posterior fontanelle closes at 3 months
  - Anterior fontanelle closes between 9 and 18 months
  - Fontanelles may provide an indirect estimate of hydration
- Sleep
  - Initially sleeps 16–18 hours per day with sleep and wakefulness evenly distributed over 24 hours
  - Gradually decreases to 14–16 hours per day with 9–10 hour concentration at night
  - Sleeps through the night at 2–4 months
  - Normal infant is easily arousable

Musculoskeletal System

- Bone growth
  - Epiphyseal plate—length
  - Growth in thickness occurs by deposition of new bone on existing bone
  - Is influenced by:
    - — Growth hormone
    - — Genetic factors
    - — Thyroid hormone
    - — General health
- Muscle weight is about 25% in infants

Dental System

- Teeth begin to erupt at 5–7 months

Growth and Development

Rapid changes occur over the first year of life.

- 2 months
  - Tracks objects with eyes
  - Recognizes familiar faces
- 3 months
  - Moves objects to mouth with hands
  - Displays primary emotions with distinct facial expressions
- 4 months
  - Drools without swallowing
  - Reaches out to people
- 5 months
  - Sleeps throughout night without food
  - Discriminates between family and strangers
- 6 months
  - Sits upright in a highchair
  - Makes one-syllable sounds; that is, ma, mu, da, di
- 7 months
  - Fear of strangers
  - Quickly changes from crying to laughing
- 8 months

- Responds to "no"
- Sits alone
- Plays "peek-a-boo"

- 9 months
  - Responds to adult anger
  - Pulls self to standing position
  - Explores objects by mouthing, sucking, chewing, and biting
- 10 months
  - Pays attention to own name
  - Crawls well
- 11 months
  - Attempts to walk without assistance
  - Shows frustration to restrictions
- 12 months
  - Walks with help
  - Knows own name

Psychosocial Development

- Family processes—Reciprocal socialization
  - Scaffolding
  - Attachment
  - Trust versus mistrust
  - Secure attachment
- Temperament—Infants may be
  - Easy child
  - Difficult child
  - Slow to warm-up child
- Crying
  - Basic cry
  - Anger cry
  - Pain cry
- Trust—based on consistent parental care
- Situational crisis—Parental separation reactions
  - Protest
  - Despair
  - Withdrawal
- Growth charts
  - Good for comparing physical development to norm

TODDLER (12–36 MONTHS)

Weight

- Rate of gain slows dramatically
- Average child gains 2 kg/year

Cardiovascular System

- Capillary beds better developed to assist in thermoregulation
- Hemoglobin levels approach normal adult levels

Pulmonary System

- Terminal airways continue to branch
- Alveoli increase in number

Renal System

- Kidneys are well developed in toddler years
- Specific gravity and other urine findings similar to adults

Immune System

- Passive immunity lost, more susceptible to minor respiratory and gastrointestinal infections
- Develops immunity to common pathogens as exposure occurs

Nervous System

- Brain 90% of adult weight
- Myelination increases cognitive development
- Development allows effortless walking and other basic motor skills
- Fine motor skills developing

Musculoskeletal System

- Muscle mass increases
- Bone density increases

Dental System

- All primary teeth have erupted by 36 months

Elimination Patterns

- Toilet training
- Physiologically capable by 12–15 months
- Psychologically ready between 18 and 30 months
- Average age for completion—28 months

Sensory

- Visual acuity—20/30 during the toddler years
- Hearing—Essential maturity at 3–4 years

Psychosocial

Cognitive

- Basics of language mastered by approximately 36 months, with continued refinement throughout childhood
- Understands cause and effect between 18 and 24 months
- Develops separation anxiety—approximately 18 months
- Develops magical thinking—between 24 and 36 months

Play

- Exploratory behavior accelerates
- Able to play simple games and follow basic rules

- Begins to display competitiveness
- Observation of play may uncover frustrations otherwise unexpressed

Sibling Relationships

- Sibling rivalry
- First-born children
- Usually maintain special relationship with parents
- Expected to exercise self-control and show responsibility in interacting with younger siblings

Peer Group Functions

- Children about the same age and maturity levels
- Provide a source of information about the outside world and other families
- Become more important to the child throughout childhood

Parenting Styles and Its Effect on Children

- Authoritarian parenting
- Authoritative parenting
- Permissive-indifferent parenting
- Permissive-indulgent parenting

Divorce Effects on Child Development

- Age
- Cognitive and social competencies
- Amount of dependency on parents
- Type of day care
- Parents' ability to respond to the child's needs

Television

- May be a cause in aggression at this age
- Careful screening of television exposure may be effective

Modeling

- Children begin to recognize the differences of sex
- Begin to model themselves based on sex

SCHOOL-AGE CHILDREN (6–12 YEARS OLD)

Growth Rate

- Average child gains 3 kg/year and 6 cm/year

Bodily Functions

- Most reach adult levels during this period
- Lymph tissues proportionately larger than adult
- Brain function increases in both hemispheres
- Loss of primary teeth and replacement with permanent teeth begins

Psychosocial

Families

- Children allowed more self regulation
- Parents still provide general supervision
- Parents spend less time with children in this age group

Develop Self-Concept

- More interaction with adults and children
- Begin comparing themselves with others
- Develop self-esteem
- Tends to be higher during early years of school than later years
- Often based on external characteristics
- Effected by peer popularity, rejection, emotional support, and neglect
- Negative self-esteem can be damaging to further development

Moral Development

- Preconventional reasoning
- Punishment and obedience
- Individualism and purpose
- Conventional reasoning
- Interpersonal norms
- Social system morality
- Postconventional reasoning
- Community rights versus individual rights
- Universal ethical principles
- Individuals move through development throughout school age and young adulthood at different paces

ADOLESCENCE (13–18 YEARS OLD)

Growth Rate

- Most experience a rapid 2–3 year growth spurt
- Begins distally with enlargement of feet and hands
- Enlargement of the arms and legs follows
- Chest and trunk enlarge in final stage
- Girls are mostly done growing by age 16; boys are mostly done growing by age 18
- Secondary sexual development occurs
- Noticeable development of the external sexual organs
- Pubic and axillary hair develops
- Vocal quality changes occur (mostly in males)
- Menstruation initiates (in females)

Endocrine Changes

- Female
  - Follicle-stimulating hormone (FSH) and luteinizing hormone (LH) release
  - Gonadotropin promotes estrogen and progesterone production
  - Other biologic changes

- Male
  - Gonadotropins promote testosterone production
  - Reproductive maturity
  - Muscle mass and bone growth nearly complete
  - Body fat decreases early in adolescence, and begins to increase later
- Females require 18–20% body fat percentage for menarche to occur
- Blood chemistry nearly equal to adult levels
- Skin toughens through sebaceous gland activity

Psychosocial

Family

- Conflicts arise
- Adolescents strive for autonomy
- Biological changes associated with puberty
- Increased idealism
- Independence and identity changes

Develop Identity

- Self-consciousness increases
- Peer pressure increases
- Interest in the opposite sex increases
- Want to be treated like adults
- Progress through various stages based on how they handle crises, etc.
- Antisocial behavior peaks around eighth or ninth grade
- Minority adolescents tend to have more identity crises than nonminority
- Body image of great concern
- Continual comparison amongst peers
- Eating disorders are common
- Self-destructive behaviors begin
- Tobacco
- Alcohol
- Illicit drugs
- Depression and suicide more common than any other age group

Ethical Development

- Develop capability for logical, analytical, and abstract thinking
- Develop a personal code of ethics

EARLY ADULTHOOD (20–40 YEARS)

- Peak physical conditioning between 19 and 26 years of age
- Adults develop lifelong habits and routines during this time
- All body systems at optimal performance
- Accidents are a leading cause of death in this age group

Psychosocial

- Experience highest levels of job stress during this time
- Love develops

- Romantic love
- Affectionate love
- Childbirth is most common in this age group
- New families provide new challenges and stress
- This period is less associated with psychological problems related to well-being

MIDDLE ADULTHOOD (41–60 YEARS)

- Body still functioning at high level with varying degrees of degradation
- Vision changes
- Hearing less effective
- Cardiovascular health becomes a concern
- Cardiac output decreases throughout this period
- Cholesterol levels increased
- Cancer strikes in this age group often
- Weight control more difficult
- Menopause in women in late 40s early 50s

Psychosocial

Adults in this group are more concerned with "social clock"

- Task oriented
- Pressed for time to accomplish lifelong goals
- Approach problems more as challenges than threats
- Empty-nest syndrome
- Often burdened by financial commitments for elderly parents as well as young adult children

LATE ADULTHOOD (61 YEARS AND OLDER)

- Life span—Maximum approximately 120 years
- Life expectancy—Average length based on year of birth

Cardiovascular Function Changes

Blood Vessels

- Thickening
- Increased peripheral vascular resistance
- Reduced blood flow to organs
- Decreased baroreceptor sensitivity
- By 80 years of age, there is approximately 50% decrease in vessel elasticity

Heart

- Increased workload causes:
  - Cardiomegaly
  - Mitral and aortic valve changes
  - Decreased myocardial elasticity
- Myocardium is less able to respond to exercise
- Fibrous tissues in sinoatrial (SA) node

- Pacemaker cells diminish, resulting in arrhythmia
- Tachycardia not well tolerated
- Blood cells
  - Functional blood volume decreased
  - Decrease in platelet count
  - Red blood cells (RBCs) diminished
  - Poor iron levels

Respiratory System

- Changes in mouth, nose, and lungs
- Metabolic changes lead to decreased lung function
- Muscular changes
- Diaphragm elasticity diminished
- Chest wall weakens
- Diffusion through alveoli diminished
- Lifelong exposure to pollutants, etc.
  - Lung capacity diminished
  - Coughing ineffective
  - Weakened chest wall
  - Weakened bone structure

Endocrine System Changes

- Decreased glucose metabolism
- Decreased insulin production
- Thyroid shows some diminished T3 production
- Cortisol diminished by 25%
- Pituitary gland 20% less effective
- Reproductive organs atrophy in women

Gastrointestinal System

- Mouth, teeth, and saliva changes
- Peristalsis decreased
- Esophageal sphincter less effective
- Gastrointestinal (GI) secretions decreased
- Vitamin and mineral deficiencies
- Internal intestinal sphincters lose tone

Renal System

- 50% nephrons lost
- Abnormal glomeruli more common
- Decreased elimination

Sensory Changes

- Loss of taste buds
- Olfactory diminished
- Diminished pain perception

- Diminished kinesthetic sense
- Visual acuity diminished
- Reaction time diminished
- Presbycusis is defined as problems with hearing

Nervous System

- Neuron loss
- Neurotransmitters diminish
- Sleep-wake cycle disrupted

Psychosocial

Terminal Drop Hypothesis

- Death preceded by a decrease in cognitive functioning over a 5-year period prior to death
- Wisdom attributed to age in some cultures
- 95% of older adults live in communities
- Challenges
- Self worth
- Declining well-being
- Financial burdens
- Death or dying of companions

CHAPTER QUESTIONS

1. A "toddler" is defined as:
   a. 12–36 months of age
   b. 36–48 months of age
   c. 1–12 months of age
   d. none of the above
2. Gonadotropins promote testosterone production in females.
   a. True
   b. False

Suggested Reading

Birren J. *The Psychology of Aging*. Englewood Cliffs, NJ: Prentice Hall; 1964.

US Department of Transportation, National Highway Traffic Safety Administration. *EMT-Paramedic: National Standard Curriculum*. Washington, DC: US Department of Transportation, National Highway Traffic Safety Administration; 1998.

Section 2

Airway

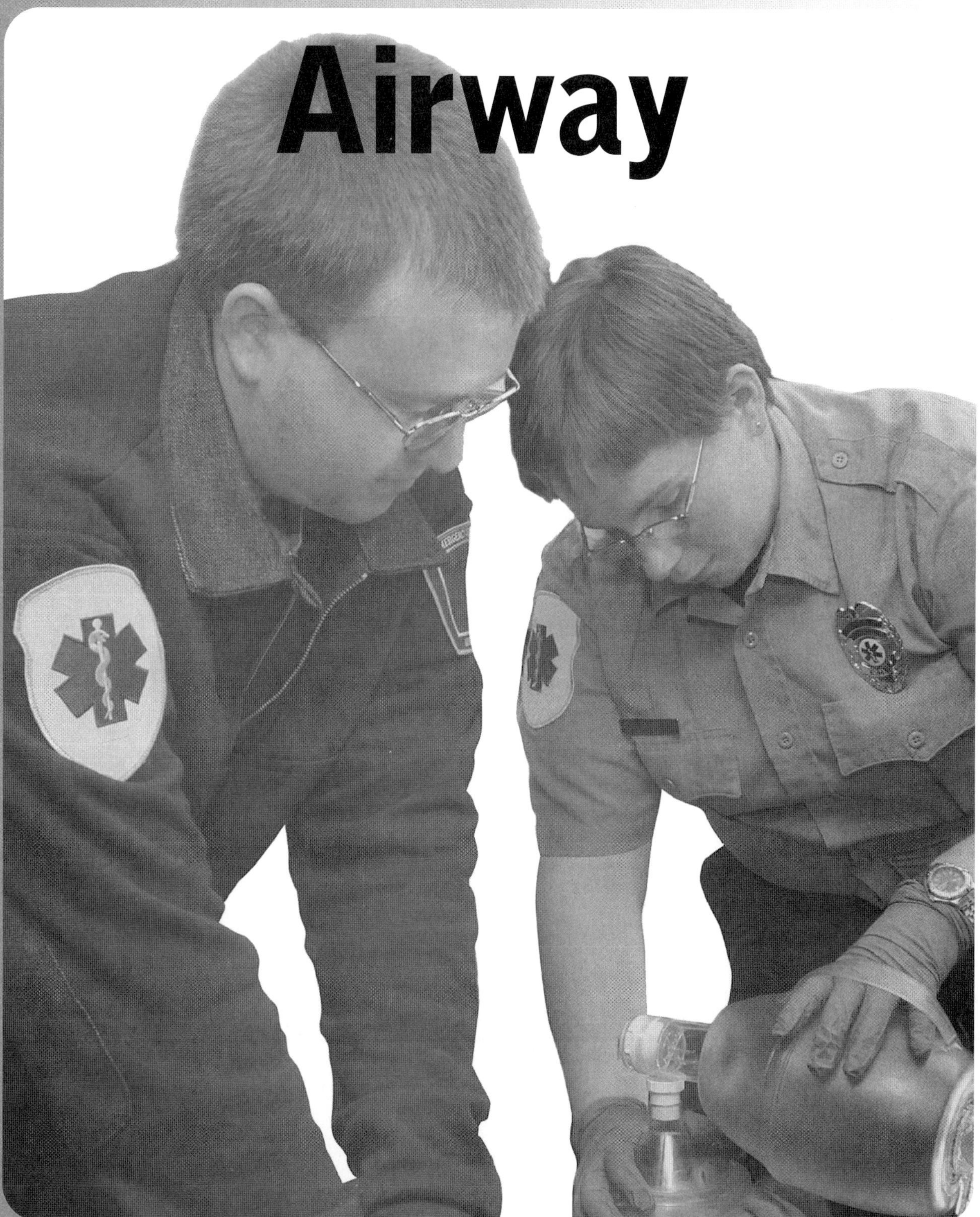

Chapter 11

Airway Management and Ventilation

Your ambulance is called to the corner of 23rd Street and 2nd Avenue for a report of a person having respiratory difficulty. Upon arrival, scene safety is established. You note an approximate middle-aged woman sitting tripod on the corner in obvious respiratory distress. The patient has obvious accessory muscle use, and can only speak in one-word sentences. The patient says, "I . . . can't . . . breathe . . . I . . . need . . . my . . . inhaler!" The patient's vital signs are as follows:

Heart Rate: 110 regular
Blood Pressure: 118/74
Respiratory Rate: 32 shallow and labored
Skin: Warm, pale, and moist
Lung Sounds: Bilateral diffuse wheezing at the bases with absent lung sounds at the apices.

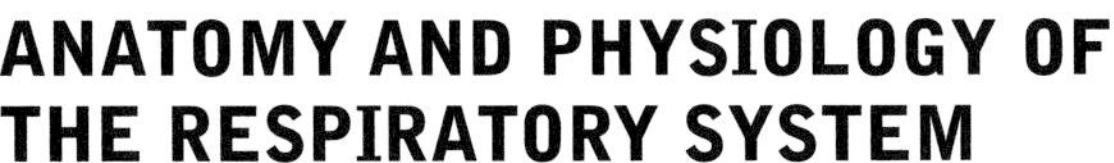

You try to elicit a past medical history, but the patient is unable to say anything other than "Asthma."

Your partner administers high concentration via nonrebreather mask and you establish a large bore intravenous (IV) line of normal saline. What should your next course of management be?

ANATOMY AND PHYSIOLOGY OF THE RESPIRATORY SYSTEM

As health-care professionals, our primary goal in emergency care is to ensure optimal ventilation, delivery of high concentration oxygen (O_2), and proper elimination of carbon dioxide (CO_2).

Anatomy of the Upper Airway

- Function of the upper airway includes warming cold air entering the respiratory tract, filtering impurities, and humidifying air entering the respiratory tract.
- Pharynx (throat).
- Nasopharynx.
  - Formed by the union of facial bones.
  - Orientation of nasal floor is toward the ear, not the eye.
  - Separated by septum (Lined with mucous membranes and cilia).

- Turbinate.
  - Parallel to the nasal floor.
  - Provides increased surface area for air entering, and allows for filtering, humidifying, and warming.
- Sinuses.
  - Cavities formed by cranial bones. Sinuses trap bacteria and act as tributaries for fluid to and from eustachian tubes and tear ducts.
  - Commonly become infected
  - Fracture of certain sinus bones may cause cerebrospinal fluid (CSF) leak.
- Tissues of the upper airway are extremely delicate and vascular.
- Improper or aggressive placement of tubes or airways will cause significant bleeding that cannot be controlled by direct pressure.

Structures of the Oropharynx

- Teeth
  - There are 32 adult teeth
  - Require significant force to dislodge
  - May fracture or avulse causing obstruction
- Tongue
  - Large muscle attached at the mandible and hyoid bone
  - Most common airway obstruction in unconscious patient
- Palate
  - Roof of mouth separates oropharynx/nasopharynx
    - — Anterior is hard palate
    - — Posterior (beyond the teeth) is soft palate
- Adenoids
  - Lymph tissue in the mouth and nose that filters bacteria
- Posterior tongue
- Epiglottis
- Vallecula
  - "Pocket" formed by the base of tongue and epiglottis
  - Important landmark for using the Macintosh blade during endotracheal intubation
- Larynx (voice box)
  - Attached to hyoid bone
  - "Horseshoe-shaped" bone between the chin and mandibular angle
  - Conducts air between the pharynx and trachea
  - Composed of muscle and cartilage
- Thyroid cartilage
  - Largest and most anterior cartilage of larynx
  - "Shield-shaped"
  - Laryngeal prominence
    - — "Adam's apple" anterior prominence of thyroid cartilage
    - — Glottic opening is located posterior to this structure
- Glottic opening
  - Narrowest part of adult trachea
  - Patency heavily dependent on muscle tone
  - Contains vocal bands

- Arytenoid cartilage
  - "Pyramid-like" posterior attachment of vocal bands
  - Important landmark for endotracheal intubation
- Pyriform fossae—"hollow pockets" along the lateral borders of the larynx
- Cricoid ring
  - First tracheal ring, completely cartilaginous
  - Compression occludes esophagus (Sellick's maneuver)
- Cricothyroid membrane
  - Fibrous membrane between the cricoid and thyroid cartilage
  - Site for surgical and alternative airway placement

Associated Structures

- Thyroid gland—Located below the cricoid cartilage and lies across the trachea and up both sides
- Carotid arteries—Branch across and lie closely alongside trachea
- Jugular veins—Branch across and lie close to trachea

Anatomy of the Lower Airway

- Function—Exchange of O_2 and CO_2
- Located from the fourth cervical vertebrae to the Xiphoid process and from the glottic opening to the pulmonary capillary membrane

Structures of the Lower Airway

- Trachea—Bifurcates at the carina into the right and left mainstem bronchi. It consists of tough C-shaped rings of cartilage that keep the trachea open.
  - The right mainstem bronchi has a lesser angle.
    - Foreign bodies and endotracheal (ET) tubes commonly displace here
  - The trachea is lined with:
    - Mucous cells
    - Beta-2 receptors—which dilate bronchioles
- Bronchi.
  - Mainstem bronchi enter the lungs at the hilum.
  - Branch into narrowing secondary and tertiary bronchi that branch into bronchioles.
- Bronchioles—Branch into alveolar ducts that end at the alveolar sacs.
- Alveoli—"grape-like" clusters.
  - The site of gas exchange.
  - Lined with surfactant.
    - Decreases the surface tension of the alveoli, facilitating ease of expansion
    - Alveoli become thinner as they expand, making diffusion of O_2/CO_2 easier
    - Alveoli collapse (atelectasis) if surfactant is decreased or the alveoli are not inflated
- Lungs.
  - The right lung has three lobes.
  - The left lung has two lobes.
  - The lobes are made of parenchymal tissue.
  - Pleura—membranous outer lining.
  - Lung capacity.

The Pediatric Airway

Pharynx

- A proportionately smaller jaw causes the tongue to encroach upon the airway.
- The epiglottis is omega shaped and floppy.
- Dentition is absent or very delicate.

Trachea

- The airway is smaller and narrower at all levels.
- The larynx lies more superior.
- The larynx is "funnel-shaped" due to narrow, undeveloped cricoid cartilage.
- The narrowest point is at the cricoid ring in children younger than 10 years of age.
- Further narrowing of the airway by tissue swelling or foreign body occlusion results in a major increase in airway resistance.

Chest Wall

- The ribs and cartilage are softer.
- The chest wall cannot optimally contribute to lung expansion.
- Infants and children depend more heavily on the diaphragm for breathing.

THE MECHANICS OF RESPIRATION

- Respiration is the exchange of O_2 and CO_2 between an organism and the environment.
- For this gas exchange to occur, air must move freely in and out of the lungs, bringing O_2 to the lungs and removing CO_2 (pulmonary ventilation).
- There are two phases of respiration:
  - External respiration—Transfer of O_2 and CO_2 between inspired air and pulmonary capillaries.
  - Internal respiration—Transfer of O_2 and CO_2 between peripheral blood capillaries and tissue cells.

Pressure Changes and Ventilation

- Gas flows from an area of higher pressure or concentration to an area of lower pressure or concentration.
- Pressure gradient.
  - Required for gas to flow into the lungs
  - Produced by differences in:
    - Atmospheric pressure:
      The pressure of gas around us
      Varies with altitude
      760 mmHg at sea level
    - Intrapulmonic pressure:
      The pressure of the gas in the alveoli
      Varies with the size of the thorax
      Usually a little above and below 760 mmHg, depending on whether it is measured during inspiration or expiration
    - Intrapleural pressure:
      Pressure in the pleural space
      Normally less than atmospheric pressure

Usually 751–754 mmHg
May exceed atmospheric pressure during coughing and straining

Inspiration

- The chest wall expands causing an increase in the size of the thoracic cavity which expands the lungs.
- The lung space increases causing a drop in intrapulmonic pressure to about 1 mmHg below the atmospheric pressure.
- The pressure gradient causes gas to flow into the lungs.
- At the end of inspiration, the thorax stops expanding.
  - The alveoli stop expanding.
  - The intrapulmonic pressure equals the atmospheric pressure.
  - Gas no longer enters the lungs.

Expiration

- The chest wall relaxes. Elastic recoil causes the thorax and lung space to decrease in size, which increases intrapulmonic pressure.
- A pressure gradient is created in the thoracic cavity, which causes:
  - A decrease in alveolar volume
  - An increase in intrapulmonic pressure to about 1 mmHg over atmospheric pressure
  - Gas to flow out of the lungs
- At the end of expiration, opposing forces and pressures become equal.

Muscles of Respiration

- Expansion of the lungs and thorax are made possible by:
  - Movement of the diaphragm.
  - Internal and external intercostal muscles.
- Inspiration (active process):
  - The diaphragm contracts and the dome of the diaphragm flattens.
    - — This increases the superior-inferior dimension of the chest cavity.
  - The internal and external intercostal muscles also contract.
    - — This raises the ribs and increases the anterior-posterior and side-to-side dimensions of the chest cavity.
- Expiration (passive motion):
  - The diaphragm and external intercostal muscles relax.
  - Elastic recoil properties of the lungs allow the size (volume) of thoracic cavity to decrease.
- Compliance is the ease with which the lungs and thorax expand during pressure changes. The greater the compliance, the easier the expansion.
- Diseases that decrease compliance and increase the work of breathing include:
  - Asthma
  - Emphysema
  - Bronchitis
  - Pulmonary edema

The Work of Breathing

- The energy required for normal, quiet breathing is 3% of the total body expenditure in healthy people.

- The energy needs for respiration may be increased by:
  - Loss of pulmonary surfactant
  - Increased airway resistance
  - Decreased pulmonary compliance

Lung Volumes and Capacities

Anatomical dead space—Refers to inspired air that fills the upper respiratory tract and lower nonrespiratory bronchioles but never reaches the alveoli for gas exchange. This accounts for approximately one-fifth of the inspired air from each breath.

Physiological dead space—Refers to the anatomical dead space plus the volume of any nonfunctional alveoli.

Anatomical and physiological dead space is nearly equal in healthy people. Destruction of alveolar walls from respiratory diseases can increase the size of the physiological dead space up to 10 times that of anatomical dead space.

Lung Volumes

Tidal volume is the volume of gas inhaled or exhaled during a normal breath.

- 500–600 mL in the adult male.
- 150 mL remains in the anatomical dead space and is exhaled during the next respiratory cycle.
- Therefore 150 mL of the atmospheric gas entering the respiratory system during each inspiration never reaches the alveoli but is merely moved in and out of the airways.

Inspiratory reserve volume is the amount of gas that can be forcefully inspired after inspiration of the normal tidal volume.

- Usually 2000–3000 mL

Expiratory reserve volume is the amount of gas that can be forcefully expired after expiration of the normal tidal volume.

- Usually less than the residual volume (~1200 mL)

Residual volume is the gas that remains in the respiratory system after forced expiration.

- Usually 1000–1200 mL
- Combined measurements of tidal volume, inspiratory reserve volume, expiratory reserve volume, and residual volume constitute the maximum volume to which the lungs can be expanded

FiO_2 is the percentage of O_2 in inspired air (increases with supplemental O_2).

- Commonly documented as a decimal (i.e., $FiO_2 = 0.85$)

Pulmonary Capacities (The Sum of Two or More Pulmonary Volumes)

Inspiratory capacity is the tidal volume plus the inspiratory reserve volume.

- The amount of gas that can be inspired maximally after a normal expiration (~3500 mL)

Functional residual capacity is the expiratory reserve volume plus the residual volume.

- The amount of gas remaining in the lungs at the end of normal expiration (~2300 mL)

Vital capacity is the volume of gas moved on the deepest inspiration and expiration or the sum of the inspiratory reserve volume, tidal volume, and expiratory reserve volume (~4600 mL).

Total lung capacity is the sum of the inspiratory and expiratory reserve volumes plus the tidal volume and the residual volume (~5800 mL).

Minute Volume and Minute Alveolar Ventilation

Minute volume is the tidal volume multiplied by the respiratory rate.

- The amount of gas inhaled or exhaled in 1 minute.
- If the minute volume is decreased, the patient is not ventilating adequately.

Minute alveolar ventilation is the amount of inspired gas that is available for gas exchange during 1 minute.

- Subtract the amount of dead space from the tidal volume and multiply this figure by the respiratory rate.
- An increase in tidal volume and/or respiratory rate increases minute volume.

MEASUREMENT OF GASES

- **Total pressure** is the amount of pressure by all gases in any mixture of gases.
- **Partial pressure** is the pressure exerted by a single gas.
- Measured in millimeters of mercury (mmHg) or torr.
- One torr equals 1 mmHg.
- Denoted by a "P" preceding the gas (PO_2).
- Atmospheric gases exert a combined partial pressure of 760 mmHg at sea level.
- Nitrogen composes 79% with a partial pressure of 597 mmHg (PN_2 of 597 torr).
- O_2 composes 21% of atmospheric gas with a partial pressure of 159 mmHg (PO_2 of 159 torr).
- **Water vapor pressure** is another partial pressure that can be measured when gas contacts water. Water molecules convert into a gas, evaporate, and exert water vapor pressure (PH_2O).

PULMONARY CIRCULATION

- Gas exchange in the lungs is the opposite of that in the tissues throughout the rest of the body.
- Blood that is low in O_2 travels through right side of the heart.
- Blood flows to either lung through the pulmonary artery, then to smaller pulmonary arterioles, and then to capillaries that surround the alveoli.
- The alveoli, filled with a high concentration of O_2 molecules and a low concentration of CO_2 from inhaled air, have the pressure gradient required for gas exchange.
- O_2 moves into surrounding capillaries as CO_2 moves into alveoli to be exhaled.
- O_2-rich blood flows through the pulmonary venules into the pulmonary veins, then through the left side of the heart, and back out through the aorta to the body's tissues.

EXCHANGE AND TRANSPORT OF GASES IN THE BODY

- In a healthy body with a constant metabolism, the relationship between tissue CO_2 production and O_2 consumption is fixed (200 mL each minute).
- 1 L of O_2 is inspired each minute.
  - 200 mL cross the alveoli into the pulmonary capillaries.
  - 800 mL are exhaled.
- The exchange of O_2 and CO_2 results from the passive process of diffusion.

Diffusion—Molecules in a solution move from an area of higher concentration to an area of lower concentration.

- The molecules of gases are in constant, random motion, which is fueled by collisions with other molecules.
- If blood is divided by a permeable barrier, such as a capillary wall or cell membrane, many gas molecules will contact and cross the barrier.
- There is a much greater likelihood that highly concentrated molecules will strike and cross the membrane than less concentrated molecules.
- The concentration of molecules across a permeable membrane tends to become balanced.
- The diffusion of gases through liquid is determined by the pressure of the gases and the solubility of the gases in liquid.
- The number of gas molecules that dissolve in the liquid is directly proportional to the pressure of the gas.
- When free gas pressure is higher than the pressure of the gas in the liquid, enough molecules dissolve in the liquid for the free gas pressure to equal the dissolved gas pressure (general gas law).
- Free gas (PO_2) in the lungs is greater than that in the bloodstream, so O_2 diffuses from the lungs to the blood.
- The PO_2 in the blood is higher than that in the peripheral tissues, so O_2 diffuses from the blood into the tissues.
- The solubility of the gases in a liquid affects the behavior of the gases.
- The ease with which gases dissolve determines the absolute number of gas molecules that diffuse through the liquid at a given pressure.

Pulmonary Circulation

Blood entering the pulmonary capillaries is systemic venous blood that is relatively high in PCO_2 and low in PO_2. O_2 molecules diffuse from the alveoli (where it is more concentrated) into the blood (where it is less concentrated). CO_2 moves from the blood (where it is more concentrated) to the alveoli (where it is less concentrated).

Respiratory Membrane

- A thin layer of tissue that separates blood flowing through the pulmonary capillaries from the alveolar air.
- Composed of the alveolar wall, interstitial fluid, and the wall of the pulmonary capillary.
- Differences in the PO_2 and PCO_2 on the two sides of the respiratory membrane result in the diffusion of O_2 into the blood and of CO_2 into the alveoli.
  - Diffusion ceases when alveolar and capillary partial pressures become equal.
- Diffusion at the capillary-alveolar level may be affected by respiratory diseases that result in:
  - Destruction and collapse of alveolar walls (atelectasis) with formation of fewer but larger alveoli, resulting in a reduction of the total area available for diffusion.
  - Decreased permeability in the alveolar capillary membrane, which forces gas molecules to travel farther, thereby decreasing the rate of diffusion.

Oxygen

- O_2 is present in the blood in two forms.
  - Physically dissolved in blood (PaO_2).
  - Chemically bound to hemoglobin (Hb) molecules (SaO_2).

- O_2 is relatively insoluble in water.
  - Only 3 mL of O_2 can be dissolved in 1 L of blood at the normal alveolar and arterial PO_2 of 100 mmHg.
  - In contrast, 197 mL of O_2 (about 98%) are carried in red blood cells (RBCs) where it is chemically bound to hemoglobin (Oxyhemoglobin).
  - Hemoglobin can unload CO_2 and absorb O_2 60 times faster than blood plasma.

Hemoglobin Molecules

- Oxyhemoglobin can carry four molecules of O_2 (fully saturated).
  - Hemoglobin nears full saturation at a PO_2 of 80–100 mmHg.
  - The extent to which hemoglobin combines with O_2 increases rapidly when the PO_2 is 10–60 mmHg.
    - About 90% of the total hemoglobin is combined with O_2 when the PO_2 is 60 mmHg.
    - Further increases in PO_2 produce only small increases in O_2 binding to hemoglobin.
    - If the PO_2 falls moderately, the amount of oxyhemoglobin decreases only slightly, still providing adequate tissue oxygenation.
- The PO_2 in the blood plasma is the most important factor in determining the extent to which O_2 combines with hemoglobin.
- Oxyhemoglobin, however, does not contribute to the PO_2 of the blood.
- Only the physically dissolved O_2 molecules can create gas pressure.
- This O_2 uptake by hemoglobin molecules removes dissolved O_2 from blood plasma and maintains a low PO_2, allowing diffusion to continue.

Carbon Dioxide

- The amount of CO_2 produced by the body is relatively constant.
- If the metabolic rate increases, more CO_2 is produced.
- Metabolic processes can also affect CO_2 production.
  - Metabolism that occurs without O_2 (anaerobic metabolism)
  - Production of ketoacids without insulin (ketoacids)
- CO_2 is transported in the blood in three major forms:
  - Plasma (8%)
  - Blood proteins (20%)
  - Bicarbonate ions (72%)
- O_2-free hemoglobin binds more readily to CO_2 than does hemoglobin bound with O_2.
- Some CO_2 that diffuses into RBCs binds to hemoglobin to form carbaminohemoglobin.
- The remainder reacts with water to form carbonic acid.
- Bicarbonate, in contrast to CO_2, is extremely soluble in water.
- Venous blood, which is rich in CO_2, is returned to the lungs. Because the blood PCO_2 is greater than that in the alveoli, CO_2 from the blood diffuses into the alveoli. From there it is expired and eliminated from the body.

Factors That Influence Blood Oxygenation

- In healthy persons, the breathing process allows blood to become fully oxygenated at the alveolar-capillary level and CO_2 to be eliminated.
- Abnormal conditions that can affect blood oxygenation include:
  - A depressed respiratory drive (narcotic overdose)
  - Paralysis of the respiratory muscles (cervical spine injury)

- An increased resistance in the respiratory airways (asthma)
- A decreased compliance of the lungs and thoracic wall (adult respiratory distress syndrome [ARDS])
- Chest wall abnormalities (flail chest)
- A decreased surface area for gas exchange (atelectasis)
- An increased thickness of the respiratory membrane (ARDS)
- Ventilation and perfusion mismatching (pulmonary embolus)
- A reduced capacity of the blood to transport O_2 (anemia)

- Hypoxia—Inadequate O_2 at the cellular level.
- Hypoxemia—A deficiency of O_2 in the arterial blood.
- Anoxia—A lack of O_2.

REGULATION OF RESPIRATION (VOLUNTARY CONTROL OF RESPIRATION)

- Breathing (an involuntary process) can be consciously altered.
  - Voluntary hyperventilation
  - Voluntary apnea
- Most often, respiratory centers override a person's conscious influence, and resume normal function.

Nervous Control of Respiration

- Inspiratory muscles (the diaphragm and intercostal muscles) are composed of skeletal muscle and cannot contract unless they are stimulated by nerve impulses.
  - The phrenic nerves are responsible for moving the diaphragm.
  - The eleven pairs of intercostal nerves are responsible for moving the intercostal muscles.
  - The nerve impulses responsible for controlling these respiratory muscles originate within neurons of the medulla.
    - — This respiratory center is bilateral, with each lateral area composed of two groups of neurons (the inspiratory and expiratory centers) that are responsible for the basic rhythm of respiration.
- Inspiratory center neurons:
  - Are spontaneously active.
  - Exhibit a pattern of activity followed by fatigue and more spontaneous activity.
  - When active, they send impulses along the spinal cord to the phrenic and intercostal nerves, stimulating the muscles of inspiration.
- Expiratory center neurons:
  - Remain inactive during quiet respiration.
  - Appear to be stimulated when activity of the inspiratory center increases (heavy or labored breathing).
  - When active, the expiratory center reciprocates with the inspiratory center, alternating forceful inspiration with forceful expiration.
- There are distinct mechanisms responsible for basic respiratory rhythm established by the inspiratory and expiratory centers, they include:
  - Vagal (Hering-Breuer reflex).
    - — Conveys sensory information from the thoracic and abdominal organs and from stretch receptors in the walls of the bronchi, bronchioles, and lungs.

—Conveys information from the vagus nerve to the medulla.

Discharges inhibitory impulses causing respirations to cease and the lungs to deflate.

Stretch receptors are no longer activated, and the inspiratory center becomes active again.

- Limits respiration and prevents overinflation of the lungs.
- Pneumotaxic center, which is located in the pons, superior to the respiratory center of the medulla. It has an inhibitory effect on the inspiratory center.
- When the inspiratory center activity ceases, inhibitory impulses no longer flow from the pneumotaxic center.
- The inspiratory center discharges impulses that initiate inspiration.
- Appears to be active only in labored breathing.
  - In quiet breathing, stretch receptors are the primary control mechanisms.
- Apneustic center
  - Located in the lower portion of the pons.
  - Stimulates the inspiratory center.
    - — Neurons are constantly active at a baseline rate.
    - — May be overridden by the pneumotaxic center when it is stimulated by a demand for increased ventilation.

Chemical Control of Respiration

- A chemoreceptive area in the medulla that contains neurons sensitive to changes in CO_2 and pH.
  - An increase or decrease in plasma PCO_2 is accompanied by changes in the hydrogen ion concentration.
  - An increased PCO_2 and the resulting decrease in pH adversely affect cellular metabolism.
    - — Excess CO_2 must be eliminated to return the pH to normal limits (accomplished by increasing ventilation).
  - A decreased PCO_2 inhibits ventilation.
    - — Allows CO_2 to accumulate and returns the PCO_2 to normal.
- These adaptive mechanisms maintain PCO_2 within a normal range of 35–45 mmHg.
- O_2 plays a smaller part in regulating respiration. If the arterial PO_2 falls and the pH and PCO_2 are held constant, ventilation increases.

Chemoreceptors

- Monitor arterial PO_2
- Located in medulla and, peripherally, in the bifurcation of the common carotid arteries in the arch of the aorta (carotid and aortic bodies)
- Carotid and aortic bodies
  - Are in intimate contact with the arterial blood of the great vessels
  - Their blood supply is greater than their use of O_2
  - The PO_2 of their tissues is close to that of arterial blood
  - Nerve fibers from these bodies enter the brain stem where they synapse with neurons of the medulla and initiate a respiratory response

Role of Oxygen

- Reduced arterial PO_2 may initiate respirations by stimulating sensory receptors of the carotid and aortic bodies.
  - Usually accompanied by metabolic acidosis secondary to anaerobic metabolism.

- In high altitudes, low barometric pressure may cause a fall in PO_2 low enough to stimulate carotid and aortic bodies.
- Chronic obstructive pulmonary disease (COPD) patients:
  - Have chronically elevated PCO_2.
  - May rely on low PO_2 as the main drive for ventilation (hypoxic drive).
  - Chemoreceptor's become less sensitive to the high CO_2 level and fails to be stimulated by it.
  - Hypoxia becomes the remaining respiratory drive.

Control of Respiration by Other Factors

- Increased body temperature:
  - Febrile illness or physical activity can affect respiratory center neurons (increasing ventilation).
  - Significant decreases (hypothermia) can lower the ventilation rate.
- Medications:
  - Some may increase ventilation (epinephrine).
  - Some may decrease ventilation (diazepam, morphine, narcotics, and barbiturates).
- Painful stimulation may stimulate ventilation.
- Expressions of emotion may increase ventilations (laughing, crying, fear, anger).
- Metabolism—Decreased physical activity may decrease ventilations.

Modified Forms of Respiration

- Cough reflex—Functions to dislodge foreign material or irritants from the respiratory passages.
- Sneezing—Expulsion of gas forced through the nasal cavity.
  - May result from:
    - — Nasal irritants
    - — Stimulation of the fifth cranial nerve in the nose
    - — Exposure to bright lights
- Sigh—Thought to be a protective mechanism that hyperventilates the lungs and reexpands alveoli that might have collapsed.
- Hiccough:
  - Results from a spasmodic contraction of the diaphragm.
  - Thought to serve no useful physiological purpose.

Considerations for Older Patients

- Pulmonary changes that result from aging:
  - Decreased vital capacity.
  - Increased physiological dead space.
- Increased ventilation-perfusion mismatching:
  - Leads to a gradually lowered PO_2.
- Changes in pulmonary physiology include:
  - Alterations in lung and chest wall compliance:
    - — Increased thoracic rigidity.
    - — Decreased elastic recoil.
  - Enlarged alveolar ducts and sacs:
    - — Fewer alveoli.
    - — Less alveolar surface for gas exchange.

- Changes in the body's ventilatory control mechanisms include:
  - The arterial PO_2 falls although there is no significant change in arterial PCO_2.
  - Thought to result from airway closure during exhalation rather than age-related changes in perfusion capacity.
- Chemoreceptor changes include:
  - Diminished ventilatory response to hypoxia, hypercapnia, and similar conditions.
  - May predispose the older patient to respiratory failure.
  - Respiratory compromise in an older patient requires immediate intervention, oxygenation, and ventilatory support.

Pathophysiology

Foreign Body Airway Obstruction (Table 11-1)

According to the National Safety Council, there are about 3000 deaths each year from foreign body airway obstruction.

- Immediate removal of an obstruction might prevent:
  - Hypoxemia
  - Unconsciousness
  - Cardiopulmonary arrest

Laryngeal Spasm and Edema

- Laryngeal spasm—Spasmodic closure of the vocal cords often results from an aggressive intubation technique. Spasm may occur immediately upon extubation, especially when the patient is semiconscious. Laryngeal spasm is best managed with:
  - Aggressive ventilation
  - Forceful upward pull of the jaw
  - Administration of muscle relaxants
- Laryngeal edema—Swelling of the glottic and subglottic tissues may lead to laryngeal closure. Possible causes include:
  - Epiglottitis
  - Croup
  - Allergic reaction
  - Thermal injury
  - Strangulation
  - Blunt trauma
  - Drowning
- The associated swelling may partially or completely obstruct the airway, making aggressive airway management mandatory for patient survival.

Fractured Larynx

- Most often caused by motor vehicle crashes.
- Signs and symptoms include:
  - Localized laryngeal pain on palpation or swallowing
  - Stridor
  - Hoarseness
  - Difficulty with speech (dysphonia)
  - Hemoptysis
- Signs of possible impending airway obstruction include:
  - Subcutaneous emphysema
  - Dysphagia
  - Throat discomfort that increases with coughing or swallowing

TABLE 11–1: AHA Foreign Body Airway Obstruction Table

Maneuver	Adult Lay rescuer: ≥8 Years HCP: Adolescent and Older	Child Lay Rescuer: 1–8 Years HCP: 1 Year to Adolescent	Infant Under 1 Year of Age
ACTIVATE Emergency Response Number (lone rescuer)	Activate when victim found unresponsive **HCP:** if asphyxial arrest likely, call after 5 cycles (2 minutes) of CPR	Activate after performing 5 cycles of CPR; for sudden, witnessed collapse, activate after verifying that victim unresponsive	
AIRWAY	Head tilt–chin lift (HCP: suspected trauma, use jaw thrust)		
BREATHS Initial	2 breaths at 1 second/breath	2 effective breaths at 1 second/breath	
HCP: Rescue breathing without chest compressions	10–12 breaths/min (approximately 1 breath every 5–6 seconds)	12–20 breaths/min (approximately 1 breath every 3–5 seconds)	
HCP: Rescue breaths for CPR with advanced airway	8–10 breaths/min (approximately 1 breath every 6–8 seconds)		
Foreign-body airway obstruction	Abdominal thrusts		Back slaps and chest thrusts
CIRCULATION **HCP:** Pulse check (≤10 sec)	Carotid (**HCP** can use femoral in child)		Brachial or femoral
Compression landmarks	Center of chest, between nipples		Just below nipple line
Compression method: Push hard and fast; allow complete recoil	**2 Hands:** Heel of 1 hand, other hand on top	**2 Hands:** Heel of 1 hand with second on top or **1 Hand:** Heel of 1 hand only	1 rescuer: 2 fingers **HCP**, 2 rescuers: 2 thumb–encircling hands
Compression depth	$1\frac{1}{2}$–2 inches	Approximately $\frac{1}{3}$–$\frac{1}{2}$ the depth of the chest	
Compression rate	Approximately 100/min		
Compression-ventilation ratio	30:2 (1 or 2 rescuers)	30:2 (single rescuer) **HCP**: 15:2 (2 rescuers)	
DEFIBRILLATION			
AED	Use adult pads. Do not use child pads/child system. **HCP:** For out-of-hospital response may provide 5 cycles/2 minutes of CPR before shock if response >4–5 minutes and arrest not witnessed	**HCP:** Use AED as soon as available for sudden collapse and in-hospital **All:** After 5 cycles of CPR (out-of-hospital); use child pads/child system for child 1–8 years if available; if child pads/system not available, use adult AED and pads	No recommendation for infants <1 year of age

Note: Maneuvers used only by health-care providers are indicated by "HCP." (Used with permission from Currents in Emergency Cardiovascular Care, Volume 16 Number 4, Winter 2005–2006. © 2005, American Heart Association.)

- Life-threatening edema may develop rapidly.
  - Rapid intervention may be required

Tracheal Trauma

A rare, but serious injury. Often associated with other injuries to the esophagus and cervical spine.

ASPIRATION BY INHALATION

- Aspiration is the active inhalation of food, a foreign body, or fluid (vomitus, saliva, blood, or neutral liquids) into the airway.
- Aspiration should always be suspected in any patient with a decreased level of consciousness.
- Aspiration may occlude the airway and cause hypoventilation of the distal lung tissue.
- Associated risk factors in children include:
  - Running with food or other objects in the mouth
  - Seizures
  - Forced feedings
- Associated risk factors in adults include:
  - Dental or nasal surgery
  - An unconscious state
  - Swallowing poorly chewed food
  - Alcohol intoxication
- Location of most aspirates:
  - 60% in right bronchus
  - 19% in left bronchus
  - 21% at the larynx or vocal cords
- Death can occur from asphyxiation within minutes.

Effects of Pulmonary Aspiration

- Severity depends on:
  - The pH of the aspirated material.
  - The volume of the aspirate.
  - The presence of food and bacterial contamination.
- Effects of pH:
  - A pH of 2.5 or less generally leads to a severe pulmonary response.
    - — Aspiration of gastric acid can be equated with chemical burns.
    - — A pH less than 1.5 generally results in death of the patient.
- Grossly contaminated aspirate (as in bowel obstruction) leads to nearly 100% mortality rate.
- Effects on lung tissue:
  - Destruction of surfactant-producing alveolar cells.
  - Alveolar collapse and destruction.
  - Destruction of pulmonary capillaries:
    - — Results in pulmonary edema
    - — Hypoventilation
    - — Shunting
    - — Severe hypoxemia
- Fluid shift from the intravascular compartment to the lungs may result in hypovolemia (requiring volume replacement).

Essential Parameters of Airway Evaluation (Rate, Regularity, and Effort)

- Rate—The normal respiratory rate in the resting adult is 12–20 bpm.
- Regularity—A steady inspiratory and expiratory pattern.
  - Breathing at rest should be effortless with only subtle changes in the rate or regularity.
- Respiratory effort—Patients in respiratory distress often assume the following positions to compensate for their inability to breathe easily:
  - Sitting upright with the head tilted back (upright sniffing position).
  - Leaning forward on the arms (tripod position).
  - Supine with the head and thorax slightly elevated (semi-Fowler's position).
  - These patients will frequently avoid lying supine.
- Respiratory distress may be caused by:
  - Upper or lower airway obstruction.
  - Inadequate ventilation.
  - Impairment of the respiratory muscles.
  - Ventilation-perfusion mismatching.
  - Diffusion abnormalities.
  - Impairment of the nervous system.
- Dyspnea is often associated with hypoxia.
- Observation techniques—Visual techniques used to recognize airway problems include:
  - Noting the patient's preferred position to facilitate breathing.
  - Assessing rise and fall of the patient's chest.
  - Other visual clues for respiratory distress include:
    - — Gasping for air
    - — Cyanosis
    - — Nasal flaring
    - — Pursed-lip breathing
- Retraction of:
  - Intercostal or subcostal muscles.
  - Suprasternal notch.
  - Supraclavicular fossa.
- Auscultation and palpation techniques.
- Evaluating air movement can be accomplished by:
  - Listening to respirations without the use of a stethoscope.
  - Using a stethoscope to assess bilateral lung fields.
  - Palpating the chest wall, which will help reveal the presence or absence of paradoxical motion.

Other Signs of Respiratory Distress

- A change in resistance (compliance) when using a bag valve mask (BVM).
  - Seen in asthma, COPD, and tension pneumothorax.
- Pulsus paradoxus.
  - A drop of 10 mmHg or more in systolic blood pressure on inspiration.
  - A change in the quality of the pulse may also be noted.
  - Sometimes seen in patients with asthma, COPD, and pericardial tamponade.

History

- Did the symptoms come on suddenly or gradually?
- If gradually, over what period of time?

- Were there any known causes or "triggers" that initiated the difficulty breathing?
- Is the respiratory distress constant or recurrent in nature?
- What makes it better?
- What makes it worse?
- Are there any associated symptoms (e.g., cough, chest pain, fever)?
- Have any medication interventions been attempted?
- Has the patient taken all medications and treatments as prescribed?

Respiratory Pattern Changes (Table 11-2)

- The breathing process should be comfortable, regular, and initiated without distress.
- Abnormal respiratory patterns may be seen in ill or injured patients.
- Recognizing abnormal breathing patterns may help determine the appropriate intervention.

Inadequate Ventilation

- Occurs when the body cannot compensate for increased O_2 demand or cannot maintain a normal range of O_2/CO_2 balance.
- Causes:
  - Infection
  - Trauma
  - Brain stem insult
  - Noxious or hypoxic atmosphere

TABLE 11-2: Respiratory Patterns

Respiratory Pattern	Description
Agonal	Slow, shallow, irregular breathing resulting from brain anoxia.
Ataxia	Irregular breathing pattern characterized by a series of inspirations and expirations. Associated with a lesion in the medullary respiratory center.
Biot's	Irregular pattern, rate, and volume with intermittent periods of apnea. Associated with intracranial pressure.
Bradypnea	Respiratory rate slower than 12 bpm. Associated with chest wall injury, respiratory failure, CVA, pulmonary infection, or narcotic overdose.
Central neurogenic hyperventilation	Deep rapid ventilation similar to Kussmaul breathing. Associated to intracranial pressure.
Cheyne-stokes	Respiratory rate and tidal volume gradually increasing followed by a gradual decrease. Associated with a brain stem insult.
Hyperventilation	Persistent rapid and deep ventilation. Usually is much slower and much deeper than tachypnea. Associated with anxiety, exercise, and diabetic ketoacidosis.
Kussmaul	Deep gasping respirations, associated with diabetic coma.
Tachypnea	Persistent respiratory rate greater than 20 bpm.

- Multiple symptoms:
  - Respiratory rate changes (up or down)
  - Respiratory pattern changes

SUPPLEMENTAL OXYGEN THERAPY (TABLES 11-3 AND 11-4)

TABLE 11-3: Oxygen Delivery Devices

Device	Description	Indications	Contraindications	Advantages	Disadvantages
Nasal canulla	Low-concentration O_2 by way of two small plastic prongs	• Long-term O_2 maintenance therapy • Low to moderate O_2 enrichment	• Mouth breathing • Severe hypoxia • Apnea • Poor respiratory effort	Well tolerated	Does not deliver a high volume/ concentration of O_2
Simple face mask	A soft, clear plastic mask that conforms to the patient's face. Can deliver O_2 concentrations of 35–60% with a flow rate of 6–8 L/min	• Long-term O_2 maintenance therapy • Low to moderate O_2 enrichment	• Mouth breathing • Severe hypoxia • Apnea • Poor respiratory effort	Higher O_2 concentrations	Delivery of volumes beyond 10 L/min does not enhance O_2 concentration
Partial rebreather mask	O_2 concentrations of 35–60% can be delivered with a flow rate that prevents the reservoir bag from collapsing completely on inspiration	• Long-term O_2 maintenance therapy • Low to moderate O_2 enrichment	• Poor respiratory effort • Apnea	• Inspired gas not mixed with room air • Higher O_2 concentrations are attainable	Delivery of volumes beyond 10 L/min does not enhance O_2 concentration
Nonrebreather mask	Delivers O_2 concentrations ranging above 95% with an adequate flow rate that keeps the reservoir bag partially inflated during inspiration	• Most commonly used in patients who require high-concentration O_2 delivery (10 to 15 L/min)	• Poor respiratory effort • Apnea	• Inspired gas not mixed with room air • Higher O_2 concentrations are attainable	
Venturi-mask	Designed to deliver O_2 concentrations of 30–40%	• Recommended for patients who rely on a hypoxic respiratory drive (e.g., COPD)		• Allows precise regulation of FiO_2 • Permits titration of O_2 for the patient with COPD so as not to exceed the patient's hypoxic drive while allowing enrichment of supplemental O_2	

TABLE 11-4: Ventilation

Delivery	Description	Indications	Contraindications	Advantages	Disadvantages
Mouth-to-mouth	Can deliver approximately 17% O_2 using the rescuer's exhalation	Apnea; when other ventilation devices are unavailable	• Conscious patients • Communicable disease concern	• Special equipment is not needed • Delivers excellent tidal volume • Delivers adequate oxygenation	• Communicable disease concerns • Direct blood/body fluid contact
Mouth-to-nose	Ventilating through the nose rather than the mouth	Apnea; injury to the mouth and lower jaw Alternative to mouth-to-mouth	Conscious patients	No special equipment is needed	• Communicable disease concerns • Direct blood/body fluid contact
Mouth-to-stoma	Ventilation through the stoma	A patient who has: • Postlaryngectomy stoma • Tracheostomy stoma	Conscious patients		
Mouth-to-mask	Used as an alternative to mouth-to-mouth	Apnea from any mechanism	Conscious patients	Eliminates direct contact with the patient • Allows the delivery of supplemental O_2 • A one-way-valve eliminates the possibility of exposure to exhaled gases	Useful only if device is available
Bag-valve-device	• May be used with a mask, ET tube, or any invasive airway device • Has a self-filling bag • Standard 15-mm to 22-mm fitting	Apnea, unsatisfactory respiratory effort	Intolerant patients	• Excellent blood, body fluid barrier • O_2 delivery from 21% to nearly 100% • Can be used with one, two, or three rescuers	• Difficult to master • Mask seal may be difficult to obtain
Flow-restricted O_2 powered ventilation devices	• Allows for positive pressure ventilation • Connects to the high pressure connection (50 psi)	• Delivery of high volume/ concentration O_2 • Awake conscious patients • Unconscious patients with caution	• Noncompliant patients • Poor tidal volume • Small children	• Can be self administered • Delivers high volume/ concentration O_2	• Lung compliance cannot be monitored • Requires an O_2 source

Rationale for Oxygen Therapy

Enriched O_2 in the atmosphere increases the O_2 content in pulmonary capillary blood. Increasing available O_2 can allow the patient to compensate without increasing the work of breathing.

Oxygen Sources

- Pure O_2 gas is the most common form of O_2 used in the prehospital setting and is delivered in liters per minute (L/min).
- O_2 in a compressed gas form is carried in stainless steel or lightweight alloy cylinders.
- Cylinders are color-coded by U.S. Pharmacopeia to distinguish various compressed gases.
- Steel green and white cylinders have been assigned to all grades of O_2.
- Stainless steel and aluminum cylinders are not painted.
- Common sizes (and their factors) used in emergency care:
  - D cylinder (400 L of O_2)—Factor: 0.16
  - E cylinder (625 L of O_2)—Factor: 0.28
  - M cylinder (3450 L of O_2)—Factor: 1.56

Liquid Oxygen (LOX)

- O_2 cooled to its aqueous state
- Converts to a gaseous state when warmed
- Used by some air medical services and other emergency medical services (EMS) agencies when weight and space that an O_2 system occupies must be considered

Regulators

High-pressure regulators are used to transfer cylinder gas from tank to tank.

- Attached to cylinder stem
- Delivers cylinder gas under high pressure

Therapy regulators are attached to a cylinder stem. Fifty pounds per square inch (psi) escape pressure is "stepped down" to 30 psi through the regulator mechanism for patient safety.

- Subsequent delivery to patient is adjustable low pressure.
- Flowmeters control the amount of O_2 delivered to the patient.
- Connected to the pressure regulator and adjusted to deliver O_2 at a certain number of liters per minute.

AIRWAY MANAGEMENT

Manual Techniques for Airway Management

Head-Tilt-Chin-Lift Method

- Preferred for opening the airway without suspected spinal injury

Indications

- Unresponsive patients who do not have a mechanism for cervical spine injury or are unable to protect their own airway

Contraindications

- Awake patients
- Possible cervical spine injury

Advantages

- No equipment required
- Simple, safe, and noninvasive

Disadvantages

- Head tilt is hazardous to patients with cervical spine injuries
- Does not protect from aspiration

Jaw-Thrust Maneuver with Head Tilt

- Used without suspected spinal injury
- Provides additional forward displacement of the mandible

Jaw-Thrust without Head-Tilt

- Head is maintained in neutral position. The patient's jaw is displaced forward at the mandibular angle.

Indications

- Unresponsive patients
- Cervical spine injury
- Patients who are unable to protect their own airway

Contraindications

- Conscious patients

Advantages

- Noninvasive, requires no special equipment
- May be used with cervical collar in place

Disadvantages

- Difficult to maintain
- Requires second rescuer for BVM ventilation
- Does not protect against aspiration

SUCTION

Fixed Units

- Mounted in patient care areas of hospitals and nursing homes and in many emergency vehicles
- Electrically powered by vacuum pumps or by the vacuum produced by the vehicle engine manifold
- Furnish an air intake of at least 30 L/min
- Provide a vacuum of more than 300 mmHg when the tube is clamped

Portable Units

- May be O_2 or air powered, electrically powered, or manually powered
- Should furnish an air intake of no less than 20 L/min to operate effectively

Suction Catheters

Whistle-Tip

- A narrow, flexible tube
- Used primarily for tracheobronchial suctioning to clear secretions through either an ET tube or the nasopharynx
- Designed with molded ends and side holes to produce minimal trauma to the mucosa
- Proximal end has a side opening that is covered with the thumb to produce suction
- Using sterile technique, the catheter is advanced to the desired location
  - Suction is applied intermittently as the catheter is withdrawn

Tonsil-Tip Suction (Yankauer)

- A rigid pharyngeal catheter
- Used to clear secretions, blood clots, and other foreign material from the mouth and pharynx
- Carefully inserted into the oral cavity under direct visualization, and slowly withdrawn while suction is activated

Potential complications

- Sudden hypoxemia secondary to decreased lung volume during suction
- Severe hypoxemia that may lead to cardiac rhythm disturbances and cardiac arrest
- Airway stimulation that may increase arterial pressure and cardiac rhythm disturbances
- Coughing that may result in increased intracranial pressure with reduced blood flow to the brain
- Increased risk of herniation in patients with head injury
- Soft tissue damage to the respiratory tract

Gastric Distension

- Results from air being trapped in the stomach
- Very common when ventilating nonintubated patients
- Stomach diameter increases and pushes against diaphragm
- Interferes with lung expansion
- Abdomen becomes increasingly distended
- Resistance to BVM ventilation

Nasogastric Decompression

Indications

- Threat of aspiration
- Need for lavage

Contraindications

- Extreme caution in esophageal disease or esophageal trauma
- Facial trauma (caution)
- Esophageal obstruction

Advantages

- Tolerated by awake patients
- Does not interfere with intubation
- Lessens frequency of recurrent gastric distention
- Helps alleviate nausea
- Patient can still talk

Disadvantages

- Uncomfortable for patient
- May cause patient to vomit during placement even if gag is suppressed
- Interferes with BVM seal

Complications

- Nasal, esophageal, or gastric trauma from poor technique
- Tracheal placement
- Supragastric placement
- Tube obstruction

Orogastric Decompression

Indications

- Same parameters as for nasogastric (NG) tube. Generally preferred for unconscious patients.

Contraindications

- Same parameters as for NG

Advantages

- May use larger tubes
- May lavage more aggressively
- Safe to pass in facial fracture
- Avoids nasopharynx

Disadvantages

- May interfere with visualization during intubation

Complications

- Same as for NG
- The patient may bite the tube

Gastric Decompression

Complications

- Uncomfortable for the patient
- May induce nausea and vomiting even when the gag reflex is suppressed
- Tubes interfere with mask seals and with visualization of airway structures during intubation
- Nasal, esophageal, or gastric trauma from poor technique
- Tracheal placement
- Supragastric placement
- Gastric tube obstruction

MECHANICAL ADJUNCTS IN AIRWAY MANAGEMENT

Nasopharyngeal Airway (Nasal Airway)

- Used to maintain an airway in a semiconscious or unconscious patient
- Should also be considered:
  - For seizure patients
  - For patients with suspected cervical spine injury
  - Before nasotracheal intubation
  - As a guide for inserting a nasogastric tube
- Soft and pliable
- Outer end is flared
- 17–20 cm in length
- Correct size is determined by selecting a tube length equal to distance between tip of patient's nose and tragus of the ear
- Recommended sizes:
  - Large adult: 8.0–9.0 mm i.d. (24–27 French)
  - Medium adult: 7.0–8.0 mm i.d. (21–24 French)
  - Small adult: 6.0–7.0 mm i.d. (18–21 French)
- The airway should rest in the posterior pharynx
  - If patient begins to gag, withdraw tube slightly or reinsert it as indicated
- Maintain displacement of the mandible when using the airway

Advantages

- Well tolerated by conscious and semiconscious patients with gag reflex
- May be inserted rapidly
- May be used when insertion of an oropharyngeal airway is contraindicated or difficult because of facial trauma or soft tissue injury

Disadvantages

- Long nasopharyngeal airways may enter the esophagus
- May precipitate laryngospasm and vomiting in patients with a gag reflex
- May injure nasal mucosa, producing bleeding and possible airway obstruction
- Small-diameter airways may become obstructed by mucus, blood, vomitus, and soft tissues of the pharynx
- Does not protect the lower airway from aspiration
- Difficult to suction through

Oropharyngeal Airway (Oral Airway)

- A plastic semicircular device designed to hold the tongue away from the posterior wall of the pharynx
- Should be used only in patients who are unconscious or semiconscious and without a gag reflex
- Two basic types:
  - Guedel (tubular in design)
  - Berman (have airway channels along each side)
- Available in various sizes (infant to adult)

- Proper size is determined by placing the airway next to the patient's face so that the flange is at the level of the central incisors and the bite block segment is parallel to the hard palate
- Should extend from the corner of the patient's mouth to the tip of the earlobe
- Recommended sizes:
  - Large adult: 100 mm (Guedel size 5)
  - Medium adult: 90 mm (Guedel size 4)
  - Small adult: 80 mm (Guedel size 3)

Advantages

- Secures the tongue forward and down away from the posterior pharynx
- Provides easy access for airway suction
- Serves as a bite block to protect an ET tube in case of convulsions

Potential complications

- Small airways may fall back into the oral cavity, occluding the airway
- Long airways may press the epiglottis against the entrance of the trachea, producing a complete airway obstruction
- May stimulate vomiting and laryngospasm in the patient with a gag reflex
- Does not protect the lower airway from aspiration
- May push the tongue back and obstruct the airway if improperly inserted

ADVANCED AIRWAY PROCEDURES

Endotracheal Intubation

Preferred technique for airway control in patients who are unable to maintain a patent airway.

Indications

- When the rescuer is unable to ventilate an unconscious patient with conventional methods such as mouth-to-mask or BVM
- When patients cannot protect their airway (e.g., due to coma or respiratory or cardiac arrest)
- When prolonged artificial ventilation is needed

Advantages

- Isolates the airway, reducing the risk of aspiration
- Facilitates ventilation and oxygenation
- Facilitates suctioning of the trachea and bronchi
- Prevents wasted ventilation and gastric insufflation during positive-pressure ventilation
- Provides route for administration for some medications (although the following drugs can be absorbed via the trachea, the IV/IO route of administration is preferred)
  - Lidocaine
  - Epinephrine
  - Atropine
  - Naloxone
  - Vasopressin (AHA class IIa)

Description

- A flexible tube that is open at each end.
- Proximal end has standard 15-mm adapter that connects to various O_2 delivery devices for positive-pressure ventilation.
- Beveled distal end to facilitate placement between the vocal cords.
- Adult (size 5.0 or larger) tube has a balloon cuff on the distal end that occludes the remainder of the tracheal lumen.
- Reduces the risk of aspiration around the tube and minimizes air leaks.
- Attached by the inflating tube to a one-way inflating valve with an inlet port (to accept a syringe for inflation).
- Specialized variations of ET tubes.
  - Armored or anode tubes that have an inner spiral of flat metal to prevent kinking or compression
  - "Trigger" tubes that have a thin cord running down the anterior wall of the tube, to which a ring is attached proximally
  - Helps maneuver the tube without a stylet
  - Medication ports for ET drug administration

Endotracheal Tube Sizes

- Markings on the ET tube show the tube's internal diameter (i.d.) in millimeters (mm).
  - Graduated sizes from 2.5 to 10.0 mm are available.
  - The length of the tube from the distal end is indicated in centimeters (cm) at several levels.
- Recommended adult sizes:
  - Females: 7.0–8.0 i.d.
  - Males: 8.0–8.5 i.d.

Pediatric Sizes

- Available cuffed or uncuffed.
- Cuffed tubes are indicated only for children older than 8–10 years of age.
- Children younger than 8–10 years of age have circular narrowing at level of cricoid cartilage.
- Serves as a functional cuff, allowing minimal air leakage at the cricoid ring.
- Uncuffed ET tubes are recommended for this age group.
- A common method of determining correct ET tube size:
  - Choose the ET tube with an outside diameter equal to the diameter of the child's little finger.
  - Regardless of the method used, appropriate ET tube selection is more reliably based on the patient's size than age.

Preparing for Intubation

- Ventilate the patient by other means before intubation.
- Hyperoxygenate the patient with 100% O_2 for at least 2 minutes before intubation.
- Examine the equipment for defects:
  - Check the cuff or inlet port for leaks.
  - Check the lightbulb after attaching the blade to the handle and make sure the bulb is secure and bright.

Anatomical Considerations

- The ET tube may be passed into the trachea through the mouth (orotracheal) or through the nose (nasotracheal).
  - The orotracheal route requires direct visualization of the glottic opening.
  - The nasotracheal route is a "blind" technique.

Important Anatomical Landmarks

- The trachea is in the midline of the neck and has its superior entry at the level of the glottic opening.
- During orotracheal intubation, the vocal cords should be visualized while passing the tube into the trachea.
- The uvula is suspended from the midline of the soft palate.
  - Used as a guide in placing the laryngoscope.
- The epiglottis is attached to the base of the tongue.
  - Should be visualized and elevated to expose the glottis and vocal cords.
  - Sellick's maneuver can occlude the esophagus (reducing the risk of regurgitation during intubation) and may help to visualize the entrance of the trachea.
- The trachea extends to the level of the second intercostal space anteriorly, before bifurcating into left and right mainstem bronchi.
  - The right main bronchus branches off to a very slight angle to the trachea.
  - The left main bronchus branches at a 45° to 60° angle.

Orotracheal Intubation for a Nontrauma (Medical) Patient

- Place the patient supine in a sniffing position to facilitate visualization.
- This position is used when the potential for cervical spine injury does not exist. The "sniffing position" is optimal hyperextension of the head with elevation of the occiput which brings the axis of mouth, pharynx, and trachea into alignment.
- Lubricate the tube.
- Have a stethoscope, stylet, and suction available.
- Hyperventilate the patient with 100% O_2 for 1–2 minutes.

Procedure for Intubation

- Position yourself at the patient's head.
- Inspect the oral cavity for secretions and foreign material (suction if needed).
- Open the patient's mouth with the fingers of your right hand.
- Retract the patient's lips on the teeth or gums to prevent pinching them in the blade.
- Grasp the patient's lower jaw with your right hand and draw it forward and upward.
  - Remove loose dentures and place padding under the adult patient's shoulders to elevate the thorax. This helps align the airway for intubation.
- Hold the laryngoscope in your left hand.
- Insert the blade in the right side of the patient's mouth, displacing the tongue to the left, identify the uvula, and avoid any pressure on the lips or teeth.
- If using a curved blade, advance the tip of the blade into the vallecula.
- If using a straight blade, insert the tip of the blade under the epiglottis.
  - Expose the glottic opening by exerting upward traction on the handle.

- Advance the ET tube through the right corner of the patient's mouth, and under direct vision, through the vocal cords.
  - Remove the stylet (if used).
  - Ensure that the proximal end of the cuffed tube has advanced past the cords about 1–2.5 cm (0.5–1 in.).
- Observe the depth markings on the ET tube during intubation.
- Inflate the cuff with 10–20 mL of air.
- Attach the tube to a mechanical airway device and begin ventilation and oxygenation.
- Confirming placement:
  - Direct revisualization (revisualize glottis).
  - Note tube depth:
    - — Average tube depth in males is 22 cm at the teeth.
    - — Average tube depth in women is 21 cm.
  - Auscultation:
    - — Epigastric area—Air entry into the stomach indicates esophageal placement.
    - — Bilateral bases—Equal volume and expansion.
    - — Apices—Equal volume.
    - — Unequal or absent breath sounds indicate:
      - Esophageal placement
      - Right mainstem placement
      - Pneumothorax
      - Bronchial obstruction

Other Methods to Confirm Tube Placement Include

- Visualization of equal chest excursion on the right and left sides
- Absent or diminished epigastric sounds with auscultation
- Positive clear tracheal sounds with auscultation
- The absence of an air leak around the cuff on bag-valve inflation of the lungs
- Improvement in the patient's color or level of consciousness
- Palpation of the balloon cuff at the sternal notch by compressing the pilot balloon
- Pulse oximetry
- O_2 saturation should increase rapidly in intubated patient with a pulse
- End-tidal CO_2 detector
- Bulb- and syringe-type esophageal detection devices
- BVM ventilation compliance
  - Increased resistance to BVM compliance may indicate:
    - — Gastric distension
    - — Esophageal placement
    - — Tension pneumothorax

Evidence of a misplaced tube (regardless of when it was last checked) must be reconfirmed.

- Confirmation must be performed
  - By multiple methods
  - Immediately after tube placement
  - After any major move

 - After manipulation of neck
 - Manipulation of neck may displace the tube up to 5 cm

Corrective Measures

- Esophageal placement
  - Ready to vigorously suction as needed
  - Likelihood of emesis is increased, especially if gastric distension is present
  - Ideally preoxygenate the patient before reintubation
  - Misplaced tube may be removed
    - — After proper tracheal placement is confirmed or
    - — Beforehand provided diligent and vigorous airway suctioning is ready

Right Mainstem Placement

- Loosen or remove securing device
- Deflate balloon cuff
- While ventilation continues, slowly retract tube while simultaneously listening for breath sounds over left chest
- Stop as soon as breath sounds are heard in the left chest
- Note tube depth
- Reinflate balloon cuff
- Secure tube

After successful intubation, insert an oropharyngeal airway in the unconscious patient.

- Note and record the tube marker at the front of the teeth.

Secure the ET tube with tape or a commercial tube holder.

- Evaluate lung sounds after taping to ensure the position of the tube.

Transillumination Technique (Lighted Stylet)

- Malleable fiberoptic stylets (or "light wands") have a high-intensity light at the distal end that is powered by a small battery housing at the operator end.

Indications

- Inability to directly visualize glottis
- Cervical spine injury

Contraindications

- Present gag reflex
- Airway obstruction
- Pediatric patient

Advantages

- Minimal manipulation of cervical spine
- Adds visual parameter to blind technique

Disadvantages

- Difficult in bright light

Method

- Rescuer should be positioned at the side of the patient's head.
- Maintain in-line spinal immobilization by a second rescuer if spinal injury is suspected.
- Ensure hyperventilation with 100% O_2 for 1–2 minutes.
- Turn on stylet.
- Insert midline into pharynx.
- Observe for focused midline glow.
- Advance ET tube additional 1–2 cm.
- Inflate the balloon cuff.
- Remove the stylet.
- Confirm placement.
- Secure the tube.

Digital or Blind Intubation

- Direct palpation of glottic structures to intubate trachea

Indications

- Apnea
- Confined space
- Inability to directly visualize from equipment failure, excessive blood, or other secretions
- Disaster situations in which equipment is in short supply

Contraindications

- Breathing patient
- Present gag reflex

Advantages

- Does not require laryngoscope
- Does not require sniffing position
- May be passed through fluid obstructions

Disadvantages

- Semiblind technique
- May only be performed on apneic patients

Method

- Rescuer should be positioned at the side of the patient's head.
- Maintain in-line spinal immobilization by a second rescuer if spinal injury is suspected.
- Ensure hyperventilation with 100% O_2 for 1–2 minutes.
- Use a bite-stick or other device to hold the patient's mouth open to protect the rescuer's fingers.
- Bend the tube/stylet combination into a J or hockey-stick shape.
- Insert gloved left middle and index fingers into the patient's mouth.
- Alternating fingers, "walk" down the patient's tongue, pulling the tongue and epiglottis away from the glottic opening.

- When a flap of cartilage covered by mucous membrane is felt with the middle finger, the epiglottis has been located.
- Maintain contact and advance the ET tube with the right hand, using the index finger of the left hand as a guide.
- The index finger maintains the tube position against the middle finger, leading the tip of the tube into the glottic opening.
- Once the cuff of the ET tube passes the tips of the paramedic's fingers, inflate the balloon cuff.
- Confirm placement.
- Secure the tube.

Potential Complications from Intubation Procedures

- Traumatic injury
  - Lacerated lips or tongue
  - Dental trauma from laryngoscope
  - Lacerated pharyngeal or tracheal mucosa
  - Tracheal rupture
  - Avulsion of an arytenoid cartilage
  - Vocal cord injury
- Vomiting and aspiration of stomach contents
- May produce significant releases of epinephrine and norepinephrine leading to the following:
  - Hypertension
  - Tachycardia
  - Cardiac rhythm disturbances
- May lead to vagal stimulation (particularly in infants and children), resulting in:
  - Bradycardia
  - Hypotension
- May increase intracranial pressure in patients with head injuries
- The esophagus may be accidentally intubated
- A bronchus may be accidentally intubated
- Cuff malfunction and air leak may occur due to:
  - Cuff rupture
  - Inflation port malfunction
  - Severance or kinking of the inflation tube

Nasotracheal Intubation

Passage of the ET tube through the nasopharynx into the trachea.

Indications

- Spontaneously breathing patient when laryngoscopy is difficult or when motion of the cervical spine must be limited
- Medication overdose
- Asthma or anaphylaxis
- Chronic obstructive pulmonary disease
- Stroke
- Seizure (status epilepticus with constant seizure activity)
- Altered mental status

Contraindications

- Apnea
- Midfacial fractures
- Suspected basal skull fractures
- Bleeding disorders
- Patients on anticoagulants (e.g., Coumadin)
- Severe nasal trauma
- Pharyngeal hemorrhage
- Acute epiglottitis
- Suspected laryngeal fracture
- Suspected increased intracranial pressure

Advantages

- Does not require laryngoscope
- Does not require sniffing position
- More easily secured
- Patient cannot bite tube

Disadvantages

- "Blind" technique.
- Can only be performed on breathing patients.
- Usually better tolerated by conscious patients than orotracheal intubation.
- Usually causes less recurrent trauma to tracheal mucosa due to less intratracheal tube movement with head motion than with orotracheal tube.
- If time permits, apply vasoconstrictor spray (phenylephrine) and topical anesthetic (lidocaine).
- Makes the procedure more comfortable for the patient.
- Decreases nasal hemorrhage secondary to the procedure.
- If time permits, insert a soft nasopharyngeal airway.
- Indicates a passable nostril.
- Compresses the mucosa to allow for less traumatic placement.

Potential complications

- Epistaxis
- Injury to the nasal septum or turbinates
- Retropharyngeal laceration
- Vocal cord injury
- Avulsion of an arytenoid cartilage
- Esophageal intubation
- Intracranial tube placement if the patient has a basilar skull fracture

Intubation With Spinal Precautions

- A second rescuer applies manual in-line stabilization from the patient's side.
- Placing his or her hands over the patient's ears, with the little fingers placed under the occipital skull and the thumbs on the face over the maxillary sinuses.
- Stabilization (without distraction) should be maintained in a neutral position throughout the procedure.
- Auscultate for bilateral breath sounds to provide a baseline measurement.

Sitting Position Method

- Position yourself at the patient's head with your legs straddling the patient's shoulders and arms (the patient's head is secured between your thighs).
- While the grip of both rescuers secures the patient's head, lean back to visualize the patient's vocal cords during the intubation procedure.
- Prone position method:
  - Lie prone at the patient's head
  - The second rescuer maintains the in-line position alone

Extubation

- Not usually indicated in the prehospital setting.
- If necessary due to the patient's intolerance of the ET tube, hyperventilate the patient with 100% O_2 if possible.
- Procedure:
  - Suction the oral cavity above the cuff before extubation
  - Deflate the cuff completely
  - Swiftly withdraw the tube on cough or expiration
  - Assess respiratory status
  - Provide high-concentration O_2 and assist ventilations as needed

Special Considerations for Pediatric Intubations

- The infant's upper airway is relatively small, and the tongue is disproportionately large.
  - Posterior displacement of the tongue easily obstructs the airway.
  - A larger tongue tends to make laryngoscopy more difficult.
- The epiglottis is omega shaped and narrower and longer in children than in adults.
  - The epiglottis is more difficult to control with a laryngoscope blade.
- The larynx lies more anteriorly in relation to the base of the tongue than in the adult, and it is also elevated under the base of the tongue.
  - Makes visualization more difficult.
- The glottic opening is at one of the following locations:
  - The third cervical vertebra in premature neonates.
  - The third to fourth cervical vertebra in term neonates.
  - The fourth to fifth cervical vertebra in adults.
- During the first few months of life, the vocal cords of the infant slope from back to front.
  - This frequently causes the ET tube to "hang up" in the angle formed by the cords.
  - This problem can be minimized by rotating the ET tube or by having a second rescuer perform the Sellick maneuver during intubation.
- The cricoid cartilage is the narrowest part of the airway in the infant and young child.
- As the child reaches 8–10 years of age, the vocal cords become the narrowest part, and this position is maintained into adulthood.
- The distance from the vocal cords to the carina varies and can be correlated with the patient's height.
  - About 4–5 cm at birth
  - 6–7 cm at age 6

Pediatric Intubation

- Laryngoscope and size-appropriate blades
  - Straight blades are preferred
  - General guidelines
    - Premature infant: 0 straight
    - Full-term infant to 1 year of age: 1 straight
    - 2 years of age to adolescent: 2 straight
    - Adolescent and older: 3 straight or curved

Appropriate Size ET Tube—General Guidelines

Age: internal diameter of tube in mm

- Premature infant: 2.5, 3.0 uncuffed
- Term infant: 3.0, 3.5 uncuffed
- 6 months: 3.5, 4.0 uncuffed
- 1 year: 4.0, 4.5 uncuffed
- 2 years: 4.5, 5.0 uncuffed
- 4 years: 5.0, 5.5 uncuffed
- 6 years: 5.5 uncuffed
- 8 years: 6.0 cuffed or uncuffed
- 10 years: 6.5 cuffed or uncuffed
- 12 years: 7.0 cuffed
- Adolescent: 7.0, 8.0 cuffed

Depth of Insertion

- 2–3 cm below the vocal cords
- Uncuffed—place the black glottic marker of the tube at the level of the vocal cords
- Cuffed—insert until the cuff is just below the vocal cords
- 3 × inside diameter: 1

General Guidelines

- Premature infant: 8 cm
- Full-term infant: 8–9.5 cm
- Infant to 1 year of age: 9.5–11 cm
- Toddler: 11–12.5 cm
- Preschool-age child: 12.5–14 cm
- School-age child: 14–20 cm
- Adolescent: 20–23 cm

Adjuncts to Aid in Confirming ET Tube Placement

End-Tidal Carbon Dioxide Detectors

- Measure capnography (the measurement of exhaled CO_2 concentrations)
- Designed to help verify ET placement and recognize inadvertent esophageal intubation
- Provides a noninvasive estimate of:
  - Alveolar ventilation
  - CO_2 production
  - Arterial CO_2 content
- Use as an adjunct to assess ET tube placement is strongly encouraged

Disposable Colorimetric Devices

- Made of white plastic.
- Contain a chemical indicator in the upper part that is sensitive to CO_2 gas.
- When the detector is attached to an ET tube, the color of the indicator changes with elevated CO_2 concentrations.
  - This would be expected in the tracheal but not in the esophageal environment.
  - Any color change indicates tracheal placement; no color change indicates esophageal intubation.

Electronic Monitor

- Use an infrared analyzer to measure the percentage of CO_2 gas at each phase of respiration.
- Information is displayed in a digital waveform on the monitor or printout.
- Both devices may be useful as an indicator of circulation during some cardiac arrest situations, since an increase in end-tidal CO_2 concentrations seem to be related to effective perfusion during external chest compression.

Bulb- and Syringe-Type Esophageal Detectors

- Esophageal detection devices are attached to the end of the ET tube.
- Operate under the principle that the esophagus is a collapsible tube.
- As such, a vacuum will be created in the bulb device (after it is compressed) or when negative pressure is applied to the syringe device, if the ET tube is in the esophagus.
- When the ET tube is correctly placed in the trachea, the bulb device will easily refill with air or the syringe device will easily be aspirated after negative pressure is applied.
- Can also be used to verify correct placement of multiple-lumen airways.

Pulse Oximetry

- Used as an adjunct in determining effective patient oxygenation.
- Measures the transmission of red and near-infrared light through arterial beds.
- Hemoglobin absorbs red and infrared light waves differently when it is bound with O_2 (oxyhemoglobin) than when it is not (reduced hemoglobin).
  - Oxyhemoglobin absorbs more infrared than red light.
  - Reduced hemoglobin absorbs more red than infrared light.
  - Pulse oximetry reveals arterial saturation by measuring this difference.
- The oximeter probe is placed on a thin tissue, such as a finger, toe, or ear lobe.
  - One side of the probe emits wavelengths of light into the arterial bed.
  - The other side detects the presence of red or infrared light.
  - Using this balance of red and infrared colors, the oximeter calculates the O_2 saturation of the blood and displays it on the monitor screen.
- The percentage of hemoglobin saturated with O_2 is denoted as SaO_2 and depends on a number of factors:
  - PCO_2
  - pH
  - Temperature
  - Normal or altered hemoglobin
- Lower range of normal for SaO_2 is between 93% and 95%
- The upper range is 99–100%.
- Once the SaO_2 falls below 90% (corresponding to a PO_2 of 60 mmHg), further decreases are associated with a marked decline in O_2 content.

- Pulse oximeters may produce false readings and should be used only as tools to assist in patient monitoring.
  - Circumstances that may produce false readings include:
    - Dyshemoglobinemia (hemoglobin saturated with compounds other than O_2 [carbon monoxide (CO), methemoglobinemia])
    - Excessive ambient light (sunlight, fluorescent lights) on the oximeter's sensor probe
    - Patient movement
    - Hypotension
    - Hypothermia/vasoconstriction
    - Patient use of vasoconstrictive drugs
    - Patient use of nail polish
    - Jaundice

Multilumen Airways

- Pharyngeal tracheal lumen (PtL) airway was introduced in 1985.
  - Esophageal tracheal combitube is similar in design.
- Allows for either esophageal or tracheal insertion.
- Uses plastic tube with twin lumen that is separated by a partition wall.
- One tube resembles an ET tube and has an open distal end.
- Second tube resembles an EOA and is blocked by an obturator at the distal end.
- Both tubes use low-pressure balloons that provide a seal for either the trachea or esophagus, depending on placement.
  - PtL airway uses an additional balloon to occlude the oropharynx.
    - Helps obviate the need for a good seal with a face mask.
    - Reduces the risk of blood or other secretions from being aspirated or swallowed.

Insertion

- Gently guide the device into the esophagus or trachea without hyperextension or flexion of the patient's head.
- Inflate the balloons and ventilate through the esophageal lumen.
- Confirm placement by auscultation of bilateral breath sounds and chest wall movement during ventilation.
- If breath sounds and chest wall excursion are absent, ventilate through the tracheal lumen and confirm placement by auscultation and observing for chest wall movement.

Necessary Equipment

- Water-soluble lubricant
- Syringes
- Bag-valve device or demand valve
- O_2 source and connecting tubing
- Suction equipment
- Stethoscope

Common Advantages to Balloon System Devices

- Airways cannot be improperly placed
- Requires little skill training or maintenance
- Requires minimal spinal movement for insertion
- Suctions easily

Common Disadvantages to Balloon System Devices

- Patient must be unresponsive without a gag reflex.
- Must be removed when the patient becomes responsive or agitated.
- Proper identification of tube location may be difficult, leading to ventilations through the wrong lumen.
- Impossible to suction trachea when tube is in esophagus.
- Should be replaced with an ET tube as soon as possible.

Common Contraindications to Balloon System Devices

- Patients under 5 ft tall or younger than 14 years of age
- Caustic ingestion
- Esophageal trauma or disease
- Presence of gag reflex

PHARMACOLOGICAL ADJUNCTS TO AIRWAY MANAGEMENT AND VENTILATION

- Sedation is sometimes used in airway management and ventilation to:
  - Reduce anxiety
  - Induce amnesia
  - Decrease the gag reflex
- Possible indications for use include:
  - Combative patients
  - Patients who require aggressive airway management but who are too alert to tolerate intubation
  - Agitated trauma patients
- Classes of medications commonly used for sedation in these situations include the following:
  - Tranquilizers
  - Barbiturates
  - Benzodiazepines
  - Narcotics

Paralytic Agents in Emergency Intubation

- Paralysis for the purpose of emergency intubation involves the use of neuromuscular blocking drugs.

Indications

- Combative patients (such as, patients with head injury)

Contraindications

- Absolute:
  - Inability to ventilate once paralyzed
- Relative:
  - Patients who will be difficult to ventilate (i.e., facial hair)
  - Patients who will be difficult to intubate (i.e., short necks, obstructions)

Pharmacology

- Neuromuscular blockers produce skeletal muscle paralysis by binding to the nicotinic receptor for acetylcholine (ACh) at the neuromuscular junction.
- The neuromuscular junction is the point of contact between the nerve ending and the muscle fiber.
- When nerve impulses pass through this junction, ACh and other chemicals are released, causing the muscle to contract.
- Two types of neuromuscular blocking drugs:
  - Depolarizing agents
  - Nondepolarizing agents

Depolarizing Agents

- Substitute themselves into the neuromuscular junction and bind to receptors for Ach.
- Because these drugs produce depolarization of the muscular membrane, they often lead to fasciculations (uncontrollable muscle twitching) and some muscular contractions.
- Example:
  - Succinylcholine (Anectine)
    - — Rapid onset of action and briefest duration of action of all neuromuscular blocking drugs, making it the drug of choice for emergency endotracheal intubation.

Nondepolarizing Agents

- Bind to receptors for Ach and block the uptake of Ach at the neuromuscular junction, without initiating depolarization of the muscle membrane
- Longer onset and duration than depolarizing agents
- Vecuronium (Norcuron)
  - Rapid onset—2 minutes
  - Short duration—45 minutes
- Pancuronium (Pavulon)
  - Rapid onset—3–5 minutes
  - Longer duration—1 hour

Rapid Sequence Induction (RSI)

- Rapid sequence induction (or rapid sequence intubation) involves virtually simultaneous administration of a potent sedative (induction) agent and a neuromuscular blocking agent for the purpose of ET intubation.
- Provides optimal intubation conditions while minimizing the risk of aspiration of gastric contents.
- RSI is indicated when:
  - Emergency intubation is warranted.
  - The patient has a "full" stomach.
  - Intubation is predicted to be successful.
  - If intubation fails, ventilation is predicted to be successful.
- Six steps of RSI (the six "Ps"):
  - Preparation.
  - Preoxygenation.
  - Pretreatment.

  - Paralysis (with induction).
  - Placement of tube.
  - Postintubation management.
- Preparation:
  - Assess the patient for difficulty of intubation (e.g., using the Mallampati score).
  - Prepare all drugs and equipment.
  - Ensure one or more patent IV lines.
  - Explain the procedure to the patient.
- Preoxygenation (to be done simultaneously with preparation):
  - Preoxygenate the patient with 100% O_2 for 5 minutes (an essential step of the "no-bagging" approach of RSI).
  - Consider use of a pulse oximeter.
- Pretreatment (to be done 3 minutes before induction):
  - Consider lidocaine (Xylocaine) to blunt a rise in intracranial pressure and to prevent laryngospasm.
  - Consider beta blockers or opioids to reduce the sympathoadrenal response to intubation.
- Paralysis (with induction):
  - Administer a sedative (per protocol) to produce unconsciousness, follow immediately with a rapid push of neuromuscular blocker.
  - Perform the Sellick maneuver as the patient loses consciousness to prevent regurgitation.
  - Do not initiate ventilations unless the patient's O_2 saturation falls below 90%.
  - Within 45 seconds after succinylcholine (Anectine) is administered, the patient will be relaxed enough for intubation.
- Placement—Perform orotracheal intubation and confirm placement.
- Postintubation management:
  - Secure the tube in place.
  - Initiate mechanical ventilation.

TRANSLARYNGEAL CANNULA VENTILATION

- Translaryngeal cannula ventilation provides high-volume/high-pressure oxygenation of the lungs through cannulation of the trachea below the glottis.
- Delivers a large volume of O_2 through a small port at high pressure to the lungs compared to other methods (50 psi vs 1 psi through a therapy regulator).
- May be valuable when:
  - A patient's airway cannot be managed by manual measures.
  - A patient cannot be intubated by oral or nasal means.
- A temporary procedure that provides oxygenation when the airway is obstructed as a result of:
  - Edema of the glottis.
  - Fracture of the larynx.
  - Severe oropharyngeal hemorrhage.
- Requires special training and authorization from medical direction.

Advantages

- Simple, inexpensive, and effective when properly performed
- Requires minimal spinal manipulation
- Least invasive of surgical procedures

- May be initiated quickly
- Does not interfere with subsequent attempts to intubate

Disadvantages

- Invasive procedure
- Requires constant monitoring
- Requires "jet ventilation"
- Does not protect the airway
- Does not allow for efficient elimination of CO_2
- May adequately ventilate the patient's lungs for only 30–45 minutes

Potential complications

- High pressure during ventilation and air entrapment may produce pneumothorax.
- Hemorrhage may occur at the insertion site, and the thyroid and esophagus can be perforated if the needle is advanced too far.
- Does not allow for direct suctioning of secretions.
- Subcutaneous emphysema may occur.

Method of removal

- Removal should follow only successful orotracheal or nasotracheal intubation or a more definitive airway (cricothyrotomy or tracheostomy).
- To remove
  - Withdraw the catheter
  - Dress the wound

CRICOTHYROTOMY

- A surgical procedure that allows rapid entrance to the airway for ventilation and oxygenation for patients in whom airway control is not possible by other means.
- Should not be performed on patients who can be orally or nasally intubated.
- The need for this procedure is rare.
- Relative indications:
  - Severe facial or nasal injuries that preclude oral or nasal intubation
  - Massive mid-facial trauma
  - Possible spinal trauma when there is an inability to provide adequate ventilation
  - Anaphylaxis
  - Chemical inhalation injuries
- Requires special training and authorization from medical direction.

Necessary Equipment (If Commercial Cricothyrotomy Kit Is Unavailable)

- Scalpel blade
- 6.0 (preferred) or 7.0 ET tube or tracheostomy tube
- Antiseptic solution
- O_2 source
- Suction device
- Bag-valve device

Potential complications

- Prolonged execution time
- Hemorrhage
- Aspiration
- Possible misplacement
- False passage
- Perforation of esophagus
- Injury to the vocal cords and carotid and jugular vessels lateral to the incision
  - The patient must be immobilized
- Subcutaneous emphysema

Contraindications

- Inability to identify anatomical landmarks
- Underlying anatomical abnormality (e.g., tumor, subglottic stenosis)
- Tracheal transection
- Acute laryngeal disease caused by trauma or infection
- Small children under 10 years of age
  - Insertion of a 12- to 14-gauge catheter over the needle may be safer than a cricothyrotomy in this patient group

Note:

Removal of adjuncts used during an emergency cricothyrotomy should not be attempted in the prehospital setting.

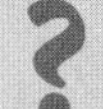

CHAPTER QUESTIONS

1. A contraindication to endotracheal tube placement is when the:
   a. glottic opening cannot be visualized
   b. patient has laryngospasm
   c. patient has had a laryngotracheotomy
   d. patient is conscious and has adequate respirations
2. All of the following are potential complications of nasotracheal intubation, except:
   a. epistaxis
   b. fracture of the cribiform plate
   c. vocal cord injury
   d. retropharyngeal laceration
3. All of the following are advantages of using a pocket mask over a BVM, except:
   a. with supplemental O_2, 80–90% O_2 can be provided
   b. there is increased ease in maintaining a mask-to-face seal
   c. a single rescuer can maintain spinal stabilization while ventilations are performed
   d. higher tidal volume can be obtained using a pocket mask
4. Correct placement of the endotracheal tube in an adult is confirmed by:
   a. the appearance of gastric contents in the endotracheal tube when managing the airway of a patient known to have aspirated
   b. an increase in heart rate
   c. checking lung fields for equal and bilateral lung sounds
   d. passing a nasogastric tube to decompress the stomach and prevent further distention

5. Following intubation with an endotracheal tube, the paramedic is able to auscultate breath sounds only on the right side. The next step is to:
   a. advance the tube a few centimeters
   b. secure the tube and ventilate
   c. withdraw the tube completely
   d. withdraw the tube a few centimeters
6. You are intubating a patient using a MacIntosh blade. This type of blade is designed to have the tip of the blade placed into the:
   a. oropharynx
   b. vallecula
   c. epiglottis
   d. glottis
7. The primary reason for performing the Sellick's maneuver during endotracheal intubation is to:
   a. prevent regurgitation
   b. decrease dead air space
   c. avoid having to hyperextend the neck
   d. make intubation easier

Suggested Readings

American Heart Association in collaboration with International Liaison Committee on Resuscitation. Guidelines 2000 for Cardiopulmonary Resuscitation and Emergency Cardiovascular Care: International Consensus on Science, Part 3. Adult Basic Life Support. *Circulation.* 2000; 102 (suppl I): I22–I59.

Circulation. 2005; 112(suppl I): IV-19 - IV-34. Published online before print November 28, 2005, doi:10.1161/CIRCULATIONAHA.105.166553.

Circulation. 2005; 112 (suppl I): IV-51 - IV-57. Published online before print November 28, 2005, doi:10.1161/CIRCULATIONAHA.105.166556.

Circulation. 2005; 112 (suppl I): IV-84 - IV-88. Published online before print November 28, 2005, doi:10.1161/CIRCULATIONAHA.105.166560.

Currents in Emergency Cardiovascular Care. 2005–2006;16(4):20.

US Department of Transportation, National Highway Traffic Safety Administration. *EMT-Paramedic: National Standard Curriculum.* Washington, DC: US Department of Transportation, National Highway Traffic Safety Administration; 1998.

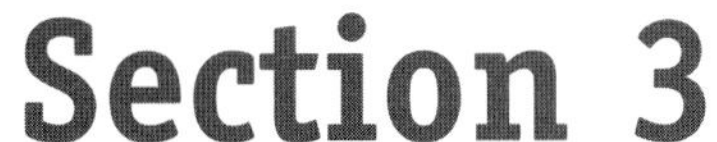

Section 3

Patient Assessment

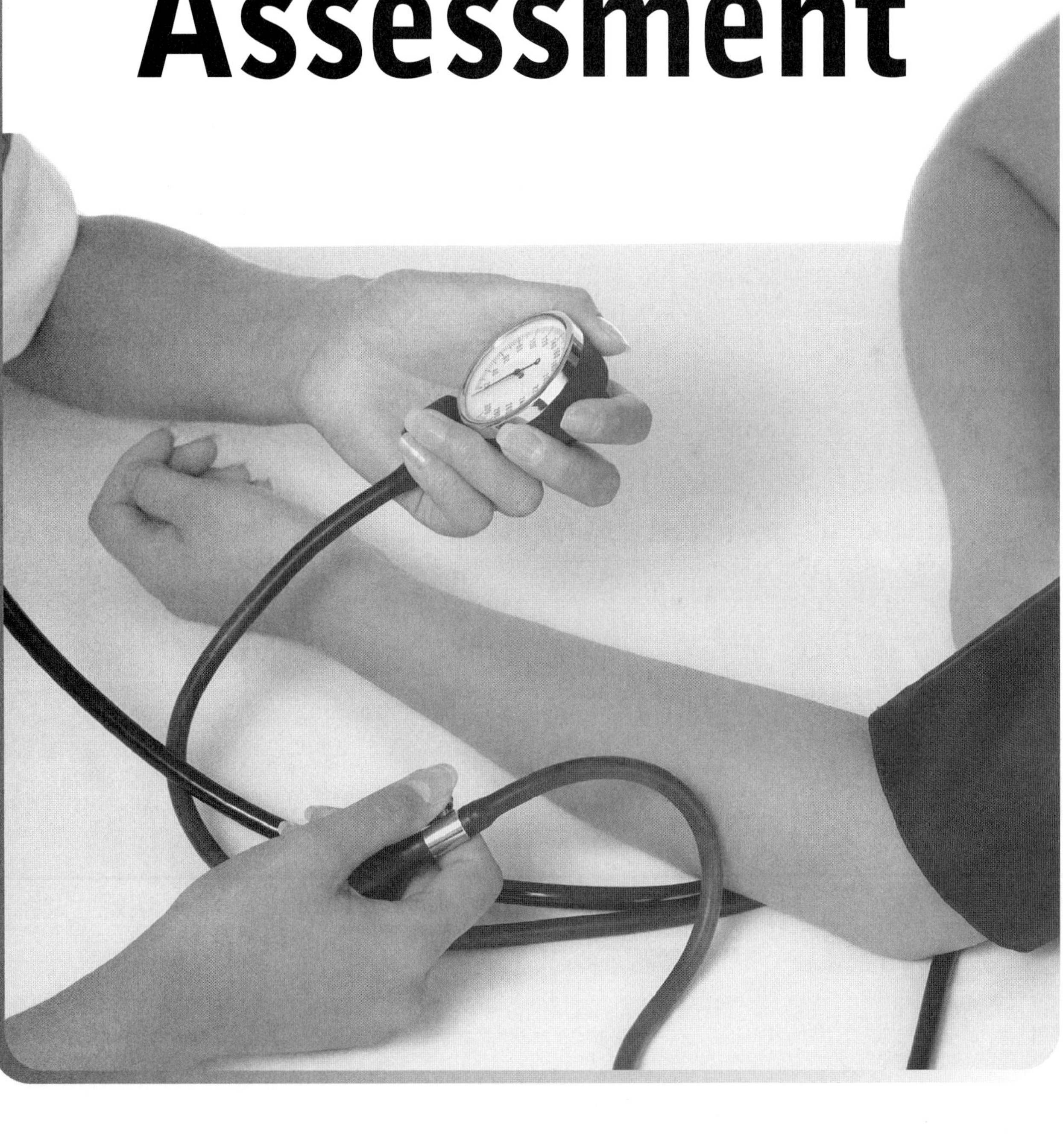

Chapter 12
Patient Assessment

On arrival at the scene of a traffic collision, you find a 21-year-old male, who was the unrestrained driver of a car that ran into a wall at approximately 50 mph. You notice the steering wheel is bent and observe "starring" on the windshield with no skid marks present. You notice air bag deployment to both the driver and passenger side, and side impact airbag curtains. The patient has a small amount of blood in his oropharynx. His breathing is labored and tachypneic at 32 breaths per minute. His pulse is thready at 154.

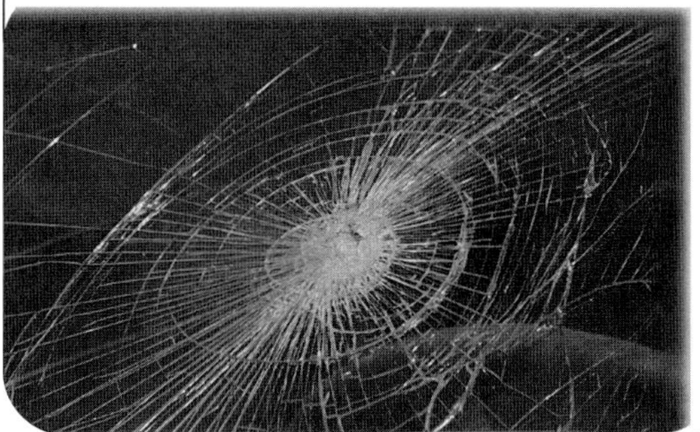

Other vitals: BP 86/64 and SpO_2 of 82%. Auscultation of his lungs reveals diminished sounds on the right side. Observation of his chest reveals some paradoxical movement, also on the right side. Palpation of his trachea at the sternal notch reveals a slight deviation to the left. He's pale and becoming restless.

SCENE ASSESSMENT

One of the critical variables in prehospital care is how the patient is found. Because the emergency scene can be different on every call, emergency medical service (EMS) personnel must have a flexible approach that allows them to adapt to the special situations they encounter.

If any aspect of the emergency setting is altered, the entire plan of action may be changed. One of the most important attributes of the streetwise prehospital care provider is having the ability to evaluate and control the emergency scene when coordinating patient care.

Scene assessment focuses on developing the following:

- Identifying and managing hazards
- Evaluating the scene to obtain essential information
- Coordinating the scene to the advantage of the provider and the patient

Dispatch Information

When the call from dispatch is received, ask the basic question:
Does the dispatch information make sense?

- The paramedic should know their response area.
- What is the location of the call?
- Potential violence?
- Police backup?
- Area known for gang activity?

Scene Size-Up

During scene size-up, the paramedic should determine:

- Safety of the scene
- Mechanism of injury (MOI) or nature of illness (NOI)
- Need for additional help
- Personnel protective equipment required, including that for infectious disease protection, body substance isolation (BSI)

Scene size-up is an ongoing process. As additional information is obtained, the prehospital provider modifies the assessment of both patient and scene requirements.

> **Note:**
>
> *In general, when emotions run high and judgement runs low, the result is often trouble. The paramedic should always maintain a high level of awareness.*

Potential Violent and Hostile Environments

- Family disturbances
- Bars and taverns
- Gang territory

Other Dangerous Environments

- Hazardous materials
- Farm emergencies
- Confined space
- Entrapments
- Industrial accidents
- Terrorism

Learning from the Scene

- Drug paraphernalia
- Beer cans and/or liquor bottles
- Medication bottles
- Cult, gang literature, or gang markings (tags)

Trauma Patients

- MOI
- Look to bystanders for information
- Consider forces involved in incident

Medical Patients

- NOI.
- Clues pertaining to medical patients are more subtle.
- Look to bystanders to provide information about facts such as how a patient was feeling (i.e., prior to losing consciousness or having a seizure).

Scene Control

Depending on where the patient is located, there are often distractions that make focusing on the patient's needs more difficult. Any aspect of the physical environment that compromises the emergency care efforts should be addressed.

Friends, Family, and Bystanders

- Can be valuable resources at the scene, but they can also cause some difficulty.
- They want to ensure their loved one is well cared for; conflict can develop if friendship interferes with patient care.
- If someone is unruly or agitating other people at the scene, control the person or have him or her removed as quickly as possible.
- Conflict detracts from the real focus of the call.
- It is always desirable to work with people when possible.
- Give family or friends a task to perform. This will help them feel useful and make the scene easier to control.
- Patients may not have divulged personal health information to friends and family such as cancer history, human immunodeficiency virus (HIV), or hepatitis status.

Infectious Disease Exposure

- Always take infection control precautions.
- When indicated, protective equipment should be in place prior to arriving on scene.
- BSI includes wearing gloves, mask, and gown to avoid exposure to airborne and blood–borne pathogens.
- High-efficiency particulate air (HEPA) masks may be needed for some airborne pathogens (e.g., tuberculosis).
- **Identifying risks is a crucial FIRST step.**

If safety issues are not identified, they are unlikely to be managed, and unmanaged safety factors compromise all other aspects of an emergency response.

INITIAL ASSESSMENT

Once the scene has been quickly surveyed and found, or made safe, the prehospital care provider can arrive at the patient's side and begin the initial assessment.

Recognizing and Managing Immediate Life Threats

Consider the mechanism of injury or the nature of illness to determine if the patient's condition is a medical or trauma event.

General Impression of the Patient

- The general impression is formed to determine priority of care and is based on the paramedic's immediate assessment of the environment and the patient's chief complaint.
  - Age
  - Sex
  - Race
  - NOI or MOI
- Assess the patient and determine if the patient has a life-threatening condition.
  - ***If a life-threatening condition is found, treat immediately.***
- Check the patient's level of consciousness.

1. Do you suspect head or neck trauma? Maintain spinal immobilization if required.
2. Is the patient responsive?

   Alert

   Verbal response to verbal stimuli

Painful response to painful stimuli

Unresponsive

3. Ask questions to determine responsiveness, adequacy of airway, and breathing.

Check the Patient's *A*irway

1. Is the airway open?
2. Is there food or fluid in the mouth?
3. Do you suspect a foreign body obstruction you cannot see?
4. Do you suspect an anatomical obstruction other than the tongue (i.e., swelling of throat tissue) or an upper airway obstruction that cannot be cleared?
5. Suction airway as needed, secure airway using an oralpharyngeal or nasopharyngeal airway.

Check the Patient's *B*reathing

1. Is the patient breathing normally?
2. Is there breathing difficulty?
3. Is the rate too slow or fast?
4. Are breath sounds absent on one side?
5. Is the trachea deviated?
6. Is there absence of breathing?
7. Ventilate the nonbreathing patient.
8. Intubate the patient if necessary.

To maintain a patent airway and provide efficient ventilation, the patient should be intubated, only after the initial assessment is complete and the patient is adequately hyperventilated.

Check the Patient's *C*irculation (Pulses and Severe Bleeding)

1. Is there a pulse? If no pulse, perform CPR for 2 minutes before analyzing for defibrillation.
2. Check and control severe bleeding.
3. Check skin color, temperature, and moisture.
4. Start intravenous (IV).
5. Administer medications as necessary.
6. Conduct the focused history and physical exam.

Summary of Airway, Breathing, Circulation Assessment

Airway

- Patent, maintainable, or nonmaintainable
- Level of conscious
- Skin: appearance, ashen, pale, grey, cyanotic, or mottled
- Airway clearance needed
- Sounds of obstruction

Breathing

- Rate and depth of respirations
- Cyanosis
- Position of trachea
- Presence of obvious injury or deformity

- Work of breathing
- Accessory muscle use
- Flaring of nostrils
- Presence of breath sounds bilaterally
- Presence of adventitious breath sounds
- Asymmetric chest movements
- Palpation of crepitus

Circulation

- Pulse, rate, and quality
- Skin appearance
- Temperature
- Level of consciousness
- Urinary output
- Blood pressure
- Cardiac monitoring

FOCUSED HISTORY AND PHYSICAL EXAMINATION

The focused history and physical examination determine additional problems that the patient may have, and may also reveal information about the severity of the patient's condition.

It includes medical history, baseline vital signs, and a rapid head-to-toe physical examination. If the patient is responsive, the prehospital care provider may ask pertinent questions and gather vital sign information.

Four Steps in Focused History and Physical Examination

1. Assess the patient's past medical history.
2. Chief complaint
3. History of present illness (HPI) or event (OPQRST)
4. Pertinent past medical history that may be relevant to current illness.

Pertinent Past History

S = Signs/symptoms
A = Allergies
M = Medications
P = Past medical history
L = Last oral intake
E = Events leading up to illness or injury

Current Health Status

- Medic alert tag or bracelet.
- Family/social history
- **If the patient's chief complaint or problem is related to pain, the OPQRST method should be used:**
  - Onset
  - Provocation

  - Quality
  - Radiation or region
  - Severity
  - Time
- Perform a physical exam, focusing on the area of the patient's chief complaint
- Obtain baseline vital signs (blood pressure; pulse—rate and quality; respirations—rate and quality)
- Skin-color, temperature, moisture

Providing emergency care should be based on signs and symptoms in accordance with local protocol and in consultation with medical control.

The Medical Patient

Emphasis is placed on patient history.

- In the responsive patient, medical history is performed before physical examination.
- Mental status is assessed during the initial assessment and is re-evaluated during the focused physical exam.

Responsive Patient

- Gather medical history first.
- Do a physical examination focusing on the chief complaint, vital signs, and symptoms.

Unresponsive Patient

- Perform a rapid physical examination (medical assessment).
- Baseline vital signs determination.
- Gather patient medical history.

The Major Trauma Patient

Emphasis is placed on *mechanism of injury*, or physical findings.

- Vehicle rollover (90° vehicle rotation or more) with an unrestrained passenger
- Ejection or partial ejection
- Death in the same passenger compartment
- Extrication time in excess of 20 minutes
- Vehicle collision resulting in 12-in. intrusion into the passenger compartment
- Motorcycle crash >20 mph or with separation of rider with motorcycle
- Falls greater than 20 ft
- Vehicle versus pedestrian or bicycle collision greater than 5 mph

Physical Findings

- Glasgow coma scale is less than or equal to 13
- Respiratory rate is less than 10 or more than 29 breaths per minute
- Pulse rate is less than 50 or more than 120 beats per minute
- Systolic blood pressure is less than 90 mmHg
- Penetrating injuries to head, neck, torso, or proximal extremities
- Two or more suspected proximal long bone fractures

- Suspected flail chest
- Amputation (except digits)
- Suspected pelvic fracture
- Open or depressed skull fracture
- Suspected spinal cord injury or limb paralysis

High-Risk Patients

- Bleeding disorders or patients who are on anticoagulant medications.
- Cardiac disease and/or respiratory disease.
- Insulin dependent diabetes patients, cirrhosis, or morbid obesity.
- Immunosuppressed patients (HIV disease, transplant patients, and patients on chemotherapy treatment).
- Age >55.
- Many medical conditions can be controlled at the scene, but patients with significant trauma need surgical intervention.
- Rapid identification of critical conditions (actual and potential) is crucial.
- Consider "load and go."
- Goal is to spend no more than 10 minutes on the scene.
- Many severe injuries are internal and are not easily identified.

Rapid Trauma Assessment

DCAP-BTLS

*D*eformities
*C*ontusions
*A*brasions
*P*enetrations or punctures
*B*urns
*T*enderness
*L*acerations
*S*welling

Continued Assessment

The initial assessment and focused history and physical examinations are completed rapidly so that serious illness or injury can be identified, intervention provided, and transportation initiated without delay. Once the patient's most serious conditions have been managed (or if none can be determined) the continued assessment is performed.

The continued assessment is a more detailed examination and always includes continued reevaluation of the patient. With serious conditions, this is done en-route to the hospital.

- Identify any missed injuries or conditions, particularly those that are life threatening.
- Assess the patient's response to care.
- Adjust the patient's management as necessary.

The detailed physical examination is specific to the patient and injury. Not all patients require a detailed physical exam. Detailed physical exam begins at the head and ends with the extremities, repeating in more depth. The detailed physical examination may reveal additional injuries or other information. Continue to observe and reevaluate the patient frequently during transportation to identify new or worsening symptoms. Complete a focused examination for the area of complaint.

Reassess and **record** the patient's mental status, airway, breathing circulation, vital signs, and effectiveness of interventions:

Stable patients = every 15 minutes

Unstable patients = every 5 minutes

Findings obtained during the continued reassessment should be compared with baseline findings obtained during the focused assessment.

Documentation

A competent prehospital report documents the nature and extent of emergency care. Well-prepared reports are an important medical/legal document.

"If it isn't written down, it wasn't done," and "if it wasn't done, don't write it down."

Health-care providers use the information from the report to trend changes in patient condition. In particular, the trending of mental status and vital signs is extremely important to physicians and nurses who assume care. The information on the report can also be used in quality assessment of emergency medical care.

The function of the prehospital care report (PCR) is:

1. Continuity of care—A form that is not read immediately in the emergency department may very well be referred to later for important information.
2. Legal document.
   a. A good report has documented what emergency medical care was provided and the status of the patient on arrival at the scene and any changes upon arrival at the receiving facility.
   b. The person who completed the form ordinarily must go to court with the form.
   c. Information should include objective and subjective information and be clear. You should not document your opinion.
3. Educational.
4. Administrative-billing and service statistics.
5. Research.
6. Evaluation and continuous quality improvement.

CHAPTER QUESTIONS

1. The patient's age, sex, race, birthplace, and occupation are included in which element of the comprehensive patient history?
   a. Past history
   b. Preliminary data
   c. Current health status
   d. None of the above
2. The mnemonic OPQRST-ASPN is a tool used during which element of the comprehensive patient history?
   a. Chief complaint
   b. Past history
   c. Present illness/injury
   d. Current health status

3. In the OPQRST mnemonic, the "P" stands for?
   a. Pertinent negatives
   b. Past medical history
   c. Prescription medications
   d. Provocative/palliative factors
4. The term "referred pain" means pain that:
   a. is not really there, as in an amputated limb
   b. is felt at a location away from its source
   c. has been relieved or not as severe as it previously was
   d. is elicited through palpation
5. The examination technique of informed observation is called:
   a. palpation
   b. inspection
   c. percussion
   d. auscultation
6. Your patient is experiencing rapid, deep respirations (gasps) with short pauses between sets. This is known as what type of respiration?
   a. Kussmaul
   b. Apneustic
   c. Cheyne-Stokes
   d. Biot's
7. The amount of air one breath moves in and out of the lungs is called:
   a. minute volume
   b. tidal volume
   c. breath volume
   d. inspired volume
8. The difference between systolic and diastolic pressures is called:
   a. pulse pressure
   b. orthostatic pressure
   c. arterial resistance
   d. pericardial range
9. Body substance isolation is a component of:
   a. scene size-up
   b. initial assessment
   c. focused history and physical exam
   d. detailed physical exam
10. While performing the initial assessment of a patient, you note an open wound to the chest. This injury should be treated:
   a. during the focused physical exam
   b. during the rapid trauma assessment
   c. during the initial assessment
   d. during the detailed physical exam

Suggested Reading

US Department of Transportation, National Highway Traffic Safety Administration. *EMT-Paramedic: National Standard Curriculum*. Washington, DC: US Department of Transportation, National Highway Traffic Safety Administration; 1998.

Section 4
Trauma

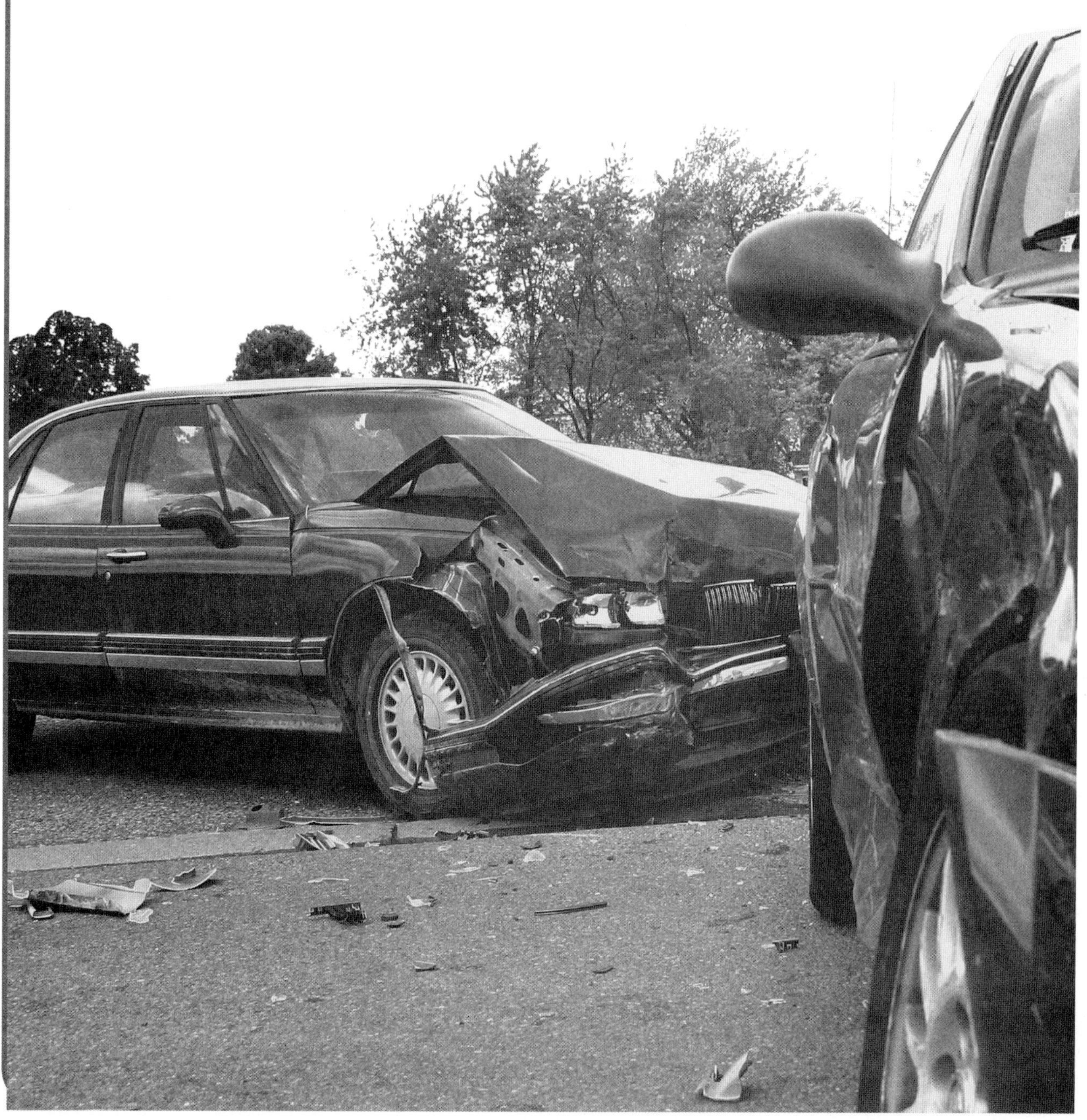

Chapter 13

Trauma Systems and Mechanism of Injury

You are transporting a patient with a chest injury that was sustained at a motor vehicle crash involving a car and semi-tractor trailer. The patient is unconscious and has significant chest trauma. Your partner has intubated the patient and is performing bag-valve-mask ventilation. He suddenly complains that the bag is becoming increasingly more difficult to squeeze. You reassess your patient and note the following:

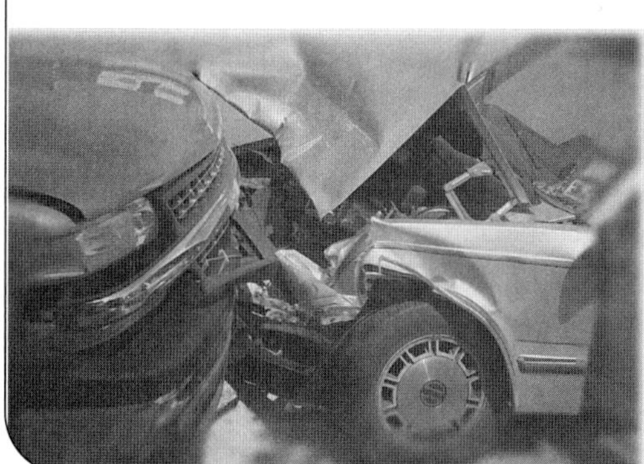

- Pronounced jugular vein distention (JVD)
- Tachycardia—124 weak and thready
- Hypotension—blood pressure 90/60
- Absent lung sounds on the entire right side
- Tracheal deviation

What is your next course of management?

INTRODUCTION TO TRAUMA SYSTEMS

- Trauma is the leading cause of death in patients 1–44 years old.
- Trauma is the fourth cause of death overall.
- 140,000 unexpected deaths/year.
- 40,000 related to automobiles.
- Understanding the mechanisms that result in patient injuries is essential to recognizing both visible and suspected (or hidden) injuries. It may also be used to determine a patient's priority status.

KINETICS OF TRAUMA

- Kinetics—Refers to motion as it pertains to material bodies.
- Kinetic energy—Refers to the amount of energy that is contained within a moving body.

Mass and Velocity

- The amount of kinetic energy a moving body contains depends upon two things:
  - The body's mass (weight)
  - The body's velocity (speed)
- An important item to note is that the velocity of an object is more important in describing kinetic energy than mass.
- During your scene size-up, try to get an idea of the travel speed of the vehicle if you're at a motor vehicle collision (MVC).
- If the mechanism is a gunshot wound (GSW), try to ascertain if it was a high- or low-velocity weapon.

Acceleration and Deceleration

- The law of inertia states that a body at rest will stay at rest, and a body in motion will stay in motion, unless acted upon by an outside force. This also applies to understanding the mechanism of injury (MOI).
- The rate at which a body in motion increases its speed is acceleration.
- The rate at which motion decreases its speed is deceleration.
- Both of these forces, which are functions of the law of inertia, play a role in the amount of force applied to a patient.

Energy Changes Form and Direction

- Energy, like rays of light, travels in a straight line unless it is deflected by some kind of interference.
- When energy from trauma impacts the body, it still tries to maintain a straight line; however, since the body is not straight, the energy becomes interrupted and a traumatic injury may result. This could result in blunt or penetrating injuries.
- An example of this is if energy is transmitted to the thorax due to impacting the steering column during a rapid deceleration injury.
- Since the energy cannot go in the curved shape of the ribs, it results in breaking of the ribcage as the energy *still* tries to travel in a straight line.
- Or if a person jumps off a roof and lands on his feet, the energy may break the thigh bone at the hip because the energy cannot turn inward to the body like the femur does.

Mechanism of Injury

- With knowledge and experience, you will be able to rapidly assess the scene and determine the type and degree of forces applied to the patient's body.
- This information, known as the mechanism of injury, is useful for identifying and anticipating certain injury patterns for a given traumatic incident.

Common MOI include:

- Vehicular collisions (most lethal)
- Falls (most common)
- Penetrating GSWs
- Penetrating knife or other sharp instrument wounds
- Explosions

Vehicle Collisions

- The greater the velocity, the greater the chance for injury (Fig. 13-1).
- Maintain a high index of suspicion with:
  - Death of another occupant of the vehicle
  - An unresponsive patient
  - A patient with an altered mental status
- These types of patients usually indicate significant forces were applied to the car, and hence, the people inside.
- Restraints—A cause of hidden injuries
  - A lap belt without a shoulder harness still allows for chest and head injuries.
  - A lap belt worn too high causes intra-abdominal injuries.
  - A lap belt worn too low can cause hip displacement.
  - A shoulder harness without a lap belt can result in severe neck injuries.
  - After an airbag deploys, any further collision events go unprotected.
  - Airbag deployment without the use of belts puts the patient too close to the deployment, and can cause additional head, neck, or chest trauma.

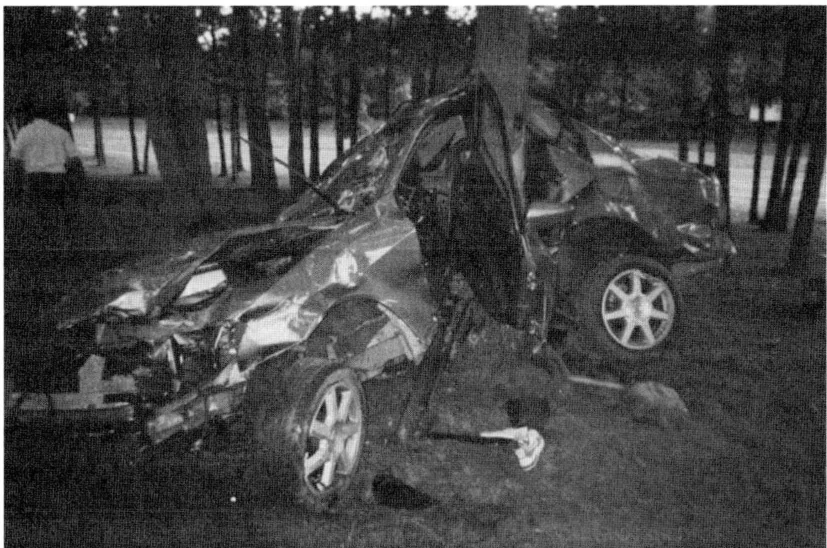

Figure 13-1 High speed single vehicle collision were the occupant died from his injuries. *(Courtesy Peter DiPrima)*

- After an airbag deploys, any further collision events go unprotected.
- Airbag deployment without the use of belts puts the patient too close to the deployment, and can cause additional head, neck, or chest trauma.

Falls

- Most common MOI
- Injuries depend upon:
  - Height of fall (>15 ft for adult and >10 ft for children considered "significant")
  - Surface landed on
  - Region of body landed on first
  - Age and general condition of the patient

Feet-First Landings

- Fractures of the heels
- Ankle injuries
- Knee joint injuries
- Possible vertebral injuries

Head-First Falls

- Injury pattern may start with arms and shoulders if they fell with their arms outstretched to "break" the fall.
- Head may be forcibly hyperextended or hyperflexed.
- Compression fractures to the cervical spine are possible.
- After landing, the torso and legs are thrown either forward or backward possibly causing truncal or lower extremity trauma.

Penetrating Injuries

- Injuries depend on velocity and the type of tissue the object (i.e., bullets, darts, nails, knives, etc.) penetrates into.
- Of all factors, the velocity of the penetrating object is what determines the greatest amount of damage.

- Penetrating injuries are classified as:
  - Low velocity
    - —Damage occurs to the immediate area of the penetration.
    - — The length of the object also determines the degree of injury.
    - — Types of objects could include knives, swords, pencils, or other similarly sharp objects used primarily by hand as an attack weapon.
  - Medium/high velocity
    - —Generally pellets or bullets.
  - Most shotguns or handguns are medium velocity.
  - High velocity usually includes rifles such as an M-16 or a 30-30 Winchester.
  - Damage is a function of the projectile's trajectory and dissipation.

Trajectory

- The path of motion of a projectile
- The higher the velocity, the flatter the trajectory

Dissipation

- How the projectile's energy is dissipated to the body

  Drag—Factors that slow a bullet down (wind or body tissue)

  Profile—Impact point of projectile

  Cavitation—Pressure wave that causes additional tissue damage beyond the pathway created by the projectile

Blast Injuries

- Result from the explosion of a volatile substance (natural gas, gasoline, fireworks, etc.)
- Every explosion has three distinct phases, each with its own pattern of injuries:
  - Primary phase—Pressure wave injuries
  - Secondary phase—Injuries from flying debris
  - Tertiary phase—Injuries from being thrown by the blast and landing against something

? CHAPTER QUESTION

1. Every explosion has three distinct phases, each with its own pattern of injuries. These phases include:
   a. tertiary phase
   b. secondary phase
   c. primary phase
   d. all of the above
   e. none of the above

Suggested Reading

US Department of Transportation, National Highway Traffic Safety Administration. *EMT-Paramedic: National Standard Curriculum.* Washington, DC: US Department of Transportation, National Highway Traffic Safety Administration; 1998.

www.traumacare.com/download/NFTC_CrisisReport_May04

Chapter 14
Hemorrhage and Shock

An elderly male has fallen 12 ft from a roof onto a concrete surface. He is complaining of head, neck, and back pain, and states he is having difficulty breathing. You note that he has fractures of the right upper arm and lower leg. He also has a 4 in. laceration to the frontal region of his forehead that is bleeding. He is conscious and alert and states he takes Digoxin and Coumadin for an irregular heartbeat. The patient's head is being stabilized by a neighbor who is a lifeguard. The patient also begins experiencing severe abdominal pain during your assessment.

What should your immediate management include?

See Table 14-1 for the stages of hemorrage.

SHOCK PATHOPHYSIOLOGY

Perfusion depends on cardiac output (CO); CO is determined by stroke volume (SV) and heart rate (HR). Blood pressure is determined by CO and systemic vascular resistance (SVR).

- $CO = HR \times SV$
- $BP = CO \times SVR$

Hypoperfusion can result from:

- Inadequate cardiac output
- Excessive systemic vascular resistance
- Inability of red blood cells to deliver oxygen to tissues

Compensation for decreased perfusion:

- Decreased perfusion can occur from blood loss, myocardial infarction, loss of vasomotor tone, tension pneumothorax, or plasma loss, to name a few.
- Baroreceptors sense decreased flow and activate the vasomotor center.
- Located in carotid sinuses and aortic arch, baroreceptors are normally stimulated between 60 and 80 mmHg systolic (lower in children).
- Arterial pressure drop decreases stretch, sending a nerve impulse through Vagus and Hering's nerve to the glossopharyngeal nerve. This impulse is then transmitted to vasomotor center. Frequency of inhibitory impulses decrease, and an increase in vasomotor activity occurs. The sympathetic nervous system is then stimulated.
- A decrease in systolic less than 80 mmHg stimulates vasomotor center to increase arterial pressure.
- Chemoreceptors are stimulated by decrease in PaO_2 and increase in $PaCO_2$.

TABLE 14-1: Stages of Hemorrhage

Stage 1	• Up to 15% intravascular loss • Compensated by constriction of vascular bed • Blood pressure maintained • Normal pulse pressure, respiratory rate, and renal output • Pallor of the skin • Central venous pressure low to normal
Stage 2	• 15–25% intravascular loss • Cardiac output cannot be maintained by arteriolar constriction • Reflex tachycardia • Increased respiratory rate • Blood pressure maintained • Catecholamines increase peripheral resistance • Increased diastolic pressure • Narrow pulse pressure • Diaphoresis from sympathetic stimulation • Renal output almost normal
Stage 3	• 25–35% intravascular loss • Classic signs of hypovolemic shock • Marked tachycardia • Marked tachypnea • Decreased systolic pressure • 5–15 mL per hour urine output • Alteration in mental status • Diaphoresis with cool, pale skin
Stage 4	• Loss greater than 35% • Extreme tachycardia • Pronounced tachypnea • Significantly decreased systolic blood pressure • Confusion and lethargy • Skin is diaphoretic, cool, and extremely pale

ADRENAL MEDULLA GLANDS SECRETE EPINEPHRINE AND NOREPINEPHRINE

Epinephrine

- Alpha-1—Vasoconstriction
  - Increase in peripheral vascular resistance
  - Increased after-load from arteriole constriction
- Alpha-2—Regulated release of alpha-1
- Beta-1
  - Positive chronotropy
  - Positive inotropy
  - Positive dromotropy
- Beta-2
  - Bronchodilation
  - Gut smooth muscle dilation

Norepinephrine

- Primarily alpha-1 and alpha-2
- Vasoconstriction
- Increase in peripheral vascular resistance
- Increased afterload from arteriolar constriction

Arginine Vasopressin (AVP)

- Also known as antidiuretic hormone (ADH)
- Is released from anterior pituitary gland

Effects

- Increases free water absorption in distal tubule and collecting ducts of kidney
- Decreases urine output
- Splanchnic vascular constriction

Renin-Angiotensin System

- Renin is released from the kidney arteriole. Renin and angiotensinogen combine in renal arteriole to produce angiotensin I.
- Angiotensin I is converted to angiotensin II by angiotensin-converting enzyme.
- Effects of angiotensin II:
  - Potent vasoconstrictor
  - Sodium reabsorption decreases urine output
  - Positive inotrope and chronotrope

Aldosterone

- Defends fluid volume
- Secreted by cells of adrenal cortex in response to stress, promotes sodium reabsorption and water retention in kidney
- Reduces urine output

Insulin

- Secretion is diminished by circulating epinephrine
  - Impaired effect on peripheral tissue
  - Contributes to hyperglycemia seen following injury and volume loss

Glucagon

- Stimulated by the release of epinephrine
- Promotes liver glycogenolysis, gluconeogenesis, amino acid uptake for conversion into glucose, and the transfer of fatty acid into mitochondria

ACTH (Adrenocorticotropic Hormone)-Cortisol System

- ACTH release stimulates the release of cortisol from the adrenal cortex of kidney. Cortisol increases glucose production by inhibiting enzymes that break down glucose.

Growth Hormone

- Secreted by anterior pituitary gland.
- Early effects of growth hormone.
- Promotes uptake of glucose and amino acids in muscle, and stimulates protein synthesis.

Failure of Compensation to Preserve Perfusion

- Preload decreases
- Cardiac output decreases
- Myocardial blood supply and oxygenation decrease
- Myocardial perfusion decreases
- Cardiac output decreases further
- Coronary artery perfusion decreases
- Myocardial ischemia

Capillary and Cellular Changes

- Ischemia
- Minimal blood flow to capillaries
- Cells go from aerobic to anaerobic metabolism

Stagnation

- Precapillary sphincter relaxes in response to:
  - Lactic acid
  - Vasomotor center failure
  - Increased carbon dioxide
- Postcapillary sphincters remain constricted
- Capillaries engorge with fluid
- Postcapillary sphincters remain constricted
- Capillaries engorge with fluid
- Anaerobic metabolism continues, increasing lactic acid production
- Aggregation of red blood cells and formation of microemboli
- Potent vasodilator
- Destroys capillary cell membrane
- Plasma leaks from capillaries
- Interstitial fluid increases
- Distance from capillary to cell increases
- Oxygen transport decreases secondary to increased capillary-cell distance
- Myocardial toxin factor released by ischemic pancreas

Washout

- Postcapillary sphincter relaxes
- Hydrogen, potassium, carbon dioxide, thrombosed—erythrocytes wash out
- Metabolic acidosis results
- Cardiac output drops further

STAGES OF SHOCK (SEE TABLE 14-2)

Etiologic Classifications of Shock

Hypovolemic Shock

- Hemorrhage
- Plasma loss
- Fluid and electrolyte loss

TABLE 14-2: Stages of Shock

Compensated or nonprogressive	• Characterized by signs and symptoms of early shock • Arterial blood pressure is normal or high • Treatment at this stage will typically result in recovery
Decompensated or progressive	• Characterized by signs and symptoms of late shock • Arterial blood pressure is abnormally low • Treatment at this stage will sometimes result in recovery
Irreversible	• Characterized by signs and symptoms of late shock • Arterial blood pressure is abnormally low • Even aggressive treatment at this stage does not result in recovery

Distributive (Vasogenic) Shock

- Increased venous capacitance
- Low resistance, vasodilation

Cardiogenic Shock

- Myocardial insufficiency
- Filling or outflow obstruction

Spinal/Neurogenic Shock

- Refers to temporary loss of all types of spinal cord function distal to injury
- Flaccid paralysis distal to injury site
- Loss of bladder and bowel control
- Priapism (male patients only)
- Loss of thermoregulation
- Does not always involve permanent primary injury
- Also called spinal vascular shock
- Temporary loss of the autonomic function of the cord at the level of injury which controls cardiovascular function

Signs and Symptoms

- Loss of sympathetic tone
- Relative hypotension
- Systolic pressure 80–100 mmHg
- Skin is pink, warm, and dry
- Due to cutaneous vasodilation
- Relative bradycardia (occurrence is rare)

Shock presentation is usually the result of hidden volume loss secondary to:

- Chest injuries
- Abdominal injuries
- Other violent injuries

Treatment

- Focus primarily on volume (fluid) replacement

Assessment—Hypovolemic Shock Due to Hemorrhage

Early or Compensated

- Narrow pulse pressure (Pulse pressure is the difference between the systolic and diastolic pressures, pulse pressure = systolic – diastolic. Pulse pressure reflects the tone of the arterial system and is more sensitive to changes in perfusion than the systolic or diastolic alone.)
- Positive orthostatic tilt test
- Tachycardia
- Pale, cool skin
- Diaphoresis
- No change in level of consciousness
- Anxious or apprehensive
- Blood pressure maintained
- Dry mucosa
- Complaints of thirst
- Weakness
- Possible delay of capillary refill

Late or Progressive

- Extreme tachycardia
- Extreme pale, cool skin
- Diaphoresis
- Significant decrease in level of consciousness
- Hypotension
- Dry mucosa
- Nausea
- Cyanosis with white waxy looking skin

Differential Shock Assessment Findings

- Shock is assumed to be hypovolemic until proven otherwise
- Cardiogenic shock—Differentiated from hypovolemic shock by one or more of the following:
  - Chief complaint (chest pain, dyspnea, tachycardia)
  - Heart rate (bradycardia or excessive tachycardia)
  - Signs of congestive heart failure (jugular vein distention, rales)
  - Dysrhythmias

Distributive Shock

- Differentiated from hypovolemic shock by presence of one or more of the following:
  - Mechanism that suggests vasodilation, such as spinal cord injury, drug overdose, sepsis, or anaphylaxis
  - Warm, flushed skin, especially in dependent areas
  - Lack of tachycardia response (not reliable, though, since significant number of hypovolemic patients never become tachycardic)

Obstructive Shock

- Differentiated from hypovolemic shock by presence of signs and symptoms suggestive of:
  - Cardiac tamponade
  - Tension pneumothorax

Advanced Life Support Management

- Airway and ventilatory support
- Ventilate and suction as necessary
- Administer high concentration oxygen
- Reduce increased intrathoracic pressure in tension pneumothorax
- Circulatory support
- Hemorrhage control
- Intravenous volume expanders:
  - Isotonic solutions
  - Hypertonic solutions
  - Synthetic solutions
  - Blood and blood products
  - Experimental solutions
  - Blood substitutes
- Consider increased rate of infusion
- External hemorrhage that can be controlled
- External hemorrhage that cannot be controlled
- Penetrating trauma (treat per local protocol)

Pneumatic antishock garment (falling out of use in prehospital care)

- Increased arterial blood pressure above garment
- Increased systemic vascular resistance
- Immobilization of pelvis and possibly lower extremities
- Increased intra-abdominal pressure

Mechanism

- Increases systemic vascular resistance through direct compression of tissues and blood vessels
- Negligible auto-transfusion effect

Indications

- Hypoperfusion with unstable pelvis
- Conditions of decreased systemic vascular resistance (SVR) not corrected by other means
- As approved locally, other conditions characterized by hypoperfusion with hypotension

Contraindications

- Advanced pregnancy (no inflation of abdominal compartment)
- Object impaled in abdomen or evisceration (inflation of abdominal compartment is contraindicated)
- Ruptured diaphragm
- Cardiogenic shock or pulmonary edema

PHARMACOLOGICAL INTERVENTIONS

Hypovolemic Shock

- Volume expanders

Cardiogenic Shock

- Volume expanders
- Positive cardiac inotropes
- Vasopressors
- Rate-altering medications

Distributive Shock

- Volume expanders
- Positive cardiac inotropes
  - Vasopressors
  - Pneumatic antishock garment (PASG) (per local protocol)

Obstructive Shock

- Volume expanders

Spinal Shock

- Volume expanders

Transport Considerations

- Indications for rapid transport to a trauma center
- Considerations for air medical transportation

CHAPTER QUESTIONS

1. Your patient has lost approximately 20% of his total blood volume. He is anxious, restless, and has cool, clammy skin. Which stage of hemorrhage is he in?
   a. Stage 1
   b. Stage 2
   c. Stage 3
   d. Stage 4
2. One step in the initial assessment of a hemorrhage/shock patient is:
   a. application of individual splints for suspected injuries
   b. initiation of IV fluid resuscitation
   c. checking skin color and condition
   d. obtaining baseline vitals
3. If a patient's blood pressure decreases when he is moved from a supine to a sitting position, he is said to have:
   a. postural vitals
   b. orthostatic hypotension

c. supine hypotension
d. a negative "tilt test"

4. Acidosis, due to lack of perfusion, causes relaxation of postcapillary sphincters, releasing lactic acid, carbon dioxide, and columns of coagulated red blood cells into the venous circulation. This is known as:
   a. a rouleaux
   b. hydrostatic pressure
   c. capillary washout
   d. angiotensin flow
5. Entry into decompensated shock is indicated by:
   a. unconsciousness
   b. thready pulse
   c. bradypnea
   d. a precipitous drop in blood pressure
6. Venous bleeding is usually:
   a. bright red and spurting in nature
   b. dark red and flowing
   c. oozing and quick-clotting
   d. dark red, forming droplets on the skin
7. The step in the clotting process in which the smooth blood vessel muscle contracts, reducing the vessel lumen is called the:
   a. platelet phase
   b. vascular phase
   c. coagulation phase
   d. aggregate phase
8. The network that forms around a wound to stop the bleeding, ward off infection, and lay a foundation for healing and repair of the wound is made up of:
   a. platelets
   b. hemoglobin
   c. fibrin
   d. plasma
9. One of the factors that can hinder the clotting process is:
   a. immobilization
   b. dehydration
   c. fever
   d. medications such as aspirin

Suggested Reading

http://www.health.state.ny.us/nysdoh/ems/nystrauma.htm. Accessed on May 1, 2007.

http://www.trauma.org/. Accessed on May 1, 2007.

US Department of Transportation, National Highway Traffic Safety Administration. *EMT-Paramedic: National Standard Curriculum.* Washington, DC: US Department of Transportation, National Highway Traffic Safety Administration; 1998.

Chapter 15
Soft Tissue Trauma

You're on the scene treating a 32-year-old construction worker who is pinned underneath heavy construction material. When evaluating the patient you notice the patient's right arm is pinned. He is complaining of pain, paresthesia, pallor, and a feeling of severe pressure, and the extremity is pulselessness distal to the crush injury. What are some of the complications of crush injuries?

SOFT TISSUE INJURIES/ANATOMY AND PHYSIOLOGY REVIEW (TABLE 15-1)

Layers of Soft Tissue (Figure 15-1)

Cutaneous Layer

- Epidermis
- Dermis

Subcutaneous Layer

- Loose connective tissue
- Fat

Deep Fascia

- Fibrous tissue
- Supportive and protective

Functions of Soft Tissue

- Protection from trauma
- Thermoregulation
- Sensory functions
- Pain, touch, temperature
- Protection from infection
- Fluid maintenance

WOUND HEALING

- Change in skin anatomy
- Initial vasoconstriction for up to 10 minutes
- Clotting process started
- Wound healing—Inflammatory phase

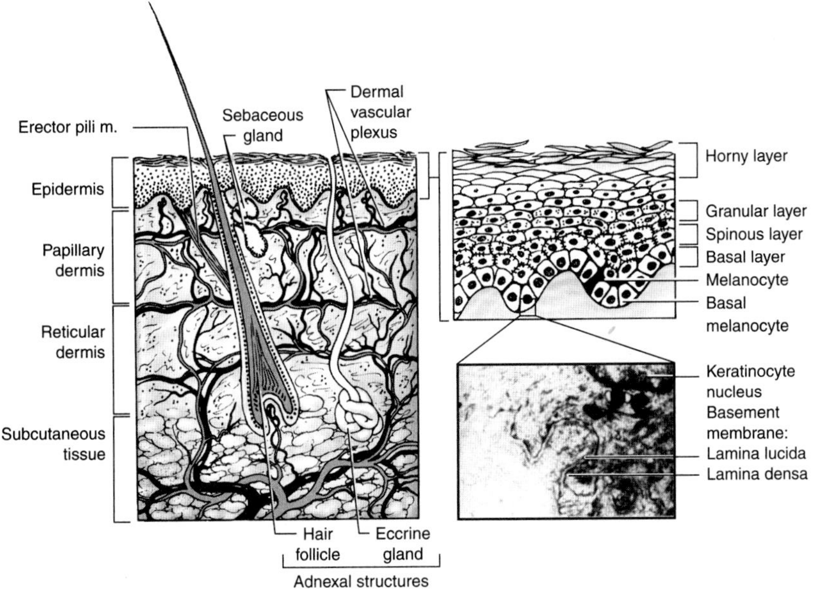

Figure 15-1 Layers of skin. *(Used with permission from Brunicardi FC, Andersen DK, Billiar TR, et al (eds).* Schwartz's Principles of Surgery, 8th Ed. *New York: McGraw-Hill, 2005, p. 430.)*

Table 15-1: Soft Tissue Injuries Review

Contusion	• Epidermis intact • Vessels in dermis are torn • Swelling and pain • Blood accumulation results in ecchymosis
Hematoma	• Collection of blood beneath skin • Larger amount of tissue damage • Larger vessels are damaged
Abrasion	• Superficial injury • Outermost skin damaged by shearing forces • Painful in proportion to degree of injury • No bleeding or minor bleeding • Contamination is primary concern
Laceration	• Skin disruption with greater depth than abrasion • Jagged wound ends bleed easily • May involve other soft tissue injuries • Caused by forceful impact with sharp object • Bleeding may be severe
Incisions	• Skin disruption with greater depth than abrasion • Similar to laceration except wound ends are smooth and even • Tend to heal better than lacerations • Caused by very sharp objects
Avulsion	• Flap of skin or tissue torn loose or pulled completely off • Avulsed tissue may or may not be viable
Amputation	• Involves extremities or body parts • Jagged skin and/or bone edges at site • Three types ◦ Complete, partial, degloving

- Granulocytes and macrophages collect debris
- Histamine release
- Wound healing—Epithelialization phase
- Within 12 hours
- Healing by establishing new skin layers

Wound Healing—Neovascularization

- New vessel formation
- Begins ~3 days after injury
- Continues for ~21 days
- Wound healing—Collagen synthesis
- Fibroblasts synthesize collagen
- Collagen binds margins together
- Remodeling—Collagen broken down and relaid

Factors Affecting Wound Healing

Drug Use

- Corticosteroids
- Nonsteroidal anti-inflammatory drugs (NSAIDs)
- Penicillin
- Colchicine (used in gouty arthritis)
- Anticoagulants
- Antineoplastics

Medical Conditions and Diseases

- Advanced age
- Alcoholism
- Acute uremia
- Hepatic failure
- Diabetes mellitus
- Hypoxia
- Severe anemia
- Malnutrition
- Chemical vapor deposition (CVD) and physical vapor deposition (PVD)
- Advanced cancer

High-Risk Wounds

- Bites—From a human or animal
- Foreign bodies contaminated with organic matter
- Injection wounds
  - Significant devitalized tissue
- Crush injury
- Immunocompromised patients
- Poor peripheral circulation

Factors Leading to Abnormal Scar Formation

- Keloid—Excessive accumulation of scar tissue beyond original wound borders. Common areas:
  - Ears
  - Extremities
  - Sternum
- Hypertrophic scar—Excessive accumulation of scar tissue within the original wound borders. Common in areas of high stress, such as:
  - Flexion creases across joints

Wounds Requiring Closure

- Cosmetic areas, such as face, lip, or eyebrow
- Gaping wounds
- Wounds over tension areas
- Degloving injuries
- Ring injuries
- Skin-tearing injuries

CRUSH INJURY AND COMPARTMENT SYNDROME

Crush Injuries

Crush injuries are caused by a crushing (compressive) force and may result in organ injury. This type of injury is often associated with severe fractures.

Causes of Crush Injuries

- Collapse of a structure onto a specific body area.
- Compressive trauma to body area.
- Prolonged compression in a chronic situation.
- Injury sustained from a compressive force sufficient to interfere with the normal metabolic function of the injured tissue may lead to:
  - rhabdomyolysis
  - electrolyte abnormalities
  - acid-base abnormalities
  - hypovolemia
  - acute renal failure

Crush Injury Assessment

- Local evidence of muscle ischemia
- Results from compressive forces in a closed space
- Maybe painful, swollen, deformed
- Little or no external bleeding
- Internal bleeding may be severe
- Reperfusion phenomenon
- Systemic effects occur after the issue is reperfused
- Oxygen-free radicals result in muscle injury
- High intracellular calcium

Rhabdomyolysis—Pathophysiology

- Muscle destroyed
- Extracellular fluid moves into muscle cells
- Increased H_20, NaCl, calcium
- Fluid from muscle moves into extracellular fluid
- Lactic acid build-up
- Myoglobin
- Potassium, phosphate
- Thromboplastin, creatine kinase, and creatinine

Rhabdomyolysis—Potential Complications

- Hypovolemia
- Hypocalcemia
- Hyperkalemia
- Increase in cardiac toxicity
- Metabolic acidosis
- Hyperuricemia
- Hyperphosphatemia
- Possible disseminated intravascular coagulopathy (DIC)
- Tissue pressure > capillary hydrostatic pressure
- Results in ischemia to muscle
- Muscle cell edema begins
- Prolonged ischemia (>6–8 hrs) leads to tissue hypoxia and cell death
- Direct soft tissue trauma also adds to edema and ischemia
- Renal failure
- Hypovolemia
- Renal tubules become obstructed
- Nephrotoxic agents present

Early Signs of Crush Syndrome

- Pain, swelling, sensory changes, weakness
- Paralysis and sensory loss to injured area
- Rigor of joint distal to the injured muscles
- May have pulses present and warm skin

Later Signs Indicating Compartment Syndrome

- 5 Ps—Pain, paresthesia, pallor, pressure, pulselessness

Wounds Requiring Transport for Evaluation

- Neural compromise
- Vascular compromise
- Muscular compromise
- Tendon/ligament compromise
- Heavy contamination or high-risk wounds
- Cosmetic complications
- Foreign body complications

SOFT TISSUE INJURY MANAGEMENT

- Tetanus vaccine
  - Caused by *Clostridium tetani*
  - Anaerobic bacteria
- Initial vaccine
- Booster q 10 years
- Every 5 years for high-risk persons
- Potential for allergic reaction
- Potential risk of infection
- Microflora common on skin surface
- Source on wound mechanism
- Is the patient immunocompromised?
- Minimize infection possibility by minimizing contamination
- Clean wound soon after injury
- Protect from further injury and contamination.

MANAGEMENT OF SPECIFIC INJURIES

Avulsion

- Airway, breathing, circulation (ABCs)
- Control bleeding
- Dress and bandage
- Package avulsed tissue for transport
- If avulsed skin is detached wrap in sterile dressing and place in plastic bag.
- Place plastic bag in bag of ice
- Transport to appropriate facility
- Consider surgery and plastic surgery capabilities

Amputation

- ABCs.
- Control bleeding.
- Do not complete partial amputations.
- Dress and bandage, wrap in sterile dressing and place in plastic bag. Place plastic bag on ice. Some EMS systems moisten the sterile dressing before placing in bag.
- Package amputated part for transport.
- Transport to appropriate facility.
- Consider surgery and plastic surgery capabilities.

Crush Injuries

- Goal is to prevent sudden death
- Prevent renal failure
- Salvage limb
- Treat early
- Fluid for hypovolemia
- Consider bolus of 1–1.5 L in 250 mL increments
- No intravascular (IV) sites distal to crush injury!!

- Alkalinize urine
- Consider $NaHCO_3$: Add 50 mEq to 1 L bag of fluid
- Goal: Urine pH > 6.5
- Controls hyperkalemia and acidosis to prevent acute myoglobinuria renal failure by changing structure of myoglobin so it passes through renal tubules
- Maintain urine output
- Diuresis of at least 300 cc/hr
- Consider Mannitol
- Avoid loop diuretics (may acidify urine)
- Ideal fluid is D5 $^1/_2$ normal saline with 50 mEq $NaHCO_3$ and Mannitol
- Treat hypovolemia
- Correct acidosis

OTHER POSSIBLE THERAPIES

- Consider insulin/glucose for severe hyperkalemia (12.5 g D50 followed by 10 units regular insulin IV)
- Amiloride
- Potassium sparing diuretic
- Hemodialysis (in-hospital treatment)

COMPARTMENT SYNDROME

- Clinical signs and symptoms may indicate need for emergency fasciotomy
- Early fasciotomy can preserve limb, avoid Volkmann's contracture and preserve sensation
- Seldom, but occasionally, performed in out-of-hospital setting
- Soft tissue injury management
- Management of specific injuries
- Hyperbaric oxygen treatment
- Shown to decrease tissue necrosis
- Inhibits formation of oxygen free radicals
- Decreases muscle edema
- Most useful if performed early

Assessment and Documentation

- Effectively assess and document
- Size, location, depth, and associated risks/complications of wound
- Neurovascular status of extremities (multiple assessments required)
- Joint involvement
- Increased risks of infection

CHAPTER QUESTION

1. The fatty layer of the skin used for insulation and absorption of energy during an injury is called:
   a. epidermis
   b. dermis
   c. subcutaneous
   d. stratum granulosum

Suggested Reading

US Department of Transportation, National Highway Traffic Safety Administration. *EMT-Paramedic: National Standard Curriculum.* Washington, DC: US Department of Transportation, National Highway Traffic Safety Administration; 1998.

Chapter 16
Burns

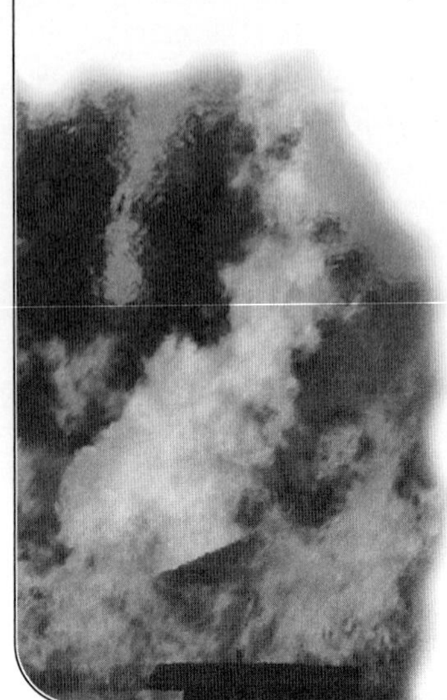

Your patient is a healthy 25-year-old city firefighter who has total body surface area (TBSA) second-degree burns of approximately 25%, and third-degree burns of approximately 10% from a flashover in a residential basement fire.

You stop the burn process, conduct an initial survey, manage the airway, and initiate cardiac monitoring and fluid resuscitation.

When assessing this patient, why is it important to monitor and control the airway early?

What are some of the signs and symptoms you may find in this particular case?

SKIN REVIEW

Functions of Skin

- Immune protection
- Physical protection
- Ultraviolet protection
- Dehydration protection
- Temperature regulation
- Sensory organ
- Excretion
- Vitamin D synthesis
- Blood reservoir

Major Regions of Skin

- Epidermis
- Dermis
- Subcutaneous (hypodermis)

COMMON CAUSES OF BURNS

- Thermal
- Electrical
- Chemical
- Radiation

Thermal Burns

Most common cause of burn injury.

- Occurs from:
  - Flame
  - Scalding
  - Contact with hot object

DETERMINING THE SEVERITY/DEPTH OF A BURN INJURY

- Superficial burn injury (first-degree burn)
- Partial thickness burn (second-degree burn)
- Full thickness burn (third-degree burn)

First degree—Superficial involvement (epidermis)

- Local pain and redness with no blistering present
- Heal spontaneously 2–5 days without scarring
- Not included when calculating percentage of TBSA

Second degree—Partial thickness burn (involves epidermal and dermal layers)

- Red, painful, and blistered skin
- Deep partial thickness presents with pale, mottled skin
- Very painful
- Infection may evolve into third degree

Third degree—Full thickness burn (involves the epidermis, dermis, subcutaneous tissue)

- White, waxy, red, brown, leathery
- Dry and painless

PATHOPHYSIOLOGY

- Injury occurs when temperature is greater than 111°F.

AREA OF BURN DAMAGE

- Zone of coagulation
- Zone of stasis
- Zone of hyperemia

JACKSON'S THEORY OF THERMAL WOUNDS

- Zone of coagulation
  - Area in a burn nearest the heat source that suffers the most damage as evidenced by clotted blood and thrombosed blood vessels
  - Central area of burn
  - Necrotic from time of exposure
- Zone of stasis
  - Area surrounding zone of coagulation characterized by decreased blood flow
  - Moderate degree of insult
  - Decreased tissue perfusion

- Vascular damage/leakage
- May progress to necrosis 24–48 hours
- Zone of hyperemia
  - Peripheral area around burn that has an increased blood flow
  - Vasodilatation
  - Inflammation
  - Viable tissue

BODY'S RESPONSE TO BURNS

Emergent Phase (Stage 1)

- Pain response which causes a catecholamine release (tachycardia, tachypnea, mild hypertension, and mild anxiety)

Fluid Shift Phase (Stage 2)

- Length 18–24 hours
- Begins after emergent phase
- Reaches peak in 6–8 hours
- Damaged cells initiate inflammatory response
- Increased blood flow to cells
- Shift of fluid from intravascular to extravascular space
- Massive edema
- Leaky capillaries

Systemic Changes

- Massive release of inflammatory mediators
- Produce vasoconstriction/dilation
- Increased capillary permeability and edema

Fluid Shifts

- Initial decrease blood flow to burned area
- Followed by increased arterial vasodilation
- Release of vasoactive substance resulting in increased capillary permeability and edema

Cardiovascular

- Loss of plasma volume
- Increased peripheral vascular resistance
- Decreased cardiac output
- Decreased blood volume
- Decreased venous return
- Increased blood viscosity
- Decreased contractility

Renal

- Decreased circulating plasma
- Increased hematocrit
- Decreased CO

- Decreased renal blood flow
- Oliguria
- Acute renal failure

Gastrointestinal

- Decreased gastrointestinal blood flow
- Increased mucosal hemorrhage

Immune System

- Depressed immune function
- Proportional to burn size
- Sepsis

Hypermetabolic Phase (Stage 3)

- Lasts for days to weeks
- Large increase in the body's need for nutrients as it repairs itself

Resolution Phase (Stage 4)

- Scar formation
- General rehabilitation and progression to normal function

Hypermetabolism

- Following severe burn and burn resuscitation
- Tachycardia
- Increased CO
- Increased oxygen (O_2) demand
- Massive proteolysis and lipolysis
- Severe nitrogen loss

Systemic Complications

- Hypothermia—Disruption of skin and its ability to thermoregulate
- Hypovolemia
- Shift in proteins, fluids, and electrolytes to the burned tissue
- General electrolyte imbalance
- Eschar—Hard, leathery product of a deep full thickness burn
  - Dead and denatured skin

Systemic Complications

- Infection
- Greatest risk of burn is infection
- Organ failure
- Release of myoglobin
- Special factors
- Age and health
- Physical abuse
- Elderly, infirm, or young

Critical Burn Areas

- Face
- Hands
- Feet
- Groin
- Joints
- Any circumferential burn

INHALATION INJURIES

- Leading cause of death in burn victims
- Caused by a closed space incident
- Presence of heavy smoke
- Toxic inhalation
- Synthetic resin combustion
- Cyanide and hydrogen sulfide

Carbon Monoxide Poisoning

- Colorless, odorless, tasteless gas
- Byproduct of incomplete combustion of carbon products
- Suspect with faulty heating unit
- 200× greater affinity for hemoglobin than O_2
- Hypoxemia and hypercarbia

Other Evidence

- Facial burns
- Profuse secretions
- Carbonaceous sputum
- Lacrimation
- Singed nasal hair
- Hoarseness
- Wheezing
- Stridor
- Edema
- Hypoxemia
- Tachycardia

Airway Thermal Burn

- Supraglottic structures absorb heat and generally prevent lower airway burns
- Injury is common from superheated steam
- Risk factors:
  - Standing in the burn environment
  - Screaming or yelling in the burn environment
  - Trapped in a closed burn environment

- Symptoms:
  - Stridor or "crowing" inspiratory sounds
  - Singed facial and nasal hair
  - Black sputum or facial burns
  - Progressive respiratory obstruction and arrest due to swelling

Types of Injuries

- Carbon monoxide poisoning
- Injury above glottis
- Injury below glottis

CO Poisoning

- Affinity for Hgb 200–250× > than O_2
- Cherry red only present at levels >40%, usually a postmortem finding
- Nausea, vomiting, headache, decreased level of consciousness (LOC), weakness, tachypnea, tachycardia
- False pulse oximetry readings
- 100% O_2 $^1/_2$ time for elimination
  - 40 min
- 21% O_2 $^1/_2$ time elimination
  - 250 minutes

Carboxyhemoglobin

- Normal—0
- Smokers, truck drivers in heavy traffic—15
- 15–40%—Neurological dysfunction
  - Weakness, dizziness, nausea, vomiting, headache
- 40–60%—Obtunded severe decreased LOC
  - Consider hyperbaric therapy—25–40%

Injury Above Glottis

- Thermal, chemical burns require early intubation

Injury Below Glottis

- Usually occurs from a chemical burn
- Respiratory distress is usually present (requires early intubation)
- Usually leads to:
  - Adult respiratory distress syndrome (ARDS)
  - Multi system organ failure (MSOF)

Estimating Percent of Body Surface Area (BSA) Burned

- Rule of palms
- Rule of nines

Body Surface Area

- Rule of nines
  - Best used for large surface areas
  - Expedient tool to measure extent of burn
- Rule of palms (a burn equivalent to the size of the patient's hand is equal to 1% BSA)
  - Best used for burns <10% BSA

Treatment

- Stop the burning process
- Airway, breathing, circulations (ABCs)
- Estimate % BSA burned
- Cool burn
- Prevent hypothermia and infection
- Pain control

Airway and Breathing

- High concentration O_2
- Acute pulmonary insufficiency can occur
- Pulmonary edema 2–3 days
- Bronchopneumonia 5–7 days
- Consider intubation—Be prepared for impending airway obstruction

Circulation

- Fluid replacement critical to survival
- Tissue destruction results in increased capillary permeability
- Profound fluid loss from the intravascular space
- Large amounts of fluid lost from loss of skin integrity due to evaporation

Parkland Formula

- 4 mL × wt kg × %BSA burned = 24-hour infusion
- 1st half over first 8 hours
- Calculated from time of injury
- 2nd/3rd degree burns only
- 4 mL × Pt wt in kg × % BSA = Amount of fluid
- Pt should receive $^1/_2$ of this amount in first 8 hours
- Remainder in 16 hours
- Consider 1 hour dose
- 0.5 mL × Pt wt in kg × % BSA = Amount of fluid

Fluid Resuscitation

- Restore effective plasma volume
- Maintain vital organ function
- Hypovolemic/renal failure—Complications
- Pulmonary edema
- Assess adequacy by urine output

Cool Burn

- Within 30 minutes
- Inhibits lactate production and acidosis
- Promotes catecholamine function and cardiovascular homeostasis
- Inhibits burn wound histamine release
- Blocks histamine mediated vascular permeability
- Minimizes edema formation
- Suppresses thromboxane a potent vasoconstrictor
- Mediator of vascular occlusion
- Progressive dermal ischemia

Hypothermia and Infection

- Cover with dry sterile sheet
- Keep warm

Pain Control

- Morphine sulfate
  - Decreases amount of protein binding
  - Rapidly eliminated
  - Small, frequent doses
  - May use up to 50 mg/hr
- Fentanyl
- Versed

Special Considerations

- Circumferential burns
  - May require fasciotomy
- Pediatrics are more susceptible to circumferential burns
- <6 months old have no shivering mechanism
- Norepinephrine converts brown fat

Burn Center

- 2nd/3rd degree burns >10% <10 years old or older than >50
- 2nd/3rd degree burns 20% TBSA
- 2nd/3rd degree burns to critical areas
- 3rd degree >5% TBSA
- Significant electrical/chemical burns
- Inhalation injury
- Circumferential burns
- Preexisting conditions—Medical or concomitant trauma

Assessment of Thermal Burns

- Scene size-up
- Is Fire Department present
- Never enter without wearing proper protective clothing and self contained breathing apparatus (SCBA)
- Initial assessment

- ABC's MUST be intact
- Consider endotracheal tube (ET) or rapid sequence intubation (RSI)
- Rapid evacuation of patient if scene is unstable
- Focused and rapid trauma assessment
- Accurately approximate extent of burn injury
- Rule of nines or rule of palms
- Depth of burn
- Area of body affected
- Any burn to the face, hands, feet, joints, or genitalia is considered a serious burn
- "Ringing" burns
- Age of patient affected

General Signs and Symptoms

- Pain
- Changes in skin condition at affected site
- Adventitious lung sounds
- Blisters
- Sloughing of skin
- Hoarseness
- Dysphasia

Management of Thermal Burns

- Local and minor burns
  - Local cooling
  - Partial thickness: <15% of BSA
  - Full thickness: <2% BSA
  - Remove clothing
  - Cool or cold water immersion
  - Consider analgesics
- Moderate to severe burns
  - Dry sterile dressings
  - Burns over IV sites
  - Place IV in partial thickness burn site.
  - Caution for fluid overload
  - Frequent auscultation of breath sounds
  - Consider analgesic for pain
  - Morphine
  - Nubain
  - Prevent infection
  - Partial thickness: >15% BSA
  - Full thickness: >5% BSA
  - Maintain warmth
  - Prevent hypothermia
  - Consider aggressive fluid therapy

Inhalation Injury

- Provide high-flow O_2 by non-rebreathing (NRB)
- Consider intubation
- Consider hyperbaric O_2 therapy
- Consider treatment for cyanide exposure
  - Sodium nitrite, amyl nitrite, sodium thiosulfate
  - Forms methemoglobin binds to cyanide
  - Nontoxic substance secreted in urine
  - Inhale 1 ampule of amyl nitrite
  - 300 mg sodium nitrite over 2–4 minutes
  - 12.5 gm of sodium thiosulfate

Lightning Injuries

- One of the top three causes of environmental death (flood, temperature extremes)
- Not alternating current (AC) or direct current (DC) but a unidirectional, massive, current impulse with several return strokes back to the cloud
- Tremendously large current impulsively flows for an incredibly short time
- Lightning bolt can raise temperature in the air by 50,000°F and contain a hundred million volts.

What Is the Difference Between Lightning and Electricity?

- Duration of exposure to current
- Internal burns and renal failure usually inconsequential
- Cardiac arrest
- Respiratory arrest
- Vascular spasm
- Neurological damage

Immediate

- Ventricular asystole
- Often spontaneously resume
- Prolonged respiratory arrest
- Results in secondary cardiac arrest
- Ischemia due to vascular spasms
- Myocardial infarction (MI), spinal artery syndromes

Long Term

- Survivors 10–20× > fatalities
- Neuropsychological and neurocognitive changes
- Chronic pain syndromes
- Chest pain
- Sympathetic nerve system dysfunction
- Sleep disorders, severe headaches (HA), cardiac effects

Demographics

- Sunday, Saturday, Wednesday
- Noon–6 pm, 6–12 pm
- May be in or outdoors
- Males, <16 years or 26–35 years

Blunt Injuries

- Muscular contractions
- Instantaneous expansion and contraction of surrounding air

Cardiac Arrest

- Only known direct cause of death
- "Cosmic defibrillation"
- Momentary asystole
- Spontaneous recovery
- Prolonged respiratory arrest
- Hypoxia
  - Secondary cardiac arrest

Neurologic

- May present only mildly disorientated
- May still sustain disabling neurocognitive deficits similar to blunt head injury
- May not be immediately apparent
- Pain
- Numbness
- Abnormal sensations
- Chronic pain syndromes may develop due to sympathetic, not significant, injury

Sympathetic Nervous System Injury

- May cause vascular spasm
- Temporary paralysis
- Mottling
- Transient hypertension
- Late problems with + tilt tests
- Vertigo/dizziness
- Pain syndromes
- Brain injury may occur
- Deep burns rare
- Superficial burns more common
- Punctate, fernlike, linear
- Secondary to metal in pockets/clothing
- Ear drum rupture common
- Direct current entry
- Concussive/explosive force
- Basilar skull fracture

Treatment

- Resuscitation
- Spinal immobilization
- NSAIDS
- Prevent long-term neurological damage
- Treat chronic pain syndromes
- Ibuprofen, ketoprofen, naproxen

Prevention

- Awareness of weather forecast
- Evacuation
- May travel >10 miles from thunderstorm, clouds/rain may not be present
- Shelter—School buses, metal top vehicles
- Avoid trees, small shelters, bleachers, fences, towers, any current-transmitting structures, pools/water, high areas
- Avoid using telephones, electronic equipment, any contact with conductive surfaces inside (plumbing, doing dishes), emergency medical service (EMS)/fire dispatch radio
- Arc electrical burn through shoe around rubber sole
- High-voltage (7600 V) alternating current

Electrical Injury

- Age-related electrical injury peaks in age groups from infancy to 4 years old.
- 20–25-year-old males—Primarily work related

Factors Affecting Severity of a Burn

- Voltage and amperage
- Resistance of body tissue
- Type and path of current
- Duration and intensity of contact

Electrical Burn Terminology

- Voltage—Difference of electrical potential between two points
- Different concentrations of electrons
- Amperes—Strength of electrical current
- Resistance (Ohms)—Opposition to electrical flow

  Ohm's Law—Defines the relationships between (P) power, (E) voltage, (I) current, and (R) resistance. One ohm is the resistance value through which one volt will maintain a current of one ampere.

  Joule's Law—States when electricity flows through a substance, the rate of evolution of heat in watts equals the resistance of the substance in ohms times the square of the current in amperes. With regard to electrical burns, the greater the current, the greater the flow through the body.

Electrical Burns

- Greatest heat occurs at the points of resistance, entrance, and exit wounds
- Dry skin = Greater resistance
- Wet skin = Less resistance

Electrical Current Flow

- Tissue of less resistance
  - Blood vessels
  - Nerve
- Tissue of greater resistance
  - Muscle
  - Bone

- Results in serious vascular and nervous injury
- Consider immobilization of muscles
- Look for flash burns

Voltage

- High voltage is classified as >1000 volts.
- Low voltage is classified as <1000 volts.
- Most household current is 110–220 volts.
- Produces low-voltage injury consistent with thermal injury.
- High voltage produces thermal injury at entry and exit as well as deep tissue injury along path.
- Amperage is better indicator of injury.

Resistance

- Current enters the body and follows the path of least resistance. Exits at ground. When current meets resistance, heat is generated and a burn injury occurs. (The greater the resistance the greater the injury.)

Complications

- Cardiac arrhythmias
- Respiratory muscle paralysis
- Thrombosis
- Renal failure
- Fractures
- DC—Direct current discrete exit
- AC—Alternating current more explosive

Current Passage Mortality

- Hand to hand—60%
- Hand to foot—20%
- Foot to foot—5%

Special Considerations

- Respiratory
- Cardiac
- Associated trauma
- Renal failure
  - Requires > fluid resuscitation

Assessment and Management of Electrical and Lightning Injuries

Electrical Injuries

- Safety of the responders is paramount
- Turn off power
- Energized lines act as whips
- Establish a safety zone

Lightning Strikes

- High voltage, high current, high energy
- Lasts fraction of a second
- No danger of electrical shock to EMS

Management of Electrical Injuries

- Assess patient for entrance and exit wounds
- Remove clothing, jewelry, and leather items
- Treat any visible injuries
- Look for thermal burns
- Electrocardiogram (ECG) monitoring (look for specific dysrhythmias such as bradycardia, tachycardia, ventricular fibrillation [VF] or asystole)
- Follow advanced cardiac life support (ACLS) algorithms
- Treat cardiac and respiratory arrest
- Aggressive airway, ventilation, and circulatory management
- Consider fluid bolus for serious burns (Parkland formula)
- Consider sodium bicarbonate: 1 mEq/kg
- Consider Mannitol: 10 g

Chemical Burns

- Strong acids cause coagulation necrosis
- Strong bases cause liquefaction necrosis (will continue burning until neutralized or diluted)
- Chemicals destroy tissue
- Acids:
  - Form a thick, insoluble mass where they contact tissue
  - Coagulation necrosis
  - Limits burn damage
- Alkalis:
  - Destroy cell membrane through liquefaction necrosis
  - Deeper tissue penetration and deeper burns
  - Oral caustic chemical burns

Degree of Damage/Toxicity of a Chemical Burn

- Chemical nature
- Amount
- Concentration
- Mechanism
- Duration

Strong Acids and Alkalis

- Strong acids and alkalis may cause burns to the mouth, pharynx, esophagus, and sometimes the upper respiratory and gastrointestinal (GI) tracts.
- Ingestions of caustic and corrosive substances generally produce immediate damage to the mucous membrane and the intestinal tract.
- Acids generally complete their damage within 1–2 minutes after exposure.
- Alkalis, particularly solid alkalis, may continue to cause liquefaction of tissue and damage for minutes to hours.

Signs and Symptoms

- Facial burns
- Pain in the lips, tongue, throat, or gums
- Drooling, trouble swallowing, hoarseness, stridor, shortness of breath
- Shock secondary to bleeding or vomiting

Management

- Establish an airway, consider intubation, or if necessary, cricothyrotomy
- Contact medical control or poison control
- Gastric lavage or charcoal administration is often contraindicated
- IV with normal saline or lactated ringers (LR)
- Rapid transport

Hydrocarbons

- A group of saturated and unsaturated compounds derived primarily from crude oil, coal, or plant substances
- Found in many household products and in petroleum distillates
- Viscosity is the most important physical characteristic in potential toxicity
- The lower the viscosity, the higher the risk of aspiration and associated complications
- Clinical features of hydrocarbon ingestion vary widely, depending on the type of agent involved
- May be immediate or delayed in onset

Signs and Symptoms

- Burns due to local contact
- Wheezing, dyspnea, hypoxia, and pneumonitis due to aspiration or inhalation
- Headache, dizziness, slurred speech, ataxia (irregular or difficult-to-control movements), and dulled reflexes
- Foot and wrist drop with numbness and tingling
- Cardiac dysrhythmias

Management

- Most are not life threatening
- Occasionally gastric lavage may be of benefit
- In seriously symptomatic patients, protect the airway and establish an IV if normal saline or LR
- Contact medical control or poison control
- Transport

Assessment and Management of Chemical Burns

- Chemical burns
  - Scene size-up
  - Hazardous materials team responsible for mitigation and decontamination of patients
  - Establish hot, warm, and cold zones
  - Prevent personnel exposure
- Specific chemicals
  - Phenol

  - Dry lime
  - Sodium
  - Riot control agents
  - Industrial cleaner

Phenol

- Alcohol dissolves phenol
- Irrigate with copious amounts of water

Dry Lime

- Strong corrosive that reacts with water.
- Brush off dry substance first, then irrigate with copious amounts of water. This prevents a reaction with the patient tissue.

Sodium

- Unstable metal
  - Reacts vigorously with water
  - Releases extreme heat
- Hydrogen gas
  - Ignition
- Decontaminate: Brush off dry chemical
  - Cover the wound with oil substance

Riot Control Agents

- Agents: Orthochlorobenzalmalonitrile (CS), alphachloroacetaphenone (CN) (Mace), oleoresin capsicum (OC, pepper spray)
- Irritation of the eyes, mucous membranes, and respiratory tract
- No permanent damage

General Signs and Symptoms

- Coughing, gagging, and vomiting
- Eye pain, tearing, temporary blindness

Management

- Irrigate eyes with normal saline

Radiation

- Decontamination is paramount
- Treated like any other burn

Radiation Injury

Transmission of energy

- Nuclear energy
- Ultraviolet light
- Visible light
- Heat
- Sound
- X-rays

- Radioactive substance
  - Emits ionizing radiation
  - Radionuclide or radioisotope

Basic Physics

- Protons—Positive charged particles
- Neutrons—Equal in mass to protons, and have no electrical charge
- Electrons—Minute electrically charged particles; when emitted from radioactive substances are termed beta particles

Radioactive Substances

Alpha Particles

- Slow moving
- Low-energy
- Stopped by clothing and paper
- Penetrate a few cell layers on skin
- Minor external hazard
- HARMFUL if ingested

Beta particles are high-energy, high-speed electrons or positrons emitted by certain types of radioactive nuclei.

Gamma Rays

- Highly energized
- Penetrate deeper than alpha or beta
- EXTREMELY DANGEROUS
- Penetrate thick shielding
- Pass entirely through clothing body
- Extensive cell damage
- Indirect damage
  - Cause internal tissue to emit alpha and beta particles
- LEAD SHIELDING is required

Effects on the body

- Geiger counter is needed to detect radiation
- R/hr: Milliroentgens per hour
- 1000 mR = 1 rad
- RAD—Radiation absorbed dose of local tissue
- REM
  - Roentgen equivalent in man
  - Injury to irradiated part of organism
  - RAD = REM for our purposes

Dose-Effect Total Body Exposure

RAD	EFFECT
• 5–25	asymptomatic, normal blood studies
• 50–75	asymptomatic, minor depression in white blood cell (WBC)

• 75–125	anorexia, nausea, vomiting, fatigue within 2 days
• 125–200	nausea, vomiting, diarrhea, anxiety, tachycardia
• 200–600	nausea, vomiting, diarrhea within several hours 50% fatal within 6 weeks, untreated
• 600–1000	severe nausea, vomiting, diarrhea within several hours, fatal 100% within 2 weeks untreated
1000+	**burning sensation within minutes, nausea and vomiting, confusion, ataxia, and prostration within 1 hour**

FATAL 100% within short time without prompt treatment!

Radiation Injury: Safety

- Clean accident
- Exposed to radiation
- Not contaminated by products
- Properly decontaminated
- Little danger to personnel
- Dirty accident
- Associated with fire at scene of radiation accident
- Trained decontamination personnel

Management

- Park upwind
- Notify radiation response or Haz-mat response team
- Look for radioactive placards
- Measure radioactivity
- Decontaminate patients before care
- Routine medical care (ABCs, etc.)

Assessment and Management of Radiation Burns

- Notify hazardous materials team
- Establish safety zones
- Hot, warm, and cold
- Personnel positioned upwind and uphill
- Use older rescuers for recovery
- Decontaminate ALL rescuers, equipment, and patients

? CHAPTER QUESTIONS

1. The most common complications of burn patients is:
   a. dehydration
   b. infection
   c. hypothermia
   d. all of the above

2. The Parkland formula used for burn resuscitation is 4 mL × wt kg × %BSA burned = 24 hr infusion. How much should the patient receive in the first 8 hours?
   a. $^1/_2$
   b. $^3/_4$
   c. all of the fluid
   d. $^1/_4$

Suggested Readings

Advanced Burn Life Support Provider Manual, Chicago, IL, 2001. American Burn Association.

American Heart Association. *Circulation.* 2005; 112 (suppl I): IV-154–155. Published online before print November 28, 2005, doi:10.1161/CIRCULATIONAHA.105.166571.

US Department of Transportation, National Highway Traffic Safety Administration. *EMT-Paramedic: National Standard Curriculum.* Washington, DC: US Department of Transportation, National Highway Traffic Safety Administration; 1998.

Chapter 17
Head and Facial Trauma

A 30-year-old male is found lying in the road after being ejected from a high-speed motor-vehicle crash. The patient does not open his eyes, verbal responses are incomprehensible, and the patient's arms appear to be flexing toward the body.

Using the Glasgow Coma Scale (Table 17-1), which of the scores best fits this patient?

HEAD AND BRAIN TRAUMA

- Approximately 4 million head injuries occur in the United States per year
- Approximately 450,000 patients require hospitalization
- Most are minor injuries
- Major head injuries are the most common cause of traumatic deaths in trauma centers (>50%)

RISK GROUPS

- Highest risk group: Males 15–24 years of age
- Very young children: 6 months to 2 years of age
- Young school-age children
- Elderly

SKULL ANATOMY REVIEW

- Cranium
  - Double layer of solid bone which surrounds a spongy middle layer
  - Frontal, occipital, temporal, parietal, mastoid
- Middle meningeal artery
  - Lies under temporal bone
  - Common source of epidural hematoma
- Foramen magnum
- Facial bones

BRAIN ANATOMY REVIEW

- The brain occupies 80% of intracranial space
- Divisions of the brain:
  - Cerebrum
  - Cerebellum
  - Brain stem

Cerebrum

- Cortex, responsible for:
  - Voluntary skeletal movement
  - Level of awareness
- Frontal lobe, responsible for personality
- Parietal lobe, responsible for:
  - Somatic sensory input
  - Memory
  - Emotions
- Temporal lobe, responsible for:
  - Speech center
  - Long term memory
  - Taste
  - Smell
- Occipital lobe, responsible for origin of optic nerve
- Hypothalamus
  - Center for vomiting, regulation of body temp and water
  - Sleep-cycle control
  - Appetite
- Thalamus, responsible for emotions and alerting or arousal mechanisms

Cerebellum

- Coordination of voluntary muscle movement
- Equilibrium and posture

Brain Stem

- Connects hemispheres, cerebellum, and spinal cord
- Responsible for vegetative functions and vital signs

Midbrain

- Relay point for visual and auditory impulses

Pons

- Conduction pathway between brain and other regions of body

Medulla Oblongata

- Cardiac, respiratory, and vasomotor control centers
- Control of vomiting and coughing

CRANIAL NERVE REVIEW

- Cranial nerve I—Olfactory nerve (smell)
- Cranial nerve II—Optic nerve (vision)
- Cranial nerve III—Oculomotor nerve (eye movement)
- Cranial nerve IV—Trochlear nerve (eye movement)
- Cranial nerve V—Trigeminal nerve (facial sensation)

- Cranial nerve VI—Abducens nerve (eye movement)
- Cranial nerve VII—Facial nerve (facial movement)
- Cranial nerve VIII—Auditory nerve (hearing and balance)
- Cranial nerve IX—Glossopharyngeal nerve (organs and taste)
- Cranial nerve X—Vagus nerve (organs and taste)
- Cranial nerve XI—Accessory nerve (shoulder shrug and head turn)
- Cranial nerve XII—Hypoglossal nerve (tongue movement)

Reticular Activating System

- Level of arousal (level of consciousness)
- Primary control along with cerebral cortex

Meninges

- Dura mater—Tough outer layer separates cerebellum from cerebral structures, landmark for lesions
- Arachnoid—Weblike, venous vessels that reabsorb cerebral spinal fluid (CSF)
- Pia mater—Directly attached to brain tissue

Cerebral Spinal Fluid

- CSF is a clear, colorless fluid that circulates through the outer layer of the brain and spinal cord and cushions and protects these structures.

Ventricles

- Center of brain, which secretes CSF by filtering blood
- Forms blood-brain barrier

BRAIN METABOLISM AND PERFUSION

- The brain has a high metabolic rate, consumes 20% of body's oxygen, and is the largest user of glucose.
- Requires thiamine.
- Cannot store nutrients.

Blood Supply

- Vertebral arteries
- Supply posterior brain (cerebellum and brain stem)
- Carotid arteries
- Most of cerebrum

Perfusion

- Cerebral blood flow (CBF)
  - Dependent upon cerebral perfusion pressure (CPP)
  - Flow requires pressure gradient
- CPP
  - Pressure moving the blood through the cranium
  - Auto regulation allows blood pressure (BP) change to maintain CPP
  - CPP = mean arterial pressure (MAP) – intracranial pressure (ICP)

- MAP
  - Largely dependent on cerebral vascular resistance (CVR) since diastolic is main component
  - Blood volume and myocardial contractility
  - MAP = diastolic + $^{1}/_{3}$ pulse pressure
  - Usually require MAP of at least 60 mmHg to perfuse brain
- ICP
  - Edema, hemorrhage
  - ICP usually 10–15 mmHg

MECHANISMS OF INJURY

- Motor vehicle crashes (MVC) are the most common cause of head trauma
  - MVC's are the most common cause of subdural hematoma
- Sports injuries
- Falls
  - Common in elderly and in presence of alcohol
  - Associated with subdural hematoma
- Penetrating trauma
  - Missiles more common than sharp projectiles

CATEGORIES OF INJURY

- Coup injury—Directly posterior to point of impact
  - More common when front of head struck
- Contra coup injury—Directly opposite the point of impact
  - More common when back of head struck
- Diffuse axonal injury (DAI)—Shearing, tearing, or stretching of nerve fibers
  - More common with vehicle occupant and pedestrian
- Focal injury—Limited and identifiable site of injury

Head Injury

- Definition—Traumatic insult to the head that may result in injury to soft tissue, bony structures, and/or the brain
- Blunt trauma
  - More common
  - Dura intact
  - Fractures, focal brain injury, DAI
- Penetrating trauma
  - Less common (gunshot wound [GSW] most common)
  - Dura and cranial contents penetrated
- Fractures, focal brain injury

Brain Injury

- A traumatic insult to the brain capable of producing physical, intellectual, emotional, social, and vocational changes
- Three broad categories:
  - Focal injury
    - — Cerebral contusion

- Intracranial hemorrhage
  - — Epidural hemorrhage
  - — Subarachnoid hemorrhage
- DAI
  - — Concussion (mild and classic form)

Causes of Brain Injury

- Direct (primary) causes
  - Impact
  - Mechanical disruption of cells
  - Vascular permeability or disruption
- Indirect (secondary or tertiary) causes
  - Secondary
    - — Edema, hemorrhage, infection, inadequate perfusion, tissue hypoxia, pressure
  - Tertiary
    - — Apnea, hypotension, pulmonary resistance, ECG changes

Pathophysiology of a Brain Injury

- As ICP ↑ and approaches MAP, CBF ↓
- Results in ↓ CPP
- Compensatory mechanisms attempt to ↑ MAP
- As CPP ↓, cerebral vasodilatation occurs to ↑ blood volume
- This leads to further ↑ ICP, ↓ CPP, and so on
- Hypercarbia causes cerebral vasodilatation
- Results in ↑ blood volume ⇨ ↑ ICP ⇨ CPP
- Compensatory mechanisms attempt to ↑ MAP
- As CPP ↓, cerebral vasodilatation occurs to ↑ blood volume
- And the cycle continues
- Hypotension results in ↓ CPP ⇨ cerebral vasodilatation
- Results in ↑ blood volume ⇨ ↑ ICP ⇨ CPP
- And the cycle continues
- Pressure exerted downward on brain
- Cerebral cortex or reticular activating system (RAS)
  - Altered level of consciousness
  - Hypothalamus
  - Vomiting
- Brain stem
  - ↑ BP and bradycardia 2° vagal stimulation
  - Irregular respirations or tachypnea
  - Unequal/unreactive pupils 2° oculomotor nerve paralysis
  - Posturing
  - Seizures dependent on location of injury
  - Herniation
  - Levels of increasing ICP
- Cerebral cortex and upper brain stem
  - BP rising and pulse rate slowing
  - Pupils reactive

  - Cheyne-Stokes respirations
  - Initially try to localize and remove painful stimuli
- Middle brain stem
  - Wide pulse pressure and bradycardia
  - Pupils nonreactive or sluggish
  - Central neurogenic hyperventilation
  - Extension
  - Levels of increasing ICP
- Lower brain stem/medulla
  - Pupil blown (side of injury)
  - Ataxic or absent respirations
  - Flaccid
  - Irregular or changing pulse rate
  - Decreased BP
  - Usually not survivable
- Herniation
  - Transtentorial herniation
  - Downward displacement of the brain
  - Uncal herniation
  - Downward displacement through the tentorial notch by a supratentorial mass exerting pressure on underlying structures including the brain stem

Head Injuries

- Scalp laceration/avulsion (most common injury)
  - Vascularity = diffuse bleeding
  - Generally does not cause hypovolemia in adults
  - Can produce hypovolemia in children
- Linear fracture
  - Usually NOT identified in field
  - 80% of all skull fractures
  - Suspect based on mechanism of injury
- Overlying soft tissue trauma
  - Usually NOT emergency
  - Temporal region = epidural hematoma
- Depressed skull fracture
  - Segment pushed inward
  - Pressure on brain causes brain injury
  - Neurological signs and symptoms evident
- Basilar skull fracture
  - Difficult to detect on x-ray
  - Signs and symptoms depend on amount of damage
  - Diagnosis made clinically by finding:
    - CSF Otorrhea
    - CSF Rhinorrhea
    - Periorbital ecchymosis
    - Battle's sign

- CSF
  - Blood clotting delayed
  - Positive Halo sign
  - Does not crust on drying
  - Positive to Dextrostick
- Basilar skull fracture
  - Do NOT pack ears
  - Let drain
  - Do NOT suction fluid
  - Do NOT instrument nose
- Open skull fracture
  - Cranial contents exposed
  - Manage like evisceration
  - Protect exposed tissue with moist, clean dressing (if possible)
  - Neurologic signs and symptoms evident

Specific Brain Injuries

Intracranial hematoma can be classified in three categories:

- Epidural
- Subdural
- Intracerebral

Epidural Hematoma

- Blood between skull and dura
- Usually occurs from an arterial tear
- Causes increase in intracranial pressure
- Unconsciousness followed by lucid interval
- Rapid deterioration (decreased level of consciousness [LOC], headache, nausea, vomiting, hemiparesis, hemiplegia)
- Unequal pupils (dilated on side of clot)
- Increased BP, decreased pulse (Cushing's reflex)

Subdural Hematoma

- Blood between the dura mater and arachnoid
- More common
- Usually caused by a venous bleed
- Bridging veins between cortex and dura
- Causes increased intracranial pressure
- Slower in onset
- Headache, decreased LOC, unequal pupils
- Increased BP, decreased pulse
- Hemiparesis, hemiplegia

Intracerebral Hematoma

- Usually due to laceration of brain
- Bleeding into cerebral substance
- Associated with other injuries

Diffuse axonal injury (DAI)—Is one of the most common and devastating types of brain injury.

- Neurological deficits depend on region involved and size
- Repetitive w/frontal lobe
- Increased ICP

Penetrating Wounds

- GSW
- Stab
- Depressed fracture
- Severe blunt trauma

Sudden Acceleration/Deceleration

- Concussion
- Transient loss of consciousness
- Retrograde amnesia, confusion
- Resolves spontaneously without deficit
- Usually due to blunt head trauma

Head Trauma

- Concussion
  - Postconcussion syndrome
    - — Headaches
    - — Depression
    - — Personality changes

Head Trauma Assessment

- The brain is enclosed in a box
- Early detection/control of increased ICP
- CPP = MAP – ICP
- LOC = best indicator
- Altered LOC = intracranial trauma
- Trauma patient unable to follow commands = 25% chance of intracranial injury needing surgery
- AVPU Scale
  - A = Alert
  - V = Responds to verbal stimuli
  - P = Responds to painful stimuli
  - U = Unresponsive
- Glasgow Scale (based on three observations) (Table 17-1)
  - Eye opening
  - Motor response
  - Verbal response
- Evaluating the eyes of a brain injury patient
  - The eyes are the window to central nervous system (CNS)
  - Evaluate pupil size, equality, and response to light
  - Unequal pupils + decreased LOC = compression of oculomotor nerve from a probable mass lesion

TABLE 17-1: Glasgow Coma Scale

Eye Opening	4 = Spontaneous 3 = To voice 2 = To pain 1 = Absent
Verbal	5 = Oriented 4 = Confused 3 = Inappropriate words 2 = Moaning, incomprehensible 1 = No response
Motor	6 = Obeys commands 5 = Localizes pain 4 = Withdraws from pain 3 = Decorticate (flexion) 2 = Decerebrate (extension) 1 = Flaccid

  - Unequal pupils + alert patient = direct blow to eye, or oculomotor nerve injury, or normal inequality

Respiratory Patterns and Locations of Insult

- Cheyne-Stokes
  - Diffuse injury to cerebral hemispheres
- Central neurological hyperventilation
  - Injury to midbrain
- Apneustic
  - Injury to pons
- Biot (cluster)
  - Injury to upper medulla
- Ataxic
  - Injury to lower medulla

Motor Response

- Is patient able to move all extremities?
- How does the patient move?
  - Decorticate posturing
  - Decerebrate posturing
- Hemiparesis or hemiplegia
- Paraplegia or quadriplegia
- Lateralized/focal signs = lateralized or focal deficits
- Altered motor function may be due to fracture/dislocation

Vital Signs

- Cushing's Triad
  - Suggests increased intracranial pressure
  - Increased BP
  - Decreased pulse

- Irregular respiratory pattern
- Isolated head injury will NOT cause hypotension in adult
- Look for other life-threatening injuries of the:
  - Chest
  - Abdomen
  - Pelvis
  - Multiple long bone fractures

Summary

- Most important sign = LOC
- Direction of changes more important than single observations
- Importance lies in continued reassessment compared with initial exam
- Altered LOC in trauma = intracranial injury

HEAD TRAUMA MANAGEMENT

Airway

- Maintain a patent airway
- Assume C-spine trauma
- Jaw thrust with C-spine control
- Clear airway—Suction as needed
- Maintain in-line stabilization and a clear airway
- Intubation if no gag reflex, or rapid sequence intubation (RSI)
- Avoid nasal intubation

Breathing

- Oxygenate—100% oxygen
- Ventilate
- No ROUTINE hyperventilation
- Hyperventilate at 20–24 breaths per minute IF:
  - Glasgow less than 8
  - Rapid neurologic deterioration
  - Evidence of herniation
- Hyperventilation—Benefits
  - Decreased $PaCO_2$
  - Vasoconstriction
  - Decreased ICP
- Hyperventilation—Risks
  - Decreased CBF
  - Decreased oxygen delivery to tissues
  - Increased edema

Circulation

- Maintain adequate BP and perfusion
- IV of lactated ringers/normal saline (LR/NS) to keep open (TKO) if BP normal or elevated

- If BP decreased
  - LR/NS bolus titrated to BP ~ 90 mmHg
  - Consider pneumatic antishock garment/medical antishock trouser (PASG/MAST) if BP below 80 (per local protocol)
  - Monitor electrocardiogram (ECG)—Do NOT treat bradycardia
  - Spinal motion restriction
- If BP normal or elevated, spine board head elevated 30°
  - Monitor for hyperthermia
  - Vasoconstriction
  - Heat retention
  - Increased cerebral oxygen demand

DRUG THERAPY CONSIDERATIONS

- Only after: Management of ABCs
- Controlled hyperventilation
- Dexamethasone (Decadron)
  - Steroid that decreases cerebral edema
  - Effects are delayed
- Mannitol (Osmitrol)
  - Osmotic diuretic that decreases cerebral edema
  - May cause hypovolemia
  - May worsen intracranial hemorrhage
  - Often reserved for herniation
- Furosemide (Lasix)
  - Loop diuretic that decreases cerebral edema
  - May cause hypovolemia
  - Often reserved for herniation
- Diazepam (Valium)
  - Anticonvulsant
  - Give if patient experiences seizures
  - May mask changes in LOC
  - May depress respirations
  - May worsen hypotension
- Glucose
  - Assess blood glucose
  - Administer only if hypoglycemic
  - Consider thiamine in malnourished

TRANSPORT CONSIDERATIONS

- Transport to a trauma center if:
  - GCS ≤12
  - Evidence of herniation
  - Unconscious
  - Multisystem trauma with head trauma

HELMET REMOVAL

- Immediate removal if the helmet interferes with priorities, such as:
  - Access to airway or airway management
  - Ventilation
  - Cervical spine motion restriction
- May only need to remove face piece to access airway
- Requires adequate assistance and proper training in the procedure
- Padding if shoulder pads left on

MAXILLOFACIAL, OPHTHALMIC AND DENTAL TRAUMA

Morbidity and Mortality

- Mortality
  - Primarily associated with brain and spine injury
  - Severe facial fractures may interfere with airway and breathing
- Morbidity
  - Disability concerns
  - Cosmetic concerns

Maxillofacial Trauma

- Most common causes:
  - MVC, home accidents, athletic injuries, animal bites, violence, industrial accidents
- Soft tissue
  - Lacerations, abrasions, avulsions
  - Vascular area supplied by internal and external carotids
- Management
  - Seldom life threatening unless the injury is affecting the airway
  - Consider spinal precautions
  - Have suction available and in control of conscious patients
  - Control bleeding

MAXILLOFACIAL ANATOMY AND PHYSIOLOGY REVIEW

- Arteries
  - Temporal artery
  - Mandibular artery
  - Maxillary artery
- Nerves
  - Trigeminal (cranial nerve V)
  - Facial (cranial nerve VII)
- Bones
  - Nasal
  - Zygoma/zygomatic arch
  - Maxilla
  - Mandible

FACIAL FRACTURES

Fracture to the mandible, maxilla, nasal bones, zygoma, and rarely the frontal bone.

Signs and Symptoms

Pain, swelling, deep lacerations, limited ocular movement, facial asymmetry, crepitus, deviated nasal septum, bleeding, depression on palpation, malocclusion, blurred vision, diplopia, broken or missing teeth.

Specific Facial Fractures

- Mandible fracture—Numbness, inability to open or close the mouth, excessive salivation, malocclusion
- Anterior dislocation—Commonly caused by extensive dental work or yawning
  - Condylar heads move forward and muscles spasm

LeFort Fractures

- Specially named facial fractures
- Usually requires significant forces especially for LeFort II and III
- LeFort I—Maxillary fracture with "free-floating" maxilla
- LeFort II—Maxilla, zygoma, floor of orbit and nose
- LeFort III—Lower $^{2}/_{3}$ of the face

Signs and Symptoms

- Often associated with orbital fractures
  - Risk of serious airway compromise (bleeding and edema)
  - Contraindication to nasogastric (NG) tube or nasotracheal intubation
- Present with:
  - Edema, epistaxis, numb upper teeth
  - Unstable maxilla, CSF rhinorrhea
  - Unusual facial appearance
  - "Donkey face" (lengthening)
  - "Pumpkin face" (edema)
  - Nasal flattening

Management

- Spinal motion restriction
- Airway is the most difficult and most critical priority
- Consider early intubation
- Surgical airway may be the only alternative but NEVER the first consideration
- Suction and control bleeding
- Critical trauma patient—transport accordingly
- NG tube or endotracheal tube placement may be HAZARDOUS!!!

Ear Trauma

- External injuries
  - Lacerations, avulsions, amputations, frostbite.
  - Control bleeding with direct pressure.

- Internal injuries
  - Spontaneous rupture of eardrum will usually heal spontaneously.
  - Penetrating objects should be stabilized, not removed!
  - Removal may cause deafness or facial paralysis.
  - Hearing loss may be result of auditory nerve damage in basilar skull fracture.

Anatomy and Physiology Review

- Ear
  - Outer ear (Pinna)
  - Cartilage
  - Little blood supply
- External ear canal
  - Mucous membrane that secretes wax for protection
- Middle ear
  - Separated from external canal by eardrum
  - Delicate structure needed for hearing

Ear Injuries

- Separation of ear cartilage
  - Treat as an avulsion
  - Dress and bandage
  - Consider disability and cosmetic concerns
- Bleeding from ear canal
  - Cover with loose dressing only

Barotitis

- Changes in pressure cause pressure buildup and/or rupture of tympanic membrane.
- Boyle's Law—At constant temperature, the volume of gas is inversely proportionate to the pressure.
- Signs and symptoms—Pain, blocked feeling in ears, severe pain.
- Equalize pressure by yawning, chewing, moving mandible, swallowing (open Eustachian tubes allowing gas to release).

Eye Anatomy

- Bony orbit
- Eyelid
- Lacrimal apparatus
- Sclera
- Cornea
- Conjunctiva
- Iris
- Pupil
- Lens
- Retina
- Optic nerve

Eye Injuries

- Penetrating
- Abrasions
- Foreign bodies (deep, superficial, impaled)
- Lacerations (deep or superficial, eyelid)
- Burns
  - Flash burn
  - Acid/alkali
- Blunt
  - Swelling
  - Conjunctival hemorrhage
  - Hyphema
  - Ruptured globe
  - Blow-out fracture of orbit
  - Retinal detachment

Blow-Out Orbital Fracture

Usually result of a direct blow to the eye.

Signs and symptoms—flatness, numbness

- Epistaxis, altered vision
- Periorbital swelling
- Diplopia
- Enophthalmos
- Impaired ocular movement

Foreign Bodies

Signs and symptoms

Sensation of something in eye, excessive tearing, burning

- Inspect inner surface of upper lid as well as sclera
- Flush with copious normal saline away from opposite eye

Corneal Abrasion

Caused by foreign body objects, eye rubbing, contact lenses.

Signs and symptoms

Pain, feeling of something in eye, photophobia, tearing, decreased visual acuity

- Irrigate, patch both eyes
- Usually heals in 24–48 hours if not infected or toxic from antibiotics

Other Globe Injuries

Contusion, laceration, hyphema, globe or scleral rupture.

Signs and symptoms

Loss of visual acuity, blood in anterior chamber, dilation or constriction of pupil, pain, soft eye, pupil irregularity.

Management

- Consider C-spine precautions due to forces required for injury
- No pressure to globe for dressing, cover both eyes
- Avoid activities that increase intraocular pressure

Mouth Injuries

- Primary concern is airway compromise secondary to bleeding, foreign body airway obstruction (FBAO) secondary to broken or avulsed teeth, or an impaled object
- Usually results from:
  - MVCs
  - Blunt injury to the mouth or chin
  - Penetrating injury due to GSW, lacerations, or punctures

Anatomy and Physiology Review

- Muscles
  - Tongue
  - Masseter muscles
- Nerves
  - Hypoglossal
  - Glossopharyngeal
  - Trigeminal
  - Facial
- Bones
  - Mandible
  - Maxilla
  - Hyoid
  - Palate
- Teeth

Management

- ABCs
- Suction as needed
- Stabilize impaled object
- Collect tissue: tongue or teeth

Dental Trauma

- 32 teeth in normal adult
- Associated with facial fractures
- May aspirate broken tooth
- Avulsed teeth can be replaced, so find them!
- Early hospital notification to find dentist
- <15 minutes, may be asked to replace the tooth in socket
- Do not rinse or scrub (removes periodontal membrane and ligament)
- Preserve in fresh whole milk
- Saline OK for less than 1 hour

Nasal Injuries

- Variety of mechanisms including blunt or penetrating trauma
- Most common injury in adults is epistaxis, and in children foreign bodies

Epistaxis

- Anterior bleeding from septum
- Usually venous
- Posterior bleeding
- Often drains to airway
- May be associated with
- Sphenoid and/or ethmoid fractures
- Basilar skull fracture

Foreign Bodies

- Variety of objects such as food or toys
- Often can be left alone and removed later

Anatomy and Physiology Review

- Nasal bone
  - Between the eyes
- Nasal cartilage
  - Provides shape to nose
- Internal
  - Septum
  - Turbinate
  - Sinuses

Nasal Injury Management

- Epistaxis
  - Direct pressure over septum
  - Upright position, leaning forward or in lateral recumbent position
- If CSF present, do not apply direct pressure allow to drain

Neck Trauma

The neck has three zones of injury:

- 1 = sternal notch to top of clavicles (highest mortality)
- 2 = clavicles or cricoid cartilage to angle of the mandible (contains major vasculature and airway)
- 3 = above angle of mandible (distal carotid, salivary, pharynx)

Transected Trachea

- Larynx separated from trachea or fractured
- Vocal cord swelling
- Altered airway landmarks
- Soft tissue edema

Vessel Lacerated or Torn

- Severe bleeding (large vessels)
- Airway compromise
- Risk of air emboli, hypoxia, or ischemia

Signs and symptoms

- Pale or cyanotic face
- Obvious external injury
- Frothy blood or sputum from wound
- Subcutaneous emphysema
- Voice change
- Feeling of fullness in throat
- Signs of stroke with air emboli

Esophageal Injury

- Especially common in penetrating trauma.
- Signs and symptoms may include subcutaneous emphysema, neck hematoma, and blood in the NG tube or posterior nasopharynx.
- High mortality rate from mediastinal infection secondary to gastric reflux through the perforation.
- Consider Semi-fowler's versus supine position unless contraindicated by MOI.

Neck Trauma Management

- ABCs
- Suction
- Intubate EARLY!!!
- May require cricothyrotomy
- Stop bleeding as best as possible
- Occlude large blood vessel quickly
- Left lateral position with occlusive dressing to wound
- Consider spinal motion restriction
- Stabilize impaled objects
- Transport to a trauma center

Cranial Nerve Hints

May not be helpful in unconscious patients, but if they happen to wake up:

- Cranial nerve I—Loss of smell, taste (basilar skull fracture hallmark)
- Cranial nerve II—Blindness, visual defects
- Cranial nerve III—Ipsilateral, dilated fixed pupil
- Cranial nerve VII—Immediate or delayed facial paralysis (basilar skull or LeFort)
- Cranial nerve VIII—Deafness (basilar skull fracture)

Ears

Note external examination (auricle and mastoid)

- Size
- Shape
- Symmetry

- Color
- Position
- Tenderness
- Odor
- Canal
- Discharge
- Scaling
- Redness
- Lesions
- Foreign bodies
- Cerumen

Eyes

External examination

- Orbital area, eyelids
- Conjunctivae/cornea
- Foreign body
- Ulcers
- Erythema/exudate
- Hyphema
- Pupils/iris

CHAPTER QUESTION

1. Blood between the dura mater and arachnoid is called:
   a. epidural hematoma
   b. subdural hematoma
   c. intracerebral hemorrhage
   d. intracerebral contusion

Suggested Readings

US Department of Transportation, National Highway Traffic Safety Administration. *EMT-Paramedic: National Standard Curriculum.* Washington, DC: US Department of Transportation, National Highway Traffic Safety Administration; 1998.

Gabriel EJ, Ghajar J, et al. US Department of Transportation, National Highway Traffic Safety Administration, Prehospital Management of Traumatic Brain Injury. *Guidelines for Prehospital Management of Traumatic Brain Injury*. Brain Trauma Foundation, New York; 2000.

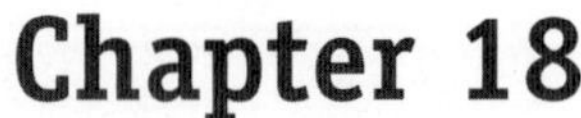

Chapter 18
Spinal Trauma

Your 12-year-old patient struck his head on the bottom of a shallow pool while diving. You suspect a possible spinal cord injury (SCI) as a result of axial loading. You observe that his ventilations are compromised, what should be your initial management sequence?

According to the National Spinal Cord Injury Association Resource Center:

- 7800 SCIs in the United States each year
- Motor vehicle accidents (44%)
- Acts of violence (24%)
- Falls (22%)
- Sports (8%) ($^{2}/_{3}$ of sports injuries are from diving)
- Other (2%)
- Falls overtake motor vehicles as leading cause of injury after age 45
- Acts of violence and sports cause fewer injuries as age increases
- Acts of violence have overtaken falls as the second most common source of SCI in the last 4 years

TRADITIONAL SPINAL ASSESSMENT CRITERIA

- Traditional criteria have focused on mechanism of injury (MOI) with spinal immobilization considerations for two specific patient groups:
  - Unconscious injury victims
  - Any patient with a "motion" injury
- Covers all patients with a potential for spinal injury
- Not always practical in the prehospital setting

PREHOSPITAL ASSESSMENT

- Prehospital assessment can be enhanced by applying clear, clinical criteria for evaluating SCI that includes the following signs and symptoms (in the absence of other injuries, altered mental status, or use of intoxicants).

MECHANISM OF INJURY OR NATURE OF INJURY

- When determining mechanism of injury in a patient who may have spinal trauma, classify the MOI as:
  - Positive

  - Negative
  - Uncertain
- When combined with clinical criteria for spinal injury, can help identify situations in which spinal immobilization is appropriate

Positive MOI

- Forces exerted on the patient are highly suggestive of SCI
- Always require full spinal immobilization
- Examples include:
  - High-speed motor vehicle crashes
  - Falls greater than three times the patient's height
  - Violent situations occurring near the patient's spine
  - Sports injuries
  - Other high-impact situations
- In the absence of signs and symptoms of SCI, some medical-direction agencies may recommend that a patient with a positive MOI not be immobilized
- Recommendations will be based on the paramedic's assessment when:
  - Patient history is reliable
  - There are no distraction injuries

Negative MOI

- Includes events where force or impact does not suggest a potential for SCI
- In the absence of SCI signs and symptoms, does not require spinal immobilization
- Examples:
  - Dropping an object on the foot
  - Twisting an ankle while running
  - Isolated soft tissue injury

Uncertain MOI

- When the impact or force involved in the injury is unknown or uncertain, clinical criteria must be used to determine need for spinal immobilization
- Examples:
  - Tripping or falling and hitting the head
  - Falls from 2–4 ft
  - Low-speed motor vehicle crashes ("fender benders")

Assessment of Uncertain MOI

- Ensure that the patient is *reliable*
- Reliable patients are calm, cooperative, sober, alert, and oriented
- Examples of *unreliable* patients:
  - Acute stress reactions from sudden stress of any type
- Brain injury
- Intoxicated
- Abnormal mental status
- Distracting injuries
- Problems communicating

SPINAL COLUMN

- Composed of 33 vertebrae (7 cervical, 12 thoracic, 5 lumbar, 5 sacrum (fused), 4 coccyx (fused)
- Anterior elements of the spine include:
  - Vertebral bodies
  - Intervertebral disks
  - Anterior and posterior longitudinal ligaments
  - Connect vertebral bodies anteriorly and inside canal
  - Each vertebra consists of:
    - — Solid body
    - — Bears most of the weight of the vertebral column
    - — Posterior and anterior arch
    - — Posterior spinous process
    - — Transverse process (in some vertebrae)
    - — Spinal cord lies in the spinal canal
    - — Spinal nerve roots pass out through the vertebral foramen

ADULT SKULL

- Sits on top of first cervical vertebra (C1) (atlas)
- Second cervical vertebra (C2) (axis) and its odontoid process allow the head to move with about 180° range of motion
- Cervical spine particularly susceptible to injury due to weight and position of the head in relation to the thin neck and cervical vertebrae

CERVICAL SPINE INJURY

- Spinal injury
- Frequent causes of spinal trauma:
  - Axial loading
  - Extremes of flexion, hyperextension, or hyperrotation
  - Excessive lateral bending
  - Distraction
- May result in stable and unstable injuries based on:
  - Extent of disruption to spinal structures
  - Relative strength of the structures remaining intact

Axial Loading (Vertical Compression)

- Results when direct forces are transmitted along the length of the spinal column
- May produce compression fracture or a crushed vertebral body without SCI
- Most commonly occur at T12–L2

Flexion, Hyperextension, and Hyperrotation

- Extremes in flexion, hyperextension, or hyperrotation may result in:
  - Fracture
  - Ligamentous injury

    - Muscle injury
    - SCI is caused by impingement into the spinal canal by subluxation of one or more cervical vertebrae

Lateral Bending

- Excessive lateral bending may result in dislocations and bony fractures of cervical and thoracic spine
- Occurs as a sudden lateral impact moves the torso sideways
- Initially, head tends to remain in place until pulled along by the cervical attachments

Distraction

- May occur if the cervical spine is suddenly stopped while the weight and momentum of the body pull away from it
- May result in tearing and laceration of the spinal cord

Less Common Mechanisms of Spinal Injury

- Blunt trauma
- Electrical injury
- Penetrating trauma

Classifications of Spinal Injury

- Sprains
- Strains
- Fractures
- Dislocations
- Sacral fractures
- Coccygeal fractures
- Cord injuries

SPINAL INJURIES

- All patients with suspected spinal trauma and signs and symptoms of SCI should be immobilized
- Avoid unnecessary movement
- An unstable spine can only be ruled out by radiography or lack of any potential mechanism for the injury

Assume Spinal Injury

- Significant trauma and use of intoxicating substances
- Seizure activity
- Complaints of pain in the neck or arms (or paresthesia in the arms)
- Neck tenderness on examination
- Unconsciousness because of head injury
- Significant injury above the clavicle
- A fall more than three times the patient's height
- A fall and fracture of both heels (associated with lumbar fractures)
- Injury from a high-speed motor vehicle crash

Spinal Injury

- Damage produced by injury forces can be further complicated by:
  - Patient's age
  - Preexisting bone diseases, congenital spinal cord anomalies
  - Spinal cord neurons do not regenerate to any great extent

Hyperflexion Sprains and Strains

- Hyperflexion sprains
- Occur when the posterior ligamentous complex tears at least partially
- Hyperextension strains (whiplash)
- Common in low-velocity, rear-end automobile collisions
- Signs and symptoms
- Management

Fractures and Dislocations

- Most frequently injured spinal regions in descending order:
  - C5–C7
  - C1–C2
  - T12–L2
- Of these, the most common are wedge-shaped compression fractures and "teardrop" fractures or dislocations

Wedge-Shaped Fractures Hyperflexion Injury

- Usually result from compressive force applied to the anterior portion of the vertebral body with stretching of the posterior ligament complex
- Commonly seen in industrial accidents and falls
- Usually occur in the mid or lower cervical segments or at T12 and L1
- Generally considered stable

Teardrop Fractures and Dislocations

- Extremely unstable injuries
- Result of severe hyperflexion and compression forces
- Commonly seen in motor vehicle crashes
- Among the most unstable injuries of the spine

Sacral and Coccygeal Fractures

- Most serious spinal injuries occur in the cervical, thoracic, and lumbar regions
- Patients frequently complain that they have "broken their tailbone"
- Experience moderate pain from the mobile coccyx
- Fractures through the foramina of S1 and S2 are fairly common and may compromise several sacral nerve elements
- May result in loss of perianal sensory motor function and in bladder and sphincter disturbances
- Sacrococcygeal joint may also be injured because of direct blows and falls

Classification of Cord Injuries

- Primary injuries occur at time of impact
- Secondary injuries occur after initial injury and can include:

  - Swelling
  - Ischemia
  - Movement of bony fragments

Cord Injuries

- The spinal cord can be concussed, contused, compressed, and lacerated
- Severity of these injuries depends on:
  - Amount and type of force that produced them
  - Duration of the injury

Cord Lesions

- Lesions (transections) of the spinal cord are classified as complete or incomplete
- Complete cord lesions
  - Usually associated with spinal fracture or dislocation
  - Total absence of pain, pressure, and joint sensation and complete motor paralysis below the level of injury
- Results in:
  - Quadriplegia—Injury at the cervical level, loss of all function below injury site
  - Paraplegia—Injury at the thoracic or lumbar level, loss of lower trunk only

Complete Cord Lesions

- Autonomic dysfunction may be associated with complete cord lesions
- Manifestations of autonomic dysfunction:
  - Bradycardia
  - Hypotension
  - Priapism
  - Loss of sweating and shivering
  - Poikilothermy
  - Loss of bowel and bladder control

Incomplete Lesions

Central cord syndrome

- Commonly seen with hyperextension or flexion cervical injuries
- Characterized by greater motor impairment of the upper extremities than of the lower extremities

Brown-sequard syndrome

- A hemi-transection of the spinal cord
- May result from:
  - A ruptured intervertebral disk
  - Encroachment on the spinal cord by a fragment of vertebral body, often after knife or missile injuries
- In the classic presentation, pressure on half the spinal cord results in:
  - Weakness of the upper and lower extremities on ipsilateral side
  - Loss of pain and temperature on contralateral side

Signs and symptoms

- Paralysis of the arms
- Sacral sparing
- Anterior cord syndrome
- Usually seen in flexion injuries
- Decreased sensation of pain and temperature below level of lesion
- Intact light touch and position sensation

Causes

- Pressure on the anterior aspect of the spinal cord by a ruptured intervertebral disk
- Fragments of the vertebral body extruded posteriorly into the spinal canal

Pharmacologic Therapy

- Benefits of pharmacologic agents in the management of incomplete cord injury are controversial
- Glucocorticoids
- Naloxone
- Calcium channel blockers
- Methylprednisolone (Solu-Medrol)

Assessment of SCI

- Spinal cord trauma should be evaluated only after all life-threatening injuries have been assessed and treated
- Priorities:
  - Scene survey
  - Assessment of airway, breathing, and circulation
  - Preservation of spinal cord function and avoiding secondary injury to the spinal cord
  - Prevent secondary injury that could result from:
    - — Unnecessary movement
    - — Hypoxemia
    - — Edema
    - — Shock

PREHOSPITAL GOALS

- Maintain a high degree of suspicion for spinal injury
- Scene survey
- Kinematics
- History of the event
- Provide early spinal immobilization
- High concentration oxygen administration
- Rapidly correct any volume deficits

Neurological Examination

- After managing life-threatening problems encountered in the initial assessment, perform a neurological exam
- May be done at the scene or en route to the hospital if the patient requires rapid transport

- Document findings
- Components of neurological examination:
  - Motor and sensory findings
  - Reflex responses

Dermatomes

- Each spinal nerve (except C1) has a specific cutaneous sensory distribution
- Dermatome refers to skin surface area supplied by a single spinal nerve
- Landmarks used for rapid sensory evaluation:
  - C2–C4 dermatomes provide a collar of sensation around the neck and over the anterior chest to below the clavicles
  - T4 dermatome provides sensation to nipple line
  - T10 dermatome provides sensation to umbilicus
  - S1 dermatome provides sensation to soles of feet

Reflex Responses

- Seldom evaluated in the prehospital setting
- Some are easily observed and may indicate autonomic injury
- Babinski's sign (also called the plantar reflex)
- Dorsiflexion of the great toe with or without fanning of toes

Other Methods of Evaluation

- Visual inspection may indicate presence of injury and its level
- Transection of the cord above C3 often results in respiratory arrest
- Lesions that occur at C4 may result in paralysis of the diaphragm
- Transections at C5–C6 usually spare the diaphragm and permit diaphragmatic breathing

SPINAL INJURY

- Absence of neurological deficits does not rule out significant spinal injury
- If a spinal injury is suspected, the patient's spine must be protected
- Patient's ability to walk should not be a factor in determining need for spinal precautions

Spinal Immobilization

- Primary goal is to prevent further injury
- Treat the spine as a long bone with a joint at either end (the head and pelvis)
- Always use *complete* spinal immobilization
- Begins in the initial assessment
- Must be maintained until the spine is completely immobilized on a long backboard

Spinal Stabilization Techniques

- Immediately on recognizing a possible or potential spine injury, manually protect the patient's head and neck
- Head and neck must be maintained in line with the long axis of the body

Rigid Cervical Collars

- Designed to protect the cervical spine from compression
- May reduce movement and some range of motion of the head, but do not by themselves provide adequate immobilization of the spine
- Must always be used with manual in-line stabilization or mechanical immobilization by a suitable device
- Available in many sizes (or are adjustable)
- Choosing the appropriate size reduces flexion or hyperextension
- Must not inhibit patient's ability to open his or her mouth or to clear his or her airway in case of vomiting
- Must not obstruct airway passages or ventilations
- Should be applied only after the head has been brought into a neutral in-line position

Short Spine Boards

- Used to splint the cervical and thoracic spine
- Vary in design and are available from many equipment manufacturers
- Generally used to provide spinal immobilization in situations in which the patient is in a sitting position or a confined space
- After short spine board immobilization, the patient is transferred to a long spine board for complete spinal immobilization

Long Spine Board

- Available in a variety of types including:
  - Plastic and synthetic spine boards
  - Metal alloy spine boards
  - Vacuum mattress splints
  - Split litters (scoop stretchers) that must be used with a long spine board

Manual In-Line Immobilization

- Should be applied without traction, applying only enough tension to relieve the weight of the head from the cervical spine
- Contraindications for moving the patient's head to an in-line position:
  - Resistance to movement
  - Neck muscle spasm
  - Increased pain
  - Presence or increase in neurological deficits during movement
  - Compromise of the airway or ventilation
  - Severe misalignment of the head away from the midline of the shoulders and body axis (rare)

Helmet Issues

- Purpose of helmets is to protect the head and brain, not the neck
- Leaves the cervical spine vulnerable to injury

Types of Helmets

- Full-face or open-face designs
- Used in motorcycling, bicycling, rollerblading, and other activities
- Helmets designed for sports such as football and motor-cross

Helmet Removal

- When determining the need to remove a helmet, consider:
  - Athletic trainers may have special equipment (and training) to remove face-pieces from sports helmets
  - Easy access to the patient's airway
  - Sports garb (e.g., shoulder pads) could further compromise the cervical spine if only the helmet were removed
  - Firm fit of a helmet may provide firm support for patient's head
- Removing a helmet from an injured patient in the prehospital setting (vs. in-hospital removal) is controversial and should be guided by medical direction
- If the patient's airway cannot be adequately accessed or secured, or if the helmet hinders emergency care procedures, the helmet should be removed in the field

Spinal Immobilization in Diving Accidents

- A supine patient should be floated to a shallow area without unnecessary movement of the spine
- A prone patient should be approached from the top of the head
- The patient should be carefully turned to a supine position and airway and breathing should be quickly assessed
- Rescue breathing may be initiated in the water
- Second rescuer slides a long spine board or other rigid device under the patient's body
- First rescuer continues to support the patient's head and neck without flexion or extension
- Apply rigid cervical collar
- Maintain manual in-line immobilization
- Spinal immobilization device should be floated to edge of water and lifted out
- Completely immobilize patient on long spine board

Extrication of a Diving Accident Victim

- Spinal shock refers to a temporary loss of all types of spinal cord function distal to the injury
- Careful handling should occur to avoid secondary injury
- Neurogenic hypotension results from blockade of vasoregulatory fibers, motor fibers, and sensory fibers

Autonomic Hyperreflexia Syndrome

- May occur after resolution of spinal shock
- Associated with patients with chronic SCI who have injuries at T6 or above

Lower Back Pain (LBP)

- Affected area between the lower rib cage and gluteal muscles
- Often radiates to thighs
- Most cases are idiopathic, making precise diagnosis difficult

Degenerative Disk Disease

- Common finding in persons over 50 years

- Biochemical and biomechanical alterations in the tissue of the intervertebral disks that occur with aging
- Associated narrowing of the disk results in variable segmental instability and occasional low back pain

Spondylosis

- Structural defect of the spine that involves the lamina or vertebral arch
- Usually occurs in the lumbar spine between superior and inferior articulating facets
- Rotational "stress" fractures are common at the affected site
- Heredity appears to be a significant factor for this condition

Herniated Intervertebral Disk

- A tear in the posterior rim of the capsule that encloses the gelatinous center of the disk
- Rupture of the disk is usually caused by:
  - Trauma
  - Degenerative disk disease
  - Improper lifting (most common)
- Disks most commonly affected:
  - L5–S1 and L4–L5
  - Occasionally seen at C5–C6 and C6–C7

Spinal Cord Tumors

- May develop from:
  - Cord compression
  - Degenerative changes in bones and joints
  - An interruption in the cord's blood supply
  - Classified by cell type, growth rate, and structure of origin
  - Signs and symptoms depend on tumor type and location
- May include:
  - Temperature dysfunction
  - Sensory changes
  - Other abnormalities
  - Paresis
  - Spasticity
  - Pain
  - Bilateral or asymmetric motor dysfunction

Nontraumatic Spinal Conditions

- Assessment and management are based on:
  - Patient's chief complaint
  - Physical examination
  - Evaluation of associated risk factors
  - Common signs and symptoms
  - Management primarily supportive to decrease pain and discomfort
  - Full spinal immobilization is not required unless the condition is a result of trauma

? CHAPTER QUESTIONS

1. The number-one cause of spinal injury in the United States is:
   a. motor vehicle collision
   b. falls
   c. acts of violence
   d. sports injuries
2. There are 33 vertebrae in the spinal column. Of these how many comprise the cervical spine?
   a. 12
   b. 5
   c. 4
   d. 7

Suggested Reading

http://www.spinalcord.org/resources/. Accessed on March 12, 2007.

US Department of Transportation, National Highway Traffic Safety Administration. *EMT-Paramedic: National Standard Curriculum*. Washington, DC: US Department of Transportation, National Highway Traffic Safety Administration; 1998.

Chapter 19
Thoracic Trauma

You are caring for a 15-year-old male who fell out of his tree house and hit the ground very hard. He presents with dyspnea and right-sided paradoxical chest movement. Vital signs are BP 100/72, HR 120, RR 30 and shallow, with diminished breath sounds bilaterally.

What is this patient suffering from?

What is the initial treatment for this patient?

CHEST INJURIES

- Directly responsible for more than 20% of all traumatic deaths
- Account for about 16,000 deaths per year in the United States

Classifications of Chest Injuries

- Skeletal injury
- Pulmonary injury
- Heart and great vessel injury
- Diaphragmatic injury

Mechanism of Injury

- Blunt thoracic injuries—Forces are distributed over a large area
  - Deceleration
  - Compression

Penetrating Thoracic Injuries

- Forces are distributed over a small area
- Organs injured are usually those that lie along the path of the penetrating object

General Types of Injury Patterns

- Open injuries
- Closed injuries
  - Thoracic cage
  - Cardiovascular
  - Pleural and pulmonary
  - Mediastinal
  - Diaphragmatic
  - Esophageal

  - Penetrating cardiac trauma
  - Blast injury (shock wave)
  - Confined spaces

ANATOMY AND PHYSIOLOGY: REVIEW OF THE THORAX

- Skin
- Bones
  - Thoracic cage
  - Sternum
  - Thoracic spine
- Muscles
  - Intercostal
  - Trapezius
  - Latissimus dorsi
  - Rhomboids
  - Pectoralis major
  - Diaphragm—chief muscle of inspiration
  - Sternocleidomastoid
- Trachea
- Bronchi
- Lungs
  - Parenchyma
  - Alveoli
  - Alveolar—capillary interface
  - Pleura
    - Visceral—located on the outer surface of each lung
    - Parietal—the membrane lining the chest wall
    - Serous fluid—secreted by the pleural membranes; allows them to slide past one another with little friction and discomfort
  - Lobes
- Vessels
  - Arteries
    - Aorta
    - Carotid
    - Subclavian
    - Intercostal
    - Innominate
    - Internal mammary
  - Veins
    - Superior vena cava
    - Inferior vena cava
    - Subclavian
    - Internal jugular
  - Pulmonary
    - Arteries
    - Veins

- Heart
  - Ventricles
  - Atria
  - Valves
  - Pericardium
- Esophagus
  - Thoracic inlet
  - Course through chest
  - Esophageal foramen through diaphragm
- Mediastinum
  - Heart
  - Trachea
  - Vena cavae
  - Pulmonary artery
  - Aorta
  - Esophagus
  - Lymph nodes

Physiology

- Ventilation—the mechanical process of moving air into and out of the lungs
  - Bellows system
  - Musculoskeletal structure
  - Intercostal muscles
- Diaphragm
  - Contracts during inspiration, increasing the length and anteroposterior diameter of the thorax
  - Passively relaxes during expiration, decreasing the size of the thorax and increasing intrapulmonary pressures, resulting in the flow of air out of the lungs
- Accessory muscles (sternocleidomastoid)
- Changes in intrathoracic pressure
- Respiration—the exchange of oxygen and carbon dioxide between the outside atmosphere and the cells of the body
- Neurochemical control
- Gas exchange
  - Alveolar-capillary interface
  - Capillary-cellular interface
  - Pulmonary circulation
  - Cardiac circulation
  - Acid-base balance
    - — Henderson-Hasselbach equation
    - — Respiratory alkalosis
    - — Respiratory acidosis
    - — Compensation for metabolic acidosis and alkalosis

General System Pathophysiology, Assessment, and Management of Thoracic Trauma

Impairments in Cardiac Output

- Blood loss
- Increased intrapleural pressures
- Blood in the pericardial sac
- Myocardial valve damage
- Vascular disruption

Impairments in Ventilatory Efficiency

- Chest bellows action is compromised
- Pain restricting chest excursion
- Air entering the pleural space
- Chest wall fails to move in unison
- Bleeding in the pleural space
- Ineffective diaphragmatic contraction

Impairments in Gas Exchange

- Atelectasis
- Contused lung tissue
- Disruption of the respiratory tract

Assessment Findings

- Pulse-deficit, tachycardia, bradycardia
- Blood pressure
  - Narrowed pulse pressure
  - Hypertension
  - Hypotension
  - Pulsus paradoxus
- Respiratory rate and effort
  - Tachypnea
  - Bradypnea
  - Labored
  - Retractions
- Possible hypothermia
- Skin
  - Diaphoresis
  - Pallor
  - Cyanosis
  - Open wounds
  - Ecchymosis
- Hemoptysis
- Neck
  - Position of trachea
  - Subcutaneous emphysema
  - Jugular venous distention
  - Penetrating wounds

- Chest
  - Contusions
  - Tenderness
  - Asymmetry
  - Lung sounds
    - Absent or decreased sounds
      Unilateral
      Bilateral
  - Location
    - Bowel sounds in hemithorax
- Abnormal percussion finding
  - Hyperresonance
  - Hyporesonance
- Heart sounds
  - Muffled
  - Distant
  - Regurgitant murmur
- Shift of apical impulse
- Open wounds
- Impaled object or penetration
- Crepitus
- Paradoxical movement of chest wall segment
- Scaphoid abdomen
- Decreased level of consciousness
- Electrocardiogram (ECG)
  - ST—T wave elevation or depression
  - Conduction disturbances
  - Rhythm disturbances
- History
- Dyspnea
- Chest pain
- Associated symptoms
  - Other areas of pain or discomfort
  - Symptoms before incident
- Past history of cardio respiratory disease
- Use of restraint in motor vehicle crash

Management of Airway and Ventilation

- High-concentration oxygen
- Endotracheal intubation
- Needle cricothyrotomy
- Surgical cricothyrotomy
- Positive-pressure ventilation
- Occlude open wounds
- Stabilize chest wall

Circulation

- Manage cardiac dysrhythmias
- Intravenous access
- Controlling major hemorrhage

Pharmacological

- Analgesics
- Antidysrhythmics

Nonpharmacological

- Needle thoracostomy
- Tube thoracostomy—in hospital management
- Pericardiocentesis—in hospital

Transport Considerations

- Appropriate mode
- Appropriate facility
- Transport to an appropriate hospital (trauma center)

SKELETAL INJURIES

Clavicular Fractures

- The clavicle is the most commonly fractured bone
- Isolated fracture of the clavicle is seldom a significant injury
- Common in the following situations:
  - Children who fall on their shoulders or outstretched arms
  - Athletes involved in contact sports

Treatment

- Usually accomplished with a sling and swathe or a clavicular strap that immobilizes the affected shoulder and arm
- Injury usually heals well within 4–6 weeks

Signs and Symptoms

- Pain
- Point tenderness
- Obvious deformity

Complications

- Injury to the subclavian vein or artery from bony fragment penetration, producing a hematoma or venous thrombosis (rare)

Rib Fractures

- Infrequent until adult life
- Most often elderly patients
- Significant force is required

Morbidity/Mortality

- Can lead to serious consequences
- Older ribs are more brittle and rigid
- There may be associated underlying pulmonary or cardiovascular injury

Pathophysiology

- Most often caused by blunt trauma—bowing effect with midshaft fracture
- Ribs 3–8 are fractured most often (they are thin and poorly protected)
- Respiratory restriction as a result of pain and splinting
- Intercostal nerve and vessel injury

Associated Complications

- First and second ribs are injured by severe trauma
  - Rupture of the aorta
  - Tracheobronchial tree injury
  - Vascular injury
- Left lower rib injury is associated with splenic rupture
- Right lower rib injury is associated with hepatic injury

Multiple Rib Fractures

- Atelectasis
- Hypoventilation
- Inadequate cough
- Over time pneumonia can set in
- Open rib fracture associated with visceral injury

Posterior Rib Fracture

- Ribs 5–9 are most frequently injured
- Lower rib fractures are associated with spleen and kidney injury

Assessment Findings

- Localized pain
- Pain that worsens with movement, deep breathing, coughing
- Point tenderness
- Crepitus or audible crunch
- Splinting on respiration
- Anteroposterior pressure elicits pain

Complications

- Splinting, which leads to atelectasis and ventilation-perfusion mismatch (ventilated alveoli that are not perfused or perfused alveoli that are not ventilated)

Management

- Airway and ventilation
  - High-concentration oxygen
  - Positive-pressure ventilation
- Encourage coughing and deep breathing

- Pharmacological
  - Analgesics
- Nonpharmacological
  - Splint—but avoid circumferential splinting
- Transport considerations

Flail Chest

- Most common cause is vehicular crash
- Falls from heights
- Industrial accidents
- Assault
- Birth trauma

Morbidity/Mortality

- Significant chest trauma
- Mortality rates 20–40% due to associated injuries
- Mortality increased with:
  - Advanced age
  - Seven or more rib fractures
  - Three or more associated injuries
  - Shock
  - Head injuries

Pathophysiology

- Two or more adjacent ribs fractured in two or more places producing a free-floating segment of chest wall
- Respiratory failure due to:
  - Underlying pulmonary contusion
  - Associated intrathoracic injury
  - Inadequate bellows action of the chest
  - Paradoxical movement of the chest
  - During inspiration, the diaphragm descends, lowering the intrapleural pressure
  - The unstable chest wall is pushed ("sucked") inward by the negative intrathoracic pressure as the rest of the chest wall expands
- During expiration, the diaphragm rises and the intrapleural pressure exceeds atmospheric pressure, causing the unstable chest wall to move outward
- May be minimal because of muscle spasm
- Must be large to compromise ventilation
- Pain
  - Reduces thoracic expansion
  - Decreases ventilation
- Pulmonary contusion
  - Decreased lung compliance
  - Intraalveolar-capillary hemorrhage
  - Alveolar hemorrhage

- Decreased ventilation
- Impaired venous return with resultant ventilation-perfusion mismatch
- Hypercapnia
- Hypoxia

Assessment Findings

- Chest wall contusion
- Respiratory distress
- Paradoxical chest wall movement
- Pleuritic chest pain
- Crepitus
- Pain and splinting of affected side
- Tachypnea
- Tachycardia
- Possible bundle branch block on ECG

Management

- Airway and ventilation
  - High-concentration oxygen
  - Positive-pressure ventilation may be needed
  - Evaluate the need for endotracheal intubation
  - Stabilize the flail segment
  - Positive end expiratory pressure (PEEP)
- Circulation—restrict fluids
- Pharmacological—analgesics
- Nonpharmacological
  - Positioning
  - Endotracheal intubation and positive-pressure ventilation for internal splinting effect
    - Intubation is usually recommended if the chest injury is associated with:
      Shock
      Other severe injuries
      Head injury
      Pulmonary disease
      Patients over the age of 65
- Transport considerations

Sternal Fractures

- Occurs in 5–8% of all patients with blunt chest trauma
- A deceleration compression injury
  - Steering wheel
  - Dashboard
- A blow to the chest; massive crush injury
- Severe hyperflexion of the thoracic cage
- Occurs at or below the manubriosternal junction

Morbidity/Mortality

- 25–45% mortality rate
- High association with myocardial or lung injury
  - Myocardial contusion
  - Myocardial rupture
  - Cardiac tamponade
  - Pulmonary contusion

Pathophysiology

- Associated injuries cause morbidity and mortality
- Pulmonary and myocardial contusion
- Flail chest
- Vascular disruption of thoracic vessels
- Intra-abdominal injuries
- Head injuries
- Rarely is fracture displaced posteriorly to directly impinge on heart or vessels

Assessment Findings

- Localized pain
- Tenderness over the sternum
- Abnormal motion or crepitus over the sternum
- Tachypnea
- ECG changes associated with myocardial contusion
- A history of significant blunt trauma to anterior chest

Management

- Airway and ventilation
  - High-concentration oxygen
- Circulation—restrict fluids if pulmonary contusion is suspected
- Pharmacological—analgesics
- Nonpharmacological—allow chest wall self-splinting
- Transport considerations

PULMONARY INJURY

Closed (Simple) Pneumothorax

- 10–30% in blunt chest trauma
- Almost 100% with penetrating chest trauma

Pathophysiology

- Caused by the presence of air in the pleural space
- A common cause of pneumothorax is a fractured rib that penetrates the underlying lung
- May occur in the absence of rib fractures from:
  - A sudden increase in intrathoracic pressure generated when the chest wall is compressed against a closed glottis (the paper-bag effect)
    - Results in an increase in airway pressure and ruptured alveoli, which lead to a pneumothorax

  - A rupture or tear of the lung parenchyma and visceral pleura with no demonstrable cause (spontaneous pneumothorax)
- Small tears self-seal, larger ones may progress
- The trachea may tug toward the effected side
- Ventilation/perfusion mismatch

Assessment Findings

- Tachypnea
- Tachycardia
- Respiratory distress
- Absent or decreased breath sounds on the affected side
- Hyperresonance
- Decreased chest wall movement
- Dyspnea
- Chest pain referred to the shoulder or arm on the affected side
- Slight pleuritic chest pain

Management

- Airway and ventilation
  - High-concentration oxygen
  - Positive-pressure ventilation if necessary
    - — If respiration rate is <12 or >28 per minute, ventilatory assistance with a bag-valve-mask may be indicated
  - Monitor for the development of a tension pneumothorax
- Nonpharmacological—needle thoracostomy
- Transport considerations
  - Position of comfort (usually semisitting) unless contraindicated by possible spine injury

Open Pneumothorax ("Sucking Chest Wound")

- Usually the result of penetrating trauma
  - Gunshot wounds
  - Knife wounds
  - Impaled objects
  - Motor vehicle collisions
  - Falls
- Severity is directly proportional to the size of the wound
- Profound hypoventilation can result
- Death is related to delayed management

Pathophysiology

- An open defect in the chest wall (>3 cm).
- If the chest wound opening is greater than two-thirds the diameter of the trachea, air follows the path of least resistance through the chest wall with each inspiration.
- As the air accumulates in the pleural space, the lung on the injured side collapses and begins to shift toward the uninjured side.
- Very little air enters the tracheobronchial tree to be exchanged with intrapulmonary air on the affected side, which results in decreased alveolar ventilation and decreased perfusion.

- The normal side also is adversely affected because expired air may enter the lung on the collapsed side, only to be rebreathed into the functioning lung with the next ventilation.
- May result in severe ventilatory dysfunction, hypoxemia, and death unless rapidly recognized and corrected.

Assessment Findings

- Air movement in and out of the defect
- A penetrating injury to the chest that does not seal itself
- A sucking sound on inhalation
- Tachycardia
- Tachypnea
- Respiratory distress
- Subcutaneous emphysema
- Decreased breath sounds on the affected side

Management

- Airway and ventilation
  - High-concentration oxygen
  - Positive-pressure ventilation if necessary
    - — Assist ventilations with a bag-valve device and intubation as necessary
  - Monitor for the development of a tension pneumothorax
- Circulation—treat for shock with crystalloid infusion
- Nonpharmacological
  - Occlude the open wound—apply an occlusive petroleum gauze dressing (covered with sterile dressings) and secure it with tape
  - Tube thoracostomy—in-hospital management
- Transport considerations

Tension Pneumothorax

- Can be caused by a penetrating injury to the chest
- Blunt trauma
  - Penetration by a rib fracture
  - A sudden decrease in intrapulmonary pressure
  - Bronchial disruption from shear forces
- Mechanical ventilation with PEEP
- A spontaneous pneumothorax with a bleb that failed to seal
- Subclavian or internal jugular venous catheter insertion

Morbidity/Mortality

- Profound hypoventilation can result
- Death is related to delayed management
- An immediate, life-threatening chest injury

Pathophysiology

- Occurs when air enters the pleural space from a lung injury or through the chest wall without a means of exit
- Results in death if it is not immediately recognized and treated

- When air is allowed to leak into the pleural space during inspiration and becomes trapped during exhalation, an increase in the pleural pressure results
- Affected, the lung collapses:
  - Lung collapse leads to right-to-left intrapulmonary shunting and hypoxia
- Increased pleural pressure produces mediastinal shift
- Mediastinal shift results in the following:
  - Compression of the uninjured lung
  - Kinking of the superior and inferior vena cava, decreasing venous return to the heart, and subsequently decreasing cardiac output

Assessment Findings

- Extreme anxiety
- Cyanosis
- Increasing dyspnea
- Difficult ventilations while being assisted
- Tracheal deviation (a late sign)
- Hypotension
- Tachycardia
- Diminished or absent breath sounds on the injured side
- Tachypnea
- Respiratory distress
- Bulging of the intercostal muscles
- Subcutaneous emphysema
- Jugular venous distention (unless hypovolemic)
- Unequal expansion of the chest (tension does not fall with respiration)

Management

- Airway and ventilation
  - High-concentration oxygen
  - Positive pressure ventilation if necessary
- Circulation—relieve the tension pneumothorax to improve cardiac output
- Nonpharmacological
  - Occlude open wound
  - Needle thoracostomy
    - — Assess the need for a second or third needle insertion
  - Tube thoracostomy—in-hospital management
- Transport considerations
- Tension pneumothorax associated with penetrating trauma
  - May occur when an open pneumothorax has been sealed with an occlusive dressing.
  - Pressure may be relieved by momentarily removing the dressing (air escapes with an audible release of air).
  - After the pressure is released, the wound should be resealed.
- Tension pneumothorax associated with closed trauma
  - Must be relieved through thoracic decompression with either a large-bore needle or commercially available thoracic decompression kit.
  - Insert a 2-in. 14- or 16-gauge hollow needle or catheter into the affected pleural space.
  - Usually the second intercostal space in the midclavicular line.

- Insert the needle just above the third rib to avoid the nerve, artery, and vein that lie just beneath each rib.
- Secure the needle or catheter in place with tape.
- If time permits, the hub of the needle can be occluded during inspiration by a one-way valve to prevent reentry of air into the pleural space. May be accomplished:
  - — By cutting the finger from a sterile glove (rinsed with sterile water), creating a small hole in the fingertip, slipping the tip over the catheter hub, and securing it with a rubber band
  - — By attaching special tubing and a flutter valve (per protocol) to the hub of the needle instead of a finger from a sterile glove

Hemothorax

- Associated with pneumothorax, blunt or penetrating trauma
- Rib fractures are a frequent cause
- A life-threatening injury that frequently requires urgent chest tube placement and/or surgery
- Associated with great vessel or cardiac injury
  - 50% of these patients will die immediately
  - 25% of these patients live 5–10 minutes
  - 25% of these patients may live 30 minutes or longer

Pathophysiology

- Accumulation of blood in the pleural space caused by bleeding from:
  - Penetrating or blunt lung injury
  - Chest wall vessels
  - Intercostal vessels
  - Myocardium
- Hypovolemia results as blood accumulates in the pleural space
- Compression of the ipsilateral lung occurs from the accumulation of blood
- Mediastinal shift can occur from compression of the contralateral lung

Assessment Findings

- Tachypnea
- Dyspnea
- Cyanosis (often not evident in hemorrhagic shock)
- Diminished or decreased breath sounds on the affected side
- Hyporesonance (dullness on percussion) on the affected side
- Hypotension
- Narrowed pulse pressure
- Tracheal deviation to the unaffected side (rare)
- Pale, cool, moist skin
- Restlessness, anxiety
- Tachycardia
- Flat (or distended) neck veins

Management

- Airway and ventilation
  - High-concentration oxygen

  - Positive-pressure ventilation if necessary
    - — Ventilatory support with bag-valve-mask, intubation, or both
- Circulation—administer volume-expanding fluids to correct hypovolemia
- Nonpharmacological—tube thoracostomy (in-hospital management)
- Transport considerations

Hemopneumothorax

- Pneumothorax with bleeding in the pleural space
- Findings and management are the same as for hemothorax
- Management is the same as for hemothorax

Pulmonary Contusion

- Blunt trauma to the chest
  - The most common injury from blunt thoracic trauma
  - 30–75% of patients with blunt trauma have pulmonary contusion
- Commonly associated with rib fracture
- High-energy shock waves from explosion
- High-velocity missile wounds
- Rapid deceleration
- A high incidence of extrathoracic injuries
- Low velocity—ice pick

Morbidity/Mortality

- May be missed due to the high incidence of other associated injuries
- Mortality—between 14% and 20%

Pathophysiology

- A blunt injury to the lung parenchyma causes intra-alveolar hemorrhage and edema, which results in a loss of alveolar-capillary integrity with subsequent interstitial edema and hemorrhage.

Three physical mechanisms:

- Inertial effect:
  - During the sudden inertial deceleration and direct impact, fixed, and mobile parts of the lung parenchyma move at different speeds.
  - Results in stretching and shearing of alveoli and intravascular structures.
- Spalding effect—This kinetic wave of energy is partially reflected at the alveolar membrane surface, with the remainder causing a localized release of energy.
- Implosion effect—Overexpansion of air in the lungs occurs after the primary energy wave has passed from low-pressure rebound shock waves that produce overstretching and damage to lung tissue.
- Alveolar and capillary damage with interstitial and intra-alveolar extravasation of blood.
- Interstitial edema:
  - Increased capillary membrane permeability.
  - Gas exchange disturbances.
  - Hypoxemia and carbon dioxide retention
  - Hypoxia causes reflex thickening of mucous secretions

- Bronchiolar obstruction.
- Atelectasis—Blood is shunted away from unventilated alveoli leading to further hypoxemia.

Assessment Findings

- Tachypnea
- Tachycardia
- Cough
- Hemoptysis
- Apprehension
- Respiratory distress
- Dyspnea
- Evidence of blunt chest trauma
- Cyanosis

Management

- Airway and ventilation
  - High-concentration oxygen
  - Positive pressure ventilation if necessary
- Circulation—restrict IV fluids (use caution restricting fluids in hypovolemic patients)
- Transport considerations

Traumatic Asphyxia

- A severe crushing injury to the chest and abdomen
  - Steering wheel injury
  - Conveyor belt injury
  - Compression of the chest under a heavy object
- Morbidity/mortality
  - Although the forces involved in this phenomenon may produce lethal injury, traumatic asphyxia alone is not life threatening (although brain hemorrhages, seizures, coma, and death have been documented as occasional sequelae).

Pathophysiology

- A sudden compression force squeezes the chest.
- An increase in intrathoracic pressure forces blood from the right side of the heart into the veins of the upper thorax, neck, and face.
- Jugular veins engorge and capillaries rupture.

Assessment

- Reddish-purple discoloration of the face and neck (the skin below the face and neck remains pink)
- Jugular vein distention
- Swelling of the lips and tongue
- Swelling of the head and neck
- Swelling or hemorrhage of the conjunctiva (subconjunctival petechiae may appear)
- Hypotension results once the pressure is released

Management

- Airway and ventilation
  - Ensure an open airway
  - Provide adequate ventilation
- Circulation
  - IV access
  - Expect hypotension and shock once the compression is released
- Transport considerations

HEART AND GREAT VESSEL INJURY

Myocardial Contusion (Blunt Myocardial Injury)

- The most common cardiac injury after a blunt trauma to the chest
- Occurs in 16–76% of blunt chest traumas
- Usually results from motor vehicle collisions as the chest wall strikes the dashboard or steering column
- Sternal and multiple rib fractures are common
- Can occur from wearing a seat belt improperly

Morbidity/Mortality

- A significant cause of morbidity and mortality in the blunt trauma patient
- Clinical findings are subtle and frequently missed due to:
  - Multiple injuries that direct attention elsewhere
  - Little evidence of thoracic injury
    - — Lack of signs of cardiac injury on initial examination

Pathophysiology

- Hemorrhage with edema and fragmented myocardial fibers
- Cellular injury
- Vascular damage may occur
- Hemopericardium may occur if the epicardium or endocardium are lacerated
- Fibrinous reaction at the contusion site may lead to:
  - Delayed rupture
  - Ventricular aneurysm
  - Areas of damage are well demarcated
  - Conduction defects

Assessment Findings

- Retrosternal chest pain
- ECG changes
  - Persistent tachycardia
  - ST elevation—T wave inversion
  - Right bundle branch block
  - Atrial flutter, fibrillation
  - Premature ventricular contractions
  - Premature atrial contractions
- New cardiac murmur

- Pericardial friction rub (late)
- Hypotension
- Chest wall contusion and ecchymosis

Management

- Airway and ventilation—high-concentration oxygen
- Circulation—IV access
- Pharmacological
  - Antidysrhythmics
  - Vasopressors
- Transport considerations

Pericardial Tamponade

- Rare in blunt trauma
- Penetrating trauma
- Occurs in less than 2% of all chest traumas

Morbidity/Mortality

- Gunshot wounds carry higher mortality than stab wounds
- Lower mortality rate if isolated tamponade is present

Anatomy and Physiology

- Pericardium:
  - A tough fibrous sac that encloses heart
  - Attaches to the great vessels at the base of the heart
- Has two layers:
  - The visceral layer forms the epicardium
  - The parietal layer is regarded as the sac itself
- Purposes:
  - Anchors the heart
  - Restricts excess movement
  - Prevents kinking of the great vessels
- The parietal layer is acutely nondistensible but can chronically distend by as much as 1000–1500 mL.
- The space between the visceral and parietal layer is the "potential space."
- The space is normally filled with 30–50 mL of straw-colored fluid secreted by visceral layer.
- Lubrication:
  - Lymphatic drainage
  - Immunologic protection for the heart

Pathophysiology

- A blunt or penetrating trauma may cause tears in the heart chamber walls, allowing blood to leak from the heart.
  - If the pericardium has been torn sufficiently, blood leaks into the thoracic cavity and the patient exsanguinates rapidly.
- The pericardium often remains intact, and blood enters the pericardial space.
  - Rapid accumulation of fluid over a period of minutes to hours leads to increases in intrapericardial pressure.

    - If 150–200 mL of blood enters the pericardial space acutely, pericardial tamponade develops.
        - Smaller volumes can also produce significant clinical changes.
- Increased intrapericardial pressure:
    - Does not allow the heart to expand and refill with blood.
    - Results in a decrease in stroke volume and cardiac output.
- Myocardial perfusion decreases due to pressure effects on the walls of the heart and decreased diastolic pressures.
- Ischemic dysfunction may result in infarction.
- Removal of as little as 20 mL of blood may drastically improve cardiac output.

Assessment Findings

- Tachycardia
- Respiratory distress
- Narrowed pulse pressure
- Pulsus paradoxus—a drop in systolic blood pressure of more than 10–15 mmHg during spontaneous inspiration
- Cyanosis of the head, neck, and upper extremities
- Beck's triad
    - Narrowing pulse pressure
    - Neck vein distention
    - Muffled heart sounds
- Kussmaul's sign—a rise in venous pressure with inspiration when spontaneously breathing
- ECG changes

Management

- Airway and ventilation—high-concentration oxygen
- Circulation—IV fluid challenge
- Nonpharmacological—pericardiocentesis (in-hospital management)
- Transport considerations

Myocardial Rupture

- Refers to an acute traumatic perforation of the ventricles or atria (including the associated cardiac structures)
- Nearly always immediately fatal but can be delayed for several weeks (after blunt trauma)
- Motor vehicle crashes are responsible for most cases of myocardial rupture
- Compression between the sternum and vertebrae
- Accounts for 15% of all fatal thoracic injuries

Other proposed mechanisms include:

- Deceleration or shearing forces that disrupt the inferior and superior vena cava
- Upward displacement of blood (causing an increase in intracardiac pressure) after abdominal trauma
- Direct compression of the heart between the sternum and vertebrae
- Laceration from a rib or sternal fracture
- Complications of myocardial contusion

Pathophysiology

- Blood-filled chambers of the ventricles are compressed with sufficient force to rupture the chamber wall, septum, or valve

Assessment

- History of significant mechanism of injury with a presentation of:
  - Congestive heart failure
  - Cardiac tamponade

Management

- Primarily supportive
- Airway and ventilatory support
- Rapid transport for definitive care

Traumatic Aortic Rupture

- Blunt trauma
  - Rapid deceleration in high-speed motor vehicle crashes
  - Falls from great heights
  - Crushing injuries
- 15% of all blunt trauma deaths

Morbidity/Mortality

- 80–90% of these patients die at the scene as a result of massive hemorrhage
- About 10–20% of these patients survive the first hour
  - Bleeding is tamponaded by surrounding adventitia of the aorta and intact visceral pleura
  - Of these, 30% have rupture within 6 hours

Pathophysiology

- Usual site of damage to the aorta is in the distal arch just beyond the takeoff of the left subclavian artery and proximal to the ligamentum arteriosum.
- The ligamentum arteriosum and descending thoracic arch are relatively fixed, whereas the transverse portion of the arch is relatively mobile.
- If shearing forces exceed the tensile strength of the arch, the junction of the mobile and fixed points of attachment may be partially torn.
- If the outer layer of tissue surrounding the aorta remains intact, the patient may survive long enough for surgical repair.

Assessment Findings

- Upper-extremity hypertension with absent or decreased amplitude of femoral pulses. Thought to result from compression of the aorta by the expanding hematoma.
- Generalized hypertension secondary to increased sympathetic discharge.
- About 25% of these patients have a harsh systolic murmur over the pericardium or interscapular region.
- Paraplegia with a normal cervical and thoracic spine (rare).
- Retrosternal or interscapular pain.
- Dyspnea.

- Dysphagia.
- Ischemic pain of the extremities.
- Chest wall contusion.

Management

- Airway and ventilation
  - High-concentration oxygen
  - Ventilatory support with spinal precautions
- Circulation—do not over hydrate
- Transport considerations

Diaphragmatic Rupture

- Blunt trauma
  - Injuries to the diaphragm account for 1–8% of all blunt injuries
  - 90% of injuries to the diaphragm are associated with high-speed motor vehicle crashes
- Penetrating trauma

Morbidity/Mortality

- Mortality rate—40%
- Morbidity rate—80%
- Mostly the result of associated injuries

Anatomy Review

- The diaphragm is a voluntary muscle that separates the abdominal cavity from the thoracic cavity.
- The anterior portion attaches to the inferior portion of the sternum and the costal margin.
- Attaches to the 11th and 12th ribs posteriorly.
- The central portion is attached to the pericardium.
- Innervated via the phrenic nerve.

Pathophysiology

- Results from high-compression forces impacting the abdomen and a sharp increase in intra-abdominal pressure.
- The pressure differences may cause abdominal contents to rupture through the thin diaphragmatic wall and enter the chest cavity.
- Rupture can allow intra-abdominal organs to enter the thoracic cavity, which may cause the following:
  - Compression of the lung with reduced ventilation
  - Decreased venous return
  - Decreased cardiac output
  - Shock
  - Very subtle signs and symptoms
  - Bowel obstruction and strangulation
  - Restriction of lung expansion
  - Hypoventilation
  - Hypoxia
  - Mediastinal shift

  - Cardiac compromise
  - Respiratory compromise

Assessment Findings

- Tachypnea
- Tachycardia
- Respiratory distress
- Dullness to percussion
- Scaphoid abdomen (hollow or empty appearance)
- If a large quantity of the abdominal contents are displaced into the chest, the following findings are possible:
  - Bowel sounds in the affected hemithorax
  - Decreased breath sounds on the affected side
  - Possible chest or abdominal pain

Management

- Airway and ventilation
  - High-concentration oxygen
  - Positive-pressure ventilation if necessary
  - Caution: positive-pressure may worsen the injury
- Circulation—IV access
- Nonpharmacological—do not place patient in Trendelenburg position
- Transport considerations

ESOPHAGEAL INJURY

- Usually the result of penetrating trauma
- Rare in blunt trauma
- Should be suspected in patients with trauma to the neck or chest
  - Specific injuries that require a high degree of suspicion of associated esophageal injury include:
    - Tracheal fracture
    - Penetrating trauma from stab or gunshot wounds
    - Ingestion of caustic substances

Morbidity/Mortality

- Could be life threatening if missed

Pathophysiology

- Missile and knife wounds penetrate the esophagus
- Can perforate spontaneously
- Violent emesis
- Carcinoma
- Anatomic distortions produced by diverticula or gastric reflux

Assessment Findings

- Pain on swallowing
- Fever
- Hoarseness
- Dysphagia

- Respiratory distress
- Cervical esophageal perforation
- Local tenderness
- Subcutaneous emphysema
- Resistance of neck on passive motion
- Intrathoracic esophageal perforation
- Mediastinal emphysema
- Mediastinitis
- Subcutaneous emphysema
- Mediastinal "crunch" sound
- Crunching sound with each heartbeat created by air surrounding the pericardial sac (Hamman's sign)
- Splinting of the chest wall
- Respiratory distress
- Shock

Management

- Airway and ventilation—high-concentration oxygen
- Circulation—IV access
- Transport considerations

TRACHEOBRONCHIAL INJURIES

- Rare injury—occurs in less than 3% of all chest traumas
- Penetrating trauma
- Blunt trauma
  - Injury secondary to blunt or penetrating trauma to the anterior neck may cause the following:
    - — Fracture or dislocation of the laryngeal and tracheal cartilages
    - — Hemorrhage
    - — Swelling of the air passages
- Rapid and judicious control of the airway can save the lives of many patients with this injury
- Maintain a high degree of suspicion for associated vascular disruption and esophageal, chest, and abdominal injury
- Injuries associated with laryngeal and tracheal trauma include:
  - Fracture of the hyoid bone resulting in laceration and distortion of the epiglottis
  - Separation of the hyoid and thyroid cartilage resulting in epiglottis dislocation, aspiration, and subcutaneous emphysema
  - Fracture of the thyroid cartilage resulting in epiglottis and vocal cord avulsion, arytenoid dislocation, and aspiration of blood and bone fragments
  - Dislocation or fracture of the cricothyroid resulting in long-term laryngeal stenosis, laryngeal nerve paralysis, and laryngotracheal avulsion
  - Fracture to the trachea resulting in tracheal avulsion, complete airway obstruction, and subcutaneous emphysema

Morbidity/Mortality

- A high mortality rate—greater than 30%

Pathophysiology

- Most major bronchial injuries occur within 3 cm of the carina
- A tear can occur anywhere along the tracheal/bronchial tree
- Rapid movement of air into the pleural space
- Tension pneumothorax refractory to needle decompression
- Continuous flow of air from the needle of a decompressed chest
- Severe hypoxia

Assessment Findings

- Tachypnea
- Tachycardia
- Massive subcutaneous emphysema
- Severe dyspnea
- Hemoptysis
- Signs of tension pneumothorax that do not respond to needle decompression

Management

- Airway and ventilation
  - Emergency airway management in these injuries is controversial and may include:
    - — Oral or nasal intubation
    - — Bag-valve-mask ventilation
    - — Cricothyrotomy
    - — Transtracheal jet insufflation
  - If penetrating trauma causes complete disruption of the laryngotracheal complex, medical direction may recommend dissection through the wound so the exposed trachea can be directly cannulated with a cuffed endotracheal (ET) tube
- Circulation
  - Control hemorrhage
  - IV access
  - Treat for shock
- Transport considerations

? CHAPTER QUESTIONS

1. A 32-year-old male has been shot in the right anterior thorax with a 0.38 caliber handgun. There is an entrance wound at the level of the 4th intercostal space (ICS) in the anterior axillary line. No exit wound is present. The patient is in acute respiratory distress. Central cyanosis is present. Air is freely moving in and out of the gunshot wound (GSW). Radial pulses are absent. A weak, rapid carotid pulse is present. Respirations are rapid and shallow. And the patient's skin is cool and diaphoretic. Your initial treatment should be:

   a. manage the patient's airway, suction as needed

   b. administer high concentration oxygen via non-rebreather

   c. seal the wound with an occlusive dressing, and prepare to perform a needle decompression

   d. all of the above

2. A 22-year-old male was struck in the left lateral thorax with a baseball bat while playing ball at the local ball park. He is in acute respiratory distress. He is anxious and combative. The patient has cyanosis of the lips and nail beds. His neck veins are distended and there is palpable deviation of the trachea to the right. There is an area of discoloration and instability of the left lateral chest wall at the level of the 5th and 6th ICS in the midaxillary line. Subcutaneous emphysema is present on the left. Breath sounds and fremitus are absent on the left. The left hemithorax is hyperresonant to percussion. The abdomen is soft and nontender. Respirations are rapid, shallow, regular. Radial pulses are present, but are rapid and thready. Initial emergency treatment will include the following:
   a. 14 gauge 1-in. and quarter angiocatheter administered in the second intercostal space midclavicular
   b. IV normal saline 14 gauge 1-in. and quarter angiocatheter administered wide-open
   c. administer oxygen 6 L/min via nasal cannula
   d. all of the above

Suggested Reading

US Department of Transportation, National Highway Traffic Safety Administration. *EMT-Paramedic: National Standard Curriculum.* Washington, DC: US Department of Transportation, National Highway Traffic Safety Administration 1998.

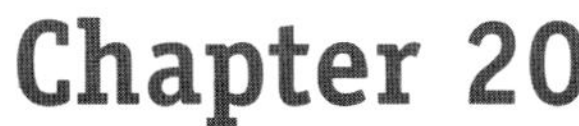

Chapter 20

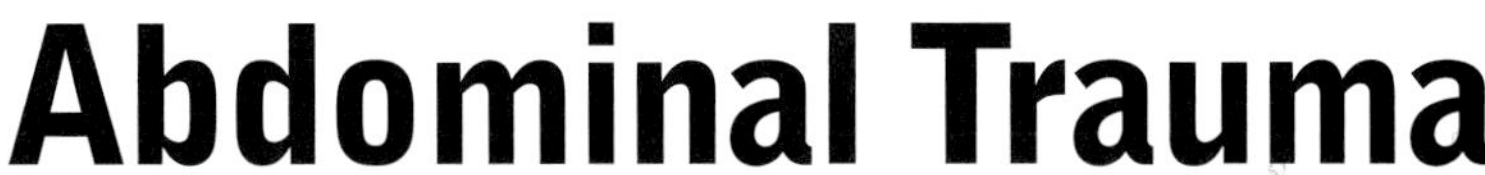

Abdominal Trauma

A male patient was skate boarding, slipped and "straddled" the top of a rale over which he was attempting to perform a trick. He has a swollen, bluish-red scrotum and bruising that extends to the medial aspects of both thighs.

You should suspect injury to what structure?

- Increased incidence of morbidity and mortality
  - Due to delay before surgical intervention
  - Death usually occurs from increased hemorrhage because of delay
    - — Solid organ injuries
    - — Hollow organ injuries
    - — Abdominal vascular injuries
    - — Pelvic fractures

ABDOMINAL TRAUMA

- May be difficult to evaluate abdominal trauma in the prehospital setting because of the following conditions:
  - Wide spectrum of potential injuries to multiple organs
  - Physical findings that are sometimes lacking or exaggerated
  - Environmental issues
  - Seat belts
  - Car seats
  - Front and side air bags
  - The paramedic must exercise a high degree of suspicion and consider the mechanism of injury and kinematics

ANATOMY REVIEW

- Boundaries of the abdomen
  - Diaphragm
  - Anterior abdominal wall
  - Pelvic bones
  - Vertebral column
  - Muscles of the abdomen and flanks

Peritoneal Cavity and Space

- Called the "true" abdominal cavity
- Surface of the abdomen is divided into four quadrants

- Quadrants are formed by drawing two lines
  - One line in the midline from the tip of the xiphoid to the symphysis pubis
  - One line perpendicular to the first at the level of the umbilicus
- Quadrants
  - Upper right
  - Upper left
  - Lower right
  - Lower left

Contents of the Abdominal Cavity

- Liver
- Spleen
- Stomach
- Small intestine
- Colon
- Gallbladder
- Female reproductive organs

Pelvic Cavity

- Surrounded by the pelvic bones
- Makes up the lower part of the retroperitoneal space
- Contains the rectum, bladder, urethra, iliac vessels, and, in women, the internal genitalia

Retroperitoneal Space

- The space or area behind the "true" abdominal cavity
- Contents
  - Abdominal aorta
  - Inferior vena cava
  - Most of duodenum
  - Pancreas
  - Kidneys
  - Ureters
  - Ascending colon
  - Descending colon
- Injuries to this area are difficult to assess and recognize
- Hemorrhage in the retroperitoneal space may go undetected

MECHANISMS OF ABDOMINAL INJURY

Blunt Trauma

- Compression or crushing forces
  - Occurs when organs of the abdomen are crushed between solid objects
  - May result in rupture with secondary hemorrhage and peritonitis
- Shearing forces
  - Shearing injuries are a form of crushing

  - May result when a restraint device is improperly worn
  - May produce a tear or rupture of the solid organs or blood vessels as they become stretched at their points of attachment (e.g., stabilizing ligaments, blood vessels)
- Deceleration forces
  - Result in movement of fixed and nonfixed parts of the body (e.g., lacerations of the liver and spleen [nonfixed structures] at sites of supporting ligaments [fixed structures])
- Degree of injury is usually related to one of the following:
  - Quantity and duration of force applied
  - Type of abdominal structure injured (fluid-filled, gas-filled, solid, hollow)
- Blunt abdominal trauma may be the result of one of the following:
  - Motor vehicle collision
    - Head-on or frontal impact
    - Down-and-under path
    - Up-and-over path
    - Rear impact
    - Lateral or side impact
    - Rotational impact
    - Rollover
    - Restrained (type of restraint) or unrestrained
    - Seat belt injuries
    - Steering wheel injuries
  - Motorcycle collisions
  - Pedestrian injuries
  - Falls
  - Assault
  - Blast injuries

Penetrating Trauma

- Caused by energy imparted to the body
- Low velocity (knife, ice pick)
- Medium velocity (gunshot wounds, shotgun wounds)
- High velocity (high-power hunting rifles, military weapons)
- Ballistics
- Trajectory
- Distance

General Pathophysiology

- Pathophysiology of abdominal injuries
- Hemorrhage
  - No external signs
  - Rapid blood loss
  - Hypovolemic shock
- Spillage of contents
  - Enzymes
  - Acids
  - Bacteria

  - Chemical irritation to peritoneum (peritonitis)
  - Localized pain sensation via somatic nerve fibers
  - Muscular spasm secondary to peritonitis (rigid abdomen)

SPECIFIC ABDOMINAL INJURIES

Solid Organ Injury

Liver

- Largest organ in the abdominal cavity
- Located in upper right quadrant of the abdomen
- Most commonly injured intra-abdominal organ
- Injury occurs more often in penetrating trauma than in blunt trauma
- Commonly injured from trauma to one of the following areas:
  - Eighth through twelfth ribs on right side of body
  - Upper central part of the abdomen
- Suspect liver injury in any patient with the following:
  - Steering wheel injury
  - Lap belt injury
- History of epigastric trauma
- After injury, blood and bile escape into the peritoneal cavity and produce signs and symptoms of shock and peritoneal irritation, respectively

Spleen

- Lies in the upper left quadrant of the abdomen
- Contains a rich blood supply
- Slightly protected by organs surrounding it medially and anteriorly and by lower portion of the rib cage
- Organ most commonly injured by blunt trauma
  - Penetrating injuries are more uncommon
- Associated intra-abdominal injuries are common
- Suspect splenic injury in the following situations:
  - Motor vehicle crashes
  - Falls or sport injuries in which there was an impact to the lower left chest, the flank, or the upper left abdomen
- Upper left quadrant pain with radiation to the left shoulder (Kehr's sign) is a common complaint associated with splenic injury; it is thought to be caused by referred pain secondary to irritation of the adjacent diaphragm from splenic hematoma or hemoperitoneum

Hollow Organ Injury

Stomach

- Not commonly injured after blunt trauma because of its protected location in the abdomen
- Penetrating trauma may cause gastric transection or laceration
- Patients exhibit signs of peritonitis rapidly from leakage of gastric contents
- Diagnosis is confirmed during surgery unless nasogastric drainage returns blood

Colon and Small Intestine

- Injury is usually the result of penetrating trauma
- Large and small bowel may also be injured by compression forces
- High-speed motor vehicle crashes
- Deceleration injuries associated with wearing personal restraints
- Bacterial contamination is a common problem with these injuries

Retroperitoneal Organ Injury

- May occur because of blunt or penetrating trauma to the following areas:
  - Anterior abdomen
  - Posterior abdomen (particularly the flank area)
  - Thoracic spine

Kidneys

- Solid organs located high on the posterior wall of the abdominal cavity in the retroperitoneal space
- Held in place by a connective tissue membrane (renal fascia)
- Cushioned by a generous layer of adipose tissue (fat)
- Partially enclosed and protected by the lower rib cage
- Injuries may involve fracture and laceration and result in hemorrhage, urine extravasation, or both
- Contusions are usually self-limiting
- Heal with bed rest and forced fluids
- Fractures and lacerations may require surgical repair

Ureters

- Hollow organs
- Rarely injured in blunt trauma because of their flexible structure
- Injury usually occurs from penetrating abdominal or flank wounds (e.g., stab wounds, firearm injuries)

Pancreas

- Solid organ that lies in the peritoneal space
- 70–75% of pancreatic injuries are due to penetrating trauma (particularly firearms)
- Blunt injury (rare) usually occurs from crushing the pancreas between the spine and a steering wheel, handlebar, or blunt weapon

Duodenum

- Lies across the lumbar spine
- Seldom injured due to its location in the retroperitoneal area, near the pancreas
- May be crushed or lacerated when great force of blunt trauma or penetrating injury occurs
- Usually associated with concurrent pancreatic trauma
- Injury is confirmed through surgery

Pelvic Organ Injury

- Usually results from motor vehicle crashes that produce pelvic fractures
- Other less frequent causes include the following:

- Penetrating trauma
- Straddle-type injuries from falls
- Pedestrian accidents
- Some sexual acts

- Because the pelvis supports and protects multiple organ systems, there is potential for associated injury
  - Urinary bladder
  - Urethra

Urinary Bladder

- Hollow organ
- May be ruptured by blunt trauma, penetrating trauma, or pelvic fracture
- Rupture is more likely if the bladder is distended at the time of injury
  - With rupture, integrity of peritoneum may be broken, and urine may extravasate into peritoneal cavity
- Suspect bladder injury in inebriated patients who have experienced lower abdominal trauma
- Gross hematuria may be present, or the patient may complain that he or she is unable to urinate

Urethra

- Urethral disruption occurs more frequently in men
- Usually secondary to blunt trauma associated with pelvic fracture
- Patient may complain of an inability to urinate and abdominal pain
- Blood at the meatus suggests urethral injury

VASCULAR STRUCTURE INJURY

Intra-Abdominal Arterial and Venous Injuries

- May be life threatening because of their potential for massive hemorrhage
- Injury usually occurs from penetrating trauma
- May also occur from compression or deceleration forces applied to the abdomen
  - Seat belt injury
  - Pelvic fracture
- Vascular injury usually presents as hypovolemia and is occasionally associated with a palpable abdominal mass
- Major vessels most frequently injured:
  - Aorta
  - Inferior vena cava
  - Renal, mesenteric, and iliac arteries and veins

Management/Treatment Plan

- Airway support
- Breathing support
- Circulatory support
- Patient packaging
- Transport

Pelvic Fractures

- Disruption of the pelvis may occur in the following situations:
  - Motorcycle crashes
  - Pedestrian-vehicle collisions
  - Direct crushing injury to the pelvis
  - Falls from heights of more than 12 feet

Pathophysiology

- Blunt or penetrating injury to the pelvis may result in the following types of injury:
  - Fracture
  - Severe hemorrhage
  - Associated injury to urinary bladder and urethra
- Suspicion of pelvic injury should be based on the following:
  - Mechanism of injury
  - Tenderness of the iliac crests on palpation
- A large amount of force is required to fracture the pelvis
- Force may be direct or indirect
  - Direct—Pelvis injured anteriorly, posteriorly, inferiorly, or laterally
  - Indirect—Forces transmitted superiorly from the acetabulum by means of the legs; force directed laterally from between the legs

Assessment

- Hemorrhage may occur rapidly
- Important physical signs:
  - Progressive perineal, groin, suprapubic, flank, or scrotal swelling or bruising
  - Pain on palpation of the pelvic ring ("pelvic squeeze")
  - Urethral, vaginal, or rectal bleeding may be present, which suggests an open pelvic fracture

Management

- Airway support
- Breathing support
- Circulatory support
- Pneumatic antishock garment (check local protocol)
- IV access (en route)
- Patient packaging
- Transport

OTHER RELATED ABDOMINAL INJURIES

Abdominal Wall Injuries

Evisceration

- An evisceration is the protrusion of an internal organ through a wound or surgical incision, especially of the abdominal wall
- Common finding with stab wounds
- May be seen, to a lesser degree, with gunshot wounds

Management/Treatment Plan

- Airway support
- Breathing support
- Circulatory support
- Patient packaging
  - Do not replace organs back into abdomen
    - Increases risk of infection
    - Complicates surgeon's evaluation of the injury
  - Protect organs from further damage
  - Cover with moistened sterile saline dressing
    - Prevents further contamination and drying
- Transport

ASSESSMENT

Focused History and Physical Examination

- Head injury and intoxicants (drugs/ethanol) mask signs and symptoms
- Hemoperitoneum (solid organ or vascular injuries)
  - An adult abdomen can hold 1.5 L with no abdominal distention
  - Often present even with a normal abdominal exam
  - Unexplained shock
    - Shock out of proportion to known injuries
- Peritonitis (hollow organ injury)
  - Pain (subjective symptom from patient)
  - Tenderness (objective sign with percussion/palpation)
  - Guarding/rigidity
  - Distention (late finding)
- Abrasions
- Ecchymosis
- Visible wounds
- Mechanism of injury
- Unexplained shock

Critical Findings

- Rapid assessment and transport
- Detailed assessment
- Ongoing assessment

Noncritical Findings

- Focused history and physical examination
- Other interventions and transport considerations

Assessment

- Vital signs
- Indications of shock

- Inspection for:
  - Abrasions
  - Ecchymosis
  - Seat belt sign
  - Distention
  - Obvious external blood loss
  - Wounds
  - Impaled object
- Evisceration
  - Auscultation
  - Percussion (tenderness)
  - Palpation
- Tenderness
- Guarding/rigidity
- Pelvic stability/tenderness
  - Absence of signs and symptoms does not rule out abdominal injuries
  - Not necessary to definitively determine if abdominal injuries are present
  - Examine the back
- Differential diagnosis and continued management

MANAGEMENT

- Initiate rapid assessment and stabilization
- Initiate shock resuscitation treatment
- Rapid packaging and transport to nearest appropriate facility
- Facility must have immediate surgical capability
- Rapid transport
- Defeated if the hospital cannot provide immediate surgical intervention
- Crystalloid fluid replacement en route to the hospital
- Airway support
- Breathing support
- Circulatory support
- Control obvious hemorrhage
- Tamponade bleeding
- Manage hypotension
- Fluid resuscitation
- Patient packaging
- Stabilize any impaled objects (if present)
- Transport
- Indications for rapid transport

Critical Findings

- Surgical intervention required to control hemorrhage or contamination
- High index of suspicion of abdominal injury
- Unexplained shock
- Physical signs of abdominal injury
- Hemorrhage continues until controlled in the operating room
- Survival determined by length of time from injury to definitive surgical control of hemorrhage

- Any delay in the field negatively impacts this period
- Indications for transport to a trauma center
- Indications for transport to acute care facility

CHAPTER QUESTIONS

1. Indicate whether the following organs are hollow (H) or solid (S).
   a. Appendix
   b. Gallbladder
   c. Liver
   d. Pancreas
   e. Stomach
   f. Sigmoid colon
   g. Spleen
   h. Right kidney
2. Indicate which quadrant each organ is found.
   a. Appendix
   b. Gallbladder
   c. Liver
   d. Pancreas
   e. Stomach

Suggested Reading

US Department of Transportation, National Highway Traffic Safety Administration. *EMT-Paramedic: National Standard Curriculum*. Washington, DC: US Department of Transportation, National Highway Traffic Safety Administration; 1998.

Chapter 21
Musculoskeletal Trauma

Your patient is a 23-year-old female who fell from a jungle gym. She is complaining of pain and tenderness in her right knee and right ankle. When you examine the affected areas, you note a deformity of the knee joint.

The leg distal to the affected joint is pale and cool. Dorsal pedal and posterior tibial pulses are weak. What problem do you suspect?

- Musculoskeletal trauma occurs in 70–80% of all patients who experience traumatic injury (occurring as an isolated injury or with other injuries)
- Usually results from:
  - Motor vehicle crashes
  - Falls
  - Acts of violence
  - Contact sports
- Upper-extremity injury contributes to long-term impairment and is rarely life-threatening
- Lower-extremity injury:
  - Associated with higher magnitudes of injury
  - More significant blood loss
  - More difficult to manage in multisystem trauma patient
  - Femur and pelvic injuries may constitute life threats

REVIEW OF MUSCULOSKELETAL ANATOMY AND PHYSIOLOGY

Primary Layers of the Skin

- Epidermis (thin outer layer)
  - "Thin skin" covers most of body surface (1–3 mm thick)
  - Most superficial layer consists of dead cells filled with keratin
    - — Stratum lucidum—Translucent layer of dead or dying cells
    - — Stratum granulosum—Contains rows of cells that are precursors to formation of keratin
    - — Stratum spinosum—Contains cells rich in RNA
    - — Stratum basale:

      Layer in which cell division takes place

      Produces all other layers

      Contains melanocytes, which secrete melanin

      Melanin stains surrounding cells, causing them to darken

- Dermis (inner layer) also called the true skin
  - Thicker layer located beneath the epidermis
  - Function:
    - — Gives strength to skin
    - — Contains collagen, which gives toughness to the skin
    - — Also contains elastic fibers to give the skin elasticity and stretch ability
    - — Serves as a reservoir storage area for water and electrolytes
    - — Rich vascular supply important in temperature regulation
    - — Receptors (specialized nerve endings) located in the dermis transmit sensations of pain, pressure, touch, and temperature to the brain
    - — Contains accessory structures including:
      Hair
      Nails
      Sweat and sebaceous glands
- Subcutaneous layer (not considered part of the skin)
  - Layer beneath the skin that carries major blood vessels and nerves to the skin
  - Composed primarily of loose connective and adipose tissue
  - Amount of adipose tissue varies depending on:
    - — Area of body
    - — Individual nutrition
  - Functions
    - — Helps insulate body from extreme temperature changes in external environment
    - — Loosely anchors skin to underlying organs/structures
- Fascia
  - Subcutaneous layer is also called superficial fascia
  - Fascia is a fibrous connective tissue membrane that covers individual skeletal muscles or certain organs

Functions of Muscular System

- Movement
- Body support and maintenance of posture
- Heat production

Properties of Muscle

- Contractility
- Excitability—Capacity of muscle fibers to respond when stimulated by a nerve impulse
- Extensibility (stretchability)—Capacity of muscle fibers to stretch beyond their relaxed length
- Elasticity—Ability to return to their original length after contraction or stretching

Types of Muscle Tissue

Skeletal Muscle

- Under conscious control
- Makes up about 40% of the total body mass
- Has two attachments

- Origin—Usually the more fixed and proximal attachment
- Insertion—More movable and distal attachment
- Contractions are rapid and forceful

Cardiac Muscle

- Called myocardium and forms the middle layer of the heart
- Innervated by the autonomic nervous system but contracts spontaneously without any nerve supply
- Contractions are strong and rhythmic

Smooth Muscle

- Found in the walls of hollow organs (urinary bladder and uterus) and in the walls of tubes (respiratory, digestive, reproductive, urinary, and circulatory systems)
- Innervated by the autonomic nervous system, regulating size of lumen of tubular structures
- Contractions are strong and slow

Structures Associated with Muscles

- Tendons
  - Bands of connective tissue binding muscles to bones
  - Muscle-tendon-bone (M-T-B)
  - Allows for power of movement across the joints
  - Supplied by sensory fibers that extend from muscle nerves
- Bursae
  - Flattened, closed sacs of synovial fluid
  - Found where a tendon rubs against a bone, ligament, or other tendon
  - Reduce friction and act as a shock absorber
  - Prone to fill with fluid when infected or injured
- Cartilage
  - Connective tissue covering the epiphysis
  - Acts as surface for articulation
  - Allows for smooth movement at joints
- Ligaments
  - Connective tissue that crosses joints and attaches bone to bone
    - — Bone-ligament-bone (B-L-B)
  - Stretch more easily than tendons
  - Allow for stable range of motion
- Fascia
  - Dense fibrous connective tissue that forms bands or sheets
  - Covers muscles, blood vessels, and nerves
  - Supports and anchors the organs to nearby structures
- Bones
  - 206 bones form the body's supporting framework
  - Protect some internal organs from mechanical injury
  - Act as points of attachment for tendons, cartilage, and ligaments
  - Act as levers on which the muscles act to produce movements permitted by joints

- Serve as a reservoir for calcium and phosphorus
- Contain and protect red bone marrow

- Joints
  - A joint is where two bones meet (articulate)
  - May be classified by the amount of movement of the joint or by structure

Classification of Movement

- Synarthrosis
  - No movement
  - Fibrous connective tissue grows between articulating bones
  - Example—Sutures of the skull; between facial bones
- Amphiarthrosis
  - Some movement but very limited
  - Cartilage connects articulating bones
  - Example—Symphysis pubis; between vertebrae
- Diathrosis
  - Free movement
  - Largest category of joints
  - Example—Knee, hip, elbow

Classification by Structure

- Fibrous joints
  - Barely movable or immovable
  - Example—Joints of the skull
- Cartilaginous joints
- Synchondroses (primary cartilaginous joints)
  - Allow no movement but growth in the length of the bone
  - Example—Epiphyseal plates
- Symphyses (secondary cartilaginous joints)
  - Slightly movable joints
  - Example—Intervertebral disks, pubic symphysis
- Synovial joints
  - Separated by a fluid-filled chamber that lubricates articular surfaces
  - Classified according to axes of movement into:
    - Plane—Allow gliding or sliding movement between two flat surfaces
    - Hinge—Allow flexion and extension only
    - Pivot—Allow rotation only
    - Condyloid—Allow flexion, extension, abduction, and adduction; do not permit axial rotation
    - Saddle—Allow flexion, extension, abduction, adduction, and circumduction; do not permit axial rotation
    - Ball and socket—Allow flexion, extension, abduction, adduction, rotation, and cumduction

SKELETAL SYSTEM

Axial skeleton (80 bones) forms the central (longitudinal) axis of the body, these structures include:

- Skull (28)
  - Cranium (8)
  - Face (14)
  - Ear bones (6)
- Hyoid bone (1)
- Vertebral column (26)
- Thoracic cage (25)

Appendicular skeleton (126 bones)

- Pectoral girdle (4)—Bones that attach the upper limbs to the axial skeleton
  - Clavicle
  - Scapula
- Upper limbs (60)—Humerus, radius ulna, carpals, metacarpals, phalanges
- Pelvic girdle (2)—Paired bones of the pelvis that attach the lower limbs to the axial skeleton, and the sacrum
- Lower limbs (60)—Femur, tibia, fibula, patella, tarsals, metatarsals, phalanges

Types of Bones (Table 21-1)

Components of a long bone

- Diaphysis
  - Main shaft of the long bone which is composed primarily of compact bone
  - Function—Provides strong support without cumbersome weight
- Medullary (or marrow) cavity
  - Tubelike, hollow space in diaphysis
  - Contains yellow (adipose) or red bone marrow depending on the age of the individual

TABLE 21-1: Types of Bones

Long bones	• Longer than they are wide • Found only in the limbs • Sustain weight of body and act in locomotion • Examples—Arms and legs
Short bones	• Shaped like cubes or are oblong • Usually grouped together to provide strength and compactness in areas of limited movement • Examples—Wrists (carpals) and ankles (tarsals)
Flat bones	• Thin, flat, and curved • Examples—Sternum, skull, ribs
Irregular bones	• Shaped differently than long, short, and flat bones • Structurally similar to short bones • Examples—Some bones of the skull, hip bones, vertebrae

- Periosteum
  - Dense, white, fibrous, connective tissue membrane that covers outside diaphysis
  - Vascular and full of nerves
  - Haversian canals allow circulation of blood
  - Functions
    - — Protects the bone
    - — Attaches tendons firmly to bones
    - — Regenerates bone after fractures
    - — Contains blood vessels that send branches into bone for nourishment
    - — Essential for bone cell survival and formation
- Epiphysis
  - Both expanded ends of a long bone with which the marrow cavity freely communicates
  - Consists of cancellous bone-filled marrow
  - Outer surface covered with articular cartilage
    - — Articular (hyaline) cartilage is located at the ends of articulating surfaces of bones and is lubricated by synovial fluid from the joint cavity
    - — Decreases friction, allowing for smooth joint movement
  - Functions
    - — Provides attachments for muscles
    - — Gives stability to joints
    - — Responsible for growth in the infant and child

Bone Markings: Terminology

- Depressions/openings
  - Foramen—Large opening through a bone; usually serves as a passageway for blood vessels, nerves, or ligaments
  - Sinus—Cavity or hollow space within a bone
  - Fossa—Depression or groove
- Projections/protrusions
  - Condyle—Large rounded bump; usually articulates with another bone
  - Crest—A pronounced ridge on a bone
  - Epicondyle—Bump located above a condyle; for muscle attachment
  - Facet—A small flat surface that forms a joint with another facet or flat bone
  - Head—Large and rounded end of a bone
  - Process—A raised area or projection
  - Spine—Slender, sharp projection
  - Tubercle—Knoblike projection
  - Tuberosity (trochanter)—Large, rough pronounced projection; larger than tubercle

Skeletal Anatomy: Appendicular Skeleton

Pectoral (Shoulder) Girdle

- Serves to attach arm to the axial skeleton of the thorax
- Place of attachment for muscles of arm and chest
- Each pectoral girdle has two bones—Scapula and clavicle

Scapula (Shoulder Blade)

- Triangular flat bon
- Glenoid fossa (glenoid cavity)
- Arm socket—Depression that receives the head of the humerus to form the shoulder joint; allows rotation of the arm at the shoulder
- Spine of scapula—Long, posterior process for muscle attachment
- Acromion—Lateral end of spine of scapula that articulates with clavicle

Clavicle (Collarbone)

- Long, slender, S-shaped bone that lies horizontally just beneath the skin
- Functions:
  - Acts as a brace that holds the upper limb away from the trunk
  - Serves to transmit forces from the upper limb to the axial skeleton
  - Provides attachment for certain muscles of neck, thorax, back, and arm
- Medial end articulates with the manubrium of sternum to form the sternoclavicular joint
- Lateral end articulates with the acromion of the scapula to form the acromioclavicular (AC) joint

Muscles Acting on the Shoulder Girdle

- Trapezius raises or lowers shoulders and shrugs them
- Rhomboid minor retracts, rotates, and fixes scapula
- Rhomboid major retracts, rotates, elevates, and fixes scapula
- Serratus anterior pulls shoulder forward and rotates it upward; holds scapula against chest wall
- Pectoralis minor pulls shoulder down and forward
- Levator scapulae elevate and retract scapula and abducts

Humerus

- Longest and largest bone of the upper extremity
- Head—Round process that articulates with the scapula at the glenohumeral joint
  - Glenohumeral joint
    - — Ball-and-socket joint
    - — Allows abduction and adduction, flexion and extension, circumduction and rotation
  - Bursae around the shoulder form a lubricating mechanism during movement of shoulder joint

Anatomical Neck

- Indentation distal to the head of the humerus
- Former site of the epiphyseal plate

Greater tubercle

- Rounded projection lateral to head on anterior surface
- Provides attachments for supraspinatus, infraspinatus, and teres minor muscles

Lesser tubercle

- Anterior projection just below anatomical neck
- Provides an insertion for subscapularis muscle

Surgical neck

- Constricted portion just distal to the tubercles
- Common fracture site

Shaft

- Capitulum—Round process superior to radius

Trochlea

- Projection with deep depression through center similar to shape of pulley
- Articulates with ulna
- Olecranon fossa—Posterior, oval depression that holds the olecranon process of the ulna when the forearm is fully extended
- Medial and lateral epicondyles
- Rough projections on either side of distal end
- Ulnar nerve winds behind medial epicondyle
- Responsive to blows or pressure that can produce temporary numbness and paralysis of muscles on the anterior surface of the forearm
- Area called the "funny bone"

Muscles That Move the Upper Arm

Trapezius

- Broad muscle on posterior neck and shoulder
- Extends head; look at the sky
- Elevates shoulder and pulls it back; shrugs shoulders

Pectoralis Major

- Large muscle that covers upper anterior chest
- Flexes upper arm
- Adducts upper arm anteriorly; draws it across the chest
- Raises ribs in forced inspiration
- Pulls shoulder forward and downward

Serratus Anterior

- Forms upper sides of chest wall below axilla
- Pulls scapula forward
- Aids in raising arms

Latissimus Dorsi

- Large broad flat muscle on mid and lower back
- Extends, adducts, and medially rotates upper arm
- "Swimmer's muscle"

Deltoid

- Covers shoulder joint
- Abducts upper arm as in "scarecrow" position

Rotator Cuff Muscles

- Group of four muscles that form a cuff over the proximal humerus
  - Supraspinatus
  - Subscapularis
  - Infraspinatus
  - Teres minor
- Attach humerus to scapula
- Rotate arm at shoulder joint

Elbow

- Forms a hinge joint between:
  - Humerus and head of radius (humeroradial joint)
  - Humerus and ulna (humeroulnar joint)
- Allows flexion and extension
- Includes radioulnar joint
  - Pivot joint that allows pronation and supination
- Innervated by radial and ulnar nerves, among others
- Cubital fossa
  - Triangular skin depression that lies in front of the elbow
  - Contains:
    - — Median nerve
    - — Bifurcation of brachial artery into radial and ulnar arteries
    - — Radial nerve
  - Cephalic and basilic veins lie in the superficial fascia covering the cubital fossa

Radius and Ulna

- Bones of forearm connected by the interosseous membrane (a flexible connective tissue)
- Articulate proximally to form a pivot joint, which with the pronator and supinator muscles, permits turning the palm up (supination) and palm down (pronation)
  - When the palm is up, the radius and ulna are parallel
  - When the palm is down, the two bones cross
- Radius
  - Bone on thumb side of forearm when palm is facing forward
  - Shorter than and lateral to the ulna
  - Head—Proximal end that articulates with humerus and ulna
  - Distal end articulates with carpal bones of wrist
  - Radial tuberosity
    - — Located on shaft of radius just below the head
    - — Site of attachment for biceps brachii muscle that flexes the forearm
- Ulna
  - The longer of the two forearm bones
  - Located on little finger side of forearm
  - Medial to radius
  - Olecranon process fits into olecranon fossa of humerus when forearm is fully extended
  - Semilunar notch—"Half-moon" depression that articulates with the trochlea of ulna

Muscles That Move the Forearm

- Biceps brachii
  - Major muscle on anterior surface of forearm
  - Flexes and supinates forearm
  - Muscle used to "make a muscle"
  - Acts synergistically with brachialis and brachioradialis
- Triceps brachii
  - Posterior surface of upper arm
  - Extends forearm
  - "Boxer's muscle"
- Brachialis
  - Deep to biceps
  - Flexes forearm
- Brachioradialis
  - Muscles of forearm
- Flexes forearm
- Pronator quadratus pronates forearm
- Pronator teres pronates and flexes forearm
- Supinator supinates forearm

Carpals-Bones of the Wrist (Carpus)

- Arranged in two rows of four bones
  - Four proximal carpals
  - Four distal carpals
- Articulate with one another at gliding joints that permit sliding and twisting
- Ligaments interconnect the carpal bones and help stabilize the wrist joint
- Radiocarpal joint (wrist)
- Forms the articulation of the radius and carpal bones
  - Synovial (condyloid) joint that permits movement in two planes
  - Permits flexion, extension, abduction, and adduction of hand
- Carpal tunnel
  - Formed by the concave anterior surface of the carpal bones
  - Contains flexor tendons of the fingers and the median nerve

Metacarpals

- Five metacarpal bones
- Miniature long bones that make up the palm of the hand
- Consist of proximal ends (bases), shafts (bodies), and distal ends (heads)
- Heads of the metacarpals form the knuckles of the hand
- Metacarpophalangeal (MCP) joint
  - Metacarpals articulate with the proximal phalanges at the MCP joints
  - These joints are synovial condyloid joints

Phalanges (Bones of the Finger)

- Miniature long bones consisting of bases, shafts, and heads
  - Each finger has three bones—Proximal, middle, and distal phalanges
  - Each thumb has only two phalanges—Proximal and distal

- Heads of proximal and middle phalanges form the knuckles
- Joints
  - Interphalangeal joints are synovial hinge joints
  - Middle phalanges articulate with the distal phalanges at the distal interphalangeal (DIP) joint
  - Proximal phalanges articulate with the middle phalanges at the proximal interphalangeal (PIP) joint
- Muscles that move the wrist, hand, and fingers
  - Flexor and extensor carpi groups flex and extend the hand
  - Flexor and extensor digitorum groups flex and extend the fingers

Pelvic Girdle

- Consists of the sacrum, coccyx, and two hip bones (os coxae or innominate bones)
- Each hip bone is formed by fusion of an ilium, ischium, and pubis on each side of the pelvis
- Functions:
  - Bears the weight of the body
  - Serves as a place of attachment for the legs
  - Protects the organs in the pelvic cavity (e.g., urinary bladder, reproductive organs)
- Ilium
  - Largest and uppermost part of the hip bone
  - Iliac crest—Upper, outer edge of ilium
- Ischium
  - Strongest and lowermost part of the hip bone
  - Ischial tuberosity—The part of the hip bone on which you sit
  - Ischial spine—Projects into the pelvic cavity and narrows the outlet of the pelvis
- Pubis—Anterior, medial portion
- Pubic symphysis
  - Cartilaginous joint between the two pubic bones
  - Softens before delivery
  - Allows expansion of the pelvic cavity to accommodate the infant's head as it exits the birth canal
- Acetabulum—Deep depression that articulates with the femur
- The two hip bones connect:
  - Posteriorly with the sacrum to form the sacroiliac joints
    - These joints are gliding synovial joints that permit slight or no movement
  - Anteriorly with each other at the symphysis pubis

Femur (Thigh Bone)

- Longest, strongest, and heaviest bone of the body
- Hip joint
  - A ball-and-socket joint between the acetabulum of the hip bone and head of the femur
  - Allows abduction and adduction, flexion and extension, and circumduction and rotation
- Head—Round process that articulates with the hip bone
- Neck—Constricted portion distal to the head

- Trochanters
  - Greater trochanter—Large lateral process for muscle attachment
  - Lesser trochanter—Medial process for muscle attachment
- Medial and lateral condyles—Rounded processes that articulate with the tibia
- Muscles that move the thigh
  - All muscles that move the thigh attach to some part of the pelvic girdle and femur
  - Gluteal group (e.g., gluteus maximus, gluteus medius, gluteus minimus)
    - Gluteus maximus

      Largest and most superficial of the gluteal muscles

      Located on posterior surface of buttocks

      Extends the thigh

      Muscle for sitting and climbing stairs
    - Gluteus medius

      Thick muscle partly behind and superior to gluteus

      Abducts and rotates the thigh
    - Gluteus minimus

      Smallest and deepest of the gluteal muscles

      Abducts and rotates the thigh
  - Iliopsoas
    - Located on anterior surface of groin
    - Crosses over hip joint to the femur
    - Flexes the thigh

      Antagonist to gluteus maximus
  - Adductor group
    - Medial inner thigh region
    - Adducts thigh
    - Muscles used by horseback riders to stay on horse

Patella (Kneecap)

- Largest sesamoid bone of the body
- Embedded in tendon of quadriceps femoris muscle
- Articulates with the femur
- Knee joint
  - Hinge-type synovial joint between the distal end of the femur and the proximal end of the tibia
  - Also includes a saddle joint between the femur and patella
  - Allows flexion, extension, and slight rotation of the tibia

Tibia (Shin Bone)

- Medial and more superficial bone of lower leg
- Articulates with femur at the knee
- Weight-bearing bone of the lower leg
- Medial malleolus
  - Distal process
  - Medial "ankle bone"

Fibula

- A slim bone of the body, proportional to its length
- Long bone on lateral side of lower leg
- Functions to increase the available area for muscle attachments in the leg
- Head articulates with lateral condyle of tibia
  - Forms tibiofibular joint
  - Gliding synovial joint
- The fibula does not:
  - Articulate with the femur
  - Play a role in the transfer of weight to the ankle and foot
- Lateral malleolus
  - Distal process
  - Lateral "ankle bone"

Muscles That Move the Leg

- Quadriceps femoris group (rectus femoris, vastus lateralis, vastus medialis, vastus intermedium)
  - Located on anterior and lateral surface of thigh
  - Form a common tendon that inserts in tibia
  - Muscle group used to extend the leg
  - Rectus femoris can flex thigh at hip joint
- Sartorius
  - Long muscle that crosses obliquely over anterior thigh
  - Permits sitting in crossed leg or lotus position
- Hamstring group (e.g., biceps femoris, semitendinosus, semimembranosus)
  - Located on posterior surface of thigh
  - Attach to tibia and fibula as a group
  - Flex leg, extend thigh
  - Antagonist to quadriceps femoris

Tarsals

- Seven tarsal bones form the ankle
- Calcaneus (heel bone)
  - Largest and strongest bone of the foot
  - Lies below the talus
  - Body weight is supported primarily by the calcaneus and talus
- Talus
  - Second largest bone of the foot
  - Articulates with calcaneus and tibia
  - Forms the talocrural joint
    - — Synovial hinge joint
    - — Allows dorsiflexion and plantar flexion
  - The only freely movable tarsal bone (has no muscle attachments)
  - Transmits body weight from the tibia toward the toes

Metatarsals

- Five long bones that form the sole (plantar surface) of the foot
- Distal ends of metatarsals form the ball of the foot

- Each metatarsal has a base, shaft, and head
  - Bases of the metatarsals articulate with the tarsal bones
  - Heads of the metatarsals articulate with the proximal phalanges
    - Form the metatarsophalangeal joints
    - The heads of the first two metatarsal bones form the ball of the foot

Phalanges—Bones Found in the Toe

- Toes contain 14 phalanges
- Great toe has two phalanges (proximal and distal); the other four toes have three phalanges each (proximal, middle, and distal)

Muscles That Move the Ankle and Foot

- Tibialis anterior
  - Anterior leg
  - Dorsiflexes foot; inversion of foot
- Peroneus
  - Lateral surface of leg
  - Plantar flexion; eversion of foot
  - Supports arch
- Gastrocnemius (calf muscle)
  - Posterior surface of leg
  - Large two-headed muscle that forms the calf
  - Plantar flexion of foot
  - "Toe-dancer" muscle
- Soleus
  - Posterior surface of leg
  - Plantar flexion of foot

Age-Associated Changes in Bones

- Morphological changes
  - Water content of intervertebral disks decreases
  - Increased risk of disk herniation
  - Loss of 1/2 to 3/4 in. in stature is common
  - Bone tissue disorders shorten the trunk
  - Vertebral column gradually assumes an arc shape
  - Costal cartilages ossify, making the thorax more rigid
  - Shallow breathing due to rigid thoracic cage
  - Facial contours change
- Fractures
  - Bones are more prone to fracture since they are more porous and brittle
  - Vertebral and femoral neck fractures are most common
  - Degree of bone disorder (osteoporosis) is related to the incidence of fracture

CLASSIFICATION OF MUSCULOSKELETAL INJURIES

- Injuries that result from application of traumatic forces to these tissues include:
  - Fractures
  - Sprains

  - Strains
  - Joint dislocations
- Problems associated with musculoskeletal injuries include:
  - Hemorrhage
  - Instability
  - Loss of tissue
  - Simple laceration and contamination
  - Interruption of blood supply
  - Nerve damage
  - Long-term disability
- Musculoskeletal injuries can result from:
  - Direct trauma—Blunt force applied to an extremity
  - Indirect trauma—A vertical fall that produces a spinal fracture distant from the site of impact
  - Pathologic conditions—Some forms of arthritis; malignancy
- Carefully evaluate the scene and consider kinematics when caring for a patient with musculoskeletal injury

Fractures (Table 21-2)

- A break in the continuity of a bone or cartilage
- May be complete or incomplete, depending on the line of fracture through the bone

TABLE 21-2: Classification of Fractures

Open	A break where a protruding bone or penetrating object causes a soft tissue injury
Closed	A break in the bone that has not yet penetrated the soft tissue or skin
Comminuted	A fracture that involves several breaks in the bone causing multiple bone fragments
Greenstick	A break in which the bone is bent, but broken only on the outside of the bend (common in children)
Spiral	A break caused by a twisting motion
Oblique	A break at a slanting angle across a bone
Transverse	A break that occurs at right angles to the long axis of the bone
Stress	A break (especially in one or more of the foot bones) caused by repeated, long-term, or abnormal stress
Pathological	A break resulting from weakness in bone tissue caused by neoplasm or malignant growth
Epiphyseal	• A break that involves the epiphyseal growth plate of a child's long bone • May result in permanent angulation or deformity • May cause premature arthritis

- May be classified as open or closed, depending on the integrity of the skin near the fracture site

Fractures of long bones may result in moderate-to-severe hemorrhage within the first 2 hours, releasing as much as:

- 550 mL of blood in the lower leg from a tibia/fibular fracture
- 1000 mL of blood in the thigh from a femur fracture
- 2000 mL of blood from a pelvic fracture

Sprain

- A partial tearing of a ligament caused by sudden twisting or stretching of a joint beyond its normal range of motion.
- Two common areas for sprains are the ankle and the knee.
- Sprains are graded by severity.
- First-degree sprain:
  - Has no joint instability because only a few ligamentous fibers are torn.
  - Swelling and hemorrhage are minimal.
  - Repeated first-degree sprains can result in ligamentous stretching.
- Second-degree sprain:
  - Causes more disruption than first-degree injuries.
  - Joint is usually intact, but there is increased swelling and ecchymosis.
- Third-degree sprain:
  - Ligaments are totally disrupted.
  - If accompanied by dislocation, nerve or vascular compromise to the extremity is possible.

Strain

- An injury to the muscle or its tendon from overexertion or overextension.
- Commonly occur in the back and arms and may be accompanied by significant loss of function.
- Severe strains may cause an avulsion of bone from the attachment site.

Joint Dislocations

- Occur when the normal articulating ends of two or more bones are displaced

Terminology

- Luxation—A complete dislocation
- Subluxation—An incomplete dislocation

Joints Frequently Dislocated

- Shoulders
- Elbows
- Fingers
- Hips
- Knees
- Ankles

Suspect a joint dislocation when a joint is deformed or does not move with normal range of motion. All dislocations can result in great damage and instability.

INFLAMMATORY AND DEGENERATIVE CONDITIONS

Bursitis

- Inflammation of a bursa (a small, fluid-filled sac that acts as a cushion at a pressure point near joints)
- Most important bursae are around the knee, elbow, and shoulder
- Bursitis is usually the result of:
  - Pressure (prolonged kneeling on a hard surface)
  - Friction
- Slight injury to the membranes surrounding the joint
- Treatment generally consists of rest, ice, and analgesics; after which the condition usually subsides
- Rarely, bursectomy may be performed

Tendonitis

- Inflammation of a tendon, often caused by injury
- Symptoms include:
  - Pain
  - Tenderness
  - Restricted movement of the muscle attached to the affected tendon
- Treatment usually includes:
  - Nonsteroidal anti-inflammatory drugs (NSAIDs)
  - Corticosteroid medications may be injected around the tendon

Arthritis

- Inflammation of a joint
- Characterized by pain, swelling, stiffness, and redness
- A joint disease (involving one or many joints) that can occur from many causes
- Varies in severity from a mild ache and stiffness to severe pain, and later joint deformity
- Osteoarthritis (degenerative arthritis) most common
  - Results from wear and tear on the joints
  - Evolves during middle age
  - Pain associated with this condition is usually managed with anti-inflammatory agents
- Rheumatoid arthritis
  - Most severe type of inflammatory joint disease
  - An autoimmune disorder
  - The body's immune system acts against and damages joints and surrounding soft tissues
  - Many joints, most commonly those in the hands, feet, and arms, become extremely painful, stiff, and deformed
  - Medications used to treat this condition include:
    - — NSAIDs to decrease pain
    - — Antirheumatic drugs and immunosuppressant agents to arrest or slow the progress of the disease
- Gouty arthritis
  - A form of joint disease in which uric acid accumulates in joints as crystals, causing inflammation
  - The first attack of this form of arthritis usually involves only one joint (the base of the big toe) and lasts a few days

  - Subsequent attacks may be more severe and may affect more joints (knee, ankle, wrist, foot, and small joints of the hand)
  - Pain and inflammation are controlled with large doses of NSAIDs or corticosteroid injections
- Other treatments may include:
  - Medications to inhibit the formation of or increase the excretion of uric acid
  - Diet modifications

SIGNS AND SYMPTOMS OF EXTREMITY TRAUMA

Patient Presentation

- Common signs and symptoms of extremity trauma include:
  - Pain on palpation or movement
  - Swelling, deformity
  - Crepitus
  - Decreased range of motion
  - False movement (unnatural movement of an extremity)
  - Decreased or absent sensory perception or circulation distal to the injury (evidenced by alterations in skin color and temperature, distal pulses, capillary refill)

Assessment

- Musculoskeletal assessment can be divided into four classes of patients:
  - Patients with life-/limb-threatening injuries or conditions, including life-/limb-threatening musculoskeletal trauma
  - Patients with other life-/limb-threatening injuries and only simple musculoskeletal trauma
  - Patients with no other life-/limb-threatening injuries and life-/limb-threatening musculoskeletal trauma
  - Patients with only isolated, non-life-/limb-threatening injuries
- Conduct the initial assessment to determine if there are any life-threatening conditions
- Care for those conditions first
- Never overlook musculoskeletal trauma
- Never allow a horrible-looking, but noncritical, musculoskeletal injury to distract from priorities of care
- Six "P's" of musculoskeletal assessment
  - Pain on palpation (tenderness) or pain on movement
  - Pallor—Pale skin or poor capillary refill
  - Paresthesia—"Pins and needles" sensation
  - Pulses—Diminished or absent
  - Paralysis—Inability to move
  - Pressure
- Evaluate an extremity's neurovascular status by assessing distal pulse, motor function, and sensation (before and after movement or splinting)
- Inspect and palpate the injured area for DCAP-BTLS:
  - Deformity
  - Contusions
  - Abrasions
  - Penetrations or punctures
  - Burns

- Tenderness
- Lacerations
- Swelling
- Compare the injured extremity with the opposite, uninjured extremity
- If extremity trauma is suspected, immobilize the injury by splinting

General Principles of Splinting

- The goal of splinting is immobilization of the injured body part
- Immobilization by splinting:
  - Helps alleviate pain
  - Decreases tissue injury, bleeding, and contamination in an open wound
  - Simplifies and facilitates transport of the patient
- Splint joints above and below, including bone ends
- Immobilize open and closed fractures in the same manner
- Cover open fractures to reduce contamination
- Check pulses, sensation, and motor function before and after splinting
- Stabilize the extremity with gentle, in-line traction to a position of normal alignment
- Immobilize long bone extremity in a straight position that can easily be splinted
- Immobilize dislocations in position of comfort; ensure good vascular supply
- Immobilize joints as found; joint injuries are aligned only if there is no distal pulse
- Apply cold to reduce swelling and pain
- Apply compression to reduce swelling
- Elevate the extremity if possible
- Types of splints
  - Rigid splints
    - — Cannot be changed in shape and require that the body part be positioned to fit the splint's design
  - Board splints
  - Soft or formable splints
    - — Can be molded into various shapes to accommodate injured body part:
      Pillows
      Blankets

UPPER-EXTREMITY INJURIES

Shoulder Injury

- Common in the older adult because of weaker bone structure
- Frequently results from a fall on an outstretched arm
- Anterior fracture or dislocation (accounting for 90% of cases)
  - Patient often positioned with the affected arm/shoulder close to the chest
  - Lateral aspect of the shoulder appears flat instead of rounded
  - Deep depression between the head of the humerus and the acromion laterally ("hollow shoulder")
- Posterior fracture or dislocation
  - Patients may be positioned with the arm above the head
  - Assessment of neurovascular status

Management

- Application of a sling and swathe.
- Application of a cold pack.
- Splinting may need to be improvised to hold the injury in place.
- Use a rolled blanket with a cravat through the center.
- Position the blanket roll under the elevated arm and secure it like a sling.
- Then swathe the arm to prevent movement.
- If the patient's arm is positioned above the head, it should be splinted in position.
- Alternatively, traction can be applied on the long axis of the arm to obtain a better position for immobilization.

Humerus Injury

- Common in older adults and children
- Often difficult to stabilize
- Radial nerve damage may be present if a fracture occurs in the middle or distal portion of the humeral shaft
- Fracture of the humeral neck may cause axillary nerve damage
- Internal hemorrhage into the joint may also be a complication

Management

- Assessment of neurovascular status
- Traction if there is vascular compromise
- Application of a rigid splint and sling and swathe or splinting the extremity with the arm extended
- Application of a cold pack

Elbow Injury

- Common in children and athletes
- Especially dangerous in children
- May lead to ischemic contracture (Volkmann's contracture) with serious deformity to the forearm and a clawlike hand
- Usually involves falling on an outstretched arm or flexed elbow
- Associated complications include laceration of the brachial artery and radial nerve damage

Management

- Assessment of neurovascular status
- Splinting in the position found with a pillow, rigid splint, or sling and swathe
- Application of a cold pack

Radius, Ulna, or Wrist Injury

- Usually result from a fall on an outstretched arm
- Wrist injuries may involve the distal radius, ulnar, or any of the eight carpal bones
- Common injury is a Colles' fracture
- Forearm injuries are common in both children and adults

Management

- Assessment of neurovascular status
- Splinting in the position found with rigid or formable splints or sling and swathe

Hand (Metacarpal) Injury

- Frequently results from:
  - Contact sports
  - Violence (fighting)
  - Crushing in industrial context
- A common injury is boxer's fracture
- Results from direct trauma to a closed fist fracturing the fifth metacarpal bone
- Injuries may be associated with hematomas and open wounds
- Hand injuries should be splinted in the position found

Management

- Assessment of neurovascular status
- Removal of jewelry if possible
- Splinting with rigid or formable splint in position of function (as with a hand grasping a football)
- Application of a cold pack and elevation

Finger (Phalangeal) Injury

- May be immobilized with foam-filled aluminum splints or tongue depressors or by taping injured finger to adjacent one ("buddy splinting")
- Finger injuries are common but should not be considered trivial
- Serious injuries include
- Thumb metacarpal fractures
- Any open fracture
- Markedly comminuted metacarpal or proximal phalanx fracture

Management

- Assessment of neurovascular status
- Splinting
- Application of a cold pack and elevation

LOWER-EXTREMITY INJURIES

Pelvic Fracture

- Blunt or penetrating injury to the pelvis may result in:
  - Fracture
  - Severe hemorrhage
  - Associated injury to the urinary bladder and urethra
- Deformity may be difficult to see since the pelvis is surrounded by heavy muscles and other soft tissues
- Suspect injury to the pelvis based on:
  - Mechanism of injury
  - Presence of tenderness on palpation of the iliac crests

Management

- High-concentration oxygen administration
- Treatment for shock (pneumatic antishock garment [PASG] per protocol)
- Full body immobilization on a long spine board (adequately padded for comfort)
- Regular monitoring of vital signs
- Rapid transport is essential

Hip Injury

- Commonly occurs in older adults because of a fall
- Also occurs in younger patients from major trauma
- If the hip is fractured at the femoral head and neck, the affected leg is usually shortened and externally rotated
- Dislocations of the hip are usually evidenced by a shortened and rotated leg

Management

- Assessment of neurovascular status
- Splinting with a long spine board and generously padding patient for comfort during transport
- Slight flexion of the knee or padding beneath the knee (may improve comfort)
- Frequent monitoring of vital signs

Femur Injury

- Usually results from major trauma (motor vehicle crashes and pedestrian accidents)
- Fairly common result of child abuse
- Fractures are usually evident from the powerful thigh muscles producing overriding of the bone fragments
- Patient generally has a shortened leg that is externally rotated and mid-thigh swelling from hemorrhage
- Bleeding may be life threatening
- Fractures should be immobilized in the field with a traction splint

Management

- High-concentration oxygen administration
- Treatment for shock
- Assessment of neurovascular status
- Application of a traction splint
- Regular monitoring of vital signs

Knee and Patella Injury

- Fractures to the knee (supracondylar fracture of the femur, intra-articular fracture of the femur or tibia) and fractures and dislocations of the patella commonly result from:
  - Motor vehicle crashes
  - Pedestrian accidents
  - Contact sports
  - Falls on a flexed knee
- The relationship of the popliteal artery to the knee joint may lead to vascular injury, particularly with posterior dislocations

Management

- Assessment of neurovascular status
- Splinting in the position found with rigid or formable splint that effectively immobilizes the hip and ankle
- Application of a cold pack and elevation, if possible

Tibia and Fibula Injury

- May result from direct or indirect trauma or twisting injury
- If associated with the knee, popliteal vascular injury should be suspected

Management

- Assessment of neurovascular status
- Splinting with a rigid or formable splint
- Application of a cold pack and elevation

Foot and Ankle Injury

- Fractures and dislocations of the foot and ankle may result from:
    - Crush injury
    - Fall from a height
    - Violent rotary force
    - Patient usually complains of point tenderness and is hesitant to bear weight on the extremity

Management

- Assessment of neurovascular status
- Application of a formable splint, such as a pillow, blanket, or air splint
- Application of a cold pack
- Elevation

Phalanx Injury

- Often caused by "stubbing" the toe on an immovable object
- Injuries are usually managed by buddy taping the toe to an adjacent toe for support and immobilization

Management

- Assessment of neurovascular status
- Buddy splinting
- Application of cold pack
- Elevation

OPEN FRACTURES

- Patients with open fractures require special care and evaluation.
- Fractures may be open in two ways:
    - From within (as when a bone fragment pierces the skin)
    - From without (after a gunshot wound)
- An open fracture may have also made contact with the skin some distance from the fracture site.

- Most are obvious because of associated hemorrhage.
- Small puncture wounds may not be immediately apparent, and bleeding may be minimal.
- Open fractures are considered a true surgical emergency because of the potential for infection.
- Most authorities agree that open wounds should be covered with sterile, dry dressings.
- They should not be irrigated in the field or soaked with any type of antiseptic solution.
- Hemorrhage should be controlled with direct pressure and pressure dressings.
- A visible bone fragment should be covered with a dry, sterile dressing and splinted.
- Bone ends that slip back into the wound during immobilization should be noted and reported to the receiving hospital so that surgical debridement can take place.

Straightening Angulated Fractures and Reducing Dislocations

- Angular fractures and dislocations may pose significant problems in splinting, patient extrication, and transportation.
- Consult with medical direction before manipulation of a fracture or dislocation to facilitate transport or to improve vascular integrity to an extremity.
- Limb-threatening injures include:
  - Knee dislocation
  - Fracture/dislocation of the ankle
  - Subcondylar fractures of the elbow
- These serious injuries require rapid transport for physician evaluation.
- As a rule, fractures and dislocated joints should be immobilized in the position of injury and the patient transported to the emergency department for realignment (reduction).
- If transport is delayed or prolonged, an attempt to reposition a grossly deformed fracture or dislocated joint should be made if circulation is impaired.
- Except for the elbow (which should never be manipulated in the prehospital setting), a grossly deformed fracture or dislocation can often be realigned if necessary without causing additional damage or extreme discomfort to the patient.

Method

- Handle the injury carefully.
- Apply gentle, firm traction in the direction of the long axis of the extremity.
- If there is obvious resistance to alignment, splint the extremity without repositioning.

Specific Techniques for Specific Joints

- Specific techniques for realigning extremity injuries:
  - Only one attempt at realignment should be made in the prehospital setting.
    - — Only if there is severe neurovascular compromise
    - — Only after consulting with medical direction
  - Manipulation (if indicated) should be performed as soon as possible after the injury.
    - — Manipulation should be avoided in the presence of other severe injuries

  - If not contraindicated by other injuries, the use of analgesics (e.g., midazolam [Versed]) for the realignment procedure should be considered.
  - Assess and document pulse, sensation, and motor function before and after manipulating any injured extremity or joint.

Finger Realignment

- Apply in-line traction along the shaft of the finger
- Continue with slow and steady traction until the finger is realigned and the patient feels relief from pain
- Immobilize the finger with a splint device or by buddy splinting

Shoulder Realignment

- Attempt only in the absence of severe back injury
- Check circulatory and sensory status
- Apply slow, gentle longitudinal traction with counter traction exerted on the axilla
- Slowly (and without force) bring the extremity to the midline and realign in the anatomical position while maintaining traction
- Immobilize with sling and swathe

Hip Realignment

- Apply in-line traction along the shaft of the femur with the hip and knee flexed at 90°
- Continue with slow and steady traction to relax the muscle spasm
- Successful realignment will be noted by:
  - A "pop" into the joint
  - Sudden relief of pain
  - Easy manipulation of the leg to full extension
- Immobilize the leg in full extension with patient positioned on long spine board; reevaluate pulses and neurovascular status
- If full extension is not achieved:
  - Immobilize the leg at a flexion not to exceed 90°
  - Immobilize the leg with pillows or blankets
  - Place the patient supine

Knee Realignment

- Apply gentle and steady traction while moving the injured joint into normal position
- Successful realignment will be noted by:
  - A "pop" into the joint
  - Loss of deformity
  - Relief of pain
  - Increased mobility
- Immobilize the leg in full extension (or slight flexion for comfort)
- Position the patient supine on a long spine board

Ankle Realignment

- Apply in-line traction on the talus while stabilizing the tibia
- Successful realignment will be noted by a sudden rotation to a normal position
- Immobilize the ankle in the same manner as a fracture

CHAPTER QUESTIONS

1. Fracture line is at a right angle to the bone's shaft.
   a. Open
   b. Transverse
   c. Closed
   d. Comminuted
2. Fracture line coils through bone like a spring.
   a. Open
   b. Transverse
   c. Closed
   d. Comminuted
   e. Spiral
3. Fracture line crosses shaft at an angle other than right angle.
   a. Open
   b. Transverse
   c. Closed
   d. Oblique
   e. Spiral
4. Bone is only partially broken on one side.
   a. Greenstick
   b. Transverse
   c. Closed
   d. Oblique
   e. Spiral

Suggested Reading

US Department of Transportation, National Highway Traffic Safety Administration. *EMT-Paramedic: National Standard Curriculum*. Washington, DC: US Department of Transportation, National Highway Traffic Safety Administration; 1998.

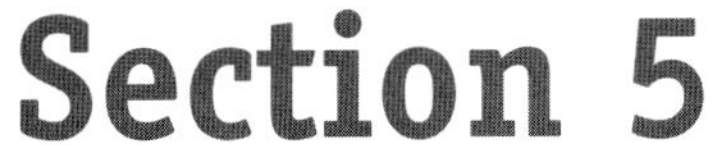

Section 5

Medical Emergencies

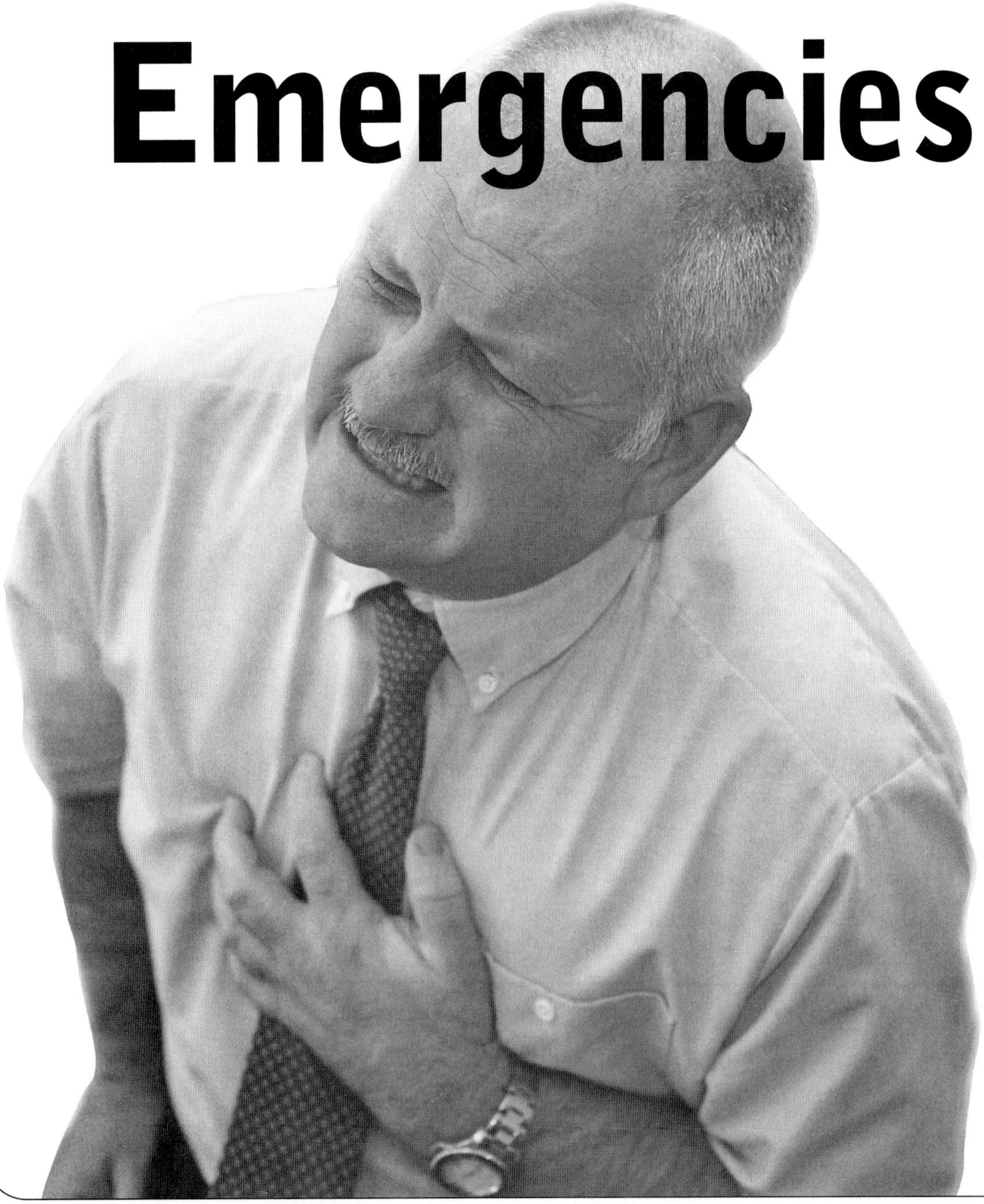

Chapter 22
Pulmonary Emergencies

An emergency medical service (EMS) unit is summoned to a patient with shortness of breath and chest pain. The patient states she is short of breath "I...can't...breathe!" Her husband describes her difficulty in breathing as increasingly getting worse over the last six hours.

Medical history includes high blood pressure, two previous myocardial infarctions, and aortic stenosis.

Social history: cigarette smoking at two packs per day and a social drinker.

Current medications include hydrochlorothiazide, Cardizem (diltiazem), Procardia (nifedipine), and nitroglycerin tablets PRN for chest pain.

Initial assessment reveals BP 210/130, HR 132, pulse is irregular, respiration is labored at 32, rales and rhonchi are heard on lung auscultation, and the skin is pale and diaphoretic. The electrocardiogram shows a sinus tachycardia with premature ventricular contractions (PVCs). The patient is sitting in the tripod position with obvious accessory muscle usage. There are audible rales noted, and the patient is complaining of impending doom.

What is your initial treatment?

What is the prehospital diagnosis of this patient?

PULMONARY

- Respiratory complaints are common in the prehospital setting, accounting for 28% of all EMS-response chief complaints.
- More than 300,000 people die of respiratory emergencies each year in the United States.

RESPIRATORY ANATOMY AND PHYSIOLOGY REVIEW

Upper Airway Structures

Nasopharynx

- Uppermost portion of the airway, just behind the nasal cavities
- Nasal septum separates right and left nasal cavities
- Warms and humidifies the nasal lining and inspired air
- Vestibule (lined with coarse hair) traps foreign substances in inspired air
- Olfactory membranes are located in the roof of the nasal cavity, contain receptors for sense of smell, and connect to the middle ear cavities through the eustachian tubes

Sinuses

- Frontal sinuses
- Maxillary sinuses
- Ethmoid sinuses
- Sphenoid sinuses

Oropharynx

- Begins at the level of the uvula and extends down to the epiglottis
- Opens into the oral cavity
- Lips
- Cheeks
- Teeth
- Tongue
- Hard and soft palates
- Palatine tonsils

Laryngopharynx

- Extends from the tip of the epiglottis to the glottis and esophagus
- Lined with mucous membrane to protect internal surfaces

Larynx

- Three main functions:
  - Air passageway between the pharynx and lungs
  - Prevents solids and liquids from entering the respiratory tree
  - Involved in speech production
- Consists of an outer casing of nine cartilages
  - Largest and most superior cartilage is the unpaired thyroid cartilage (Adam's apple)
  - Most inferior cartilage is the unpaired cricoid cartilage (only complete cartilaginous ring in the larynx)
  - Third unpaired cartilage is the epiglottis
- U-shaped hyoid bone lies beneath the mandible (the only bone of the human body that does not articulate with another bone), and helps suspend the airway by anchoring muscles to the jaw
- Cricothyroid membrane joins the thyroid and cricoid cartilages
- Vestibular folds (false vocal cords)
  - Not directly involved in speech production
  - Formed by the superior pair of ligaments extending from the anterior surface of the largest inferior cartilages (arytenoid cartilages)
- Vocal cords (true vocal cords)
  - Participate directly in voice production
  - Formed by the inferior pair of ligaments extending from the arytenoid cartilages

Lower Airway Structures

Trachea

- Air passage from the larynx to the lungs
- Composed of dense connective tissue reinforced with 15–20 C-shaped pieces of cartilage that form an incomplete ring
  - Protects the trachea
  - Maintains an open air passage

- Located anterior to the esophagus
- Extends from the larynx to the fifth thoracic vertebra (in adults)
- Lined with ciliated epithelium that contains goblet cells
- Protect lower airway by sweeping mucus, bacteria, and foreign substances toward the larynx

Bronchial Tree

- May be thought of as an inverted tree
  - Subdivides until termination at the alveoli
  - Trachea divides into right and left primary bronchi at the carina
  - Right primary bronchus is shorter, wider, and more vertical
  - Both are lined with ciliated epithelium and supported by C-shaped cartilage rings
  - Extend from the mediastinum to the lungs
- Primary bronchi divide into secondary bronchi as they enter the right and left lungs
- Secondary bronchi divide into the tertiary segmental bronchi
  - Extend to individual segments of each lobe (lobule)
  - Eventually become bronchioles

Bronchioles

- Walls are devoid of cartilage
- Muscles are sensitive to circulating hormones (epinephrine)
- Contraction and relaxation of these muscles alter resistance to air flow
- May constrict forcefully (as in asthma)
- Divide to form terminal bronchioles, and finally respiratory bronchioles
- Respiratory bronchioles form alveolar ducts, ending in grapelike clusters of alveoli

Alveoli

- Functional units of respiratory system
- Primary constituent of lung tissue
- 300 million alveoli in the two lungs

Alveolar Walls

- Consist of single layer of epithelial cells and elastic fibers
- Permit stretching and contracting during breathing
- Location of respiratory gas exchange
- Each alveolus is surrounded by a network of blood capillaries
- Air in alveolus is separated from blood contained in the alveolar capillaries by a thin respiratory membrane with a large surface area
- Surface area may be decreased by respiratory diseases
  - Emphysema
  - Lung cancer
  - Decreased surface area restricts gas exchange
- Pulmonary surfactant
  - Thin film that coats alveoli
  - Prevents alveoli from collapsing

Lungs

- Large, paired spongy organs whose principal function is respiration
- Attached to the heart by pulmonary arteries and veins
- Separated by the mediastinum and its contents
- Adult lung weighs less than 2 lb
- Base of each lung rests on the diaphragm, with its apex extending 2.5 cm above each clavicle
- Left lung is slightly smaller than right and is divided into two lobes (divided into lobules)
  - Nine lobules in left lung
  - Ten lobules in right lung
- Separate pleural cavity surrounds each lung
- Attached to each other only at the point of entry of the bronchi, vessels, and nerves of each lung
- Composed of two layers (visceral and parietal)
- Layers are separated by pleural fluid
- Serves as a lubricant to allow the pleural membranes to slide past each other during respiration

Pleural Space

- Potential space between the two pleurae
- May become filled with air (pneumothorax) or blood (hemothorax) with significant chest wall injury or pulmonary pathology
- Other fluid may accumulate in the pleural space due to congestive heart failure, infections, etc.

Physiology

- Respiratory system functions as a gas exchange system
- 10,000 liters of air are filtered, warmed, humidified, and exchanged daily in adults
- Oxygen is diffused into the bloodstream for use in cellular metabolism by the body's 100 trillion cells
- Wastes, including carbon dioxide, are excreted from the body via the respiratory system

PATHOPHYSIOLOGY

- A variety of problems can impact the pulmonary system's ability to achieve gas exchange to provide for cellular needs and the excretion of wastes.
- Specific pathophysiologies responsible for respiratory emergencies include those related to ventilation, diffusion, and perfusion.

Risk Factors Associated with the Development of Respiratory Disease

Intrinsic Factors

- Genetic predisposition
  - Asthma
  - Obstructive lung disease
  - Cancer

- Cardiac or circulatory pathologies
  - Pulmonary edema
  - Pulmonary emboli
- Stress may increase:
  - Severity of respiratory complaints
  - Frequency of exacerbations of asthma and chronic obstructive pulmonary disease (COPD)

Extrinsic Factors

- Smoking increases:
  - Prevalence of COPD and cancer
  - Severity of virtually all respiratory disorders
- Environmental pollutants increase:
  - Prevalence of COPD
  - Severity of all obstructive airway disorders

Physiology

Ventilation

- Ventilation refers to the process of air movement in and out of the lungs.
- In order for ventilation to occur, the following must be intact:
  - Neurological control to initiate ventilation
  - Nerves between the brain stem and the muscles of respiration
  - Functional diaphragm and intercostal muscles
  - Patent upper airway
  - Functional lower airway
  - Alveoli that is functional and noncollapsed
- Specific pathophysiologies associated with ventilation:
  - Upper and lower airway obstruction
  - Chest wall impairment
  - Problems in neurological control
- Emergency interventions of ventilation problems:
  - Ensuring that the upper and lower airways are open and unobstructed
  - Providing assisted ventilation

Diffusion

- Diffusion refers to the process of gas exchange between the air-filled alveoli and the pulmonary capillary bed
- Gas exchange is driven by simple diffusion where gases move from areas of high concentration to areas of low concentration (until the concentrations are equal)
- In order for diffusion to occur, the following must be intact:
  - Alveolar and capillary walls that are not thickened
  - Interstitial space between the alveoli and capillary wall that is not enlarged or filled with fluid
- Specific pathophysiologies associated with diffusion:
  - Inadequate oxygen concentration in ambient air
  - Alveolar pathology

  - Interstitial space pathology
  - Capillary bed pathology
- Emergency interventions for diffusion problems:
  - Providing high-concentration oxygen
  - Taking measures to reduce inflammation in the interstitial space

Perfusion

- Process of circulating blood through the pulmonary capillary bed
- In order for perfusion to occur, the following must be intact:
  - Adequate blood volume
  - Adequate hemoglobin within the blood
  - Pulmonary capillaries that are not occluded
  - Properly functioning left heart that provides smooth flow of blood through the pulmonary capillary bed
- Specific pathophysiologies associated with perfusion:
  - Inadequate blood volume
  - Impaired circulatory blood flow
  - Capillary wall pathology
- Emergency interventions for perfusion problems:
  - Ensuring adequate circulating volumes and hemoglobin levels
  - Optimizing left heart function as necessary

ASSESSMENT FINDINGS

- Pulmonary complaints may be associated with exposure to a variety of toxic environments that have deficient ambient oxygen.
- During scene size-up, ensure a safe environment for all EMS personnel before initiating patient contact.
- Rescue personnel with specialized training and equipment should be used as necessary to ensure scene safety.

Initial Assessment

- Major focus of the initial assessment is the recognition of life-threatening conditions
  - Variety of pulmonary conditions offer a great risk for patient death
  - Recognition of life threats and initiation of resuscitation takes priority over detailed assessment
- Signs of life-threatening respiratory distress in adults include:
  - Alterations in mental status
  - Severe cyanosis
  - Absent breath sounds
  - Audible stridor
  - One- or two-word dyspnea
  - Tachycardia
  - Pallor and diaphoresis
  - Retractions and/or the use of accessory muscles to assist with breathing

Focused History and Physical Exam

- Ascertain the patient's chief complaint
  - Dyspnea
  - Chest pain
  - Cough
    - Productive
    - Nonproductive
    - Hemoptysis
  - Wheezing
- Signs of infection
- Fever/chills
- Increased sputum production
- Get patient's history
  - Previous experiences with similar/identical symptoms.
  - Patient's subjective description of acuity is an accurate indicator of the acuity of this episode if the pathology is chronic.

Known Pulmonary Diagnosis

- If the diagnosis is not known, make an effort to learn whether it is primarily related to ventilation, diffusion, perfusion, or a combination.
- History of previous intubation is an accurate indicator of severe pulmonary disease and suggests that intubation may be required again.

Medication History

- Current medications
- Medication allergies
- Pulmonary medications
  - Sympathomimetic
    - Inhaled
    - Oral
    - Parenteral
  - Corticosteroid
    - Inhaled
    - Oral (daily versus during exacerbations only)
    - Cromolyn sodium
  - Methylxanthines (theophylline preparations)
- Antibiotics
- Cardiac-related drugs

History of the Present Episode

- Exposure/smoking history
- Do a physical exam
- General impression
  - Position
  - Sitting
  - "Tripod" position
  - Feet dangling
  - Mentation (Confusion is a sign of hypoxemia or hypercarbia.)

- Restlessness and irritability may be signs of fear and hypoxemia
- Severe lethargy or coma is a sign of hypercarbia
- Ability to speak one to two word dyspnea versus ability to speak freely
  - Rapid, rambling speech as a sign of anxiety and fear
- Respiratory effort
  - Hard work indicates obstruction
  - Retractions
  - Use of accessory muscles
  - Color
  - Pallor
  - Diaphoresis
  - Cyanosis
  - Central/peripheral

Vital Signs

Pulse

- Tachycardia is a sign of hypoxemia and the use of sympathomimetic medications.
- In the face of a pulmonary etiology, bradycardia is an ominous sign of severe hypoxemia and imminent cardiac arrest.

Blood Pressure

- Hypertension may be associated with sympathomimetic medication use.

Respiratory Rate

- The respiratory rate is not a very accurate indicator of respiratory status unless it is very slow.
- Trends are essential in evaluating the chronic patient.
- Slowing rate in the face of an unimproved condition suggests exhaustion and impending respiratory insufficiency.
- Respiratory patterns
  - Eupnea
  - Tachypnea
  - Cheyne-Stokes
  - Central neurogenic hyperventilation
  - Kussmaul
  - Ataxic (Biot's)
  - Apneustic
  - Apnea
- Head/neck
  - Pursed lip breathing
  - Use of accessory muscles
- Sputum
  - Increasing amounts suggests infection.
  - Thick green or brown sputum suggests infection and/or pneumonia.
  - Yellow or pale gray sputum may be related to allergic or inflammatory etiologies.
  - Frank hemoptysis often accompanies severe tuberculosis or carcinomas.
  - Pink, frothy sputum is associated with severe, late stages of pulmonary edema.

- Jugular venous distention may accompany right-sided heart failure, which may be caused by severe pulmonary obstruction.
- Chest
  - Signs of trauma
  - Barrel chest demonstrates the presence of long-standing chronic obstructive lung disease
  - Retractions
  - Symmetry of the chest
  - Breath sounds
    - Normal sounds
      - Bronchial
      - Bronchovesicular
      - Vesicular
    - Abnormal sounds
      - Stridor
      - Wheezing
      - Rhonchi (low wheezes)
      - Rales (crackles)
      - Pleural friction rub
- Extremities
  - Peripheral cyanosis
  - Clubbing
  - Carpopedal spasm

Prehospital Diagnostic Testing

Pulse Oximetry

- Used to evaluate or confirm the adequacy of oxygen saturation
- May be inaccurate in the presence of conditions that abnormally bind hemoglobin, including:
  - Carbon monoxide poisoning
  - Methemoglobinemia

Peak Flow

- Provides a baseline assessment of airflow for patients with obstructive lung disease

Capnometry

- Provides ongoing assessment of endotracheal tube position
- End-tidal CO_2 drops immediately when the tube is displaced from the trachea

OBSTRUCTIVE AIRWAY DISEASE

- Obstructive airway disease is a major health problem in the United States, affecting 17 million Americans.
- Obstructive airway disease is a triad of distinct diseases that often coexist:
  - Chronic bronchitis and emphysema (together called chronic obstructive pulmonary disease or COPD)
  - Asthma
- Different degrees of each condition are frequently present in the same patient.

- Predisposing factors to obstructive pulmonary disease
  - Smoking
  - Environmental pollution
  - Industrial exposures
  - Various pulmonary infectious processes

Chronic Bronchitis (see Table 22-1)

- A clinical description that refers to inflammatory changes and excessive mucus production in the bronchial tree that affects about 20% of adult males in the United States.
- Characterized by hyperplasia and hypertrophy of mucus-producing glands that result from prolonged exposure to irritants (most commonly, cigarette smoke).
- Clinically diagnosed by the presence of a cough with sputum production occurring on most days for at least 3 months in the year and for at least 2 consecutive years.
- Alveoli are not seriously affected, and diffusion remains relatively normal.
- Patients have a low oxygen pressure (PO_2) because of altered ventilation-perfusion relationships in the lung, and hypoventilation.
- Leads to hypercapnia, hypoxemia, and increases in arterial carbon dioxide pressure (PCO_2).
- Frequent respiratory infections eventually result in scarring of lung tissue.
- In time, irreversible changes occur in the lung, which may lead to emphysema or bronchiectasis (an abnormal dilation of the bronchi caused by a pus-producing infection of the bronchial wall).

Emphysema (see Table 22-1)

- Anatomical description of pathological changes in the lung.
- The end stage of a process that progresses slowly for many years.
- Characterized by:
  - Permanent abnormal enlargement of the air spaces beyond the terminal bronchioles
  - Destruction of the alveoli
  - Failure of the supporting structures to maintain alveolar integrity
- Results in:
  - Reduced alveolar functional surface area
  - Reduced elasticity, leading to trapping of air
    - — Residual volume increases while vital capacity remains relatively normal

TABLE 22-1: Signs and Symptoms of Emphysema and Chronic Bronchitis

Emphysema	Chronic Bronchitis
Thin, barrel chest appearance	Typically overweight
Nonproductive cough	Productive cough with sputum
Wheezing and rhonchi	Coarse rhonchi
Pink complexion	Chronic cyanosis
Extreme dyspnea on exertion	Mild, chronic dyspnea
Prolonged inspiration (purse-lipped breathing)	Resistance on inspiration and expiration

- Associated reduction in arterial PO_2 leads to increased red blood cell production and polycythemia (an elevated hematocrit).
  - This elevation in hematocrit is much more common in chronic bronchitis due to chronic hypoxemia.
- Decrease in alveolar membrane surface area and in the number of pulmonary capillaries decreases the area for gas exchange and increases resistance to pulmonary blood flow.
- Patients with emphysema have some resistance to airflow in and out of the lungs.
  - Most of the hyperexpansion results from air trapping secondary to the loss of elastic recoil.
- Normally an involuntary act, expiration becomes a muscular act in patients with COPD.
  - Over time, the chest becomes rigid (barrel shaped), and the patient must use accessory muscles of the neck, chest, and abdomen to breathe.
  - Full deflation of the lungs becomes more difficult and finally impossible.
- Emphysema patients are often thin because of:
  - Poor dietary intake
  - Increased caloric consumption required for the work of breathing
- Patients with emphysema often develop bullae (thin-walled cystic lesions in the lung) from the destruction of alveolar walls.
  - When bullae collapse, they increase the diffusion defect seen with these patients and can lead to pneumothorax.

Assessment

- Patients with COPD are generally aware of and have adapted to their illness.
- A request for emergency care usually indicates that a significant change has occurred.
- Patients usually present with:
  - An acute episode of worsening dyspnea (even at rest)
  - An increase or change in sputum production
  - An increase in the malaise that accompanies the disease
  - Nocturnal awakening with dyspnea and wheezing
  - Frequent headaches
- Patient is likely to be in respiratory distress:
  - Will often be sitting upright and leaning forward to facilitate breathing
  - Using pursed-lip breathing to maintain positive airway pressure
  - Using accessory muscles
- Increases in hypoxemia and hypercarbia may be evidenced by:
  - Tachypnea
  - Diaphoresis
  - Cyanosis
  - Confusion
  - Irritability
  - Drowsiness
- Other physical findings include:
  - Wheezes
  - Rhonchi
  - Crackles

- Breath sounds and heart sounds may be diminished because of:
  - Reduced air exchange
  - Increased diameter of the thoracic cavity
- Late stages of decompensation may result in:
  - Peripheral cyanosis
  - Clubbing of the fingers
  - Signs of right-sided heart failure
  - Cardiac dysrhythmias or signs of atrial enlargement

Management

- The primary goal is correction of hypoxemia through improved airflow with oxygen administration and pharmacological therapy.
- Both can produce serious side effects and complications, particularly if the patient has used medication before EMS arrival.
- Obtain a thorough medical history regarding:
  - Medication use
  - Home oxygen use
  - Drug allergies
- Establish an intravenous (IV) line.
- Apply an electrocardiogram (ECG) monitor.
- If the patient has a productive cough, encourage coughing.
  - Collect any sputum and transport it with the patient for laboratory analysis.
- Administer supplemental oxygen
  - Consider the use of pulse oximetry to measure oxygen saturation
  - Assisted ventilation may be needed
  - Intubate as necessary
- Medications used in the prehospital setting to relieve bronchospasm and reduce constricted airways are beta agonists such as metaproterenol (Alupent) and albuterol (Proventil).
- Other medications that may be given after physician evaluation include:
  - Steroids (methylprednisolone)
  - Nebulized anticholinergics (atropine)
  - Occasionally, methylxanthines (aminophylline) for bronchodilation and stimulation of the respiratory drive

Asthma

- Also called reactive airway disease.
- According to the American Lung Association, approximately 20.5 million Americans (6.2 million children) had asthma in 2004.
- Most common in 5–17 years of age.
- Can occur in any decade of life, but the prevalence decreases with age.
- Exacerbating factors tend to be extrinsic in children and intrinsic in adults.
- Childhood asthma often improves or resolves with age, but adult asthma is usually persistent.

Pathophysiology of an Asthma Exacerbation

- Generally occurs in acute episodes of variable duration, between which the patient is relatively symptom free.
- Characterized by reversible airflow obstruction caused by:
  - Bronchial smooth muscle contraction
  - Hypersecretion of mucus, resulting in bronchial plugging
  - Inflammatory changes in the bronchial walls
- With increased resistance to airflow there is:
  - Alveolar hypoventilation
  - Marked ventilation-perfusion mismatching (leading to hypoxemia)
  - Carbon dioxide retention (stimulating hyperventilation)
  - Air trapping
  - Excessive demand on the muscles of respiration
  - Greater accessory muscle use
  - Increasesed potential for respiratory fatigue
- If labored breathing continues, excessive positive intrathoracic pressure may decrease left ventricular preload.
- The result is a transient reduction in cardiac output and systolic blood pressure, with the subsequent physical findings of pulsus paradoxus.
- If the episode continues, hypoxemia and the hemodynamic alterations may lead to death.

Assessment

- Patient is usually sitting upright, leaning forward with hands on knees (tripod position), and using accessory muscles to breathe.
- Respiratory distress is obvious.
- Rapid, loud respirations.
- Audible wheezing may be present.
- Monitor the patient's mental status closely; lethargy, exhaustion, agitation, and confusion are ominous signs of impending respiratory failure.
- Quickly obtain an initial history.
- Questions regarding onset, relative severity, medication use, allergies, and precipitating cause of the exacerbation should be specific and to the point.
- Auscultation may reveal a prolonged expiratory phase, usually with wheezing from the movement of air through the narrowed airways.
- Inspiratory wheezing suggests secretions in large airways.
- A silent chest may indicate such severe obstruction that flow rates are too low to generate breath sounds.
- Other signs of severe asthma include:
  - Diaphoresis and pallor
  - Retractions
  - Inability to speak after only one or two words
  - Pulse rate greater than 130 bpm
  - Respirations greater than 30 bpm
  - Pulsus paradoxus greater than 20 mmHg
  - Altered mental status

Management

- Ensure adequate airway
- Provide high-concentration supplemental oxygen

Reversing the Bronchospasm

- Pharmacological therapy is based on the patient's age and medication use before EMS arrival
- Initial medications prescribed by medical direction will probably be those with a short onset of action
- Medical direction may prescribe IV fluids for rehydration
- Transport in a position of comfort to maximize the use of respiratory muscles
- Monitor for cardiac rhythm disturbances

Pulmonary Function Tests

- Measure peak expiratory flow rate (PEFR)
- Help determine the severity of an asthma exacerbation
- Evaluate the effectiveness of treatment in reversing airway obstruction

Peak Flow Meters

- Requires a cooperative patient (who can make a maximal respiratory effort) and coaching by the paramedic.
- To determine baseline airflow (before drug administration), instruct the patient to fully inflate the lungs and forcefully exhale into the flow meter.
- Compare the reading with standard tables based on height, gender, and race.
- Repeat the measurement throughout treatment to evaluate the patient's response to drug therapy.

Status Asthmaticus

- Severe, prolonged asthma exacerbation that has not been broken with repeated doses of bronchodilators
- May be of sudden onset (resulting from spasm of the airways), or it may be more insidious
- Is frequently precipitated by a viral respiratory infection or prolonged exposure to allergen(s)
- True emergency that requires early recognition and immediate transport
- Patients in imminent danger of respiratory failure

Management

- Treatment guidelines are the same as those for acute asthma exacerbations, but the urgency of rapid transport is more important.
- These patients are usually dehydrated and require IV fluid administration.
- Closely monitor the patient's respiratory status.
- Administer high-concentration oxygen and anticipate the need for intubation and aggressive ventilatory support.
- Continuous bronchodilator therapy may be ordered.

Differential Considerations

- Although wheezing commonly is associated with asthma, it also may be present with other diseases that cause dyspnea.

- Tachypnea, wheezing, and respiratory distress may suggest:
  - Heart failure
  - Pneumonia
  - Pulmonary edema
  - Pulmonary embolism
  - Pneumothorax
  - Toxic inhalation
  - Foreign body aspiration
- Only through gathering a complete history and performing a thorough patient assessment can appropriate emergency care decisions be made.

PNEUMONIA

- Seventh most common cause of death from infectious disease in the United States. According to the American Lung Association, 63,241 people died of pneumonia in 2003.
- Not a single disease, but a group of specific infections that causes an acute inflammatory process of the respiratory bronchioles and the alveoli.
- Caused by bacterial, viral, fungal infection, or aspirated food, liquid, or gases.
- May be spread by:
  - Droplets or contact with infected persons
  - Aspiration of bacteria from one's own nasopharynx
- May be classified as viral, bacterial, mycoplasma, or aspiration pneumonia.
- Frequency of community-acquired pneumonia has risen in recent years due to:
  - Increased percentage of population over age 65
  - Increasing number of patients taking immunosuppressive drugs for the treatment of malignancy, transplantation, or autoimmune disease
- Risk factors:
  - Cigarette smoking
  - Alcoholism
  - Exposure to cold
  - Very young and very old

Viral Pneumonia

- Accounts for 50% of all pneumonia cases.
- Influenza A is the most common type of viral pneumonia.
- Often occurs as epidemics in populations of small groups.
  - School children
  - Army recruits
  - Nursing home residents
- Interstitial infection caused by the virus predisposes the patient to secondary bacterial pneumonia.

Signs and Symptoms

- Productive cough
- Pleuritic chest pain
- Fever that produces "shaking chills"
- May also present with nonspecific complaints (particularly in the elderly and debilitated patients) that include:

- A nonproductive cough
- Headache
- Fatigue
- Sore throat (atypical pneumonia)

Bacterial Pneumonia

- Twenty-five to thirty-five percent of the overall cases of pneumonia.
- The pneumococcus bacillus (Streptococcus pneumoniae) accounts for 90% of all bacterial pneumonias.
- Affects 1 in 500 persons annually.
- Peak incidence in winter and early spring.
- A vaccine now available is 80–90% effective against this type of pneumonia in adults.
- Begins with infection in the alveoli that progressively fills the alveoli with fluid and purulent sputum.
- As the infection spreads from alveolus to alveolus, large areas of the lung, sometimes entire lobes, can become consolidated (filled with fluid and cellular debris).
- Consolidation reduces the available surface area of respiratory membranes and decreases the ventilation-perfusion ratio, both of which may lead to hypoxemia.
- Can result from aspiration of oropharyngeal contents.
- Predisposing risk factors:
  - Coma
  - Seizures
  - Suppressed cough reflex
  - Increased secretion
  - Infection
  - Upper respiratory infection (URI) (influenza)
  - Postoperative infection
  - Foreign body aspiration
  - Alcohol or other drug addiction
  - Cardiac failure
  - Stroke
  - Syncope
  - Pulmonary embolism
  - Chronic illness
    - — Chronic respiratory disease
    - — Diabetes mellitus
    - — Congestive heart failure
  - Prolonged immobilization of patients
  - Compromised immune status

Signs and Symptoms

- Acute shaking chills
- Tachypnea
- Tachycardia
- Cough
- Sputum production
  - Rust colored (classic for pneumococcus)
  - More commonly is yellow, green, or gray
- Malaise

- Anorexia
- Flank or back pain
- Vomiting

If the disease is uncomplicated and treated with antibiotics, the patient begins to recover within 3–5 days, although antibiotics are usually continued for a total of 7–10 days.

Mycoplasmal Pneumonia

- Accounts for 20% of all pneumonia cases
- Caused by infection with Mycoplasma pneumoniae
- Exposure causes mild URI in school-age children and young adults
- Transmission is believed to be through infected respiratory secretions
- Spreads quickly among family members
- Can be treated effectively with antibiotics

Aspiration Pneumonia

- An inflammation of the lung parenchyma resulting from introduction of foreign material into the tracheobronchial tree
- Aspiration syndrome is common in patients who have an altered level of consciousness from:
    - Head injury
    - Seizure activity
    - Use of alcohol or other drugs
    - Anesthesia
    - Infection
    - Shock
    - Intubated patients
    - Patients who have aspirated foreign bodies
- Factors common to victims of aspiration include:
    - Depression of the cough or gag reflex
    - Inability of the patient to handle secretions or gastric contents
    - Alterations in physiological mechanisms to protect the airway
- Aspiration pneumonia may be:
    - Nonbacterial
        - After aspiration of:
            Stomach contents
            Toxic materials
            Inert substances
        - Typically called pneumonitis to distinguish it from infectious pneumonia
    - Bacterial (as a secondary complication)
        - Has a poor prognosis, even with antibiotic therapy

Signs and Symptoms

- Chest pain
- Cough
- Fever

- Dyspnea
- Occasionally, hemoptysis
- General malaise
- Upper respiratory and gastrointestinal (GI) symptoms
- Wheezing
- Fine crackles

If uncomplicated, symptoms usually subside in 7–10 days.

- The physiological effects of aspiration pneumonia are based on the volume and pH of the aspirated substances.
- If the pH is below 2.5 (e.g., aspiration of stomach contents), atelectasis, pulmonary edema, hemorrhage, and cell necrosis may occur.
- Alveolar-capillary membrane may be damaged, leading to exudation and, in severe cases, adult respiratory distress syndrome.
- Patient presentation varies with the scenario and the severity of the insult (i.e., near-drowning, foreign body aspiration, aspiration of gastric contents).

Management

Prehospital care for patients with pneumonia includes:

- Airway support
- Oxygen administration
- Ventilatory assistance as needed
- IV fluids to support blood pressure and to thin and loosen mucus
- Cardiac monitoring
- Transportation for physician evaluation
- Bronchodilator therapy (may be suggested for some patients)
- Suctioning of the airway (may be required in cases of aspiration)

ADULT RESPIRATORY DISTRESS SYNDROME

- Adult respiratory distress syndrome (ARDS) is a form of respiratory failure characterized by acute lung inflammation and diffuse alveolar-capillary injury.
- All disorders that result in ARDS cause severe pulmonary edema.
- Develops as a complication of injury or illness such as:
  - Trauma
  - Gastric aspiration
  - Cardiopulmonary bypass surgery
  - Gram-negative sepsis
  - Multiple blood transfusions
  - Oxygen toxicity
  - Toxic inhalation
  - Drug overdose
  - Pneumonia
  - Infections
- Increased capillary permeability (high-permeability noncardiogenic pulmonary edema) results in a clinical condition in which the lungs are:
  - Wet and heavy
  - Congested

  - Hemorrhagic
  - Stiff
- Decreased perfusion capacity across alveolar membranes requires higher airway pressure for each breath.
- Pulmonary edema associated with ARDS leads to:
  - Severe hypoxemia
  - Intrapulmonary shunting
  - Reduced lung compliance
  - Irreversible parenchymal lung damage (in some cases)
- Unique to this syndrome is that most patients who develop this condition have healthy lungs before the event that caused the disease.
- Complications include:
  - Respiratory failure
  - Cardiac dysrhythmias
  - Disseminated intravascular coagulation
  - Barotrauma
  - Congestive heart failure
  - Renal failure

Management

- Airway management
- High-concentration oxygen administration
- Depending on the underlying cause of ARDS, prehospital management may include:
  - Fluid replacement to maintain cardiac output and peripheral perfusion
  - Drug therapy to support mechanical ventilation
  - Use of pharmacological agents
    - — Corticosteroids to stabilize pulmonary capillary and alveolar walls
    - — Diuretics (all of which are controversial)
- 12–72 hours after the initial injury, patients with ARDS usually have:
  - Tachypnea
  - Labored breathing
  - Impaired gas exchange
- Most patients with moderate-to-severe respiratory distress require mechanical ventilatory support with positive end expiratory pressure (PEEP) or continuous positive airway pressure (CPAP).
  - Both provide positive pressure ventilation
  - Both increase PO_2 by decreasing intrapulmonary shunting and ventilation-perfusion mismatch
  - Both may produce adverse circulatory effects including:
    - — Decreased venous return
    - — Decreased cardiac output
    - — Pulmonary barotrauma
  - This type of ventilatory support requires special training and authorization from medical direction

PEEP

- Maintains a degree of positive pressure at the end of exhalation to keep alveoli open and to push fluid from the alveoli back into the interstitium or capillaries.
- Ventilatory support with PEEP can be accomplished through intubation and the use of a Boehringer valve, a cylinder in which a metal ball is suspended.
  - Boehringer valve is connected to the expiratory port of a bag-valve device and creates PEEP by forcing the patient to exhale against the weight of the metal ball
  - Available in 5-, 10-, and 15-cm water pressures

CPAP

- Transmits positive pressure into the airways of a spontaneously breathing patient throughout the respiratory cycle
- Increase in airway pressure allows for better diffusion of gases and reexpansion of collapsed alveoli, resulting in:
  - Improvement of gas exchange
  - Reduction in the work of breathing
- Can be applied:
  - Invasively (via an endotracheal [ET] tube, creating PEEP)
  - Noninvasively via a face or nose mask
    - Mask CPAP is provided through a tight-fitting face mask connected to a battery-operated breathing circuit with an adjustable FiO_2 and PEEP valve that delivers 5- to 10-cm water pressure
- Reduces the inspiratory work of breathing and lowers mean airway pressures
- Besides managing patients with pulmonary congestion, may also benefit patients with acute blunt and penetrating pulmonary injury and those with obstructive airway disease
- Patients who receive CPAP require much coaching and reassurance

BiPAP (Biphasic Positive Airway Pressure)

- BiPAP conceptually combine partial ventilatory support and CPAP.
- BiPAP is applied by face or nose mask through a noninvasive ventilator device with two settings; the device provides a 5-cm water pressure difference between inspiratory positive airway pressure (IPAP) and expiratory positive airway pressure (EPAP).
- The leak-tolerant system (CPAP is not) allows IPAP and EPAP settings to be titrated to reach a desired PEEP range.
- In selected patients with respiratory distress caused by COPD, pulmonary edema, pneumonia, and asthma, BiPAP may avert the need for ET intubation.

PULMONARY THROMBOEMBOLISM (PULMONARY EMBOLISM OR PE)

- Refers to the blockage of a pulmonary artery by a clot or other foreign material that has traveled there from another place of origin, usually the lower extremities.
- A relatively common disorder that affects about 650,000 individuals each year in the United States. Of this number, about 50,000 (less than 10%) of the patients die of the emboli, 10% within the first hour after blockage.
- PE is responsible for 5% of all sudden deaths.
- Usually begins as a venous disease.

- Most often caused by migration of a thrombus from the large veins of the lower extremities.
  - Can also occur because of fat, air, sheared venous catheters, amniotic fluid, or tumor tissue
- Clot or embolus dislodges and travels through the venous system to the right side of the heart.
  - From there it migrates to the pulmonary arteries, obstructing blood supply to a section of lung
- Most common sites for thrombus formation are the deep veins of the legs and pelvis.
- Contributing factors for the development of venous thrombosis
  - Venostasis
  - Extended travel
  - Prolonged bed rest
  - Obesity
  - Advanced age
  - Burns
  - Varicose veins
  - Venous injury
  - Surgery of the thorax, abdomen, pelvis, or legs
  - Fractures of the pelvis or legs
  - Increased blood coagulability
  - Malignancy
  - Oral contraceptives
  - Congenital or acquired coagulopathies
  - Pregnancy
- Disease
  - Chronic lung disease
  - Congestive heart failure
  - Sickle cell anemia
  - Cancer
  - Atrial fibrillation
  - Myocardial infarction
  - Previous pulmonary embolism
  - Previous deep-vein thrombosis
  - Infection
  - Diabetes mellitus
  - Multiple trauma
    - — Long-bone fracture
    - — Pelvic fracture
- When one or more pulmonary arteries occlude, the embolism produces an area of lung that is ventilated but hypoperfused.
- In response, a reflex bronchoconstriction results from local hypocarbia and the release of various mediators (most notably, histamine and serotonin) from the clot formation.
- Causes blood vessels to constrict.
- If the vascular obstruction is severe (60% or greater blockage of the pulmonary vascular supply), hypoxemia, acute pulmonary hypertension, systemic hypotension, and shock may rapidly occur, with subsequent death.

Signs and Symptoms

- Pulmonary embolus may be small, moderate, or massive.
- Signs and symptoms depend on the location and size of the clot and may include:
  - Dyspnea
  - Cough
  - Hemoptysis (rare)
  - Pain
  - Anxiety
  - Syncope
  - Hypotension
  - Diaphoresis
  - Tachypnea
  - Tachycardia
  - Fever
  - Distended neck veins
  - Chest splinting
  - Pleuritic pain
  - Pleural friction rub
  - Crackles
  - Localized wheezing
- Consider a PE in any patient who has cardiorespiratory problems that cannot be otherwise explained, particularly when the risk factors are present.

Management

- Supplemental high-concentration oxygen
- ECG monitoring
- Pulse oximetry
- Establish IV of normal saline (NS) or lactated ringers (LR)
- Transport patient in a position of comfort
- Definitive care requires hospitalization and thrombolytic or heparin therapy

UPPER RESPIRATORY INFECTION

- URIs affect the nose, throat, sinuses, and larynx.
- They are among the most common of all illnesses, affecting nearly 80 million persons each year.
- These illnesses (which include the common cold, pharyngitis, tonsillitis, sinusitis, laryngitis, and croup) are rarely life threatening.
- They often exacerbate underlying pulmonary conditions and may lead to significant infections in patients with suppressed immune function.
- A variety of bacteria and viruses can cause URIs:
  - Group A streptococci are responsible for 20–30% of cases.
  - 50% have no demonstrated bacterial or viral cause.

Signs and Symptoms

- Sore throat
- Fever
- Chills

- Headache
- Facial pain (sinusitis)
- Purulent nasal drainage
- Halitosis
- Cervical adenopathy
- Erythematous pharynx

Management

- Most URIs are self-limiting and require little prehospital intervention.
- Prehospital care is symptomatic and is based in part on the presence of underlying pulmonary conditions (in which oxygen administration may be appropriate).
- Administration of bronchodilators or corticosteroids may be indicated.
- Throat cultures (if obtained at the scene) require family notification of results and physician follow-up (follow local protocol).

SPONTANEOUS PNEUMOTHORAX

- A primary spontaneous pneumothorax usually results when a subpleural bleb (a cystic lesion on a lobe of the lung) ruptures, allowing air to enter the pleural space from within the lung.
- May occur in apparently healthy persons, usually between 20 and 28 years of age.
  - Often, these persons are males who are tall and thin and have long, narrow chests.
  - In contrast, a secondary spontaneous pneumothorax may sometimes develop from an underlying disease process such as COPD.
- In recent years, the number of spontaneous pneumothoraces has increased in some populations.
  - These groups include people with AIDS who have pneumonia and drug abusers who deeply inhale freebase cocaine, marijuana, or inhalants (such as glue or solvents).
- Most primary spontaneous pneumothoraces are well tolerated by the patient if the pneumothorax does not occupy more than 20% of the hemithorax (partial pneumothorax).

Signs and Symptoms

- Include shortness of breath and chest pain that is often sudden in onset, pallor, diaphoresis, and tachypnea
- In severe cases where the pneumothorax occupies more than 20% of the hemithorax, the following signs and symptoms may be present:
  - Altered mentation
  - Cyanosis
  - Tachycardia
  - Decreased breath sounds on the affected side
  - Local hyperresonance to percussion
  - Subcutaneous emphysema

Management

- Prehospital care is based on the patient's symptoms and degree of respiratory distress.
- High-concentration oxygen administration is indicated to help resolve the pneumothorax.
- Airway, ventilatory, and circulatory support may be required in severe cases.

- Transport in a position of comfort for physician evaluation and possible decompression of the pleural space.
- In some cases, surgery may be indicated to allow for lung reexpansion or to prevent recurrence.

HYPERVENTILATION SYNDROME

- Refers to abnormally deep or rapid breathing that results in excessive loss of carbon dioxide (producing respiratory alkalosis)
- The syndrome produces hypocarbia that leads to:
  - Cerebrovascular constriction
  - Reduced cerebral perfusion
  - Paresthesias
  - Dizziness
  - Feelings of euphoria
- Causes include:
  - Anxiety
  - Hypoxia
  - Pulmonary disease
  - Cardiovascular disorders
  - Metabolic disorders
  - Neurological disorders
  - Drugs
  - Fever
  - Infection
  - Pain
  - Pregnancy

Signs and Symptoms

- Dyspnea with rapid breathing and high minute volume
- Chest pain
- Circumoral tingling
- Carpopedal spasm
- Other assessment findings will vary, based on the cause of the syndrome

Management

- If the syndrome clearly is caused by anxiety (psychogenic dyspnea—a diagnosis of exclusion), prehospital care will primarily be supportive, consisting of calming measures and reassurance.
- If the paramedic suspects that the syndrome is a result of illness (e.g., diabetes, renal disease) or drug ingestion, emergency care also may include oxygen administration, and airway and ventilatory support.
- All patients who are hyperventilating should be calmed, and the paramedic should coach the patient's ventilations.
- If the hyperventilation is severe or complicated by illness or drug ingestion, transport for physician evaluation (consult with medical direction).

LUNG CANCER

- Lung cancer is an epidemic in the United States, with an estimated 150,000 new cases being reported each year.
- Most lung cancer develops in persons between the ages of 55 and 65.
- Of the new cases reported, most will die of the disease within 1 year:
  - 20% will have local lung involvement
  - 25% will have cancer that has spread to the lymph system
  - 55% will have distant metastatic cancer

Risk Factors

- Cigarette smoking (most common cause)
- Passive smoking (exposure to someone else's cigarette smoke)
- Exposure to:
  - Asbestos
  - Radon gas
  - Dust
  - Coal products
  - Ionizing radiation
  - Other toxins

Pathophysiology

- Lung cancer is uncontrolled growth of abnormal cells.
  - At least a dozen different cell types of tumors are associated with primary lung cancer.
- The two major cell types of lung cancer are small-cell lung cancer and non–small-cell lung cancer (which is further divided into squamous cell carcinoma, adenocarcinoma, and large cell carcinoma).
  - Each cell type has a different growth pattern and a different response to treatment.
  - Most abnormal cell growth begins in the bronchi or bronchioles.
- The lung is also a fairly common site of metastasis of non-lung primary cancers (breast cancer).

Signs and Symptoms

- Early-stage disease signs and symptoms are often nonspecific and attributed by the person to the effects of smoking, including:
  - Coughing
  - Sputum production
  - Lower airway obstruction (noted by wheezing)
  - Respiratory illness (e.g., bronchitis)
- As the disease progresses, signs and symptoms may include:
  - Cough
  - Hemoptysis (which may be severe)
  - Dyspnea
  - Hoarseness or voice change
  - Dysphagia
  - Weight loss/anorexia
  - Weakness

Management

- Most lung cancer patients are aware of their disease.
- Prehospital management includes:
  - Airway, ventilatory, and circulatory support
  - Oxygen administration (based on symptoms and pulse oximetry)
  - Transport for physician evaluation
- Depending on the severity of the patient's condition, medical direction may recommend:
  - IV fluids to improve hydration and to thin sputum
- Some patients will have an indwelling vascular access device in place
  - Consult with medical direction regarding the use of these devices for vascular access
- Pharmacological agents such as bronchodilators and corticosteroids to improve breathing
  - Analgesics to relieve pain
- End-stage patients may have advance directives or do not resuscitate orders (DNRs).
- In these cases, emotional support will also be required for family and loved ones.

? CHAPTER QUESTIONS

1. Your 80-year-old female patient has been a three-pack-a-day smoker since age 15, and has chronic bronchitis. She called you today because she has not felt well for about a week and says she is tired of fighting for every breath. You notice she is cyanotic, and has a productive cough. Her cardio respiratory system relies on ______ as the main drive for respiration.
   a. oxygen pressure (PaO_2)
   b. alkalemia
   c. carbon dioxide pressure ($PaCO_2$)
   d. acidemia
2. Over time, patients with severe emphysema or chronic bronchitis rely on _______ as the only remaining respiratory drive.
   a. hypercapnia
   b. hypocapnia
   c. hypoxemia
   d. hypocarbia
3. Sighing with a slow, deep inspiration followed by a prolonged expiration is thought to be a protective reflex to prevent:
   a. hypoxia
   b. pulmonary hypertension
   c. apnea
   d. atelectasis
4. A 22-year-old male is recovering from a fractured femur sustained while snow skiing in New Jersey. Shortly after his friends drove him home, 911 was called because he experienced a sudden onset of shortness of breath and chest pain. His respiratory rate is 32. You suspect:
   a. a pulmonary embolus
   b. pleurisy
   c. a spontaneous pneumothorax
   d. a myocardial infarction

5. As a general rule, application of high-flow oxygen should routinely be applied to all the following, except:
   a. an asthmatic with bilateral wheezing
   b. a chronic obstructive pulmonary disease patient with unilateral rhonchi
   c. an intubated patient with spontaneous respirations
   d. none of the above
6. A factor which increases carbon dioxide blood levels in healthy people is:
   a. digestion
   b. exercise
   c. sleep
   d. hyperventilation
7. Factors which can alter oxygen levels in the blood include all of the following, except:
   a. pulmonary embolus
   b. head injury
   c. hypertension
   d. tuberculosis

Suggested Readings

American Heart Association. *Circulation.* 112 [Suppl I]: IV-51–57; published online before print November 28, 2005, doi:10.1161/CIRCULATIONAHA.105.166556. Accessed on April 22, 2007.

US Department of Transportation, National Highway Traffic Safety Administration. *EMT-Paramedic: National Standard Curriculum.* Washington, DC: US Department of Transportation, National Highway Traffic Safety Administration 1998.

Chapter 23
Cardiology

A 65-year-old male is complaining of sudden onset of palpitations and anxiety. Initial assessment reveals a blood pressure of 102/76, pulse rate of 180, with normal respiration and skin examination. The electrocardiogram shows uncontrolled atrial fibrillation.

Medical history includes high blood pressure, aortic valve replacement, and a prior myocardial infarction.

What is your initial treatment modality?

HEART ANATOMY

- The heart is a two-sided muscular pump consisting of four chambers:
  - Two atria
  - Two ventricles
- The heart is cone-shaped, located in the mediastinum of the thoracic cavity, and is approximately the size of a closed fist (the patient's fist).
- Two-thirds of the heart's mass lies left of midline of sternum.

Pericardium

- Consists of a fibrous outer layer, and a thin inner layer that surrounds the heart.
- Cavity between the two layers contains pericardial fluid that reduces friction as heart moves within pericardial sac.

Coronary Vessels

- Seven large veins carry blood to the heart:
  - Four pulmonary veins carry oxygenated blood from the lungs to the left atrium.
  - Superior and inferior vena cavae carry deoxygenated blood from the body to the right atrium.
  - Coronary sinus carries deoxygenated blood from the walls of the heart to the right atrium.
- Two arteries exit the heart:
  - Aorta carries oxygenated blood from left ventricle to body.
  - Pulmonary trunk carries deoxygenated blood from right ventricle to lungs.
  - Right and left coronary arteries exit aorta and supply heart muscle with oxygen and nutrients.

Heart Chambers and Valves

- Right and left chambers are separated by a septum.
- Interatrial septum separates the right and left atria and the interventricular septum separates the two ventricles.

Atrioventricular Valves

- Allow blood to flow from atria into ventricles, and prevent blood from flowing back to the atria
- Tricuspid valve—Located between the right atrium and right ventricle
- Mitral (bicuspid) valve—Located between the left atrium and left ventricle

Semilunar Valves

- Aortic and pulmonary semilunar valves
- Blood flowing out of ventricles pushes against each valve, forcing it open
- Blood flowing back from aorta or pulmonary trunk toward ventricles causes valves to close

BLOOD FLOW THROUGH THE HEART

Blood from the body is carried into the heart's right atrium by the inferior vena cava (blood from the legs and the lower part of the body) and the superior vena cava (blood from the head, neck, and arms). When the right atrium fills with blood, it contracts, sending blood to the right ventricle through the tricuspid valve.

When the right ventricle fills with blood, it contracts, sending blood to the lungs through the pulmonic semilunar valve into the blood vessels called the pulmonary arteries (deoxygenated blood). In the lungs, blood picks up oxygen, and then returns to the heart's left atrium through blood vessels called the pulmonary veins (oxygenated blood). When the left atrium contracts, it sends blood through the mitral valve to the left ventricle. From the left ventricle, blood is pumped through the aortic semilunar valve out to the aorta and through the body. This cycle occurs over and over.

THE CAPILLARY NETWORK

- Blood is supplied to each capillary network by arterioles.
- Blood flows through the capillary network into venules.
- Flow is regulated by smooth muscle cells (precapillary sphincters).
- Major function is exchange of nutrients and waste products.

Arteries and Veins

- Three layers of elastic tissue comprise all blood vessel walls (except capillaries and venules):
  - Tunica intima (inner layer)
  - Tunica media (middle layer)
  - Tunica adventitia (outer layer)

Types of Arteries

- Conducting arteries (large elastic arteries)
- Distributing arteries (small to medium-sized arteries)
- Arterioles (smallest arteries)

Venules

- Similar in structure to capillaries, collect blood from capillaries and transport blood to small veins.
- Nutrient exchange occurs across the walls of venules.

Veins

- Walls are a continuous layer of smooth muscle cells.
- Medium-sized and large veins carry blood to the venous trunks and then to the heart.
- Large veins have valves that allow blood to flow to, but not from, the heart.
- Prevents backflow of blood, especially in dependent tissues.

Arteriovenous Anastomoses (AV Shunts)

- Allow blood to flow from arteries to veins without passing through capillaries.
- Natural AV shunts occur in the sole of the foot and nail beds where they regulate body temperature.
- Pathological shunts may result from injury or tumors.

Coronary Arteries

- Exclusive suppliers of arterial blood to the heart muscle.
- Left coronary artery carries about 85% of the blood supply to the myocardium.
- Right coronary artery carries the remainder.
- Originate just above the aortic valve where the aorta exits the heart.

Left coronary artery

- Subdivides into left anterior descending and circumflex arteries.
- Left anterior descending (LAD) supplies:
  - Anterior wall of left ventricle and the interventricular septum
- Circumflex supplies:
  - Lateral and posterior portions of left ventricle and part of right ventricle

Right coronary artery

- Right coronary artery supplies:
  - Most of the right atrium and ventricle and the inferior aspect of the left ventricle
- Anastomoses between arterioles of coronary arteries provide collateral circulation.

Coronary Capillaries

- Permit exchange of nutrients and metabolic wastes
- Merge to form coronary veins
- Deliver most of the blood to the coronary sinus, which empties directly into right atrium

Coronary sinus

- Major vein draining myocardium

PHYSIOLOGY

- The heart can be thought of as two pumps in one:
  - A low-pressure pump (right atrium and right ventricle) supplying pulmonary vasculature
  - A high-pressure pump (left atrium and left ventricle) supplying systemic vasculature

NERVOUS SYSTEM CONTROL OF THE HEART

- Extrinsic control by parasympathetic and sympathetic nerves of autonomic nervous system is a major factor influencing:
  - Heart rate
  - Conductivity
  - Contractility
  - Atria supplied with many sympathetic and parasympathetic nerve fibers
  - Ventricles supplied mainly by sympathetic nerves

Sympathetic Control

- Postganglionic sympathetic fibers release norepinephrine.
  - Inotropic effect on myocardium
  - Dromotropic effect on myocardium
  - Chronotropic effect on myocardium
- Sympathetic stimulation of the heart causes dilation of coronary blood vessels along with the constriction of peripheral vessels.
- Ensures that increased oxygen demands of the heart are met by an increase in blood and oxygen supply.
- Cardiac effects of norepinephrine result from stimulation of alpha and beta adrenergic receptors.
- Strong sympathetic stimulation of the heart may significantly increase heart rate.

Parasympathetic Control

- Parasympathetic innervation of the heart is through the vagus nerve.
- Has a continuous inhibitory influence on the heart primarily by decreasing heart rate and, to a lesser extent, contractility.

Hormonal Regulation of the Heart

Sympathetic impulses are transmitted to the adrenal medulla at the same time they are transmitted to all blood vessels, causing the adrenal medulla to secrete epinephrine and norepinephrine.

Epinephrine

- Epinephrine has essentially the same effect on cardiac muscles as norepinephrine, increasing the rate and force of contraction.
- Epinephrine also causes:
  - Constriction of blood vessels in the skin, kidneys, gastrointestinal (GI) tract, and other viscera
  - Dilation of skeletal and coronary vessels

Norepinephrine

- Causes constriction of peripheral blood vessels in most areas of the body
- Stimulates cardiac muscle

Role of Electrolytes

- Myocardial cells are bathed in an electrolyte solution
- Major electrolytes that influence cardiac function:
  - Calcium (Ca+)
  - Potassium (K+) largest intracellular cation
  - Sodium (Na+) largest extracellular cation
  - Magnesium (Mg+)

Electrophysiology of the Heart

- Two basic groups of cells within the myocardium:
  - Specialized cells of the electrical conduction system which are responsible for the formation and conduction of electric current
  - Working myocardial cells that possess the property of contractility

Electrical Activity of Cardiac Cells

- Ions are charged particles that are electrically positive or negative, depending on their ability to accept or donate electrons.
- Cations are ions that have a positive electric charge.
- Anions are negatively charged ions.
- Electrically charged particles may be thought of as small magnets.
- Require energy to push them apart if they have opposite charges.
- Require energy to push them together if they have like electrical charges.

Membrane Potentials

- The electrical magnetic-like attraction gives separated particles of opposite charges potential energy.
- Establishes a membrane potential between the inside and the outside of the cell.
- Electrical charge between the inside and outside of cells is expressed in millivolts (mV).

Resting Membrane Potential

- When the cell is in its "resting" state, the electrical charge difference is called a resting membrane potential (RMP).
- The inside of the cell is negative compared with the outside of the cell membrane.
- RMP is primarily established by the difference between the intracellular potassium ion level and the extracellular potassium ion level.

Depolarization

- Sodium is a positively charged ion on the outside of the cell which has a chemical and electrical gradient.
- Depolarization (electrical conduction) takes place when sodium rushes into the cell, making it more positive on the inside compared with the outside.

Diffusion Through Ion Channels

- The cell membrane:
  - Is relatively permeable to potassium and less permeable to calcium chloride
  - Is minimally permeable to sodium
  - Appears to have individual protein-lined channels that allow passage of a specific ion or group of ions
- Permeability is influenced by:
  - Their electrical charge
  - Their size
  - The proteins that open and close the channels (gating proteins)

Sodium-Potassium Pump

- Actively pumps sodium ions out of the cell and potassium ions in
- Normally transports three sodium ions out for every two potassium ions taken in
- Returns the cell to its resting state

Sodium-Potassium Exchange Pump

Channels

- In cardiac muscle, sodium and calcium ions can enter the cell through two separate channel systems in the cell membrane:
  - Fast channels
  - Slow channels
- Fast channels are sensitive to small changes in membrane potential.
- As the cell drifts toward threshold level (the point at which a cell depolarizes), fast sodium channels open.
- Results in a rush of sodium ions intracellularly and in very rapid depolarization.
- Slow channel selectively permeable to calcium and, to a lesser extent, sodium.

Action Potential

- Rapid depolarization creates a local area of current known as the action potential. After one patch of membrane is depolarized, the electrical charge spreads along the cell surface, opening more channels.
- The cardiac action potential can be divided into five phases (phases 0 through 4) (Fig 23-1).
  - Phase 0 (rapid depolarization phase)
  - Phase 1 (early rapid depolarization phase)
  - Phase 2 (plateau phase)
  - Phase 3 (terminal phase of rapid repolarization)
  - Phase 4

Action Potential of Myocardial Cells

Propagation of action potential

- An action potential at any point on the cell membrane acts as a stimulus to adjacent regions of the cell membrane.
- The excitation process, once started, is spread along the length of the cell and on to the next. A stimulus strong enough to cause a cell to reach the threshold and depolarize (action potential) starts a cascade of depolarization from one cell to another.
- All-or-none principle—A stimulated muscle contracts a nerve impulse either completely or not at all.

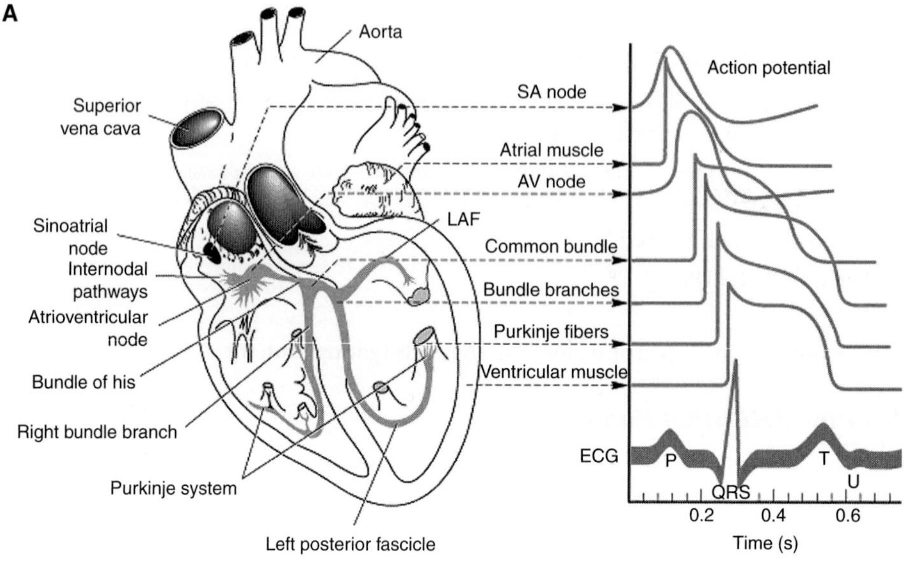

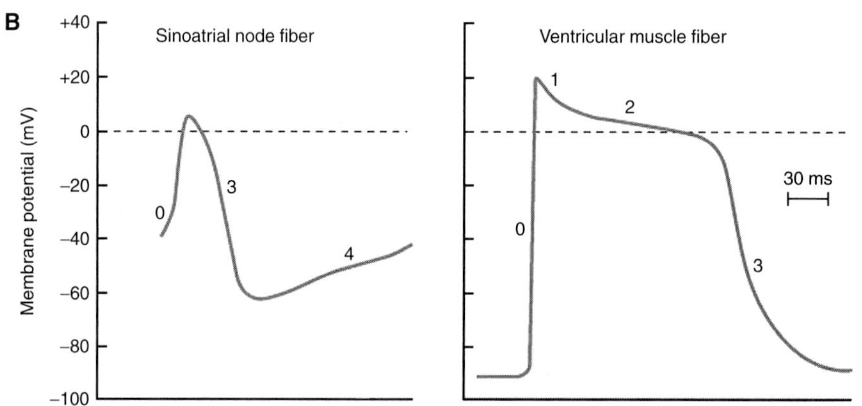

Figure 23-1 Action potential phases. (*Used with permission from Ganong WF: Review of Medical Physiology, 20th ed. McGraw-Hill, 2001.*)

Absolute Refractory Period

During the absolute refractory period, the cardiac muscle cell is completely insensitive to further stimulation. The refractory period of the ventricles is of about the same duration as that of the action potential.

Relative Refractory Period

During the relative refractory period, the muscle cell is more difficult than normal to excite, but it can still be stimulated.

Electrical Conduction System

- Sinoatrial node (SA node)
- Atrioventricular (AV) junction
- AV node
- Bundle of His

- Right and left bundle branches
- Left anterior fascicle
- Left posterior fascicle
- Perkinje system

Characteristics of Myocardial Cells

- Automaticity
- Excitability
- Conductivity
- Contractility

Intrinsic Rates

- SA node (60–100/min)
- AV junctional tissue (40–60/min)
- Ventricles—Bundle branches and Purkinje fibers (20–40/min)

Ectopic Electrical Impulse Formation

- An ectopic beat results when pacemaker function is assumed for one beat by cells other than those in SA node.
- Sometimes called premature beats because they occur early in diastole before the SA node is normally scheduled to discharge.
- Depending on the location of the ectopic focus, the premature beats may be of:
  - Atrial origin—Premature atrial complexes (PACs)
  - Junctional origin—Premature junctional complexes (PJCs)
  - Ventricular origin—Premature ventricular complexes (PVCs)
- Two basic mechanisms by which ectopic electrical impulses can be generated in the heart:
  - Enhanced automaticity
  - Reentry

Enhanced Automaticity

- Caused by an acceleration in depolarization
- Commonly results from an abnormally high leakage of sodium ions into the cells
- Causes the cells to reach threshold prematurely
- As a result, the rate of electrical impulse formation in potential pacemakers increases beyond their inherent rate
- Responsible for dysrhythmias in Purkinje fibers and other myocardial cells
- May occur secondary to:
  - Excess catecholamines (i.e., norepinephrine, epinephrine)
  - Digitalis toxicity
  - Hypoxia
  - Hypercapnia
  - Myocardial ischemia or infarction
  - Increased venous return (preload)
  - Hypokalemia or other electrolyte abnormalities
  - Atropine administration

Reentry

- The reactivation of myocardial tissue for the second or subsequent time by the same impulse
- Occurs when the progression of an electrical impulse is delayed, blocked, or both in one or more segments of the heart's electrical conduction system
- Can occur in the SA node, atria, AV junction, bundle branches, or Purkinje fibers

Delayed Impulses

- Common causes of delayed or blocked electrical impulses:
  - Myocardial ischemia
  - Certain drugs
  - Hyperkalemia

Chief Complaint

- Cardiovascular disease may present with a variety of symptoms.
- Common chief complaints include:
  - Chest pain or discomfort, including shoulder, arm, neck, or jaw pain or discomfort
  - Dyspnea
  - Syncope
  - Abnormal heart beat or palpitations

Chest Pain or Discomfort

- Most common chief complaint of patients with myocardial infarction
- Many causes of chest pain are unrelated to cardiac disease:
  - Pulmonary embolus
  - Pleurisy
  - Reflux esophagitis
- A history of chest pain is important
- Use the OPQRST method (or a similar method) to obtain information when possible

Dyspnea

- Often associated with myocardial infarction
- Primary symptom of pulmonary congestion caused by heart failure
- Common causes of dyspnea that may be unrelated to heart disease include:
  - Chronic obstructive pulmonary disease
  - Respiratory infection
  - Pulmonary embolus
  - Asthma
- Historical factors important in differentiating breathing difficulties:
  - Duration and circumstances of onset of dyspnea
  - Anything that aggravates or relieves the dyspnea, including medications
  - Previous episodes
  - Associated symptoms
  - Orthopnea
  - Prior cardiac problems

Syncope

- Caused by a sudden decrease in cerebral perfusion.
- Cardiac causes of syncope result from events that decrease cardiac output.
- The most common cardiac disorders associated with syncope are dysrhythmias.
- Other causes of syncope in the medical patient include:
  - Stroke
  - Drug or alcohol intoxication
  - Aortic stenosis
  - Pulmonary embolism
  - Hypoglycemia

Syncope History

- Presyncope aura (nausea, weakness, lightheadedness)
- What were the circumstances with this occurence
- Patient's position before the event
- Severe pain
- Emotional stress
- Duration of syncopal episode
- Symptoms before syncopal episode (palpitation, seizure, incontinence)
- Previous episodes of syncope

Palpitations

- Palpitations are sometimes a normal occurrence but may also indicate a serious dysrhythmia.
- Important information to obtain includes:
  - Pulse rate (if obtained)
  - Regular versus irregular rhythm (if obtained)
  - Circumstances of occurrence
  - Duration
  - Associated symptoms (chest pain, diaphoresis, syncope, confusion, dyspnea)
  - Previous episodes, frequency
  - Medications (drug stimulant or alcohol use)

Significant Past Medical History

- Is the patient taking prescription medications, particularly cardiac medications?
- Is the patient being treated for any other illness?
- Has the patient ever had any of the following?
  - Myocardial infarction or episodes of angina pectoris
  - Coronary artery bypass procedure or angioplasty
  - Implanted pacemaker or implantable cardioverter-defibrillator (ICD)
  - Heart failure
  - Hypertension
  - Diabetes
  - Chronic lung disease
- Does the patient have any allergies?
- Are there any other associated risk factors for a cardiac event?

Physical Examination

- The "classic presentation" of myocardial infarction is pain or discomfort beneath the sternum that lasts more than 30 minutes.
- Associated signs and symptoms:
  - Apprehension
  - Diaphoresis
  - Dyspnea
  - Nausea and vomiting
  - Sense of impending doom
- Presentation may also be atypical. A thorough medical history and physical examination are important.

Initial Assessment

- Level of consciousness
- Respirations
- Pulse (rate, regularity)
- Blood pressure

"Look-Listen-Feel" Approach

Look

- Skin color, capillary refill, skin moisture
- Indications of adequate hemoglobin oxygenation (pulse oximetry)
- Indications of cardiac function (peripheral perfusion)
- Jugular vein distention (JVD)
  - Should be evaluated with the patient's head elevated at 45°
  - May be difficult to assess in obese patients
  - Peripheral and presacral edema
    - — Caused by chronic back-pressure in systemic venous circulation
    - — Most obvious in dependent areas (ankles and sacral region in bedridden patients)
  - May be:
    - — Nonpitting—Minimal or no depression of tissue after removal of finger pressure
    - — Pitting—Depression of tissue remains after removal of finger pressure
- Additional indicators of cardiac disease
  - Nitroglycerin patch
  - Midsternal scar from coronary surgery
  - Implanted pacemaker or automatic ICD (left upper chest; abdominal wall)
  - Medic alert information

Listen

- Lung sounds
- Assess for equality
- Assess for adventitious sounds that may indicate pulmonary congestion or edema
- Heart sounds

- May be auscultated for:
  - Frequency (pitch)
  - Intensity (loudness)
  - Duration
  - Timing in the cardiac cycle
- Auscultating heart sounds
  - Aortic—Second intercostal space to the right of the sternum
  - Pulmonic—Second intercostal space to the left of the sternum
- Tricuspid
  - Fifth left intercostal space close to the sternal border
- Mitral
  - Fifth intercostal space just medial to the left midclavicular line
  - Directly over the left ventricle
  - Sometimes called the apical area or apex
- S1
  - The lub of the lub-dub sound produced by the heart
  - Occurs as the mitral and tricuspid valves close
  - Marks the beginning of ventricular systole
  - Best heard with the diaphragm of the stethoscope at the apex of the heart (fifth intercostal space)
- S2
  - The dub of the lub-dub sound
  - Occurs as the aortic and pulmonic valves close
  - Marks the end of ventricular systole
  - Best heard with the diaphragm of the stethoscope at the second intercostal space to the right and left of the sternum (aortic and pulmonic areas)
- S3
  - An extra heart sound associated with rapid ventricular filling
  - Common in children, athletes, and young adults
  - The presence of a third heart sound is considered abnormal in persons over age 30
  - Best heard at the apex with the bell of the stethoscope
  - Sounds like Ken-Tuck-Y with the emphasis on Tuck
  - Ken = S1, Tuck = S2, Y = S3
  - May be a warning sign of impending congestive heart failure
- S4
  - Thought to be due to the last of ventricular filling, tensing of the atrioventricular valves, and atrial contraction
  - Heard just before S1
  - Best heard at the apex with the bell of the stethoscope
  - Sounds like Ten-Nes-See with the emphasis on Ten
  - Ten = S4, Nes = S1, See = S2

Feel

- Peripheral or presacral edema
- Pulse rate
- Regularity

- Equality
- Pulse deficit
- Pulsus paradoxus
- Pulsus alternans
- Skin
  - Diaphoretic pale skin is an indicator of peripheral vasoconstriction and sympathetic stimulation.
  - Cyanosis is an indicator of poor oxygenation.
  - Fever is usually an indicator of infection.

Point of Maximal Impulse (PMI)

- Apical impulse
- Visible and palpable force produced by the contraction of the left ventricle
- Pulse deficits can be noted by palpating or auscultating the apical impulse and the carotid pulse simultaneously

ECG Monitoring

- The electrocardiogram (ECG) is a graphic representation of the heart's electrical activity generated by depolarization and repolarization of the atria and ventricles.
- Valuable diagnostic tool for identifying cardiac abnormalities including:
  - Abnormal heart rates and rhythms
  - Abnormal conduction pathways
  - Hypertrophy or atrophy of portions of the heart
  - Approximate location of ischemic or infarcted cardiac muscle
- The ECG tracing is only a reflection of the heart's electrical activity.
- It does not provide information regarding mechanical events such as force of contraction or blood pressure.
- The summation of all the action potentials transmitted through the heart during the cardiac cycle can be measured on the surface of the body.
- This measurement is obtained by applying electrodes on the body's surface connected to an ECG machine.
- Voltage changes are fed to the machine, amplified, and displayed visually on the oscilloscope, graphically on ECG paper, or both.

Voltage

- Positive—Seen as an upward deflection on the ECG tracing
- Negative—Seen as a downward deflection on the ECG tracing
- Isoelectric—No electrical current detected is seen as a straight baseline on the ECG

ECG Leads

- An ECG lead consists of two surface electrodes of opposite polarity.
- Bipolar lead
  - Two electrodes of opposite polarity
  - Constitutes the standard limb leads (I–III)
- Unipolar lead

- ◦ Single positive electrode and reference point
- ◦ Make up the:
  - — Augmented limb leads (aVR, aVL, and aVF)
  - — Precordial leads (V1–V6)
- Each lead assesses electrical activity from a different angle

Waveforms

- The various leads produce different ECG tracings.
- If the wave of depolarization moves toward a positive electrode, the ECG shows an upward deflection.
- If the wave moves away from a positive electrode, a negative deflection appears on the ECG.

Rule of Electrical Flow

Standard Limb Leads

- Record the difference in electrical potential between the left arm, the right arm, and the left leg electrodes.
- Represent the axis (the average direction of the heart's electrical activity) of the standard limb leads.

Axis

- If the axis is moved so that they cross a common midpoint without changing their orientation, they form three intersecting lines of reference.

Triaxial reference system

- Lead I is a lateral (leftward) lead—Assesses the heart's electrical activity from a vantage point defined as 0° on a circle divided into an upper negative 180° and a lower positive 180°.
- Leads II and III are inferior leads—Assess the heart's electrical activity from vantage points of +60° and +120°, respectively.

Bipolar Lead Placement

- The electrodes of the three bipolar leads are placed on the following areas of the body:
  - ◦ Augmented limb leads
    - — Use the same set of electrodes as the standard limb leads.
    - — Record the difference in electrical potential between the respective extremity. lead sites and a reference point with zero electrical potential at the center of the electrical field of the heart.
    - — The axis of each lead is formed by the line from the electrode site (on the right arm, left arm, or left leg) to the center of the heart.
    - — The aVR, aVL, and aVF leads intersect at different angles than the standard limb leads and produce three other intersecting lines of reference.
    - — With the standard limb leads, these leads make up the hexaxial reference system.
    - — Measure an axis between the two bipolar leads by electronically combining the negative electrodes.

Lead aVR

- Distant recording electrode
- Looks down at heart from right shoulder

Lead aVL

- Acts as a lateral lead
- Records the heart's electrical activity from a vantage point that looks down from the left shoulder (–30°)

Lead aVF

- Acts as an inferior lead
- Records the heart's electrical activity from a vantage point that looks up from the left lower extremity (+90°)

Limb Leads

- Modified lead recording
- Limb lead placement can be altered to mimic the precordial leads (V1–V6)
- Called modified chest leads and become MCL1 through MCL6
- These leads may help:
  - Distinguish between supraventricular tachycardia with aberration and ventricular tachycardia
  - Diagnose conduction blocks in the bundle branches

MCL1

- Positive electrode is placed in the V1 position (in the fourth intercostal space, just to the right of the patient's sternum)
- Negative electrode is placed anteriorly, just below the lateral end of the left clavicle

MCL6

- Positive electrode is placed on the left midaxillary line at the level of the fifth intercostal space (as for lead V6).
- Negative electrode is placed anteriorly, just below the left shoulder.

Routine ECG Monitoring

- Usually obtained in lead II or MCL1
- Best leads to monitor for dysrhythmias because of their ability to visualize P waves

Single-Lead ECG Monitoring

- Information that can be gathered from a single monitoring lead:
  - Heart rate
  - Regularity of heart beat
  - Length of conduction in different parts of the heart
- Limitations—May fail to reveal various abnormalities (particularly ST-segment changes that signal myocardial injury or infarction)

12-Lead ECG Monitoring

- Obtained through 10 electrodes:
  - Four limb leads (right arm, right leg, left arm, left leg)
    - — Provide readings of leads I, II, and III, and aVF, aVL, and aVR

- Six chest leads (V1–V6)
  - Each lead views the left ventricle from the position of its positive electrode
- Can be used to help:
  - Identify ST- and T-wave changes relative to myocardial ischemia, injury, and infarction
  - Identify ventricular tachycardia (VT) in wide-complex tachycardia
  - Determine electrical axis and the presence of fascicular blocks
  - Determine the presence and location of bundle branch blocks

Precordial Leads

- The six precordial leads used in 12-lead (and 9-lead) ECG monitoring are projected through the anterior chest wall toward the patient's back (the negative end of each chest lead).
- These positive leads are placed on the chest in reference to the thoracic landmarks.
- Record the heart's electrical activity in the transverse or horizontal plane.
- Leads V1 and V2 are septal leads.
- V2–V4 are anterior leads.
- V4–V6 are lateral precordial leads.

Application of Monitoring Electrodes

- Electrodes are pregelled, stick-on disks that can easily be applied to the chest wall.
- When applying electrodes:
  - Cleanse the area with alcohol to remove dirt and body oil.
  - Use the inner surfaces of the arms and legs when attaching electrodes to extremities.
- When applying electrodes:
  - Trim excess body hair (if necessary) before placing the electrodes.
  - Attach the electrodes to the prepared site.
  - Attach the ECG cables to electrodes.
  - Turn on the ECG monitor and obtain a baseline tracing.

Monitoring Electrodes

- If the signal is poor, recheck the cable connections and electrode contact with the patient's skin.
- Other causes of a poor signal include:
  - Excessive body hair
  - Dried conductive gel
  - Poor electrode placement
  - Diaphoresis

12-Lead Electrode Application

- From a standard 3-lead monitor, enable the machine's diagnostic setting (if available).
- Run leads I, II, and III.
- Obtain a representative sample of each lead and label it.

- Leave the monitor in lead III (the negative electrode at the left shoulder) and move the left leg cable (the red lead wire) to each of the MCL positions (from V1–V6) to obtain a readout.
- Label each sample.

ECG Graph Paper

- ECG graph paper is standardized to allow comparative analysis of an ECG wave.
- Divided into squares 1 mm in height and width.
- Further divided by darker lines every fifth square, both vertically and horizontally.
- Each large square is 5 mm high and 5 mm wide.
- As the graph paper moves past the stylus of the ECG machine, it measures time and amplitude.
- Time is measured on the horizontal plane (side to side).
- When the ECG is recorded at the standard paper speed of 25 mm/sec:
  - Each small square equals 1 mm (0.04 second)
  - Each large square (the dark vertical lines) equals 5 mm (0.20 second)
  - Amplitude is measured on the vertical axis (top to bottom) of the graph paper
  - Each small square of the graph paper equals 0.1 mV
  - Each large square (five small squares) equals 0.5 mV

Calibration

- The sensitivity of the 12-lead ECG machine is standardized.
- When properly calibrated, a 1-mV electrical signal produces a 10-mm deflection (two large squares) on the ECG tracing.

Time Interval Markings

- Denoted by short vertical lines on the ECG graph paper.
- At standard speed, the distance between each short vertical line is 75 mm (3 seconds).

Relationship of ECG to Electrical Activity

- Each waveform represents the conduction of an electrical impulse through a specific part of the heart.
- All waveforms begin and end at the isoelectric line.
- The isoelectric line represents the absence of electrical activity in cardiac tissue.
- A deflection above the baseline is positive.
  - Indicates electrical flow toward positive electrode
- A deflection below the baseline is negative.
  - Indicates electrical flow away from positive electrode
- The normal ECG consists of a P wave, a QRS complex, and a T wave.
- Other components that should be evaluated:
  - PR interval
  - ST segment
  - QT interval
- The combination of these waves represents a single heartbeat or one complete cardiac cycle.

P Wave

- First positive (upward) deflection on ECG
- Represents atrial depolarization
- Usually rounded and precedes the QRS complex
- Begins with first positive deflection from baseline
- Ends at point where wave returns to baseline
- Duration normally 0.10 second or less
- Amplitude normally 0.5–2.5 mm
- Usually followed by a QRS complex unless conduction disturbances are present

PR Interval

- Represents the time it takes for an electrical impulse to be conducted through the atria and the AV node up to the instant of ventricular depolarization.
- Measured from the beginning of the P wave to the beginning of the next deflection on the baseline (the onset of the QRS complex).
- Normal is 0.12–0.20 second.
- A normal PR interval indicates that the electrical impulse has been conducted through the atria, AV node, and bundle of His normally and without delay.

QRS Complex

- Generally composed of three individual waves: the Q, R, and S waves.
- Begins at the point where the first wave of the complex deviates from the baseline.
- Ends where the last wave of the complex begins to flatten at, above, or below the baseline.
- Direction of the QRS complex may be:
  - Predominantly positive (upright)
  - Predominantly negative (inverted)
  - Biphasic (partly positive, partly negative)
- The normal QRS complex is narrow and sharply pointed.
- Duration is generally 0.08–0.10 second or less.
- Amplitude normally varies from less than 5 mm to more than 15 mm.

Q Wave

- The first negative (downward) deflection of the QRS complex on the ECG
- May not be present in all leads
- Represents depolarization of the interventricular septum

R Wave

- First positive deflection after the P wave.
- Subsequent positive deflections in the QRS complex that extend above the baseline and that are taller than the first R wave are called R prime (R′), R double prime (R″).

S Wave

- Negative deflection that follows the R wave.
- Subsequent negative deflections are called S prime (S′), S double prime (S″), and so on. R and S waves represent the sum of electrical forces resulting from depolarization of the right and left ventricles.

QRS Complex

- Follows the P wave
- Marks the approximate beginning of mechanical systole of the ventricles, which continues through the onset of the T wave
- Represents ventricular depolarization
- Conduction of an electrical impulse from the AV node through the bundle of His, Purkinje fibers, and the right and left bundle branches

ST Segment

- Represents the early phase of repolarization of the right and left ventricles.
- Immediately follows the QRS complex and ends with the onset of the T wave.
- The point at which the ST segment "takes off" from the QRS complex is called the J point.
- The position of the ST segment is commonly judged as normal or abnormal using the baseline of the PR or TP interval as a reference.
- ST segment elevation.
- ST segment depression.
- Abnormal ST segments may be seen in:
  - Infarction
  - Ischemia
  - Pericarditis
  - After digitalis administration

T Wave

- Represents repolarization of ventricular myocardial cells.
- Occurs during the last part of ventricular systole.
- May be above or below the isoelectric line and is usually slightly rounded and slightly asymmetrical.
- Deep and symmetrically inverted T waves may suggest cardiac ischemia.
- A T wave elevated more than half the height of the QRS complex (peaked T wave) may indicate a new onset of myocardial ischemia or hyperkalemia.

QT Interval

- The period from the beginning of ventricular depolarization (onset of the QRS complex) until the end of ventricular repolarization, or the end of the T wave.
- From the peak of the T wave onward, the conduction system is in a relative refractory period in which premature impulses may depolarize the heart while it is vulnerable.

Artifact

- A series of deflections on the ECG display or tracing produced by factors other than the heart's electrical activity
- Common causes of artifact:
  - Improper grounding of the ECG machine
  - Patient movement
  - Loss of electrode contact with the patient's skin
  - Patient shivering or tremors
  - External chest compressions

- Muscle tremors
- AC (60 cycle) interference
- Loose electrode
- Biotelemetry

Rhythm Analysis

- Five questions that must be asked to determine the presence or potential for life-threatening rhythm disturbances:
  - Is the patient sick?
  - What is the heart rate?
  - Are there normal-looking QRS complexes?
  - Are there normal-looking P waves?
  - What is the relationship between P waves and QRS complexes?

Step 1: Analyze the QRS Complex

- Analyze the QRS complex for regularity and width.
- Supraventricular QRS complexes are less than or equal to 0.10 second wide.
- Are the QRS complexes normal?
- Normal QRS complexes
  - Complexes that are equal to or greater than 0.12 second wide indicate either:
    - — A conduction abnormality in the ventricles
    - — A focus that originates in the ventricles and is abnormal
- When evaluating an abnormal QRS width, identify the lead with the widest QRS complex because part of the QRS complex may be blended with the baseline in some leads.

Step 2: Analyze the P Waves

- Are P waves present?
- Are the P waves regular?
- Is there one P wave for each QRS complex, and is there a QRS complex following each P wave?
- Are they upright or inverted?
- Do they all look alike?

Step 3: Analyze the Rate

- If the rate is below 60, it is considered a bradycardia.
- If the rate is equal to or greater than 100, it is considered a tachycardia.

Heart rate rulers

- Available from a number of manufacturers.
- Reasonably accurate if the rhythm is regular.
- A mechanical device or tool should not be solely relied on to determine heart rate since one may not be readily available.
- Heart rate calculator ruler
  - Triplicate method
    - — Requires memorizing two sets of numbers: 300-150-100 and 75-60-50
  - R-R method 1
    - — Measure the distance in seconds between the peaks of two consecutive R waves.
    - — Divide this number into 60 to obtain heart rate.

- R-R method 2
  - Count the large squares between the peaks of two consecutive R waves.
  - Divide this number into 300 to obtain the heart rate.
- R-R method 3
  - Count the small squares between the peaks of two consecutive R waves.
  - Divide this number into 1500 to obtain the heart rate.
- Six-second method
  - Least accurate method of determining heart rate.
  - May be used to quickly obtain an approximate rate in regular and irregular rhythms.
  - Count number of QRS complexes in a 6-second interval and multiply number by 10.

Step 4: Analyze the Rhythm

- To analyze ventricular rhythm, compare R-R intervals systematically from left to right.
- If distances between the R waves are equal or vary by less than 0.16 sec, the rhythm is regular.
- If the shortest and longest R-R intervals vary by more than 0.16 second, the rhythm is "irregular."
- Determining the rhythm:
  - Regular rhythm
  - Regularly irregular rhythm—Patterned irregularity or "group beating"
  - Occasionally irregular—Only one or two R-R intervals are unequal to the others
  - Irregularly irregular—Totally irregular; no relationship between R-R intervals

Step 5: Analyze the PR Interval

- Indicates the time it takes for an electrical impulse to be conducted through the atria and AV node
- Should be constant across the ECG tracing
- Prolonged PR interval
  - Indicates a delay in the conduction of the impulse through the AV node or bundle of His and is called an AV block
- Short PR interval
  - Indicates that the impulse progressed from the atria to the ventricles through pathways other than the AV node

Causes of Cardiac Dysrhythmias

- Myocardial ischemia or necrosis
- Autonomic nervous system imbalance
- Distention of heart chambers
- Acid-base abnormalities
- Hypoxemia
- Electrolyte imbalance
- Drug effects or toxicity

- Electrical injury
- Hypothermia
- Central nervous system (CNS) injury

Classification of Dysrhythmias

- Classification of dysrhythmias can be based on a number of factors, including:
    - Changes in automaticity versus disturbances in conduction
    - Cardiac arrest (lethal) rhythms and noncardiac arrest (nonlethal) rhythms
    - Site of origin

Dysrhythmias Originating in the SA Node

- Sinus bradycardia
- Sinus tachycardia
- Sinus dysrhythmia
- Sinus arrest

Dysrhythmias Originating in the Atria

- Wandering pacemaker
- Premature atrial complex (PAC)
- Paroxysmal supraventricular tachycardia (PSVT)
- Atrial flutter
- Atrial fibrillation

Dysrhythmias Originating in the AV Node

- Premature junctional complex (PJC)
- Junctional escape complexes or rhythms
- Accelerated junctional rhythm

Dysrhythmias Originating in the Ventricles

- Ventricular escape complexes or rhythm
- PVC
- VT
- Ventricular fibrillation (VF)
- Asystole
- Artificial pacemaker rhythm

Disorders of Conduction

- AV blocks
- First-degree AV block
- Second-degree AV block Type I (Wenckebach)
- Second-degree AV block Type II
- Third-degree AV block
- Disturbances of ventricular conduction
- Pulseless electrical activity (PEA)
- Preexcitation syndrome: Wolff-Parkinson-White (WPW) syndrome

Treatment Guidelines

- First, treat the patient, not the monitor!
- Apply different interventions whenever appropriate indications exist.
- Adequate airway, ventilation, oxygenation, chest compression, and defibrillation are more important than administration of medications and take precedence over initiating an IV line or administering pharmacological agents.
- Several medications can be administered via the endotracheal tube:
  - epinephrine
  - lidocaine
  - atropine
  - narcan
  - vasopressin
- Use an endotracheal dose 2–2.5 times the intravenous dose for adults.
- After each IV medication, give a 20- to 30-mL bolus of IV fluid.
- Last, treat the patient, not the monitor.

Dysrhythmias Originating in the SA Node

- Most sinus dysrhythmias result from increases or decreases in vagal tone.
- The SA node generally receives sufficient inhibitory parasympathetic impulses from the vagus nerve to keep the heart rate well below the intrinsic discharge rate of the pacemaker cells.
- If vagal discharge increases, the heart rate becomes bradycardic.
- If vagal discharge decreases, sympathetic stimulation results in sinus tachycardia.
- ECG features common to all SA node dysrhythmias:
  - Normal duration of QRS complex (in the absence of bundle branch block)
  - Upright P waves in lead II
  - Similar appearance of all P waves
  - Normal duration of PR interval (in the absence of AV block)

Sinus bradycardia

- Results from slowing of the pacemaker rate of the SA node

Sinus tachycardia

- Results from an increase in the rate of sinus node discharge

Sinus dysrhythmia

- Present when the difference between the longest and shortest R-R intervals is greater than 0.16 second

Sinus arrest

- Results from a marked depression in SA node automaticity.
- Failure of the sinus node causes short periods of cardiac standstill until lower-level pacemakers discharge (escape beats) or the sinus node resumes its normal function.

Dysrhythmias Originating in the Atria

- May originate in the tissues of the atria or in the internodal pathways
- Common causes of atrial dysrhythmias:
  - Ischemia

- Hypoxia
- Atrial dilation caused by:
  - — Congestive heart failure
  - — Mitral valve abnormalities
  - — Increased pulmonary artery pressures
- ECG features common to all atrial dysrhythmias (provided there is no ventricular conduction disturbance):
  - Normal QRS complexes
  - P waves (if present) that differ in appearance from sinus P waves
  - Abnormal, shortened, or prolonged PR intervals

Wandering Atrial Pacemaker

- The passive transfer of pacemaker sites from the sinus node to other latent pacemaker sites in the atria and AV junction.
- The shift in the site is usually transient, back and forth along the SA node, atria, and AV junction.

Multifocal Atrial Tachycardia

- A variant of wandering atrial pacemaker
- Resembles wandering pacemaker but is frequently associated with rates in the 120–150 per minute range (always considered pathological)
- Most often found in patients with severe chronic obstructive pulmonary disease (COPD) and may respond to treatment of this underlying disorder

Premature Atrial Complex

- A single electrical impulse originating in the atria, outside the sinus node.
- PACs may originate from a single ectopic pacemaker site or from multiple sites in the atria.
- Probably results from enhanced automaticity or a reentry mechanism.

SVT and PSVT

- Supraventricular tachycardias (SVTs) include:
  - Paroxysmal supraventricular tachycardia (PSVT)
  - Nonparoxysmal atrial tachycardia
  - Multifocal atrial tachycardia
  - Junctional tachycardia
  - Atrial flutter
  - Atrial fibrillation

PSVT

- A supraventricular tachycardia that begins abruptly
- Can originate in the atria (paroxysmal atrial tachycardia [PAT]) or AV junction (paroxysmal junctional tachycardia [PJT])
- Results from rapid atrial or junctional depolarization that overrides the SA node

Atrial flutter

- Usually the result of a rapid atrial reentry focus

Atrial fibrillation

- Results from multiple areas of reentry within the atria or ectopic atrial pacemakers outside the SA node
- Electrical activity results in chaotic impulses too numerous for all to be conducted by the AV node through the ventricles
- AV conduction is random
- Ventricular response is irregular but usually rapid unless the patient is on medication (digoxin) to slow the ventricular rate

Dysrhythmias of the AV junction

- When the SA node and the atria cannot generate the electrical impulses needed to begin depolarization, the AV node or the area surrounding the AV node may assume the role of the secondary pacemaker.
- May occur because of:
  - Hypoxia
  - Ischemia
  - Myocardial infarction
  - Drug toxicity
  - Usually a benign dysrhythmia, but must be assessed to determine the patient's tolerance of the rhythm disturbance

Premature junctional complex

- Results from a single electrical impulse originating in the AV junction, which occurs before the next expected sinus impulse

Junctional escape complex or rhythm

- An isolated impulse or rhythm (series of impulses)
- Results when rate of primary pacemaker (usually the SA node) falls below that of AV junction

Accelerated junctional rhythm

- Results from increased automaticity of the AV junction, causing it to discharge faster than its intrinsic rate (40–60 beats per minute), overriding the primary (SA node) pacemaker

Dysrhythmias Originating in the Ventricles

- Ventricular rhythms usually considered life threatening
- Generally result from failure of the atria, AV junction, or both, to initiate an electrical impulse
- Are secondary to enhanced automaticity or reentry phenomena in the ventricles
- May lead to PVCs, VT, and even VF
- Often associated with myocardial ischemia or infarction
- Least efficient pacemaker of the heart

Ventricular escape complexes or rhythms

- An isolated impulse or rhythm (series of complexes)
- Also known as idioventricular rhythm

- Results when impulses from higher pacemakers fail to fire or to reach the ventricles or when the rate of discharge of higher pacemakers falls to less than that of the ventricles
- Serves as a compensatory mechanism to prevent cardiac standstill

Ventricular escape rhythm

- "Dying heart" or agonal rhythm
- PVCs
- A single ectopic impulse arising from an irritable focus in either ventricle (bundle branches, Purkinje fibers, or ventricular muscle)
- Occurs earlier than the next expected sinus beat
- A common dysrhythmia that can occur with any underlying cardiac rhythm
- Results from enhanced automaticity or a reentry mechanism

PVCs

Compensatory pause

- Confirmed by measuring the interval between the R wave before the PVC and the R wave after it
- If the pause is compensatory, the distance equals at least twice the R-R interval of the underlying rhythm
- Interpolated PVC
    - A PVC that falls between two sinus beats without interrupting the rhythm

Unifocal and multifocal PVCs

- Unifocal PVCs originate from a single site within the ventricles and look alike.
- Multifocal PVCs originate from different ventricular sites and have varying shapes and sizes.

Fusion beats

- PVCs that occur at the same time as ventricular activation by the underlying rhythm can cause ventricular depolarization to occur simultaneously in two directions.
- This fusion beat results in a QRS complex that has the characteristics of the PVC and the QRS complex of the underlying rhythm.

Grouped beating

- PVCs frequently occur in patterns of grouped beating:
    - Bigeminy occurs when every other complex is a PVC.
    - Trigeminy occurs when every third complex is a PVC.
    - Quadrigeminy occurs when every fourth complex is a PVC.

Salvos or couplet PVCs

- Consecutive PVCs that are not separated by a complex of the underlying rhythm can also occur on the ECG:
    - Couplets are two PVCs in a row
    - Three or more sequential PVCs at a rate of 100 per minute or more = a run of VT

Causes of PVCs

- Occur in healthy individuals without apparent cause and are usually of no significance
- Pathological PVCs are usually a result of:
    - Myocardial ischemia
    - Hypoxia
    - Acid-base and electrolyte imbalance
    - Hypokalemia
    - Congestive heart failure
    - Increased catecholamine and sympathetic tone (as in emotional stress)
    - Ingestion of stimulants (alcohol, caffeine, tobacco)
    - Drug toxicity
    - Sympathomimetic drugs

Ventricular Tachycardia

- A dysrhythmia defined by three or more consecutive ventricular complexes occurring at a rate of more than 100 beats per minute, which overrides the primary pacemaker.
- Generally starts suddenly, triggered by a PVC.
- During VT, the atria and ventricles are asynchronous.
- If the rhythm disturbance is sustained, the patient's condition may become unstable, possibly leading to unconsciousness and occasionally even to loss of a perfusing pulse.

Criteria for VT

- If extreme right axis deviation is not present, assess the QRS deflection in MCL1 (V1) and MCL6 (V6).
- Regardless of the QRS deflection in leads I, II, and III, positive QRS deflections with either a single peak, a taller left "rabbit ear," or an RS complex with a fat R wave or slurred S wave in MCL1 (V1) indicate VT.
- A negative QS complex, a negative RS complex, or any wide Q wave in MCL6 (V6) also indicates VT.
- Note "rabbit ear."
- If right axis deviation is present (negative QRS complex in lead I; positive QRS complex in leads II and III) and the QRS complex is negative in MCL1 (V1), it indicates VT.
- Right axis deviation and a downward MCLI indicate VT.
- If all precordial leads (V leads) are either positive or negative (precordial concordance), it indicates VT.

VT-concordance

- If the RS interval is greater than 0.10 second in any V lead (increased ventricular activation time), it indicates VT.
- VT (RS interval is 0.16 sec).

Ventricular fibrillation

- A chaotic ventricular rhythm that results in quivering ventricular movements and pulselessness
- Coarse and fine VF
- Refers to absence of all ventricular activity

Artificial Pacemaker Rhythms

- Artificial pacemakers generate a rhythm by regular electrical stimulation of the heart through an electrode implanted in the heart.
- Fixed rate or asynchronous pacemakers.
- Demand pacemakers.
- Atrial synchronous ventricular pacemakers.
- AV sequential pacemakers.
- Rate-responsive pacemakers.

Potential Causes of Pacemaker Malfunction

- Battery failure
- Runaway pacemaker
- Failure of the sensing device in demand pacemaker
- Failure to capture

Heart Blocks

- Partial delays or complete interruptions in cardiac electrical conduction
- Can occur anywhere in the atria, between the SA node and the AV node, or in the ventricles between the AV node and the Purkinje fibers
- May be caused by pathology in the conduction system or by a physiological block, as occurs in atrial fibrillation or atrial flutter
- AV junctional ischemia
- AV junctional necrosis
- Degenerative disease of the conduction system
- Electrolyte imbalances (hyperkalemia)
- Drug toxicity, especially with digitalis

Heart Blocks—Classifications

- Conduction blocks may be classified by several characteristics:
  - Site of block
  - Degree of block
  - Category of AV conduction disturbances

First-degree AV block

- Not a true block but rather a delay in conduction, usually at the level of the AV node. Not considered a rhythm in itself because it is usually superimposed on another rhythm. Underlying rhythm must be identified.

Second-degree AV block type I (wenckebach)

- An intermittent block that usually occurs at the level of the AV node
- Conduction delay progressively increases from beat to beat until conduction to the ventricle is blocked
- Produces a characteristic cyclical pattern in which the PR intervals get progressively longer until a P wave occurs that is not followed by a QRS complex

Second-degree AV block type II

- An intermittent block that occasionally occurs when atrial impulses are not conducted to the ventricles
- Characterized by consecutive P waves being conducted with a constant PR interval before a dropped beat
- Usually occurs in a regular sequence with the conduction ratios (P waves to QRS complexes) such as 2:1

Third-degree heart block

- Results from complete electrical block at or below the AV node (infranodal)
- SA node serves as the pacemaker for the atria, and an ectopic focus serves as a pacemaker in the ventricles
- P waves and QRS complexes occur rhythmically, but the rhythms are unrelated to each other (AV dissociation)

Ventricular conduction disturbances

- Delays or interruptions in the transmission of electrical impulses that occur below the bifurcation of the bundle of His

Bundle Branch Blocks and Hemiblocks

- Common causes of bundle branch block:
  - Ischemic heart disease
  - Acute heart failure
  - Acute myocardial infarction
  - Hyperkalemia
  - Trauma
  - Cardiomyopathy
  - Aortic stenosis
  - Infection
- Bundle branch anatomy
  - Bundle of His begins at the AV node and divides to form the left and right bundle branches
  - Right bundle branch continues toward the apex and spreads throughout right ventricle
  - Left bundle branch subdivides into the anterior and posterior fascicles and spreads throughout the left ventricle
  - Conduction of electrical impulses through the Purkinje fibers stimulates the ventricles to contract
  - Major divisions of ventricular conduction system and possible sites of block and the conduction deficits that may be produced
  - With normal conduction, the first part of the ventricle to be stimulated is the left side of the septum
  - The electrical impulse then traverses the septum to stimulate the other side
  - Shortly after that, the left and right ventricles are simultaneously stimulated

Bundle Branch Block

- When an electrical impulse is blocked from passing through either the right or left bundle branch, one ventricle depolarizes and contracts before the other because ventricular activation is no longer simultaneous; the QRS complex widens, often with a slurred or notched appearance known as "rabbit ears."
- The characteristic of a bundle branch block is a QRS complex that is equal to or greater than 0.12 second.

Two criteria for bundle branch block recognition:

- A QRS complex equal to or greater than 0.12 second
- QRS complexes produced by supraventricular activity
- Best identified by monitoring leads MCL1 and MCL6 (or by monitoring V1 and V6 with a 12-lead machine)
- These leads permit the easiest differentiation of the right and left bundle branch blocks
- Normal conduction
- During normal conduction, MCL1 is predominantly negative, and the QRS complex is usually 0.08–0.10 wide

Right bundle branch block

- In right bundle branch block, the left bundle branch performs normally, activating the left side of the heart before the right
- Initial negative deflection (S wave)
- RSR-prime pattern
- QRS (or in this case, RSR) duration at least 0.12 second

Left bundle branch block

- In left bundle branch block, the fibers that usually fire the interventricular septum are blocked
- This alters normal septal activation and sends it in the opposite direction
- ECG characteristics:
  - Initial Q wave in MCL1
  - R wave in MCL1
  - Deep, wide S wave (QS pattern)
  - QRS duration at least 0.12 second

Anterior Hemiblock

- Occurs more frequently than posterior hemiblock.
- The anterior fascicle of the left bundle branch is a longer and thinner structure, and its blood supply comes primarily from the left anterior descending (LAD) coronary artery.
- Anterior hemiblock is characterized by left axis deviation in a patient who has a supraventricular rhythm.
- Other ECG findings associated with an anterior hemiblock include:
  - A normal QRS complex (less than 0.12 second) or a right bundle branch block
  - A small Q wave followed by a tall R wave in lead I
  - A small R wave followed by a deep S wave in lead III
- These patients are at high risk of developing complete heart block.

Posterior Hemiblock

- Identified by right axis deviation with a normal QRS complex or a right bundle branch block
- Other ECG findings that indicate the presence of a posterior hemiblock:
  - A small R wave followed by a deep S wave in lead I
  - A small Q wave followed by a tall R wave in lead III

Bifascicular Block

- Blockage of two out of three pathways for ventricular conduction
- Occurs in the presence of right bundle branch block with anterior or posterior hemiblock, and in left bundle branch block
- Compromises myocardial contractility and cardiac output
- Patients may develop complete heart block suddenly and without warning

Multilead Determination of Axis and Hemiblocks

- Identifying axis can be useful in determining the presence of hemiblocks
- Best evaluated by looking at the QRS complexes in leads I, II, and III

Axis is considered:

- Normal when the QRS deflection is positive (upright) in all bipolar leads
- Physiologic left (which may be normal in some patients) when the QRS deflection is:
  - Positive in leads I and II
  - Negative (inverted) in lead III
  - Pathological left when the QRS deflection is:
    - — Positive in lead I
    - — Negative in leads II and III (indicating an anterior hemiblock)
  - Right axis when the QRS deflection is:
    - — Negative in lead I, negative or positive in lead II
    - — Positive in lead III (pathologic in any adult)
  - Indicative of a posterior hemiblock
  - Extreme right ("no man's land") when the QRS deflection is negative in all three leads (indicating the rhythm is ventricular in origin)

Pulseless Electrical Activity

- PEA is the absence of a detectable pulse and the presence of some type of electrical activity other than VT or VF.
- Prognosis for PEA invariably is poor unless an underlying cause can be identified and corrected.
- The highest priority of care is to maintain circulation for the patient with basic and advanced life support techniques while searching for a correctable cause.
- Correctable causes:
  - Cardiac tamponade
  - Tension pneumothorax
  - Hypoxemia
  - Acidosis
  - Hyperkalemia
  - Hypothermia
  - Drug overdoses

- Less correctable causes:
  - Massive myocardial damage from infarction
  - Prolonged ischemia during resuscitation
  - Profound hypovolemia
  - Massive pulmonary embolism
  - Patients in profound shock of any type

Preexcitation Syndromes

- Preexcitation syndrome (anomalous or accelerated AV conduction) is a clinical condition associated with an abnormal conduction pathway between the atria and ventricles that bypasses the AV node and/or bundle of His.
- Allows the electrical impulses to initiate depolarization of the ventricles earlier than usual.
- Premature ventricular activation may occur through one of several accessory pathways.
- Most common preexcitation syndrome is WPW syndrome.

Wolff-Parkinson-White Syndrome

Etiology

- P waves—Normal
- Rate—Normal unless associated with rapid supraventricular tachycardia
- Rhythm—Regular
- PR interval—Usually less than 0.12 second, since the normal delay at the AV node does not occur
- Three characteristic ECG findings in WPW:
  - A short PR interval
  - A delta wave
  - QRS widening
- Usual appearance of WPW syndrome in leads where QRS complex is predominantly upright
- Appearance of WPW syndrome with QRS complex predominantly negative

Atherosclerosis

- A disease process characterized by progressive narrowing of the lumen of medium and large arteries
- Results in the development of thick, hard atherosclerotic plaque called atheromas or atheromatous lesions which are most commonly found in areas of turbulent blood flow

Effects of Atherosclerosis

Two major effects on blood vessels:

- The disease disrupts the intimal surface, causing a loss of vessel elasticity and an increase in thrombogenesis.
- The atheroma reduces the diameter of the vessel lumen and thus decreases the blood supply to tissues.

Angina Pectoris

- A symptom of myocardial ischemia
- Literally means "choking pain in the chest"

- Caused by an imbalance between myocardial oxygen supply and demand
- Results in an accumulation of lactic acid and carbon dioxide in ischemic tissues of the myocardium
- These metabolites irritate nerve endings that produce anginal pain
- Most common cause is atherosclerotic disease of the coronary arteries
- A temporary occlusion caused by spasm of a coronary artery with or without atherosclerosis (Prinzmetal's angina) can also cause angina pectoris
- Pain is usually described as a pressure, squeezing, heaviness, or tightness in the chest
- 30% of patients feel pain only in the chest
- Others describe the pain as radiating to the shoulders, arms, neck, and jaw and through to the back
- Associated signs and symptoms:
  - Anxiety
  - Shortness of breath
  - Nausea or vomiting
  - Diaphoresis

Stable Angina

- Usually precipitated by physical exertion or emotional stress
- Pain typically lasts 1–5 minutes but may last as long as 15 minutes
- Relieved by rest, nitroglycerin, or oxygen
- "Attacks" are usually similar in nature and are always relieved by the same mode of therapy

Unstable Angina

- Also called preinfarction angina
- Denotes an anginal pattern that has changed in its ease of onset, frequency, intensity, duration, or quality
- Includes any "new-onset" anginal chest pain
- May occur during periods of light exercise or at rest
- Pain usually lasts 10 minutes or more
- Less promptly relieved with cessation of activity or nitroglycerin than the stable anginal pattern
- The early thrombus has not completely obstructed coronary flow
- Causes an intermittent ischemic episode that may eventually result in complete occlusion and AMI

Myocardial Infarction

- Occurs when there is a sudden and total occlusion or near-occlusion of blood flowing through an affected coronary artery to an area of heart muscle
- Results in ischemia, injury, and necrosis of the area of myocardium distal to the occlusion
- Most often associated with atherosclerotic heart disease (ASHD)

Types and Locations of Infarcts

- Infarction develops distally to the occluded artery.
- Size of the infarct determined by:
  - Metabolic needs of the tissue supplied solely or predominantly by the occluded vessel

  - Presence of collateral circulation
  - Duration of time until flow is reestablished
- Emergency management is aimed at:
  - Increasing oxygen supply by administering supplemental oxygen
  - Decreasing the metabolic needs and providing collateral circulation
  - Reestablishing perfusion to the ischemic myocardium as quickly as possible after the onset of symptoms
- Most AMIs involve the left ventricle or interventricular septum, which is supplied by either of the two major coronary arteries.
- Some patients sustain damage to the right ventricle.
- Anterior, lateral, or septal wall infarction is usually the result of left coronary artery occlusion.
- Inferior wall infarction (of the inferior-posterior wall of the left ventricle) is usually the result of right coronary artery occlusion.
- Infarction can be classified into one of three ischemic syndromes based on the rupture of an unstable plaque in an epicardial artery:
  - Unstable angina
  - Non-ST-elevation myocardial infarction
  - ST-elevation myocardial infarction

Non-ST-Elevation MI

- Evident only with ST-segment depression or T-wave abnormalities

ST-Elevation MI

- Formerly called Q-wave MI
- Diagnosed by development of abnormal Q waves
- Pathologic Q waves
- Greater than 5 mm in depth or greater than 0.04 sec in duration in two or more contiguous leads

Death of Myocardium

- When blood flow to the myocardium ceases, cells switch from aerobic to anaerobic metabolism.
- This contributes to produce ischemic pain (angina).
- As cells lose their ability to maintain their electrochemical gradients, they begin to swell and depolarize.
- If collateral flow and reperfusion are inadequate, much of the muscle distal to the occlusion dies.

Area of Infarction

- Deaths secondary to myocardial infarction usually result from:
  - Lethal dysrhythmias such as VT or VF
  - Cardiac standstill
  - Pump failure
  - Cardiogenic shock
  - CHF
  - Myocardial tissue rupture
  - Rupture of the ventricle, septum, or papillary muscle

Signs and Symptoms

- Pain is similar to anginal pain and may radiate to the arms, neck, jaw, or back
- Dyspnea
- Anxiety
- Agitation
- Sense of impending doom
- Nausea and vomiting
- Diaphoresis
- Cyanosis
- Palpitations
- Chest pain associated with AMI is often constant and is not altered or alleviated by nitroglycerin or other cardiac medications, rest, changes in body position, or breathing patterns
- Onset of pain in over half of all patients with AMI occurs during rest
- Most patients have experienced warning anginal pain (preinfarction angina) hours or days before the attack

Common ECG Findings

- A damaged heart muscle is unable to contract effectively and remains in a constant depolarized state.
- The flow of current between the pathologically depolarized and normally repolarized areas produce abnormal ST-segment elevation on the ECG.
- ST-segment elevation greater than 0.1 mV in at least two contiguous ECG leads suggests AMI.
- ST-segment elevation likely with acute injury.
- ST-elevation and infarct location.
- Multilead assessment of the heart.

Left Ventricular Failure (LVF) and Pulmonary Edema

- LVF occurs when the left ventricle fails to function as an effective forward pump, causing a back-pressure of blood into the pulmonary circulation.
- May be caused by a variety of forms of heart disease including ischemic, valvular, and hypertensive heart disease.
- Untreated, significant LVF culminates in pulmonary edema.

Signs and Symptoms

- Severe respiratory distress
- Severe apprehension, agitation, confusion
- Cyanosis (if severe)
- Diaphoresis
- Adventitious lung sounds
- JVD
- Abnormal vital signs

Right Ventricular Failure (RVF)

- Occurs when the right ventricle fails as an effective forward pump, causing back-pressure of blood into the systemic venous circulation

- Can result from:
  - Chronic hypertension (in which LVF usually precedes RVF)
  - COPD
  - Pulmonary embolism
  - Valvular heart disease
  - Right ventricular infarction
  - RVF most commonly results from LVF

Signs and Symptoms

- Tachycardia
- Venous congestion
- Engorged liver, spleen, or both
- Venous distention; distention and pulsations of the neck veins
- Peripheral edema
- Fluid accumulation in serous cavities
- Chest pain, hypotension, and distended neck veins

Cardiogenic Shock

- The most extreme form of pump failure
- Occurs when left ventricular function is so compromised that the heart cannot meet the metabolic needs of the body
- Usually caused by extensive myocardial infarction, often involving more than 40% of the left ventricle, or by diffuse ischemia

Cardiac tamponade

- Impaired diastolic filling of the heart caused by increased intrapericardial pressure and volume.
- As the volume of pericardial fluid encroaches on the capacity of the atria and ventricles to fill adequately, ventricular filling is mechanically limited and stroke volume is decreased.

Thoracic and Abdominal Aortic Aneurysms

- Aneurysm is a nonspecific term meaning "dilation of a vessel"
- May result from:
  - Atherosclerotic disease (most common)
  - Infectious disease (primarily syphilis)
  - Traumatic injury
  - Certain genetic disorders (such as, Marfan's syndrome)
  - Signs and symptoms of a leaking or ruptured AAA

Pathogenesis of Dissecting Aneurysms

- Medial and intimal degeneration in anotic wall
- Hemodynamic forces produce tear
- Dissecting hematoma propagated by pulse wave

Acute Arterial Occlusion

- A sudden blockage of arterial flow most commonly caused by:
  - Trauma
  - Embolus
  - Thrombosis

- Severity of the ischemic episode depends on:
  - Site of occlusion
  - Quality of collateral circulation around the blockage

Signs and Symptoms

- Pain in the extremity that may be severe and sudden onset or be absent from paresthesia
- Pallor (skin may also be mottled or cyanotic)
- Lowered skin temperature distal to occlusion
- Changes in sensory and motor function
- Diminished or absent pulse distal to the injury
- Bruit over affected vessel
- Slow capillary filling

Venous Thrombosis

- Predisposing factors:
  - History of trauma
  - Sepsis
  - Stasis or inactivity
  - Recent immobilization
  - Pregnancy
  - Birth control pills
  - Malignancy
  - Coagulopathies
  - Smoking
  - Varicose veins

Acute Deep Vein Thrombosis (DVT)

- Occlusion of the deep veins is a serious, common problem.
- May involve any portion of the deep venous system but is much more common in the lower extremities.

Common Causes of Atherosclerotic Occlusive Disease

- Hypertension—Often defined by a resting BP consistently greater than 140/90 mmHg
- There are several categories of hypertension based on level of blood pressure, symptoms, and urgency of need for intervention
- Chronic hypertension—Conditions commonly associated with chronic, uncontrolled hypertension:
  - Cerebral hemorrhage and stroke
  - Myocardial infarction
  - Renal failure (secondary to vascular changes in the kidney)
- Development of thoracic and/or abdominal aortic aneurysm

Hypertensive Emergencies

- Conditions in which a blood pressure increase leads to significant, irreversible end-organ damage within hours if not treated.
- Organs most likely to be at risk are the brain, heart, and kidneys.

Causes

- Myocardial ischemia with hypertension
- Aortic dissection with hypertension
- Pulmonary edema with hypertension
- Hypertensive intracranial hemorrhage
- Toxemia
- Hypertensive encephalopathy

Signs and Symptoms

- Paroxysmal nocturnal dyspnea (PND)
- Shortness of breath
- Altered mental status
- Vertigo
- Headache
- Epistaxis
- Tinnitus
- Changes in visual acuity
- Nausea and vomiting
- Seizures
- ECG changes

Hypertensive Encephalopathy

- Unremitting hypertension produces hypertensive encephalopathy and cerebral hypoperfusion with loss of the integrity of the blood-brain barrier
- Results in fluid exudation into brain tissue
- May progress over several hours from initial symptoms of severe headache, nausea, vomiting, aphasia, hemiparesis, and transient blindness to seizures, stupor, coma, and death
- Adult witnessed cardiac arrest: If a defibrillator is readily available, defibrillation should occur. Unwitnessed cardiac arrest: 2-minutes of CPR should be performed prior to analysis and defibrillation.

Defibrillation

- The delivery of electrical current through the chest wall to terminate VF and pulseless VT.
- The shock depolarizes a large mass of myocardial cells at once.
- If about 75% of these cells are in the resting state (depolarized) after the shock is delivered, a normal pacemaker may resume discharging.
- Early defibrillation is supported by the following rationale:
  - The most frequent initial rhythm in sudden cardiac arrest is VF.
  - The most effective treatment for VF is electrical defibrillation.
  - The probability of successful defibrillation diminishes rapidly over time.
- VF tends to convert to asystole within a few minutes.

> **Note:**
> **Adult witnessed cardiac arrest:** If a defibrillator is readily available, defibrillation should occur. **Unwitnessed cardiac arrest:** 2-minutes of CPR should be performed prior to analysis and defibrillation.

Paddle Electrodes

- Designated by location of use as "apex" or "sternum."
- Place the paddles so that the heart (primarily the ventricles) is in the path of the current, and the distance between the electrodes and the heart is minimized.

Stored and Delivered Energy

- Electrical energy is measured in joules (watt seconds).
- Delivered energy is about 80% of stored energy because of:
  - Losses within the circuitry of the defibrillator and resistance to the flow of current across the chest wall
- As a rule, 80% of stored energy approximates the amount of joules delivered to the patient.

Monophasic Versus Biphasic Defibrillation

- When defibrillating with a monophasic defibrillator start with a joule setting of 360.
- When defibrillating with a biphasic truncated exponential waveform defibrillator the ideal dose is 150-200 joules.
- When defibrillating with a biphasic rectilinear defibrillator the initial dose should be 120joules, second dose of 150 joules, and subsequent dose of 200 joules.
- When it is unknown what type of biphasic defibrillator, a default dose of 200 joules should be used.

Defibrillator Safety

- Clear all personnel from the patient, bed, and defibrillator before a defibrillation attempt.
- Do not make contact with the patient except through the defibrillator paddle handles.
- Do not use excessive gel or coupling material that can become a contact between the patient's chest and the paddle handles.
- Do not discharge paddles over a pacemaker or ICD generator or nitroglycerin paste.
- Remove nitroglycerin patches before defibrillation.
- To prevent gel from the patient's chest being transferred to the paddle handles, do not have one person perform CPR and defibrillation alternately.
- Apply gel or paste before turning on the defibrillator.
- Do not "open air" discharge the defibrillator to get rid of an unwanted charge.
- Turn the defibrillator off to "dump" the charge.
- Do not fire the defibrillator with the paddles placed together.
- Do not touch the metal electrodes or hold the paddles to your body when the defibrillator is on.
- Clean the paddles after use.
- Routinely check the defibrillator (including batteries) to make sure the equipment is functioning properly.

Defibrillator Use in Special Environments

- Patient's chest should be kept dry between the defibrillator electrode sites
- Operator's hands and paddle handles should be kept as dry as possible

Implantable Cardioverter-Defibrillators

- Commonly are implanted through a median sternotomy incision although other approaches are also used
- The ICD functions by monitoring the patient's cardiac rhythm, rate, and QRS morphology

Synchronized Cardioversion

- Used to terminate dysrhythmias other than VF and pulseless VT
- Designed to deliver the shock about 10 minutes after the peak of the QRS complex, avoiding the "vulnerable" relative refractory period

- May reduce the energy required to end the dysrhythmia
- May decrease the potential for development of secondary complicating dysrhythmias

Transcutaneous Cardiac Pacing (TCP)

- Also called external cardiac pacing; utilized in the treatment algorithms for bradycardia and asystole.

CHAPTER QUESTIONS

1. The upper chambers of the heart are called:
   a. ventricles
   b. atria
   c. SA node
   d. AV node
2. The intrinsic firing rate for the SA node is?
   a. 40–60
   b. 20–40
   c. 60–100
   d. None of the above
3. Which valve(s) are considered a semilunar valve?
   a. Mitral
   b. Tricuspid
   c. Pulmonic
   d. Aortic
   e. Both c and d
4. Which valve(s) are considered an atrioventricular valve?
   a. Mitral
   b. Tricuspid
   c. Pulmonic
   d. Aortic
   e. Both a and b

Suggested Readings

Circulation 2005 112 [Suppl I]: IV-51–57; published online before print November 28, 2005, doi:10.1161/CIRCULATIONAHA.105.166556.

Circulation 2005 112 [Suppl I]: IV-58–66; published online before print November 28. 2005, doi:10.1161/CIRCULATIONAHA.105.166557.

Circulation 2005 112 [Suppl I]: IV-67–77; published online before print November 28, 2005, doi:10.1161/CIRCULATIONAHA.105.166558.

Circulation 2005 112 [Suppl I]: IV-84–88; published online before print November 28, 2005, doi:10.1161/CIRCULATIONAHA.105.166560.

Currents in Emergency Cardiovascular Care. 2005–2006; 16(4):16.

US Department of Transportation, National Highway Traffic Safety Administration. *EMT-Paramedic: National Standard Curriculum*. Washington, DC: US Department of Transportation, National Highway Traffic Safety Administration; 1998.

Chapter 24
Neurology

Your unit responds to a report of a patient unresponsive in a local grocery store. Upon arrival, the scene is determined to be safe. You are escorted by an employee who states one of their regular customers was found sitting on the floor by the poultry department. They were unable to ascertain what is wrong because the "patient is unable to speak clearly." As you approach the patient you notice a middle aged woman leaning/sitting against a display unit listing to the left. As you try to determine the patient's mental status, the patient looks at you with a blank stare. You begin assessing the patient and get the following vital signs:

Cincinnati Pre-hospital Stroke scale: Slurred speech, left arm drift, and facial drooping are noted.

B/P: 240/110

Pulse: 82 regular

Respiratory rate: 16 regular, with equal expansion of the chest wall

Skin: warm, dry

Oxygen is administered via nonrebreather at 12 L/min. What treatment should be established? What questions should be elicited from bystanders?

ANATOMY AND PHYSIOLOGY OF THE NERVOUS SYSTEM

- The nervous system is divided into two parts:
  - Central nervous system (CNS)
  - Peripheral nervous system (PNS)
- The human body's ability to maintain a state of homeostasis results primarily from the nervous system's regulatory and coordinating activities.
- The CNS consists of the brain and spinal cord, both of which are encased in and protected by bone (vertabrae).
- 43 pairs of nerves originate from the CNS to form the PNS:
  - 12 pairs of cranial nerves originate from the brain.
  - 31 pairs of spinal nerves originate from the spinal cord.

Cells of the Nervous System

- Cells of the nervous system include the following:
  - Neurons—Fundamental units of the nervous system
  - Neuroglias—Connective tissue cells that protect and hold functioning neurons together
- Each neuron consists of three main parts:
  - The *cell body,* which contains a single, relatively large nucleus with a prominent nucleolus; one or more branching projections called *dendrites;* and a single elongated projection known as an *axon.*
- Dendrites transmit impulses to the neuron cell bodies.

- Axons transmit impulses away from the cell bodies.
  - Axons are surrounded by supportive and protective sheaths formed by the cytoplasmic extensions of neuroglial cells in the CNS (unmyelinated axons) and by the Schwann's cells in the PNS (myelinated axons).
  - Bundles of parallel axons with their associated sheaths are white in color (white matter).
  - The action potential initiated in the neuron body is transmitted forward through the axons via conduction pathways (nerve tracts) from one area of the CNS to another.
- In the PNS, bundles of axons and their sheaths are called nerves.
  - Collections of nerve cells are more gray in color (gray matter).
  - Gray matter is the site of integration within the nervous system.
  - The outer surfaces of the cerebrum and the cerebellum consist of gray matter, which comprises the cerebral cortex and the cerebellar cortex.

Types of Neurons

- Neurons are classified by the direction in which they transmit impulses.
  - *Sensory neurons* transmit impulses to the spinal cord and brain from all parts of the body. They are also called afferent neurons.
  - *Motor neurons* transmit impulses away from the brain and spinal cord (in the opposite direction of sensory neuron transmission) and only to muscle and glandular epithelial tissue. They are also called efferent neurons.
  - *Interneurons* conduct impulses from sensory neurons to motor neurons. They are also called central or connecting neurons.

Impulse Transmission

- Impulse transmission in the nervous system is similar to the conduction of electrical impulses through the heart.
  - In its resting state, the neuron is positively charged on the outside and negatively charged on the inside.
  - When the neuron is stimulated by pressure, temperature, or chemical changes, the permeability of the neuron's membrane to sodium ions increases. As a result, positively charged sodium ions rush into the interior of the neuron.
  - This inward movement begins a wave of depolarization that travels down the axon and results in the propagation of an action potential.
- In unmyelinated axons, action potentials are propagated along the entire axon membrane.
- Myelinated axons, however, have interruptions in the myelin sheaths that are known as nodes of Ranvier.
  - These nodes allow nerve impulses to "jump" from one node to the next without propagation along the entire length of the cell.
  - Myelinated axons conduct action potentials more rapidly than unmyelinated axons.

Synapse

- The synapse is the membrane-to-membrane contact that separates the axon endings of one neuron (presynaptic neuron) from the dendrites of another neuron (postsynaptic neuron).
- The synapse is composed of the following pieces:
  - A presynaptic terminal
  - A synaptic cleft
  - A plasma membrane of the postsynaptic neuron

- Within each presynaptic terminal are synaptic vesicles that contain neurotransmitter chemicals.
- Each action potential arriving at the presynaptic terminal initiates a series of specific events that results in the release of the neurotransmitter substance.
  - The neurotransmitter chemical rapidly diffuses the short distance across the synaptic cleft and binds to specific receptor molecules on the postsynaptic membrane.
  - After an impulse is generated and a conduction by postsynaptic neurons is initiated, neurotransmitter activity ends rapidly.
- Well-known neurotransmitters include the following:
  - Acetylcholine
  - Norepinephrine
  - Epinephrine
  - Dopamine

Reflexes

- A reflex is the basic functional unit of the nervous system that can receive a stimulus and generate a response.
- Reflexes allow unidirectional conduction of impulses and have several basic components:
  - A sensory receptor
  - A sensory neuron
  - Interneurons
  - A motor neuron
  - An effector organ
- Individual reflexes vary in complexity.
  - Some function to remove the body from painful stimuli or prevent the body from suddenly falling or moving because of external forces.
  - Others are responsible for maintaining relatively constant levels of the following:
    - — Blood pressure
    - — Body fluid pH
    - — Blood carbon dioxide
    - — Water intake
- All reflexes are homeostatic; they function to maintain healthy survival.
- Action potentials initiated in sensory receptors are propagated along sensory axons within the PNS to the CNS, where they synapse with interneurons.
- Interneurons synapse with motor neurons in the spinal cord, and then send their axons out of the spinal cord and through the PNS to muscles or glands, thereby causing an effector organ to respond.

Blood Supply

- Arterial blood supply to the brain comes from the vertebral and internal carotid arteries.
- The right and left vertebral arteries (supplying the cerebellum) enter the cranial vault through the foramen magnum and unite to form the midline basilar artery.
  - The basilar artery branches to supply the pons, cerebellum, and bifurcates to form the posterior cerebral arteries, which supply the posterior portion of the cerebrum.
- The internal carotid arteries enter the cranial vault through the carotid canals.
  - These vessels give rise to the anterior cerebral arteries, which supply blood to the frontal lobes of the brain.

  - They terminate by forming the middle cerebral arteries, which supply blood to a large portion of the lateral cerebral cortex.
  - A posterior communicating artery branches off of each internal carotid artery and connects with the ipsilateral posterior cerebral artery.
  - The two posterior cerebral arteries are connected at their common origin from the basilar artery.
  - The anterior cerebral arteries are connected by an anterior communicating artery and thus complete a circle around the pituitary gland and the brain (circle of Willis).
- The circle of Willis provides an important safeguard to help ensure the supply of blood to all parts of the brain in the event of a blockage in the vertebral or internal carotid arteries.
- Veins that drain blood from the head form the venous sinuses (spaces within the dura mater surrounding the brain) and eventually drain into the internal jugular veins.
  - These veins exit the cranial vault and receive several venous tributaries that drain the external head and face.
  - The internal jugular veins join the subclavian veins on each side of the body.

Ventricles

- Each cerebral hemisphere contains a large space filled with cerebrospinal fluid; these spaces are called the lateral ventricles.
- The lateral ventricles are connected posteriorly with the third ventricle, which is located in the center of the diencephalon between the two halves of the thalamus.
- The two lateral ventricles communicate with the third ventricle through two interventricular foramina.
- The third ventricle communicates with the fourth ventricle (located in the superior region of the medulla) by way of a narrow canal known as the cerebral aqueduct.
- The fourth ventricle is continuous with the central canal of the spinal cord.

Divisions of the Brain

- Major divisions of the adult brain:
  - Brainstem
    - — Medulla
    - — Pons
    - — Midbrain
    - — Site of the reticular formation
  - Cerebellum
  - Diencephalon
    - — Hypothalamus
    - — Thalamus
  - Cerebrum

NEUROLOGICAL PATHOPHYSIOLOGY

- Some neurological emergencies affect cerebral blood flow (CBF) because of the following:
  - Structural changes or damage
  - Circulatory changes
  - Alterations in intracranial pressure (ICP)

- Three structures occupy the intracranial space:
  - Brain tissue
  - Blood
  - Water
- Brain tissue contains mostly water, which is found both intracellularly and extracellularly.
- Blood is contained within the following vessels:
  - The major arteries in the base of the brain
  - The arterial branches, arterioles, capillaries, venules, and veins within the substance of the brain
  - The cortical veins and dural sinuses
- Water is located in the following vessels and substances:
  - The ventricles of the brain
  - Cerebrospinal fluid
  - Extracellular and intracellular fluid
- Normally the volumes of brain tissue, blood, and water are such that the pressure inside the skull is maintained within a millimeter of mercury above atmospheric pressure.

Cerebral Perfusion Pressure (CPP)

- Cerebral blood flow depends on cerebral perfusion pressure, which is the pressure gradient across the brain.
- Cerebral blood flow remains constant when the CPP is between 50 and 160 mmHg.
- If the CPP falls below 30 mmHg, the cerebral blood flow (CBF) declines and critically affects cerebral metabolism.
  - The CPP is estimated as mean arterial pressure (MAP) minus intracranial pressure.
  - With mild-to-moderate elevation of ICP, mean arterial pressure usually rises.
  - The rise in MAP causes cerebral blood vessels to constrict and prevents the increase in blood volume and CBF that would normally occur.
  - If the MAP falls, the cerebral arteries dilate and increase cerebral blood flow.
- Between a MAP of about 60 and 150 mmHg, CBF may be maintained in a constant state.
- When ICP elevations are marked (i.e., greater than 22 mmHg), perfusion of brain tissue often decreases despite a rise in systemic arterial pressure.

Assessment of the Nervous System

- As with every patient encounter, care begins with the initial assessment.
- Maintain a systematic approach to avoid overlooking signs and symptoms that may suggest the development of an urgent condition.
- Goals of emergency care:
  - Airway control
  - Stabilization and support of the cardiovascular system
  - Intervention to interrupt ongoing cerebral injury
  - Protection of the patient from further harm

Initial Assessment

- Determine the patient's level of consciousness.
- Ensure an open and patent airway.
- If the patient is unconscious when EMS arrive and there is reason to suspect a cervical spine injury, open the airway with spinal precautions.

- Immobilize the cervical spine.
- Provide ventilatory support and supplemental oxygen for any patient experiencing a neurological emergency.
- Remember that unconscious patients are unable to maintain their airways.
- Airway adjuncts, including tracheal intubation with appropriate spinal precautions, may be indicated.
- Closely monitor the patient for respiratory arrest.
- Respiratory arrest may result from increased ICP and vomiting or aspiration of stomach contents. Suction should be readily available!
- Increased carbon dioxide pressure (PCO_2) or decreased oxygen pressure (PO_2) results in dilation of the blood vessels, presumably in response to greater cerebral metabolic needs.
  - As PCO_2 is lowered, blood volume and flow to the brain are reduced.
  - Controlled hyperventilation may be indicated to maintain the patient's PCO_2 at about 30 mmHg and PO_2 at greater than 80 mmHg.

Physical Examination

- The patient with neurological illness may be difficult to assess if his or her mental function is impaired.
- Important elements of the physical examination that may provide clues to the nature of the neurological emergency include the following:
  - Patient history
  - History of the event
  - Vital signs
  - Respiratory patterns

History

- Attempt to gather a thorough history of the event from the patient or from family members or bystanders.
- Important elements of the patient history:
  - Chief complaint
  - Details of the presenting illness
  - Pertinent underlying medical problems:
    - — Cardiac disease
    - — Lung disease
    - — Neurological disease (multiple sclerosis)
    - — Previous stroke
    - — Chronic seizures
    - — Diabetes
    - — Hypertension
    - — Drug or alcohol use
    - — Previous history of similar symptoms
    - — Recent injury (particularly head trauma)
- If loss of consciousness was involved, ascertain the events that preceded the unconscious state:
  - Patient position, such as sitting, standing, lying down
  - Complaints of a headache
  - Seizure activity

- Fall
- If no history is available, assume the onset of unconsciousness was acute and that an intracranial hemorrhage is likely.

Vital Signs

- Vital signs should be checked and recorded frequently because they often change rapidly in patients with a neurological emergency.
- Monitor the ECG for dysrhythmias, which are common.
- Cushing's triad may be noted in the early stages of increased ICP:
  - An increase in systolic pressure (widening pulse pressure)
  - A decrease in pulse rate
  - Irregular respiratory pattern
- In the terminal stages, as ICP continues to rise and brain tissue is compressed, body temperature usually remains elevated, but the pulse rate generally decreases and the blood pressure falls, particularly after herniation occurs.

Respiratory Patterns

- Respiratory patterns may be normal or abnormal.
- Abnormalities of rate and rhythm may give clues to the mechanisms responsible for the neurological emergency and the level of neurological dysfunction.
- Acute respiratory arrest usually results from involvement of the medullary respiratory center (brainstem compression or infarct).
- Neural pathway involvement (anywhere from the cortex down to the medulla) is more often associated with disturbances of respiratory rhythm rather than with respiratory arrest.
- Abnormal respiratory patterns include the following:
  - Cheyne-Stokes respiration
  - Central neurogenic hyperventilation
  - Ataxic respiration
  - Apneustic respiration
  - Diaphragmatic breathing

Neurological Evaluation

- AVPU scale and the Glasgow coma scale may be used to determine patient's baseline neurological status and to allow comparisons during future treatment.
- Evaluation should be repeated and recorded frequently so changes in the patient's mental state may be detected early. Report and record patient information with descriptive terms specific to responses to certain stimuli.

Posturing, Muscle Tone, and Paralysis

- Significant neurological emergencies may be associated with abnormal or unusual posturing, paralysis of a limb or several limbs, or both.
- Generally disturbances of posture result from the following:
  - Flexor spasms
  - Extensor spasms
  - Flaccidity
- Decorticate rigidity is the abnormal flexor response of one or both arms with extension of the legs. It is thought to result from structural impairment of certain cortical regions of the brain.
- Decerebrate rigidity is the abnormal extensor response of the arms with extension of the legs. It has a worse prognosis than decorticate rigidity. The condition is thought to result from impairment of certain subcortical regions of the brain.

- Flaccidity is usually caused by brainstem or cord dysfunction. It usually involves a poor prognosis. Abnormal reflexes may also be present.
- Positive Babinski's sign—Loss of or diminished Achilles tendon reflex.
- Relaxation of sphincter tone with evacuation of the bowels or bladder.

Pupillary Reflexes

- Pupil examination is important in the unconscious patient.
- Diagnosis of drug intoxication can be suspected on the basis of pupillary appearance and reaction.
- If deviations from normal are observed, note whether these deviations are unilateral or bilateral. If both pupils are dilated and do not react to light:
  - The brainstem has probably been affected
  - The patient has suffered severe cerebral anoxia
- Pupillary constriction is controlled by parasympathetic fibers that originate in the midbrain and accompany the oculomotor nerve.
- Pupillary dilation involves fibers that descend into the entire brainstem and ascend into the cervical sympathetic chains.
- Midbrain failure interrupts both pathways and generally results in fixed, mid-size pupils.
- Compression of the third cranial nerve interrupts parasympathetic tone and is manifested by a unilateral, fixed, dilated pupil.
- Any unconscious patient who suddenly develops a fixed, dilated pupil probably has suffered a significant brain event.
- This type of injury requires immediate transport to an appropriate medical facility.
- Extraocular movements—Conscious patients should be able to move their eyes in full directional ranges. Evaluate extraocular movements by asking the patient to follow the finger movements of the paramedic: to the extreme left, then up and down, to the extreme right, then up and down.
- Record any deviations from normal. Deviation of both eyes to either side (conjugate gaze) at rest implies a structural lesion.
- An "irritative focus" causes the eyes to look away from the lesion.
- A "destructive focus" causes the eyes to look toward the lesion.
- Deviation of the eyes to opposite sides (dysconjugate gaze) at rest implies a structural brainstem dysfunction in the pathways that traverse the brainstem from the upper midbrain to at least the level of the lower pons.

PATHOPHYSIOLOGY AND MANAGEMENT OF SPECIFIC CNS DISORDERS

Coma

- An abnormally deep state of unconsciousness from which the patient cannot be aroused by external stimuli.
- Two mechanisms produce coma:
  - Structural lesions (tumor, abscess) that depress consciousness by destroying or encroaching on the ascending reticular activating system in the brainstem
  - Toxic metabolic states that involve the presence of circulating toxins or metabolites or the lack of metabolic substrate (e.g., oxygen, glucose)
- Either mechanism may cause diffuse depression of both cerebral hemispheres with or without depression of the ascending reticular activating system.

- Within these two mechanisms, there are six general causes of coma.
  - Structural causes include:
    - — Intracranial bleeding
    - — Head trauma
    - — Brain tumor or other space-occupying lesions
  - Metabolic causes include:
    - — Anoxia
    - — Hypoglycemia
    - — Diabetic ketoacidosis
    - — Thiamine deficiency
    - — Kidney and liver failure
    - — Postictal phase of seizure
  - Drugs
    - — Barbiturates
    - — Narcotics
    - — Hallucinogens
    - — Depressants (alcohol)
  - Cardiovascular system
    - — Hypertensive encephalopathy
    - — Shock
  - Dysrhythmias
    - — Stroke
  - Respiratory system
    - — Chronic obstructive pulmonary disease
    - — Toxic inhalation (carbon monoxide poisoning)
  - Infection
    - — Meningitis
    - — Sepsis
- A mnemonic aid that may be useful in remembering the common causes of coma is "AEIOU TIPS."
  - A—Acidosis or alcohol
  - E—Epilepsy
  - I—Infection
  - O—Overdose
  - U—Uremia
  - T—Trauma
  - I—Insulin
  - P—Psychosis
  - S—Stroke

Structural Versus Toxic-Metabolic Coma

- Coma caused by structural causes
  - Focal (asymmetrical) neurological signs
  - Sudden onset
  - Unresponsive or asymmetrical pupillary responses
  - Follows a progressive pattern of deterioration caused by focal pressure or compression

  - Asymmetrical secondary examination (e.g., hemiparesis)
  - As a rule, lesions affect the ascending reticular activating system by virtue of increased ICP and herniation
    - Require rapid surgical correction
- Coma of toxic metabolic origin
  - Neurological findings often symmetrical
  - Often slow in onset
  - Preserved pupillary responses

Assessment and Management

- Whatever the cause of coma, prehospital care is directed at the following:
  - Support of the patient's vital functions
  - Prevention of further deterioration of the patient's condition
  - Administration of medications, IV fluids, or both to treat potentially reversible causes of coma
- Airway maintenance and ventilatory support with supplemental high-concentration oxygen are the priorities in patient stabilization.
- The unconscious patient with no gag reflex should be intubated.
- Establish an IV line to keep the vein open or to manage hypotension (if present).
- Monitor the patient's ECG.
- Draw a blood sample for laboratory analysis (per protocol).
  - If hypoglycemia is suspected, measure serum glucose level
  - Administer 50% dextrose if indicated (per protocol)
  - If alcohol is suspected as the cause of coma, consider thiamine administration before glucose administration (per protocol)
  - If the patient does not respond to glucose, administer naloxone per protocol to rule out or reverse narcotic depression
- If the patient remains in a comatose state, transport the patient in a lateral recumbent position (if not contraindicated) so that the following occur:
  - Drainage of secretions
  - Reduction in the risk for aspiration of stomach contents
- Closely monitor the patient's airway and have suction readily available.
- Protect the patient's eyes from corneal drying by gently closing them and covering the lids with moist gauze pads.

Stroke and Intracranial Hemorrhage

- Stroke (CVA or "brain attack") is a sudden interruption in blood flow to the brain that results in a neurological deficit.
  - Affects more than 500,000 Americans each year
  - Associated with a 30-day mortality rate of about 10–15%
  - Third leading cause of death in the United States
  - Frequently leaves survivors severely debilitated

Risk Factors

- Modifiable risk factors:
  - High blood pressure
  - Cigarette smoking
  - Transient ischemic attacks
  - Heart disease

  - Diabetes mellitus
  - Hypercoagulopathy
  - High red blood cell count and sickle cell anemia
  - Carotid bruit
- Nonmodifiable risk factors:
  - Age
  - Gender
  - Race (African Americans are at greater risk than whites)
  - Prior stroke
  - Heredity

Pathophysiology

- Blood reaches the brain through four major vessels:
  - Two carotid arteries, which supply of cerebral blood flow
  - Two vertebral arteries
    - — Combine to form the single basilar artery
    - — Supply the remaining 20% of cerebral blood flow
  - These two systems are interconnected at various levels, primarily the circle of Willis.
- There are individual variations of extensive collateral blood flow supplied through facial anastomoses between scalp vessels and vessels of the dura and arachnoid.
  - Beyond this, there is no collateral circulation in the depths of the brain.
  - Occlusion of any one of the more distal vessels may result in ischemia and infarction.
- Normally cerebral blood flow is maintained through autoregulation of cerebral vessels that constrict or dilate to preserve perfusion pressure, even with systemic hypotension.
  - Cerebral perfusion is also regulated at the arteriolar level by the level of oxygen and glucose supplied.
  - Sudden cessation of circulation to a portion of the brain that results from vessel occlusion or hemorrhage cannot be readily corrected by these autoregulatory mechanisms.
  - Uncorrected ischemia that occurs within a short time leads to neuronal dysfunction and death.
- The onset and symptoms of the stroke depend on the area of the brain involved.

Types of Stroke

- Stroke refers to the neurological manifestations of a critical decrease in blood flow to a portion of the brain, regardless of the cause.
- Strokes are classified as ischemic or hemorrhagic (Table 24-1).
  - Both forms of stroke can be life threatening.
  - Ischemic stroke rarely leads to death within the first hour.
  - Hemorrhagic stroke can be rapidly fatal.

Ischemic Stroke

- About 80–85% of strokes are ischemic.
- They are caused by a cerebral thrombosis, which occurs as a result of the following:
  - Atherosclerotic plaques
  - Extrinsic pressure from a mass within the brain itself

TABLE 24-1: Differentiating between Ischemic and Hemorrhagic Strokes

Ischemic Strokes	Hemorrhagic Strokes
Most common	Least common
Usually result from atherosclerosis or tumor within the brain	Usually result from cerebral aneurysms, AV malformations, hypertension
Develop slowly	Develop abruptly
Long history of vessel disease	Commonly occur during stress/exertion
May be associated with valvular heart disease and atrial fibrillation	May be associated with cocaine and other sympathomimetic amines
History of angina, previous strokes	May be asymptomatic before rupture

- Onset of stroke from cerebral thrombosis is usually associated with a long history of vessel disease.
- Most patients with stroke are older and have evidence of atherosclerotic disease in other areas of the body.
- Signs and symptoms of thrombotic stroke (usually slower to develop than those of cerebral hemorrhage):
  - Hemiparesis or hemiplegia on the side of the body opposite the lesion
  - Numbness (or decreased sensation) on the side of the body opposite the lesion
  - Aphasia
  - Confusion or coma
  - Convulsions
  - Incontinence
  - Diplopia (double vision)
  - Numbness of the face
  - Dysarthria (slurred speech)
  - Headache
  - Dizziness or vertigo

Cerebral Embolus

- A stroke caused by an embolus results from an occlusion of any intracranial vessel by a fragment of a foreign substance arising outside of the CNS.
- Common sources of cerebral emboli:
  - Atherosclerotic plaques (originating from large vessels of the head, neck, or heart)
  - Thrombi that develop on the valves or in the chambers of the heart; common in patients with valvular heart disease and atrial fibrillation
  - Air embolism after thoracic injury (rare)
  - Fat embolism after long bone injury (rare)
  - Bacterial and fungal endocarditis (rare)
- Women taking oral contraceptives and patients with sickle cell disease are also at increased risk of developing a stroke (both by thrombotic and perhaps embolic origin).

Signs and symptoms

- Similar to those of thrombotic stroke, but usually develop more quickly
- Often associated with an identifiable cause (e.g., atrial fibrillation, valvular heart disease)

Hemorrhagic Stroke

- Hemorrhagic stroke accounts for 15–20% of all strokes.
- Hemorrhage may occur anywhere within the cranial vault, including the epidural, subdural, subarachnoid, intraparenchymal, and intraventricular spaces.
- Most common causes of hemorrhagic stroke:
    - Cerebral aneurysms
    - Arteriovenous (AV) malformations
    - Hypertension

Cerebral aneurysms and AV malformations

- Congenital anomalies that can be familial.
- Often asymptomatic until time of rupture.
- Cerebral hemorrhages are fatal in 50–80% of cases.
- Commonly occur during stress or exertion.
- Cocaine and other sympathomimetic amines may also contribute to intracranial hemorrhage by drug-induced rapid elevation of blood pressure.

Signs and symptoms

- Presentation is abrupt.
    - Often begins with a headache (sometimes described as the worst headache of the patient's life)
    - Nausea/vomiting
    - Progressive deterioration in mental status from alert to lethargic
- At time of hemorrhage, patient often loses consciousness or experiences a seizure.
- As hemorrhage expands and ICP increases, patient becomes comatose, with increasing hypertension and bradycardia (Cushing's reflex).

Transient Ischemic Attacks (TIA)

- TIA are episodes of focal cerebral dysfunction that last from minutes to several hours from which the patient returns to normal within 24 hours without permanent neurological deficit.
- They are thought to be the most important indication of impending stroke.
- About 5% of patients with a TIA will develop completed stroke within 1 month if they do not seek treatment.

Signs and symptoms

- Weakness
- Paralysis
- Numbness of the face
- Speech disturbances
- Most patients who experience a TIA are hospitalized for close observation, evaluation, and treatment of vascular disease (e.g., endarterectomy, anticoagulant therapy)

Assessment

- Emergency care priorities are directed at the following:
  - Maintaining a patent airway
  - Providing adequate ventilatory support with supplemental high-concentration oxygen
  - Obtaining a thorough history if the patient is conscious and able to converse

History

- Important components of the patient history:
  - Previous neurological symptoms (TIA)
  - Previous neurological deficits
  - Initial symptoms and their progression
  - Alterations in level of consciousness
  - Precipitating factors
  - Dizziness
  - Palpitations
- Significant past medical history
  - Hypertension
  - Diabetes mellitus
  - Cigarette smoking
  - Oral contraceptive use
  - Cardiac disease
  - Sickle cell disease
  - Previous stroke

Cincinnati Prehospital Stroke Scale

- Using this scale can help identify a stroke patient who requires rapid transport to a hospital, and it enables pre-arrival notification of the receiving hospital.
- The Cincinnati Prehospital Stroke Scale evaluates three major physical findings:
  - Facial droop
  - Arm drift
  - Speech

Facial Droop

- Ask patient to "Show me your teeth" or "Smile for me"
- Normal—Both sides of face move equally well
- Abnormal—One side of face does not move at all

Arm Drift (Weakness)

- Ask patient to extend arms out in front of him or her 90° (if sitting) or 45° (if supine)
- Normal—Both arms move the same OR both arms do not move at all
- Abnormal—One arm either does not move OR one arm drifts down compared to the other
- Drift is scored if the arm falls before 10 seconds

Speech

- Ask patient to say "You can't teach an old dog new tricks"
- Normal—Phrase is repeated clearly and correctly
- Abnormal—Words are slurred (dysarthria) or abnormal (aphasia) or patient is mute

Management

- After the diagnosis of a stroke is suspected, time in the field must be minimized, because there is limited time to initiate therapy.
- Less than 3 hours from symptom onset is required for thrombolytic therapy.
- Prehospital care is directed at managing the patient's airway, breathing, and circulation and monitoring vital signs.

Airway

- Paralysis of the muscles of the throat, tongue, and mouth can lead to partial or complete airway obstruction.
- Frequent suctioning of the oropharynx and nasopharynx is required to prevent aspiration of pooled saliva.

Breathing

- Inadequate ventilation should be managed with supplemental oxygen and positive pressure ventilation.
- Respiratory arrest from severe coma-producing brain injuries should be managed with intubation and assisted ventilations.

Circulation

- Cardiac arrest is uncommon, but may follow respiratory arrest.
- Cardiac dysrhythmias are frequent.
- The patient's ECG and blood pressure require constant monitoring.
- Treatment of hypertension in the prehospital setting is not recommended for suspected stroke patients.
- Other supportive measures.
- If the patient's condition permits, the patient should be kept supine, with the head elevated 15° to facilitate venous drainage.
- Other patient care measures that can be initiated en route to the receiving hospital include the following:
  - Initiate an IV line of lactated Ringer's solution or normal saline at 30 mL/hr.
  - Draw a blood sample for laboratory analysis (per protocol).
  - Perform serum glucose analysis and administer 50% dextrose if indicated.
  - Protect paralyzed extremities.
  - Provide comforting measures and reassurance.
  - Provide gentle transportation to the receiving hospital.

Seizure Disorders

- A seizure is a temporary alteration in behavior or consciousness caused by abnormal electrical activity of one or more groups of neurons in the brain.
- The annual incidence of seizure is estimated to be about 0.5% of the U.S. population, with the highest incidence of seizures among feverish children less than 5 years old.
- Seizures are generally believed to result from alterations in neuronal membrane permeability secondary to a structural lesion or metabolic derangement. Increased membrane permeability to sodium and potassium ions enhances the ability of the neurons to depolarize and emit an electrical charge, which sometimes results in seizure activity.

- Seizures may be caused by multiple factors, including the following:
  - Stroke
  - Head trauma
  - Toxins, including alcohol
  - Alcohol or other drug withdrawal
  - Hypoxia
  - Hypoperfusion
  - Hypoglycemia
  - Infection
  - Metabolic abnormalities
  - Brain tumor or abscess
  - Vascular disorders
  - Eclampsia
  - Drug overdose

Types of Seizures

- All seizures are pathological.
- They may arise from almost any region of the brain and therefore have many clinical manifestations.
- The two most common seizure types are generalized and partial (focal).

Generalized Seizures

- Generalized seizures do not have a definable origin (focus) in the brain, although focal seizures may progress to a generalized seizure.
- Term includes petit mal (absence seizures) and grand mal (tonic-clonic) seizures.

Petit mal seizures

- Occur most often in children between the ages of 4 and 12
- Characterized by brief lapses of consciousness without loss of posture
- Often there is no motor activity, although some children exhibit the following behaviors:
  - Eye blinking
  - Lip smacking
  - Isolated clonic activity
- Usually last less than 15 seconds, during which the patient is unaware of his or her surroundings; this is followed by immediate return to normal environmental contact
- Most patients have remission by age 20, but they may subsequently develop grand mal seizures

Grand mal seizures

- Common and associated with significant morbidity and mortality
- May be preceded by an aura (olfactory or auditory sensation), which is often recognized by the patient as a warning of the imminent convulsion
- Seizure is characterized by the following:
  - Loss of consciousness associated with loss of organized muscle tone.
  - Tonic phase—Sequence of extensor muscle tone activity (sometimes flexion) and apnea. Lasts only a few seconds.

  - Clonic phase—Bilateral rigidity alternating with relaxation. Usually lasts 1–3 minutes. During this phase there is a massive autonomic discharge that results in hyperventilation, salivation, and tachycardia.
  - Postictal phase—After the seizure, the patient usually experiences drowsiness or unconsciousness. Resolves over minutes to hours. Patient is often confused and fatigued. May demonstrate a transient neurological deficit. Grand mal seizures may be prolonged or recur before the patient regains consciousness. When this occurs, the patient is said to be in status epilepticus.

Partial Seizures

- Arise from identifiable cortical lesions and may be classified as simple or complex.

Simple partial seizures

- Result mainly from seizure activity in the motor or sensory cortex
- Simple motor seizures
- Usually manifest in clonic activity limited to one specific body part (e.g., one hand, one arm or leg, one side of the face)
- Simple sensory seizures
- Result in symptoms such as tingling or numbness of a body part or abnormal visual, auditory, olfactory, or taste symptoms
- Patients generally do not lose consciousness, and they maintain a relatively normal mental status
- Seizure focus may spread and lead to a generalized tonic-clonic seizure

Jacksonian seizure

- Partial seizure activity that spreads in an orderly fashion to surrounding areas

Complex partial seizures

- Arise from focal seizures in the temporal lobe (psychomotor) and manifest primarily as changes in behavior
- Classic complex partial seizure
- Preceded by an aura
- Followed by abnormal repetitive motor behavior (automatisms):
  - Lip smacking
  - Chewing
  - Swallowing
- Patient is amnestic
- Seizures are typically brief (less than 1 minute)
- Patient usually regains normal mental status quickly
- Complex partial seizures may progress to a generalized tonic-clonic seizure

Hysterical Seizures (Pseudoseizures)

- Can mimic a true seizure but stem from psychological causes
- Not considered true seizures because they have no organic origin and do not respond to normal treatment modalities
- Can usually be terminated by sharp commands or painful stimuli (e.g., a sternal rub)
- These maneuvers may help provide a differential aid in distinguishing between pathological and psychogenic seizure activity

Assessment of the Seizure Patient

- Commonly the patient's seizure activity has ceased before EMS arrival.
- If possible, the assessment should include a thorough history and a physical examination that includes a neurological evaluation.

History

- History of seizures
  - Frequency
  - Compliance in taking prescribed medications
- Description of seizure activity
  - Duration of seizure
  - Typical or atypical pattern of seizure for the patient
  - Presence of aura
  - Generalized or focal
  - Incontinence
  - Tongue biting
- Recent or past history of head trauma
- Recent history of fever, headache, nuchal rigidity (suggests meningeal irritation)
- Past significant medical history
  - Diabetes
  - Heart disease
  - Stroke

Physical Examination

- Maintain a patent airway.
- Be alert to signs of trauma that may have occurred before or during the seizure activity.
  - Head and neck trauma
  - Tongue injury
  - Oral lacerations
- Inspect the patient's gums for gingival hypertrophy (swelling of the gums), which is a sign of chronic phenytoin (Dilantin) therapy.
- Other components of the physical examination include the following:
  - Determination of the level of sensorium
    - — Including the presence or absence of amnesia
  - Cranial nerve evaluation, particularly pupillary findings
  - Motor and sensory evaluation, including coordination
    - — Abnormalities may be caused by the following:
      - Metabolic disturbances
      - Meningitis
      - Intracranial hemorrhage
      - Drug use
  - An evaluation for hypotension and hypoxia
  - Presence of urine or feces (suggesting bladder or bowel incontinence)
  - Automatisms
  - Cardiac dysrhythmias

Syncope Versus Seizure (Table 24-2)

- May be difficult to determine which has occurred
- Main differentiating characteristics are in the symptoms before and after the event

Management

- Prevent the patient from sustaining physical injury.
  - Best accomplished by removing obstacles in the patient's immediate area or, if necessary, moving the patient to a safe environment (e.g., a carpeted or soft, grassy area)
- At no time should a patient with seizure activity be restrained, and no objects should be forced between the patient's teeth to maintain an airway.
  - Restraining activity may harm the patient or the EMS crew.
  - Forcing objects into the oral cavity to secure an airway or prevent the patient from biting his or her tongue may evoke vomiting, aspiration, or spasm of the larynx.
- Most patients with an isolated seizure can be appropriately managed in the postictal phase by placing them in a lateral recumbent position to allow drainage of oral secretions and to facilitate suctioning (if needed).
- Administer supplemental oxygen with a nonrebreather mask.
- Move the patient to a quiet environment and away from onlookers.
  - Patients commonly are embarrassed or self-conscious after a seizure, particularly if incontinence has occurred.
  - Be sensitive to the physical and emotional needs of the patient.
- All seizure patients should be transported to the emergency department for physician evaluation.
  - Medical direction may recommend that an IV line be established if medication therapy becomes necessary.
  - Few patients who experience an isolated seizure require pharmacological agents in the prehospital setting.

Status Epilepticus

- Status epilepticus is defined as continuous seizure activity lasting 30 minutes or longer, or a recurrent seizure without an intervening period of consciousness. This condition is a true emergency. Without immediate treatment, status epilepticus can result in the following:
  - Permanent neurological damage
  - Respiratory failure
  - Death

TABLE 24-2: Differentiating Characteristics of Syncope and Seizure

Characteristics	Syncope	Seizure
Position	Usually starts in standing position	May start in any position
Warning	Usually a warning period of lightheadedness	Little or no warning
Level of consciousness	Usually regains consciousness immediately on becoming supine; fatigue, confusion, headache last less than 15 min	May remain unconscious for minutes to hours; fatigue, confusion, headache last more than 15 min
Clonic-tonic activity	Clonic movements (if present) are of short duration	Tonic-clonic movements occur during unconscious state
ECG analysis	Bradycardia caused by increased vagal tone	Tachycardia caused by muscular exertion

- Associated complications
  - Aspiration
  - Brain damage
  - Fracture of long bones and spine
- Most common precipitating cause in adults is failure to take prescribed anticonvulsant medications

Management

- Manage the airway and provide ventilatory support.
- Protect the patient from injury.
- Transport the patient to a medical facility for physician evaluation.
- Stop the seizure activity with anticonvulsant medications (per protocol).
  - Diazepam (Valium)
  - Lorazepam (Ativan)
  - Phenobarbital (Luminal)
  - Phenytoin (Dilantin)
- Secure the airway with oral or nasal adjuncts (or intubate the patient's trachea during the flaccid period between seizures).
- Administer high-concentration oxygen.
- Support ventilations with a bag-valve device.
- Establish an IV line to keep open and secure well with tape and roller bandage.
- Draw blood for laboratory analysis (per protocol).
- Per medical direction, the following medications may be administered:
  - 50% dextrose slow IV infusion (controversial unless hypoglycemia is suspected) to replace blood glucose lost during seizure activity or correct hypoglycemia that caused the seizure
  - Administration of lorazepam (Ativan) IV or diazepam (Valium) IV to stop the spread of the seizure focus
    - Seizure activity may require phenytoin (Dilantin) or phenobarbital (Luminal)
  - During administration of anticonvulsants, closely monitor the patient's blood pressure and respiratory status
    - Be prepared for aggressive airway control and ventilatory assistance
    - Stop drug therapy if the patient's blood pressure begins to fall or if the respiratory rate or effort decreases

Headache

- Most headaches are minor health concerns and are easily treated with analgesics. Headaches are categorized according to their underlying cause:
  - Tension headaches
  - Migraine headaches
  - Cluster headaches
  - Sinus headaches
- Therapies that may be useful include the following:
  - Prescription and over-the-counter medications
  - Herbal remedies
  - Meditation
  - Acupressure
  - Aromatherapy

- Headaches are a common medical complaint.
  - Thirty percent of all Americans will have what they consider to be a serious headache at some point during their lives.
  - Tension headaches—Pain associated with these headaches is a result of muscle contractions of the face, neck, and scalp.
- Causes include the following:
  - Stress
  - Persistent noise
  - Eyestrain
  - Poor posture

Characteristics of Tension Headache Pain

- Usually described as dull, persistent, and nonthrobbing
- May last for days or weeks
- Can cause variable degrees of discomfort
- Can be short lived and infrequent or chronic in nature

Management

- Analgesics such as aspirin, acetaminophen, or ibuprofen

Migraines

- Are severe, incapacitating headaches
- Often preceded by visual disturbances, GI disturbances, or both
- Usually begin with an intense, throbbing pain on one side of the head, which then may spread
- Often accompanied by nausea and vomiting
- Symptoms are associated with constriction and dilation of blood vessels
  - May be brought on by an imbalance of serotonin or hormone fluctuations
- Can also be triggered by the following:
  - Excessive caffeine use
  - Various foods
  - Changes in altitude
  - Extremes of emotions

Management

- Wide range of medications are prescribed for migraines and include the following:
  - Beta blockers
  - Calcium channel blockers
  - Antidepressants
  - Serotonin-inhibiting drugs

Cluster Headaches

- Occur in bursts (clusters)
- Often begin several hours after a person falls asleep
- Pain may be severe, usually located in and around one eye
  - Generally accompanied by nasal congestion and tearing
  - Episode often lasts 30 minutes to 2 hours, then diminishes or disappears, and then recurs a day or so later
  - May occur every day for weeks or months before going into a long period of remission

- Cluster headaches are also known as histamine headaches because they are associated with the release of histamine from the body tissues and marked by the following symptoms:
  - Dilated carotid arteries
  - Fluid accumulation under the eyes
  - Tearing or lacrimation
  - Rhinorrhea

Management

- Generally treated with antihistamines, corticosteroids, and calcium channel blockers

Sinus Headaches

- Characterized by pain in the forehead, nasal area, and eyes
- Often produce a feeling of pressure behind the face
- Usually a result of allergies, inflammation, or infection of the membranes lining the sinus cavities

Management

- Headaches seldom require prehospital emergency care measures.
- Obtain a thorough history of the headache to help identify patients who may have a more serious cause of headaches, such as aneurysm or stroke.
- Important assessment findings include the following:
  - Patient's general health
  - Previous medical conditions
  - Medication use
  - Previous experience with headaches
  - Time of onset
- After gathering a patient history and performing a neurological examination, prehospital care for patients with tension headaches, migraines, cluster headaches, and sinus headaches is primarily supportive.
- Consult with medical direction to determine the appropriate disposition for the patient.
- Patient transportation for physician evaluation may be indicated.

Brain Neoplasm and Brain Abscess

- Brain tumor or neoplasm refers to a mass in the cranial cavity that can be either malignant or benign.
- Brain tumor risk factors include the following:
  - Genetics
  - Exposure to radiation
  - Tobacco use
  - Dietary habits
  - Some viruses
  - Use of some medications
- Effects of the tumor depend on the following:
  - Tumor size
  - Location
  - Evidence of hemorrhage or edema
  - Rate of growth

- Brain tumors may cause local and generalized manifestations.
- Local effects are caused from the destructive action of the tumor on a particular site in the brain and compression, which causes decreased cerebral blood flow. These effects are varied and may include the following:
  - Seizures
  - Visual disturbances
  - Unstable gait
  - Cranial nerve dysfunction
- Lesions inside the cranial vault produce pain by distending or stretching the arteries and other pain-sensitive structures of the head and neck.
  - Headache may be present, but it is often a late finding in the absence of hemorrhage, which may cause a sudden onset of pain
- The principal treatment for a cerebral tumor is surgical or radiosurgical excision or surgical decompression if total excision is not possible.
  - Chemotherapy and radiation may also be used

Brain Abscess

- A brain abscess is an accumulation of purulent material (pus) surrounded by a capsule within the brain. It develops from a bacterial infection (usually one that originated in the nasal cavity, the middle ear, or the mastoid cells).
- It may also follow surgery or penetrating cranial trauma, particularly when bone fragments are retained in cranial tissue.
- Clinical manifestations of a brain abscess are associated with intracranial infection and an expanding intracranial mass.
- Headache is the most frequent early symptom of a brain abscess.

Management

- Prehospital care for a patient with a brain neoplasm or abscess may range from providing comfort and emotional support during patient transport to managing seizure activity and providing airway, ventilatory, and circulatory resuscitation.
- If the patient's condition permits, obtain a focused history and perform a neurological evaluation.

DEGENERATIVE NEUROLOGICAL DISEASES

Muscular Dystrophy

- An inherited muscle disorder of unknown cause in which there is a slow but progressive degeneration of muscle fibers.
- Different forms of the disease are classified by the following:
  - Patient's age when the symptoms appear
  - Rate at which the disease progresses
  - Way in which the disease is inherited
- Duchenne muscular dystrophy
  - Most common type of muscular dystrophy
  - Affects about 1 or 2 out of every 10,000 male children
  - Inherited through a recessive sex-linked gene so that only males are affected; only females pass on the disease
  - Often first diagnosed by a child's physician, who will observe that the child is slow in learning to sit up and walk
  - The disease is confirmed through the following means:

  - — Blood tests that reveal high levels of enzymes released from damaged muscle cells
  - — Nerve conduction studies
  - — Muscle biopsy (relatively rare)
- Rarely diagnosed before child reaches age 3.
- As the disease progresses, the following characteristics will appear:
  - The child tends to walk with a waddle and has difficulty climbing stairs.
  - Muscles (especially those in the calves) become bulky as wasted muscle is replaced by fat.
  - By about age 12, affected children are no longer able to walk, and few will survive their teenage years.
  - Death usually results from pulmonary infections and heart failure.
- There is no effective treatment for muscular dystrophy.
- Parents or siblings of an affected child should receive genetic counseling.
- Some types of muscular dystrophy can be diagnosed before birth through blood analysis and amniocentesis.

Multiple Sclerosis (MS)

- MS is a progressive central nervous system disease in which scattered patches of myelin in the brain and spinal cord are destroyed.
- The cause of MS remains unknown, but it is thought to be an autoimmune disease in which the body's defense system begins to treat the myelin in the central nervous system as foreign, gradually destroying it (demyelination) and causing subsequent scarring and nerve fiber damage.
- Most common acquired disease of the nervous system in young adults.
  - Affects about 1 in every 1000 people
  - The ratio of women to men sufferers is 3:2

Symptoms

- Condition may be active briefly in early adult life and resume years later.
- Condition varies with which parts of the brain and spinal cord are affected.
- Physical effects range from numbness and tingling to paralysis and incontinence.
- Duration may be from several weeks to several months.
- Damage to the white matter in the brain may lead to the following:
  - Fatigue
  - Vertigo
  - Clumsiness
  - Unsteady gait
  - Slurred speech
  - Blurred or double vision
  - Facial numbness or pain
- Some patients may have mild relapses and long symptom-free periods throughout life. Others may gradually become disabled from the first attack and then become bedridden and incontinent in early middle life.
- Diagnosis is usually made by exclusion of all other possible conditions.
- Affected patients are managed with the following:
  - Medications to control symptoms of an acute episode and to prevent exacerbations
  - Physical therapy to maintain mobility and independence
- There is presently no cure.

Dystonia

- Refers to local or diffuse alterations in muscle tone (usually abnormal muscle rigidity) that cause the following:
  - Painful muscle spasms
  - Unusually fixed postures
  - Strange movement patterns
- Localized dystonia may result from the following:
  - Torticollis (painful neck spasm)
  - Scoliosis (abnormal curvature of the spine)
- Generalized dystonia results from the following:
  - Parkinson's disease
  - Stroke
- May also be a feature of schizophrenia or a side effect of some antipsychotic drugs.
- After physician evaluation, dystonia is sometimes managed with medications such as benztropine (Cogentin) or diphenhydramine (Benadryl) to reverse the symptoms and to prevent recurrent symptoms.

Parkinson's Disease

- Is caused by degeneration or damage of unknown origin to nerve cells within the basal ganglia in the brain which causes a lack of dopamine that prevents the basal ganglia from modifying nerve pathways that control muscle contraction. The result is muscles that are overly tense and cause tremor, joint rigidity, and slow movement.
- Affects about 130 out of 100,000 people, with 50,000 new cases diagnosed in the United States each year. If left untreated, the disease progresses over a course of more than 10–15 years to severe weakness and incapacitation.
- Leading cause of neurological disability in people who are more than 60 years old. There are currently about 500,000 people in the United States with the disease.
- Usually begins as a slight tremor in one hand, arm, or leg.
  - In early stages, the tremor is worse while the limb is at rest.
  - In later stages, the disease affects both sides of the body and causes stiffness, weakness, and trembling of the muscles.
  - Other symptoms include the following:
    - Unusual walking pattern (shuffling) that may break into uncontrollable and tiny running steps
    - Constant trembling of the hands, sometimes accompanied by shaking of the head
    - A permanent rigid stoop
    - Unblinking and fixed facial expression
  - Late in the disease, intellect may be affected, and speech becomes slow and hesitant. Depression is common.
- Initially managed with counseling, exercise, and special aids in the home.
- As the disease progresses, treatment may include various combinations of drugs such as levodopa (Dopar, L-Dopa), which is converted by the body into dopamine (anticholinergic agents), to provide relief from specific symptoms.
- Other treatments may include:
  - Brain surgery to reduce tremor and rigidity

Central Pain Syndrome

- Refers to infection or disease of the trigeminal nerve (cranial nerve V).
- Tic douloureux (trigeminal neuralgia).

  - Common form of the syndrome
  - Patient complains of paroxysmal episodes of excruciating pain (often described as recurrent bursts of an electric shock) that affect the cheek, lips, gums, or chin on one side of the face
  - Episode is usually very brief (lasting only a few seconds to minutes), but it may be so intense that the person is debilitated during the attack
  - Pain often causes wincing, hence the name tic douloureux (literally, "painful twitch")
- Central pain syndrome is unusual in people less than 50 years old, but it may be associated with MS in younger people.
- Attacks occur in bouts that may last weeks at a time.
- The pain of trigeminal neuralgia usually begins from a "trigger point" on the face and can be set off by touching, washing, shaving, eating, drinking, or talking.
- Treatment is difficult, because the cause of the syndrome is uncertain.
- Management includes the use of drugs to inhibit nerve impulses (commonly carbamazepine [Epitol, Tegretol]), and sometimes surgery is used, if the cause is a tumor or lesion.

Bell's Palsy (Facial Palsy)

- Refers to paralysis of the facial muscles due to inflammation of the seventh cranial nerve.
- Usually one-sided and temporary and often develops suddenly.
- Most common cause of facial paralysis; affects 1 out of 60 to 70 people in a lifetime. The cause of inflammation is uncertain, but it has been associated with many past or present infectious processes that include Lyme disease, herpes viruses, mumps, and HIV.
- Usually causes the eyelid and corner of the mouth to droop on one side of the face and is sometimes associated with numbness and pain.
- Depending on which branches of the nerve are affected, taste may be impaired, or sounds may seem unusually loud.
- Treatment involves the use of corticosteroid drugs (controversial) to reduce inflammation of the nerve; these will be used in addition to analgesics.
- Recovery is usually complete within 2 weeks to 2 months.
- An important component of therapy is to protect the affected eye from corneal drying and injury that may result from paralysis of eyelid closure; this is accomplished through the use of lubricating ointments and eye patches.

Amyotrophic Lateral Sclerosis (ALS; Lou Gehrig's Disease)

- One of a group of rare disorders (motor neuron diseases) in which the nerves that control muscular activity degenerate within the brain and spinal cord.
- Motor neuron diseases may involve deterioration of both the upper and lower neuron tracts.
  - When only muscles of the tongue, jaw, face, and larynx are involved, the term *progressive bulbar palsy* is used.
  - When only corticospinal processes are affected, the term *primary lateral sclerosis* is used.
  - When only lower motor neurons are affected, the term *progressive spinal muscular atrophy* is used.
  - ALS is used to describe neuron signs that predominate in the extremities and trunk.
- ALS usually affects people over age 50.
- It is more common in men than women.

  - One or two cases of ALS are diagnosed annually per 100,000 people in the United States.
  - About 10% of ALS cases are familial disease in origin.
- Patients with ALS often first notice weakness in the hands and arms that is accompanied by involuntary quivering (fasciculations).
  - The disease progresses to involve the muscles of all of the extremities and of those involved in respiration and swallowing.
  - In the final stages of the disease, patients are often unable to speak, swallow, or move, even though awareness and intellect are maintained.
  - Death usually follows within 2–4 years after diagnosis because of involvement of the respiratory muscles, aspiration pneumonia, and general inanition (i.e., starvation, failure to thrive).
  - In some cases life can be prolonged through the use of feeding tubes and ventilators.
  - Care generally is aimed at providing emotional support and easing discomfort.

Peripheral Neuropathy

- Peripheral neuropathy refers to diseases and disorders affecting the peripheral nervous system, particularly the following areas:
  - Spinal nerve roots
  - Cranial nerves
  - Peripheral nerves
- Most neuropathies arise from damage or irritation either to the axons or their myelin sheaths that slow or completely block the passage of electrical signals.
- The various types of peripheral neuropathy are classified according to the site and distribution of damage.
  - Damage to sensory nerve fibers may cause numbness, tingling, and sensations of cold or pain that often start at the hands and feet and spread toward the central body.
  - Damage to motor nerve fibers may cause muscle weakness and muscle wasting.
  - Damage that occurs to the nerves of the autonomic nervous system may result in blurred vision, impaired or absent sweating, fluctuations in blood pressure (and associated syncope), gastrointestinal disorders, incontinence, and impotence.
  - Some peripheral neuropathies have no identifiable cause.
  - Others may be related to specific causes, including the following:
    - Diabetes
    - Dietary deficiencies (especially of vitamin B)
    - Alcoholism
    - Uremia
    - Leprosy
    - Lead poisoning
    - Drug intoxication
    - Viral infection (Guillain-Barré syndrome)
    - Rheumatoid arthritis
    - Systemic lupus
    - Malignant tumors (lung cancer)
    - Lymphomas
    - Leukemias
    - Inherited neuropathies (peroneal muscular atrophy)
- When possible, treatment is aimed at the underlying cause.
  - Blood sugar control in a diabetic patient
  - Correction of a nutritional deficiency

- If treatment is successful and the cell bodies of the damaged nerves have not been destroyed, full recovery from the neuropathy is possible.

Myoclonus

- Refers to rapid and uncontrollable muscular contractions (jerking) or spasms of muscle(s) that occur at rest or during movement
- May be associated with the following:
  - Disease of nerves and muscles
  - Brain disorder (encephalitis)
  - Seizure disorder
- May occur in healthy people
  - For example, a limb jump that is sometimes experienced just before falling asleep

Spina Bifida

- Spina bifida is a congenital defect in which one part of one (or more) vertebrae fails to develop completely, leaving a portion of the spinal cord exposed. This condition can occur anywhere on the spine, but it is most common in the lower back.
- Cause is unknown.
- Occurs in about 1 out of every 1000 births.
- More likely to occur with extremes in maternal age.
- A woman who has had one spina bifida birth is 10 times more likely than the average of giving birth to another affected child; this indicates the need for genetic counseling.

Types of Spina Bifida

- Severity depends on how much nerve tissue is exposed after neural tube closure.
- Four types of spina bifida:
  - Spina bifida occult
  - Meningocele
  - Myelocele
  - Encephalocele

Spina bifida occult

- Most common and least serious form
- Little external evidence of the defect

Meningocele

- Nerve tissue of the spinal cord is usually intact and covered with a membranous sac of skin
- Usually does not cause functional problems, but it requires surgical repair early in life

Myelocele

- Most severe form of spina bifida
- Often results in a child who is severely handicapped
- There is a raw swelling over the spine and a malformed spinal cord that may or may not be contained in a membranous sac
- The legs of these children are often deformed
- There is partial or complete paralysis and loss of sensation in all areas below the level of the defect

- Associated abnormalities include the following:
  - Hydrocephalus (excess cerebrospinal fluid within the skull) with brain damage
  - Cerebral palsy
  - Epilepsy
  - Mental retardation

Encephalocele

- Very rare
- Protrusion of brain through the skull occurs
- Severe brain damage is common with this condition

Polio (Poliomyelitis)

- This condition is caused by poliovirus hominis.
- The virus attacks with variable severity ranging from unapparent infection to a febrile illness without neurological sequela to aseptic meningitis and finally to paralytic disease (including respiratory paralysis) and possible death.
- Incidence has declined in the United States and Europe since the development of the Salk and Sabin vaccines in the 1950s.
- May affect nonimmune adults and indigent (particularly immigrant) children. Remains a serious risk for anyone not vaccinated and traveling in southern Europe, Africa, or Asia.
- People infected with the polio virus can pass large numbers of virus particles in their feces where they may be spread directly or indirectly by fingers to food to infect others, and by airborne transmission.
- Signs and symptoms of polio differ in the nonparalytic and paralytic forms.
- Fever, headache, sore throat, and malaise are common to both forms.
- The paralytic form of polio is also associated with generalized pain, weakness, muscle spasms, and the paralysis of limbs and other muscles.
  - If the infection spreads to the brainstem, the result may be difficulty or inability to swallow or breathe
- Recovery from nonparalytic polio is complete.
- Of those who become paralyzed, more than half eventually make a full recovery.
- Some patients may develop "post-polio deterioration," which involves new weakness and pain from recovered muscles.

? CHAPTER QUESTIONS

1. The lowest Glasgow Coma Scale score possible is ______; the highest possible score is _______.
   a. 2/14
   b. 3/15
   c. 4/16
   d. 0/15
2. During the postictal phase following a seizure, the highest priority of care is to:
   a. restrain the patient to further prevent injury
   b. establish an intravenous line
   c. move the patient to a quiet environment
   d. manage the airway and administer oxygen

3. Your patient is a 20-year-old female who has a history of seizure activity. Her friend called 911 when she observed her having a second seizure before she awoke from the first. Upon your arrival, she is actively seizing. Priority treatment should consist of:
   a. administering naloxone (Narcan) while closely monitoring her blood sugar
   b. immediately administering diazepam (Valium) while closely monitoring her level of consciousness
   c. checking her blood sugar and administering diazepam (Valium)
   d. closely monitoring her respirations and blood pressure
4. You suspect your unresponsive patient has a history of seizures. Which of the following medications might you expect to find in her medicine cabinet?
   a. Tegretol
   b. Prozac
   c. Zestril
   d. Inderal

Suggested Readings

Circulation 2005 112 [Suppl I]: IV-111–120; published online before print November 28, 2005, doi:10.1161/CIRCULATIONAHA.105.166562.

US Department of Transportation, National Highway Traffic Safety Administration. *EMT-Paramedic: National Standard Curriculum.* Washington, DC: US Department of Transportation, National Highway Traffic Safety Administration; 1998.

Chapter 25
Endocrinology

Paramedics will encounter patients with endocrine system disorders that range from barely detectable to life threatening. It is important to understand endocrine gland function and how it relates to the body as a system.

ANATOMY AND PHYSIOLOGY OF THE ENDOCRINE SYSTEM

- The endocrine system consists of ductless glands and tissues that produce and secrete hormones.
- Major endocrine glands include the following:
  - Pituitary gland
  - Thyroid and parathyroid glands
  - Adrenal cortex and medulla
  - Pancreatic islets
  - Ovaries and testes
- Other specialized groups of cells that secrete hormones are found in the kidneys and in the mucosa of the gastrointestinal tract.

Endocrine Gland Functions

- Endocrine glands secrete their hormones directly into the bloodstream.
  - They exert a regulatory effect on various metabolic functions
- Because the products of endocrine glands travel by means of the blood or tissue fluids, they are able to exert their effects at widespread sites.
- The release of hormones occurs in response to the following:
  - An alteration in the cellular environment
  - The process of maintaining a regulated level of certain hormones or substances
- This integrated chemical and coordination system enables reproduction, growth and development, and the regulation of energy.
- The specificity of this complex system is determined by the affinity of receptors on target organs and body tissues to a particular hormone.

Hormone Receptors

- Most hormones can be categorized as one of the following:
  - Proteins
  - Polypeptides
  - Derivatives of amino acids
  - Lipids

- Each hormone may affect a specific organ or tissue, or may have a general effect on the entire body.
- Hormones may also be classified as steroid or nonsteroid.
- Steroid hormones are manufactured by endocrine cells from cholesterol.
  - They include cortisol, aldosterone, estrogen, progesterone, and testosterone.
- Nonsteroid hormones are synthesized primarily from amino acids.
  - They include insulin and parathyroid hormone.
- Hormones affect only cells with appropriate receptors. They then act on these cells to initiate specific cell functions or activities.
  - Hormone receptor sites may be in one of two locations:
    - — On the cell membrane
    - — In the interior of the cell
  - Cells with fewer receptor sites will bind with less hormone than cells with many receptor sites.
  - Abnormalities in or the presence of specific hormone receptors can cause a pathologic state as a result of complete rejection of that receptor site's hormone by the target cells.

Regulation of Hormone Secretion

- All hormones operate within feedback systems (either negative or positive) to maintain an optimal internal environment.
  - Negative feedback system is the most common feedback mechanism.
    - — This term usually refers to an increase in the serum level of hormone or hormone-related substances that suppress further hormone output.
    - — Hormone production is stimulated when the serum levels fall.

DISORDERS OF THE ENDOCRINE SYSTEM

Causes of disorders of the endocrine system include an imbalance in the production of one or more hormones or an alteration in the body's ability to use the hormones produced.

Diabetes Mellitus

- A systemic disease of the endocrine system.
- Usually occurs as a result of pancreatic dysfunction.
- Complex disorder of fat, carbohydrate, and protein metabolism.
- According to the American Diabetes Association, there are 20.8 million children and adults in the United States, or 7% of the population, who have diabetes. While an estimated 14.6 million have been diagnosed with diabetes, unfortunately, 6.2 million people (or nearly one-third) are unaware that they have the disease.
- Can predispose the patient to several kinds of true medical emergencies.

Anatomy and Physiology of the Pancreas

- The pancreas is important in the absorption and use of carbohydrates, fat, and protein. It is a principal regulator of blood glucose concentration.
- It is located retroperitoneally adjacent to the duodenum on the right and extending to the spleen on the left.
- The healthy pancreas has both exocrine and endocrine functions.
- The exocrine portion of the pancreas consists of acini (glands that produce pancreatic juice) and a duct system that carries the pancreatic juice to the small intestine.

- The endocrine portion of the pancreas consists of pancreatic islets (islets of Langerhans) that produce hormones.

Islets of Langerhans and Pancreatic Hormones

- There are 500,000 to 1 million pancreatic islets dispersed among the ducts and the acini of the pancreas.
- Each islet is composed of the following:
  - Beta cells that secrete insulin (at a daily average of 0.6 units/kg of body weight)
  - Alpha cells that secrete glucagon
  - Other cells of questionable function, some of which are delta cells that secrete the hormone somatostatin, which inhibits the secretion of growth hormone
- Nerves from both divisions of the autonomic nervous system (ANS) that innervate these islets. Each islet is surrounded by a well-developed capillary network.

Insulin

- Insulin is a small protein released by the beta cells that respond to elevated blood glucose levels. Primary function of insulin is to:
  - Increase glucose transport into cells
  - Increase glucose metabolism by cells
  - Increase liver glycogen levels
  - Decrease blood glucose concentration toward normal levels

Glucagon

- Glucagon is a protein released by the alpha cells that respond when blood glucose levels fall. Two major effects of glucagon:
  - An increase of blood glucose levels caused by the stimulation of the liver to release glucose stores from glycogen and other glucose storage sites (glycogenolysis).
  - A stimulation of gluconeogenesis (glucose formation) through the breakdown of fats and fatty acids, thereby maintaining a normal blood glucose level.

Growth hormone (GH)

- GH is a polypeptide hormone produced and secreted by the anterior pituitary gland. GH secretion is triggered by many physiological stimuli including:
  - Exercise
  - Stress
  - Sleep
  - Hypoglycemia
- GH acts as an insulin antagonist. By decreasing insulin actions on cell membranes; it reduces the capacity of muscles and adipose and liver cells to absorb glucose.

Effects of Insulin and Glucagon on Target Tissues (Table 25-1)

Under normal conditions, the body maintains a range of serum glucose concentration that varies between 60 and 120 mg/dL.

Dietary Intake

- There are three main organic components of food:
  - Carbohydrates
  - Fats
  - Proteins

TABLE 25-1: Effects of Insulin and Glucagon on Target Tissues

Target Tissue	Response to Insulin	Response to Glucagon
Skeletal muscle, cardiac muscle, cartilage, joints, bone, fibroblasts, leukocytes, mammary glands	Increased glucose uptake and glycogen synthesis; increased uptake of certain amino acids	Little effect
Liver	Increased glycogen synthesis; increased use of glucose for energy (glycolysis)	Causes rapid increase in breakdown of glycogen to glucose (glycogenolysis) and release of glucose into the blood; increased formation of glucose (gluconeogenesis) from amino acids and, to some degree, from fats; increased metabolism of fatty acids, resulting in increased ketones in the blood
Adipose cells	Increased glucose uptake, glycogen synthesis, fat synthesis, and fatty acid uptake; increased glycolysis	High concentrations cause breakdown of fats (lipolysis); probably unimportant under most conditions
Nervous system	Little effect except to increase glucose uptake in the satiety center	No effect

Carbohydrates

- Carbohydrates are found in all sugary, starchy foods.
- They are a ready source of near-instant energy.
- Carbohydrates are the first food substances to enter the blood stream after a meal is ingested.
- They yield the simple sugar glucose.
- If not "burned" for immediate energy, glucose will be used in one of the following ways:
  - It will be stored in the liver and muscles as glycogen for short-term energy needs.
  - It will be converted into fat by adipose tissue and stored for intermediate and long-term needs.

Process of digestion

- Before food compounds can be used by body cells, they must be digested and absorbed into the blood stream. Digestion begins in the mouth and is accomplished by physical forces (chewing) and by chemical forces (enzymatic; e.g., salivary amylase).
- Chewing and saliva begin the process that reduces the food to soluble molecules and particles small enough to be absorbed.
- After food is swallowed, it enters the stomach; at this point, various nutrients including glucose, salts, and water, as well as other substances (alcohol and certain other drugs), are absorbed into the circulatory system.
  - The remaining chyme is shunted from the stomach and into the small intestine for further digestion.
- The duodenum signals the release of hormones that mobilize the pancreas, to contribute its molecule-splitting enzymes, and the gallbladder, to release its bile salts.
- Carbohydrates are absorbed as simple sugars, fats are absorbed as fatty acids, and proteins are absorbed as amino acids.

- Nutrients are carried from the intestine to the liver by way of the portal vein; water and remaining salts are absorbed from food residues that reach the colon.
- The liver synthesizes the following substances:
  - Glycogen from absorbed glucose
  - Lipoproteins from absorbed fatty acids
  - Many proteins required for health from absorbed amino acids

Carbohydrate metabolism

- Insulin secretion is under chemical, neural, and hormonal control.
- An increased concentration of blood glucose, parasympathetic stimulation, and gastrointestinal hormones involved with the regulation of digestion cause beta cells of the pancreas to release insulin after the dietary intake of carbohydrates.
- Insulin travels through the blood to target tissues where it combines with specific chemical receptors on the surface of cell membranes to permit glucose to enter the cell. This allows the body cells to use glucose for energy. It also prevents the breakdown of alternative energy sources (proteins and fat cells).
- Insulin promotes the uptake of glucose into the liver, where it is converted to glycogen for storage. When blood glucose levels begin to fall, the liver releases glucose back into the circulating blood.
- The liver removes glucose from the blood when it is present in excess after dietary intake, and returns it to blood when it is needed between meals.
- Normally about 60% of the glucose taken in during a meal is stored in the liver as glycogen and released later.
- If muscles are not exercised after a meal, much of the glucose transported into the muscle cells by insulin is stored as muscle glycogen.
- Muscle glycogen differs from liver glycogen in that it cannot be reconverted into glucose and released into the circulation.
- The stored glycogen must be used by the muscle for energy.
- Insulin has little or no effect on the uptake or use of glucose by the brain.
- The cells of the brain do not have adequate storage capacities.
- Because the brain normally uses only glucose for energy, it cannot depend on stored supplies of glycogen.
- It is essential that serum glucose be maintained at a level that provides adequate energy to these tissues. When serum glucose falls too low, signs and symptoms of hypoglycemia can develop quickly; they include the following:
  - Progressive irritability
  - Altered mental states
  - Fainting
  - Convulsions
  - Coma

Fat metabolism

- A third of the glucose that passes through the liver is converted to fatty acids.
- Under the influence of insulin, fatty acids are converted to triglycerides (storable fats) and stored in adipose tissue.
- Without insulin, the stored fat is broken down and the plasma concentration of free fatty acids rapidly increases.
  - Relative insulin deficiency can result in a high circulating concentration of triglycerides and cholesterol (as lipoproteins) in the plasma, and this is thought to contribute to the development of atherosclerosis in patients with serious diabetes.

- If needed (in the absence of insulin), fatty acids in the liver can be metabolized and used for energy.
  - A byproduct of the breakdown of fatty acids in the liver is acetate, which is converted to acetoacetic acid and beta-hydroxybutyric acid (released in the circulating blood as ketone bodies).
  - Ketone bodies may cause acidosis and coma (diabetic ketoacidosis) in the diabetic patient.

Protein metabolism

- Insulin causes proteins, carbohydrates, and fats to be stored.
- Amino acids are actively transported into various cells of the human body.
  - Most amino acids are used as building blocks to form new proteins (protein synthesis).
  - Some amino acids enter the metabolic cycle by being converted to glucose after their initial breakdown in the liver.
- In the absence of insulin, protein storage stops and protein breakdown (particularly in muscle) begins. This releases large quantities of amino acids into the circulation, which are then used directly for energy or as substrates for gluconeogenesis.
  - The degradation of amino acids leads to increased urea excretion in the urine.
- This "protein wasting" has serious effects in diabetic patients because it leads to extreme weakness and dysfunction in many organs.

Glucagon and its functions

- Glucagon has several functions that are the opposite of those of insulin, the most important of which is its ability to increase blood glucose concentration.
- Major effects of glucagon on glucose metabolism:
  - Breakdown of liver glycogen
  - Increased gluconeogenesis
- As the serum glucose level returns to normal (several hours after dietary intake), insulin secretion is decreased with continued fasting, and blood sugar levels begin to drop.
- As a result, glucagon, cortisol, GH, and epinephrine are secreted, thereby initiating the release of glucose from glycogen and other glucose-storage sites.
- Glycogen is converted back to glucose and released into the blood.
- The uptake of glucose by most tissues helps maintain blood glucose at levels necessary for normal function.
- The four mechanisms for achieving blood glucose regulation:
  - The liver functions as a glucose-buffer system, removing glucose from the blood when it is present in excess (storing it as glycogen) and returning glucose to the blood when glucose concentration and insulin secretion decline.
  - Insulin and glucagon production function as a feedback control system to maintain normal serum glucose concentrations.
  - When serum glucose levels rise, insulin is secreted to lower them toward normal levels.
  - When serum glucose levels fall, glucagon is secreted to raise serum glucose levels toward normal levels.
  - Low serum glucose levels stimulate the sympathetic nervous system to secrete epinephrine.
  - Epinephrine and norepinephrine (to a lesser degree) have glucagon-like effects that promote liver glycogenolysis.
  - GH and cortisol play a role in the less-immediate regulation of serum glucose levels.

— They are secreted in response to more prolonged hypoglycemic episodes (late overnight fast).

— These two substances tend to increase the rate of glucose production (gluconeogenesis) and decrease the rate of glucose use.

Pathophysiology of Diabetes Mellitus

- Diabetes mellitus is characterized by a deficiency of insulin or an inability of the body to respond to insulin. It is often associated with the following:
  - Increased intake of fluid (polydipsia)
  - Excretion of large quantities of urine that contains glucose (polyuria, glucosuria)
  - Weight loss
- Diabetes mellitus is generally classified as type 1 or type 2.

Type 1 diabetes mellitus

- Type 1 diabetes mellitus is characterized by the inadequate production of biologically effective insulin. This type of diabetes affects 1 in every 10 diabetics. Onset may occur any time after birth, but it usually occurs in teenagers and young adults. This type of diabetes has a genetic component, and might be an autoimmune phenomenon resulting from a genetic abnormality or susceptibility that causes the body to destroy its own insulin-producing cells. It requires lifelong treatment with insulin injections, exercise, and diet regulation. Signs and symptoms of type 1 diabetes mellitus usually present suddenly and include the following:
  - Polyuria
  - Polydipsia
  - Dizziness
  - Blurred vision
  - Rapid, unexplained weight loss

Type 2 diabetes mellitus

- Type 2 diabetes mellitus is usually characterized by a decreased production of insulin by the beta cells of the pancreas and diminished tissue sensitivity to insulin. It occurs most often in adults who are more than 31 years old and overweight. Other populations at an increased risk for this disease include the following:
  - Native Americans
  - Hispanics
  - African Americans
- Most patients with this condition require oral hypoglycemic medications, exercise, and dietary regulation to control their illness.
- Some patients require insulin injection.
- Warning signs (if present) are gradual and include all of those associated with type 1 diabetes:
  - Fatigue, changes in appetite, and tingling, numbness, and pain in the extremities are also indicators

Effects of Diabetes Mellitus

- Most effects of diabetes mellitus can be attributed to:
  - Decreased use of glucose by the body cells, with a resultant increase in serum glucose.
  - Markedly increased mobilization of fats from the fat storage areas, which causes abnormal fat metabolism; may result in the short term in ketoacidosis and in the long term in severe atherosclerosis.
  - Depletion of protein in the tissues of the body and muscle wasting.

Loss of glucose in the urine

- When the quantity of glucose entering the kidney tubules in the glomerular filtrate rises above the threshold for reabsorption of glucose by the tubules (typically 80 mg/dL), a significant portion of the glucose "spills" into the urine.
- The loss of glucose in the urine causes diuresis because the osmotic effect of glucose in the tubules prevents tubular reabsorption of fluid (osmotic diuresis); the effect is dehydration of the extracellular and intracellular spaces.

Acidosis in diabetes

- The shift from carbohydrate to fat metabolism results in the formation of ketone bodies (ketoacids).
- Ketone bodies are strong acids, and their continuous production leads to metabolic acidosis, which is often at least partially compensated for by respiratory alkalosis (manifested by Kussmaul's respirations).
- The body's mechanism for clearing the acid load by the kidneys is overwhelmed by the continuous production of ketone bodies, and profound acidosis eventually occurs.
- Acidosis, along with the usually severe dehydration that occurs as a result of the osmotic diuresis, can lead to death.
- Treatment of this condition can be lifesaving.
- Diabetes mellitus is a systemic disease with many long-term complications that include the following:
  - Blindness—5000 diabetics lose their sight each year
  - Kidney disease—10% of all diabetics develop some form of kidney disease, including end-stage kidney failure, which requires dialysis or kidney transplant
  - Peripheral neuropathy—Results in nerve damage to the hands and feet and increased incidence of foot infections
  - Autonomic neuropathy
    - — Causes damage to nerves that control voluntary and involuntary functions
    - — May affect bladder and bowel control and blood pressure
  - Heart disease and stroke
    - — High blood glucose and blood fat contribute to atherosclerosis
    - — Diabetics are 2–4 times as likely to develop heart disease
    - — Diabetics are 2–6 times as likely to have a stroke

Management

- Management of diabetes mellitus consists of drug therapy (insulin or oral hypoglycemic agents), diet regulation, and exercise to enable the patient's metabolism to be as nearly normal as possible.
- Insulin—Genetically engineered human insulin (Humulin) is available in rapid-, intermediate-, and long-acting preparations.
  - A patient with type 1 diabetes usually self-administers a single dose of a long-acting insulin preparation each day and additional quantities of rapid-acting insulin (which lasts only a few hours) for those times of day when the serum glucose would be elevated.
  - Insulin may also be self-administered by an insulin-infusion pump that administers a continuous dose of insulin and is adjusted so that the level of blood glucose is constantly controlled.
  - Regular monitoring of glucose levels (blood or urine testing) by the patient is necessary to ensure adequate medication control.

— Medication balance is delicate.
— The same dosage of insulin that appears correct on one occasion may be too much or too little on another, depending on various factors (exercise, infection).

Characteristics of oral hypoglycemic agents

- Stimulate the release of insulin from the pancreas
- Effective only in patients who have functioning beta cells
- Commonly prescribed oral hypoglycemic agents include the following:
  - Chlorpropamide (Diabinese)
  - Tolazamide (Tolinase)
  - Tolbutamide (Orinase)
  - Acetohexamide (Dymelor)
  - Glipizide (Glucotrol)
  - Glyburide (Micronase)

Diabetic Emergencies

- Three life-threatening conditions may result from diabetes mellitus:
  - Hypoglycemia
  - Hyperglycemia (diabetic ketoacidosis or DKA)
  - Hyperosmolar hyperglycemic nonketotic (HHNK) coma

Hypoglycemia

- Hypoglycemia is a syndrome related to blood glucose levels below 80 mg/dL.
- Symptoms usually occur at levels less than 60 mg/dL or at slightly higher blood glucose levels if the drop in level has been rapid.
  - May also occur in nondiabetic patients
- Hypoglycemia is usually a result of one of the following:
  - Excessive response to glucose absorption
  - Physical exertion
  - Alcohol or drug effects
  - Pregnancy and lactation
  - Decreased dietary intake
- In diabetics, hypoglycemic reactions are usually caused by one of the following:
  - Too much insulin (or oral hypoglycemic medication)
  - Decreased dietary intake (a delayed or missed meal)
  - Unusual or vigorous physical activity
  - Emotional stress
- Less common causes and predisposing factors include the following:
  - Chronic alcoholism (alcohol depletes liver glycogen stores)
  - Adrenal gland dysfunction
  - Liver disease
  - Malnutrition
  - Tumor of the pancreas
  - Cancer
  - Hypothermia
  - Sepsis
  - Administration of beta blockers (propranolol)

- Administration of salicylates in ill infants or children
- Intentional overdose with insulin, oral hypoglycemic agents, or salicylates

Signs and symptoms

- Rapid onset (often within minutes)
- In early stages, the patient may complain of extreme hunger and demonstrate one or more of the signs and symptoms secondary to decreased glucose availability to the brain:
  - Nervousness, trembling
  - Irritability
  - Psychotic (combative) behavior
  - Weakness, lack of coordination
  - Confusion
  - Appearance of intoxication
  - Weak, rapid pulse
  - Cold, clammy skin
  - Drowsiness
  - Seizures
  - Coma (in severe cases)

Diabetic Ketoacidosis (DKA)

- DKA results from an absence of or resistance to insulin.
- The low insulin level prevents glucose from entering the cells and causes glucose to accumulate in the blood.
  - Cells become starved for glucose and begin to use other sources of energy (principally fat).
  - The metabolism of fat generates fatty acids and glycerol.
  - Glycerol provides some energy to the cells, but the fatty acids are further metabolized to form ketoacids, resulting in acidosis.
- DKA increases the transport of potassium from the intracellular space into the intravascular space.
  - The subsequent diuresis results in high potassium concentration in the urine and a total body potassium deficit.
  - The sodium concentration in the extracellular fluid usually decreases through osmotic dilution and is replaced by increased quantities of hydrogen ions, thus adding greatly to the acidosis.
- As blood sugar rises, the patient undergoes massive osmotic diuresis, which, with vomiting, causes dehydration and shock.
  - Associated electrolyte imbalances may cause cardiac dysrhythmias and altered neuromuscular activity (including seizures).

Signs and symptoms

- The signs and symptoms of DKA are usually related to diuresis and acidosis, are usually slow in onset (over 12–48 hours), and include the following:
  - Diuresis
  - Warm, dry skin
  - Dry mucous membranes
  - Tachycardia, thready pulse
  - Postural hypotension

  - Weight loss
  - Polyuria
  - Polydipsia
  - Acidosis
  - Abdominal pain (usually generalized)
  - Anorexia, nausea, vomiting
  - Acetone (fruity) breath odor
  - Kussmaul's respirations in an attempt to reduce carbon dioxide levels
  - Decreased level of consciousness

Hyperosmolar Hyperglycemic Nonketotic Coma (HHNK)

- HHNK is a life-threatening emergency that frequently occurs in older patients with type 2 diabetes or in undiagnosed diabetics.
- HHNK differs from DKA in that residual insulin may be adequate to prevent ketogenesis and ketoacidosis but not enough to permit glucose use by peripheral tissues or to decrease gluconeogenesis by the liver.
- Hyperglycemia produces the following effects:
  - CNS dysfunction
  - A hyperosmolar state followed by an osmotic diuresis
  - Dehydration
  - Electrolyte losses
- Patients with this condition typically have greater hyperglycemia because they are more dehydrated and have less ketone formation.
  - The presence of insulin in the liver directs free fatty acids into nonketogenic pathways, resulting in less acidemia than is found in patients with DKA.
- Precipitating factors of HHNK:
  - Type 2 diabetes
  - Advanced age
  - Preexisting cardiac or renal disease
  - Inadequate insulin secretion or action
  - Increased insulin requirements (e.g., stress, infection, trauma, burns, myocardial infarction)
  - Medication use (thiazide and thiazide diuretics, glucocorticoids, phenytoin [Dilantin], sympathomimetics, propranolol [Inderal], immunosuppressives)
  - Supplemental parenteral and enteral feedings

Signs and symptoms

- Weakness
- Thirst
- Frequent urination
- Weight loss
- Extreme dehydration
- Flushed, dry skin
- Dry mucous membranes
- Decreased skin turgor
- Postural hypotension
- Altered levels of consciousness
- Tachycardia

- Hypotension
- Tachypnea

Assessment of the Diabetic Patient

- Diabetic emergency may mimic more commonly encountered conditions; maintain a high degree of suspicion for diabetes-related illness.
- Besides the patient assessment measures appropriate for any emergency patient encounter (initial assessment, physical examination, and treatment of life-threatening illness or injury), be alert for thc following:
  - Medic alert information
  - Presence of insulin syringes
  - Diabetic medications (often kept in the refrigerator)
- Important components of the diabetic patient history to consider when dealing with a patient with possible HHNK:
  - Onset of symptoms
  - Food intake
  - Insulin or oral hypoglycemic use
  - Alcohol or other drug consumption
  - Predisposing factors such as exercise, infection, illness, stress

Management of the Conscious Diabetic Patient

- Obtain a pertinent history while assessing airway, breathing, and circulation.
- Administer high-concentration oxygen.
- Administer glucose if appropriate.
- Medical direction may recommend drawing a blood sample for analysis before administering glucose.
- Some EMS services use field glucose testing with Dextrostix, Chemstrips, or a Glucometer. Any patient with a glucose reading of less than 80 mg/dL and signs and symptoms consistent with hypoglycemia should receive dextrose.
- Some patients who have experienced a diabetic reaction may be treated at the scene and released if protocol permits.
  - Others may need to be transported for physician evaluation
  - Consult with medical direction or follow established protocol
- Methods of glucose administration vary by protocol.
- A conscious patient who is alert, has a gag reflex, and can swallow may be administered sugar orally in one of the following forms:
  - Candy bar
  - Glass of orange juice mixed with sugar
  - Nondiet soft drink
  - Sublingual or buccal glucose gel preparation
- An alternate method is to slowly administer dextrose 50% through a stable peripheral vein.

Management of the Unconscious Diabetic Patient

- Prehospital management of any unconscious patient should be directed at airway management, high-concentration oxygen administration, and ventilatory support.
- Establish an IV line of lactated Ringer's or normal saline solution to replenish fluids and electrolytes (flow rate to be guided by the patient's blood pressure and heart rate).
- Obtain a blood sample for laboratory analysis before IV fluids or D50 is administered.

- If alcoholism or other drug abuse is suspected, medical direction may recommend the administration of thiamine, naloxone, or both before the administration of glucose.
- If an IV line cannot be established, IM glucagon can help raise serum glucose levels by stimulating the breakdown of liver glycogen; however, glucagon is ineffective in chronic alcoholics and those with liver disease.
- Definitive treatment for patients with DKA or HHNK requires administration of insulin, fluid replacement, electrolyte monitoring, and in-hospital observation.

Differential Diagnosis

- Differentiating the origin of a diabetic emergency is sometimes difficult in the prehospital setting.
- When in doubt as to the cause, all diabetic patients should receive glucose if indicated by testing.

THYROTOXICOSIS

- Thyrotoxicosis refers to any toxic condition that results from thyroid hyperfunction.
- Hyperthyroidism and thyrotoxicosis are designations for common, milder forms of the disease.
- Thyroid storm is a heightened and life-threatening manifestation of thyroid hyperfunction, and it is a relatively rare condition.
- Thyroid storm may occur spontaneously or be precipitated by one of the following:
  - Infection
  - Stress
  - Thyroidectomy
  - Toxic diffuse goiter (Grave's disease)
- Grave's disease—A type of excessive thyroid activity characterized by a generalized enlargement of the gland (goiter), leading to a swollen neck and often to protruding eyes (exophthalmos).
  - Most frequently occurs in young women
  - May be due to an autoimmune process in which an antibody stimulates the thyroid cells

Anatomy and Physiology of the Thyroid Gland

- The thyroid gland is located in the front of the neck, just blow the larynx.
- It consists of two lobes, one on each side of the trachea.
  - It is joined by a narrower portion of tissue called the isthmus.
- Thyroid tissue is composed of two types of secretory cells:
  - Follicular cells
  - Parafollicular cells (C cells)

Follicular Cells

- Follicular cells make up most of the gland.
- They are arranged in the form of hollow, spherical follicles.
- They secrete the iodine-containing hormones thyroxine (T4) and triiodothyronine (T3).

Parafollicular Cells

- Parafollicular cells are found individually or in small groups in the spaces between the follicles and secrete the hormone calcitonin, which helps regulate the level of calcium in the body.

Thyroid Hormones

- Thyroid hormones play an important role in controlling body metabolism.
- They are essential in children for normal physical growth and mental development.
- The secretion of T3 and T4 is controlled by a feedback system involving the pituitary gland and hypothalamus.
- The secretion of calcitonin is regulated directly by the level of calcium in the blood and independently of the pituitary gland or hypothalamus.

Thyroid Gland Disorders (Table 25-2)

- Disorders of the thyroid gland may be a result of defects of the gland itself or a disruption of the hypothalamic-pituitary hormonal control system.
- Causes of thyroid gland disorders:
  - Congenital defects
  - Genetic disorders
  - Infection (thyroiditis)
  - Tumors (benign or malignant)
  - Autoimmune disorders
  - Hormonal disorders during puberty or pregnancy
  - Nutritional disorders
- Thyroid disorders advance slowly (with nonspecific signs and symptoms over months to years) and may culminate in an acute episode.
- Nonspecific signs and symptoms of hyperthyroidism include the following:
  - Fatigue
  - Anxiety
  - Palpitations
  - Sweating
  - Weight loss
  - Diarrhea
  - Intolerance of heat
- In acute episodes of thyroid storm, signs and symptoms may include:
  - Severe tachycardia
  - Heart failure

TABLE 25-2: Signs and Symptoms of Thyroid Disorders

Hyperthyroidism	Hypothyroidism
Exophthalmos	Facial edema
Goiter	JVD, sometimes goiter
Warm, flushed skin	Cool skin
Agitation/psychosis	Coma
Hyperactivity	Weakness
Weight loss	Weight gain
Common Medications	**Common Medications**
Iodine	Levothyroxine (Synthroid)
Methimazole (Tapazole)	Liothyronine (Cytomel)
Propylthiouracil (Propacil)	Liotrix (Euthroid)

  - Cardiac dysrhythmias
  - Shock
  - Hyperthermia
  - Restlessness
  - Agitation and paranoia
  - Abdominal pain
  - Delirium

Management

- Mild hyperthyroidism requires no emergency therapy and is best managed with physician follow-up.
- Thyroid storm is a true emergency that requires immediate intervention.
- Emergency care efforts are directed at providing airway, ventilatory, and circulatory support and rapid transport to an appropriate medical facility.
- In-hospital care will focus on the following:
  - Inhibiting hormone synthesis
  - Blocking hormone release and the peripheral effects of thyroid hormone with antithyroid drugs
  - Providing general support of the patient's vital functions

MYXEDEMA

- Myxedema (severe hypothyroidism) is a condition that results from a deficiency in thyroid hormone.
- It may be associated with the following:
  - Inflammation of the thyroid gland (Hashimoto's thyroiditis)
  - Atrophy of the thyroid gland
  - Treatment for hyperthyroidism
- Myxedema causes the accumulation of mucinous material in the skin and results in the thickening and coarsening of the skin and other body tissues (most notably the lips and nose).
- Myxedema is most common in adults (especially women) who are more than 31 years old.

Signs and Symptoms

- Hoarse voice
- Fatigue
- Weight gain (mild)
- Cold intolerance
- Depression
- Dry skin
- Hair loss
- Infertility
- Constipation
- Heavy or extended menstruation

Myxedema coma

- Is a rare illness characterized by the following:
  - Hypothermia
  - Mental obtundation

- It is a medical emergency that may be precipitated by the following:
  - Exposure to cold
  - Infection (usually pulmonary)
  - Congestive heart failure
  - Trauma
  - Drugs (sedatives, hypnotics, anesthetics)
  - Stroke
  - Internal hemorrhage
  - Hypoxia
  - Hypercapnia
  - Hyponatremia
  - Hypoglycemia

Management

- Prehospital care is directed at managing life-threatening conditions (airway, ventilatory, and circulatory compromise) and providing rapid transport to an appropriate medical facility for physician evaluation.
- After other causes of the coma are ruled out and the patient's vital functions are stabilized, treatment of myxedema involves the oral administration of thyroxine, which must be continued for life.

CUSHING'S SYNDROME

- Cushing's syndrome is caused by an abnormally high circulating level of corticosteroid hormones, which are produced naturally by the adrenal glands.
- Cushing's syndrome may be produced in the following ways:
  - Directly by an adrenal gland tumor (causing excessive secretion of corticosteroids)
  - By prolonged administration of corticosteroid drugs (used to treat conditions such as rheumatoid arthritis, inflammatory bowel disease, and asthma)
  - By enlargement of both adrenal glands due to a pituitary tumor
- Cushing's syndrome is a rare disease. It primarily affects women who are between 30 and 50 years old.
- People with Cushing's syndrome have a characteristic appearance:
  - Face appears round ("moon-faced") and red
  - Trunk tends to become obese from disturbances in fat metabolism
  - Limbs become wasted from muscle atrophy
  - Acne develops
  - Purple stretch marks may appear on the abdomen, thighs, and breasts
  - Skin often thins and bruises easily
  - Bones become weak and have an increased risk of fracture
- Other features of the disease include the following:
  - Increased body and facial hair
  - Hump on the back of the neck ("Buffalo hump")
  - Supraclavicular fat pads
  - Weight gain
  - Hypertension
  - Psychiatric disturbances such as depression or paranoia
  - Insomnia
  - Diabetes mellitus

Signs and Symptoms

- Progressive weakness
- Progressive weight loss
- Progressive anorexia
- Skin hyperpigmentation (the pituitary increases production of the hormone that stimulates melanin)
- Hypotension
- Hyponatremia
- Hyperkalemia
- Gastrointestinal disturbances

Management

- Prehospital care is primarily supportive.
- The disease is diagnosed with the use of the following measures:
  - Measurement of adrenocorticotropic hormone (ACTH) levels in the blood and corticosteroid levels in the blood and urine.
  - Radiologic imaging (CT scan).
- If the cause of the syndrome is overtreatment with corticosteroid drugs, the condition is usually reversible with modification of drug treatment.
- If the cause is a tumor or overgrowth of the adrenal gland, surgical removal may be necessary.
- If the tumor lies in the pituitary gland, it is treated with surgery or irradiation and medication.
- Successful treatment is usually followed by regression of the clinical manifestation of the disease.
- Lifelong hormonal replacement therapy is required for patients with this condition.

ADDISON'S DISEASE

- Addison's disease is a rare, potentially life-threatening disorder caused by a deficiency of the corticosteroid hormones cortisol and aldosterone, which are normally produced by the adrenal cortex.
- This condition can be caused by any disease process that destroys the adrenal cortices (adrenal hemorrhage or infarction, fungal infections, autoimmune diseases).
- The most common cause of Addison's disease is idiopathic atrophy of adrenal tissue, in which case the production of corticosteroid hormones is inadequate to meet the metabolic requirements of the body.
- Addison's disease generally has a slow onset and a chronic course, with symptoms developing gradually over months to years.
- Acute episodes (addisonian crisis) may be precipitated by emotional and physiological stresses such as:
  - Surgery
  - Alcohol intoxication
  - Hypothermia
  - Myocardial infarction
  - Severe illness
  - Trauma
  - Hypoglycemia
  - Infection

- During these events, the adrenal glands cannot increase the production of the corticosteroid hormones to help the body cope with stress; this can result in the following:
  - A drop in blood glucose levels
  - The body's loss of the ability to regulate the content of sodium, potassium, and water in body fluids (causing dehydration and extreme muscle weakness)
  - A drop in blood volume and blood pressure
  - Inability to maintain efficient circulation
- In these situations, airway, ventilatory, and circulatory support will be required in the prehospital setting.

Signs Symptoms

- Progressive weakness
- Progressive weight loss
- Progressive anorexia
- Skin hyperpigmentation (the pituitary increases production of the hormone that stimulates melanin)
- Hypotension
- Hyponatremia
- Hyperkalemia
- Gastrointestinal disturbances

Management

- In-hospital care will be directed at maintaining the patient's vital functions and at correcting the sodium deficiency and dehydration.
- After managing the life-threatening episode, the treatment of Addison's disease consists of the administration of the deficient corticosteroids.
- The patient is often advised to increase the dosage of these medications during times of emotional and physiologic stress.

? CHAPTER QUESTIONS

1. A release of insulin causes what change in blood glucose levels?
   a. Increase
   b. Decrease
   c. No change
   d. None of the above
2. A release of glucagon causes what change in blood glucose levels?
   a. Increase
   b. Decrease
   c. No change
   d. None of the above

Suggested Readings

American Diabetes Association. Available at http://www.diabetes.org/type-1-diabetes/treatment-conditions.jsp. Accessed on April 11, 2007.

US Department of Transportation, National Highway Traffic Safety Administration. *EMT-Paramedic: National Standard Curriculum.* Washington, DC: US Department of Transportation, National Highway Traffic Safety Administration; 1998.

Chapter 26
Allergies and Anaphylaxis

Your patient was stung by a bee. She is very agitated and shows all of the signs and symptoms associated with anaphylaxis. She tells you she thinks she is going to die. While you begin to treat her symptoms, she deteriorates further, exhibiting loss of consciousness and seizure activity.

Why is this patient deteriorating so fast?

Anaphylaxis is an immediate, systemic, life-threatening allergic reaction associated with major changes in the cardiovascular, respiratory, and cutaneous systems. Prompt recognition and appropriate drug therapy are crucial to patient survival.

ANTIGEN-ANTIBODY REACTION

Antigens

- An antigen is a substance that induces the formation of antibodies.
- Antigens can enter the body by injection, ingestion, inhalation, or absorption.
- Examples of common antigens associated with anaphylactic reactions:
  - Drugs (penicillin, aspirin)
  - Envenomation (wasp stings)
  - Foods (seafood, nuts)
  - Pollens

Antibodies

- Protective protein substances developed by the body in response to antigens
- Bind to the antigen that produced them
- Facilitate antigen neutralization and removal from the body

Normal Antigen-Antibody Reaction

- Protects the body from disease by activating the immune response.
- Immune responses are normally protective. But they can become oversensitive or be directed toward harmless antigens to which we are often exposed. When this occurs, the response is termed allergic.
  - The antigen or substance causing the allergic response is called an allergen.
- Common allergens include drugs, insects, foods, and animals.

IMMUNE RESPONSE

- A healthy body responds to an antigen challenge through a collective defense system known as immunity, which is:
  - Natural, present at birth
  - Acquired, resulting from exposure to a specific antigenic agent or pathogen
  - Artificially induced, such as that resulting from inoculation (immunization) against certain infectious diseases, for example, diphtheria and measles

Immunity May Be Active or Passive

- In passive immunization, antibodies are injected and provide immediate but short-lived protection against specific disease-causing bacteria, viruses, or toxins.
  - Active immunization primes the body to make its own antibodies against such microorganisms and confers longer-lasting immunity.
  - Whether natural, acquired, or artificially induced, active immunity produces physiologically similar responses precipitated by the immune system.

Components of Immune System

- Lymphatic system
- Leukocytes
- Lymphocytes
- Immunoglobulins
- Mediators

Lymphatic System

- Every tissue supplied by blood vessels (excluding the brain and placenta) contains lymphatic vessels, which vary in size. The lymphatic system "cleans house" and carries foreign material to the correct "disposal site."
- Lymph fluid—Originates in the blood and enters the interstitial spaces by virtue of hydrostatic pressure in the capillaries.
  - Picks up organisms, cellular debris, or other foreign matter in tissue and carries it back through the lymphatic vessels, including the lymph nodes.
  - Foreign material is processed inside the nodes and presented to B or T lymphocytes where an immune response to one or more specific antigens on the foreign material is activated.
- Lymph nodes are strategically clumped in areas that might be exposed to large amounts of antigens.

Leukocytes

- The blood component associated with the immune response.
- Most of the leukocytes in the peripheral blood consist of polymorphonuclear granulocytes, which are further divided into neutrophils, eosinophils, and basophils.
  - Circulating lymphocytes account normally for about one-third of the peripheral white blood cell count (may vary considerably with infection).
- A third circulating leukocyte is the monocyte (essentially a circulating macrophage), which is capable of phagocytosis and is instrumental in processing antigens so that lymphocytes can recognize them and produce antibodies.
  - The monocytes gobble up the antigens and change them.
- Neutrophils and monocytes are the primary cells involved in phagocytosis; they can migrate out of blood vessels to sites where antigenic stimulation from a foreign body or infection has occurred.

Lymphocytes

- Undergo a maturation process that depends on their lymphoid tissue of origin.
- Two classes of lymphocytes that are principal players in the immune response are T lymphocytes (T cells) and B lymphocytes (B cells).
  - T—Thymus
  - B—Bone marrow

T lymphocytes

- Make up 80% of all lymphocytes and are produced in the thymus.
- Help defend against foreign cells or viruses that enter the body.
- Each T lymphocyte possesses receptors for a specific antigen that allows it to "recognize" and attach to the antigen.
- Once stimulated by its specific antigen, the T lymphocyte proliferates and produces many clone cells that contain identical antigen receptors.
- Within 48 hours, the clone cells further specialize with different receptors and travel to the designated site of action.
- Some clones (known as killer T cells) act directly to destroy the invading pathogens with enzymes.
- Others remain in lymph tissue as "memory cells" and facilitate a much more rapid response if a subsequent exposure to the same antigen occurs.
- T lymphocytes can be further divided into helper and suppressor cells.
  - A reduction in the ratio of helper to suppressor cells or a loss of T lymphocyte function is the primary physiological alteration in the acquired immunodeficiency syndrome (AIDS) and is responsible for these patients' susceptibility to unusual infections and tumors.

B lymphocytes

- Account for the remaining 20% of lymphocytes (developed in the bone marrow). Like T lymphocytes, B lymphocytes are equipped with antigen-specific receptors. They split apart, like troops in the military, and specialize into active forces (antibodies) and reserves (memory cells).
- When activated, B lymphocytes clone to form two types of cells:
  - Antibody-secreting plasma cells that bind to antigens on the organism and allow phagocytic cells and T lymphocytes to destroy the pathogen
  - Memory cells reserved for future encounters with the same antigen—The basis for developing acquired immunity

Immunoglobulins (Ig)

- Immunoglobulins = antibodies.
- Large glycoprotein molecules produced in large numbers by plasma cells (activated B lymphocytes) in response to antigenic stimulation.
- Five distinct classes of immunoglobulins are produced in humans; these consist of different subunits and perform different functions.
- Each antibody has a variable portion and a constant portion—The variable portion binds to the antigen and the constant portion binds complement in some circumstances and phagocytic cells in others.
  - Complement is a complex of at least 20 serum enzymatic proteins that mediate the inflammatory reaction and amplify a specific immune response.

Mediators

- Proteins that cause many physiological responses
- Most of these substances are present throughout the body and remain inactive until triggered by an immune response
- All have different properties and most perform several functions
- These substances are classified as follows:
  - Vasoactive substances cause small vessels to dilate and become more permeable.
  - Leukocytosis promoters stimulate the release of leukocytes from bone marrow and the production of new leukocytes.
  - Chemotactic substances cause the attraction of phagocytic cells toward or away from the pathogenic agent.
  - Leukotactic substances attract leukocytes to the pathogenic agent.
  - Opsonins bind phagocytes to the invading microorganism, which promotes phagocytosis.

ALLERGIC REACTION

- Marked by an increased physiological response to an antigen after a previous exposure (sensitization) to the same antigen
- Initiated when a circulating antibody (IgG or IgM) combines with a specific foreign antigen, resulting in hypersensitivity reactions
- Or to antibodies bound to mast cells or basophils (IgE)
- Hypersensitivity reactions are divided into four distinct types:
  - Type I (IgE-mediated allergic reactions)
    - — Type I or immediate hypersensitivity reaction is the most dramatic and may lead to life-threatening anaphylaxis
  - Type II (tissue-specific reactions)
  - Type III (immune-complex-mediated reactions)
  - Type IV (cell-mediated reactions)

Causative Agents

Drugs and Biological Agents

- Antibiotics
- Local anesthetics
- Cephalosporins
- Chemotherapeutics
- Aspirin
- Nonsteroidal antiinflammatory agents
- Opiates
- Muscle relaxants
- Anticancer agents
- Vaccines
- Insulin

Insect Bites and Stings

- Wasps
- Bees
- Fire ants

Foods

- Peanuts, soybeans
- Cod, halibut, shellfish
- Egg white
- Strawberries
- Food additives
- Wheat and buckwheat
- Sesame and sunflower seeds
- Cottonseed
- Milk
- Mango

Patients who have known sensitivity to these or other agents should avoid exposure.

Localized Allergic Reaction

- Localized allergic reactions (type IV) do not manifest multisystem involvement.
- In these situations, the mast cell and basophil mediator release is limited to the site of antigenic contact.
- Common signs and symptoms of localized allergic reaction include:
    - Conjunctivitis
    - Rhinitis
    - Angioedema
    - Urticaria
    - Contact dermatitis
- Localized allergic reactions are best managed with drugs that compete at receptor sites with histamines to prevent their physiological actions.
    - Common antihistamines include over-the-counter oral and nasal decongestants, and prescription and nonprescription diphenhydramine (Benadryl).
    - Other medications that may be useful for some local reactions include steroids and topical creams.

ANAPHYLAXIS

- It is the most extreme form of an allergic reaction, accounting for 400–800 deaths per year. Anaphylaxis has a mortality rate of 3%.
- Rapid recognition and aggressive therapy are essential.

Causative Agents

- Almost any substance can cause anaphylaxis.
- Antigenic agents most frequently associated with anaphylaxis are:
    - Penicillin (by ingestion or injection)
    - Envenomation by stinging insects
- Regardless of the offending antigen, the risk of anaphylaxis in sensitive individuals increases with the frequency of exposure and to a lesser extent the length of exposure.

Pathophysiology

- Person must first be exposed to a specific antigen to develop type I hypersensitivity. In the first exposure, the antigen enters the body by injection, ingestion, inhalation, or absorption and activates the immune system. In susceptible individuals, large amounts of IgE antibody are produced.

- IgE antibodies leave the lymphatic system and bind to the cell membranes of basophils circulating in the blood and to mast cells in tissues surrounding the blood vessels.
- They remain there, inactive, until the same antigen is introduced into the body a second time.
- With subsequent exposure to the specific antigen, the allergen cross-links at least two of the cell-bound IgE molecules.
  - Resulting in degranulation (release of internal substances) of the mast cells and basophils and the onset of an anaphylactic reaction
- Degranulation of the target cell is associated with the release of pharmacologically active chemical mediators inside the affected basophils and mast cells. These chemicals include the following:
  - Histamines
  - Leukotrienes
  - Eosinophil chemotactic factor of anaphylaxis
  - Heparin
  - Kinins
  - Prostaglandins
  - Thromboxanes
- Histamines promote vascular permeability and cause dilation of capillaries and venules and contraction of nonvascular smooth muscle, especially in the GI tract and bronchial tree.
  - There is an associated increase in gastric, nasal, and lacrimal secretions, resulting in tearing and rhinorrhea.
  - Increased capillary permeability allows plasma to leak into the interstitial space.
    - Decreases intravascular volume available for the heart to pump
  - The profound vasodilation that results further decreases cardiac preload, compromising stroke volume and cardiac output.
  - These physiological effects lead to:
    - Cutaneous flushing
    - Urticaria
    - Angioedema
    - Hypotension
  - Very rapid onset of action of histamines
    - Effects are short lived because histamines are quickly broken down by plasma enzymes
- Leukotrienes—The most potent bronchoconstrictors whose chemical mediators cause:
  - Wheezing
  - Coronary vasoconstriction
  - Increased vascular permeability
- Eosinophils
  - Process of anaphylaxis attracts eosinophils to the site of allergic inflammation.
  - Exact mechanism of action is unknown, but it is believed that eosinophils contain an enzyme that can deactivate leukotrienes.
- Remaining chemical mediators (heparin, neutrophil chemotactic factor, and kinins) exert varying effects, which may include:
  - Fever
  - Chills

  - Bronchospasm
  - Pulmonary vasoconstriction
- These complex chemical processes can rapidly lead to:
  - Upper airway obstruction and bronchospasm
  - Dysrhythmias and cardiac ischemia
  - Circulatory collapse and shock

Assessment Findings

- An accurate history and physical assessment are necessary to differentiate severe allergic reactions from other medical conditions that may mimic anaphylaxis (Table 26-1).
- Disease entities that may present with similar signs and symptoms of anaphylaxis include the following:
  - Severe asthma with respiratory failure
  - Upper airway obstruction
  - Toxic or septic shock
  - Pulmonary edema (with or without myocardial infarction)
  - Drug overdose
  - Hypovolemic shock
  - Respiratory effects
- Initial signs of respiratory involvement associated with anaphylaxis may range from sneezing and coughing to complete airway obstruction (secondary to laryngeal and epiglottic edema).
- The patient may complain of throat tightness and dyspnea, and stridor or voice changes may be evident.
- Lower airway bronchospasm and associated hypersecretion of mucus may produce wheezing and significant respiratory distress.
- Symptoms can develop with startling rapidity.
- Cardiovascular effects:
  - Cardiovascular manifestations of allergic reactions range from mild hypotension to vascular collapse and profound shock in anaphylaxis.
  - Dysrhythmias are common.
    - — May be related to severe hypoxia and intervascular hypovolemia
  - Patient may complain of chest pain if myocardial ischemia is present.

TABLE 26-1: Conditions That May Mimic Anaphylaxis

Signs and Symptoms	Possible Causes
Stridor	Upper airway obstruction, foreign body aspiration, epiglottitis
Bronchospasm	Asthma, chronic obstructive pulmonary disease (COPD), bronchitis
Syncope	Vasovagal syncope
	Seizure
	Hypoglycemia
	Cardiac dysrhythmias
Hypotension	Shock from any cause
Urticaria	Infection

- Gastrointestinal effects—Nausea, vomiting, diarrhea, and severe abdominal cramping may be present.
  - Increased GI activity is related to:
    - Smooth muscle contraction
    - Increased mucus production
    - Outpouring of fluid from the gut wall into the intestinal lumen, initiated by chemical mediators
- Nervous system effects:
  - Are largely caused by the impaired gas exchange and shock associated with anaphylaxis.
  - Initially, the patient may be agitated and speak of a sense of impending doom.
- As hypoxia worsens, neurological function may deteriorate, resulting in confusion, weakness, headache, syncope, seizures, and coma.
- Cutaneous effects:
  - Perhaps the most visible signs that distinguish anaphylaxis from other medical conditions
  - Signs are secondary to vasodilation induced by histamine release from the mast cells
  - Initially, the patient may complain of warmth and pruritus
  - Physical examination often reveals diffuse erythema and urticaria that result in well-circumscribed wheals of 1 to 6 cm, which may be more reddened or paler than the surrounding skin and often accompanied by severe itching
  - Marked swelling of the face and tongue and angioedema may be present, reflecting involvement of deeper capillaries of the skin and mucous membranes
  - As hypoxia and shock continue, cyanosis may be evident

Initial Assessment

- As in any critical emergency, initial patient care measures are directed at providing adequate airway and ventilatory and circulatory support.
  - Pharmacological therapy is often the definitive treatment, so drug administration should be expedited in anaphylaxis.
- Airway assessment is critical; most deaths from anaphylaxis are directly related to upper airway obstruction.
  - Evaluate the conscious patient for voice changes, stridor, or a barking cough.
  - Complaints of tightness in the neck and dyspnea suggest impending airway obstruction.
  - Airway of unconscious patient should be evaluated and secured.
  - If airflow is impeded, endotracheal intubation should be performed.
  - If there is severe laryngeal and epiglottic edema, surgical or needle cricothyrotomy may be indicated to provide airway access.
- Monitor the patient closely for signs of respiratory distress as indicated by:
  - Pulse oximetry
  - Skin color
  - Accessory muscle use
  - Wheezing
  - Diminished breath sounds
  - Abnormal respiratory rates
- Circulatory status may deteriorate quickly.
  - Pulse quality, rate, and location should frequently be assessed.

History

- May be difficult to obtain but is critical to rule out other medical emergencies that may mimic anaphylaxis.
- Question the patient regarding the chief complaint and the rapidity of onset of symptoms. Signs and symptoms of anaphylaxis usually appear within 1 minute to 30 minutes of introduction of the antigen.
- Significant medical history to obtain includes the following:
  - Previous exposure and response to the suspected antigen
  - Method of introduction of the antigen
  - Injection frequently produces the most rapid and severe response
  - Chronic or current illness and medication use
  - Preexisting cardiac disease or bronchial asthma
  - Allergic reaction may lead to severe complications in the cardiopulmonary system
  - Use of certain medications (beta-blockers) may diminish the patient's response to epinephrine and necessitate administration of other drugs
  - Determine whether the patient has been prescribed an emergency epinephrine (Adrenalin) drug kit (Epi Pen) and whether the medication was administered before the arrival of emergency medical service (EMS) personnel

Physical Examination

- Assess and frequently reassess vital signs.
  - Initially, most patients are tachycardic, tachypneic, and hypotensive if deterioration to cardiac arrest has not occurred.
- Inspect the patient's face and neck for angioedema, hives, tearing, and rhinorrhea, and note the presence of erythema or urticaria on other body regions.
- Assess lung sounds frequently to evaluate the clinical progress of the patient and to monitor the effectiveness of interventions.
- Monitor electrocardiogram (ECG).

Drug Therapy

- Ventilatory support and the parenteral administration of epinephrine (adrenalin) are the most specific interventions in the management of anaphylaxis, along with fluid resuscitation in the presence of hypovolemia.
- If manifestations are mild or moderate and the adult patient is alert, the SQ/IM administration of 0.3 mL of 1:1000 epinephrine is generally recommended.
  - Pediatric dose for epinephrine is 0.01 mL/kg of 1:1000 solution
- If the antigen was injected by an insect sting, medical direction may recommend that 0.15–0.25 mL of 1:1000 epinephrine be injected into the site after the initial dose of epinephrine (with the exception of fingers, toes, ear, nose, and penis).
  - Applying ice to the affected area and applying a constricting band (released for 1 minute of every 10 minutes) to an affected extremity may help decrease antigen absorption.
  - The affected limb also should be splinted to limit movement.
- In the presence of circulatory collapse, IV fluid therapy with a volume-expanding solution should be initiated.
- Alternative drug routes:
  - The subcutaneous administration of epinephrine is usually effective in managing anaphylaxis.
  - In some situations, however, the IV, IO, or sublingual administration of epinephrine may be indicated (controversial).

  - Consult with medical direction before administering epinephrine by any alternative route.

Additional Drug Therapy

- Additional drug therapy may be helpful, but epinephrine is the only drug that can immediately reverse the life-threatening complications of anaphylaxis.
- Pharmacological agents that may be used with epinephrine include the following:
  - Antihistamines to antagonize the effects of histamine
  - Diphenhydramine (Benadryl)
  - Hydroxyzine (Atarax, Vistaril)
  - Promethazine (Phenergan)
  - Cimetidine (Tagamet)
  - Ranitidine (Zantac)
  - Beta agonists to improve alveolar ventilation
  - Albuterol (Ventolin, Proventil)
  - Metaproterenol (Alupent)
  - Isoetharine (Bronkosol)
  - Corticosteroids to prevent a delayed reaction
  - Methylprednisolone (Solu-Medrol)
  - Hydrocortisone (Solu-Cortef)
  - Dexamethasone (Decadron)
  - Antidysrhythmics
  - Lidocaine (Xylocaine) and others
  - Vasopressors to manage protracted hypotension
  - Dopamine (Intropin)
  - Norepinephrine (Levophed)
- After pharmacological therapy and stabilization, the patient should be rapidly transported to the receiving hospital.

CHAPTER QUESTIONS

1. A 24-year-old female was stung by a bee. She is complaining of urticaria on her arms and legs. What medication would you administer to reduce the histamine release?
   a. Albuterol 0.083%
   b. Solumedrol 125 mg
   c. Diphenhydramine 50 mg
   d. Atropine 1 mg
2. The patient described in question 1 is now complaining of angio edema and states, "I feel like my throat is closing." What is the primary drug of choice for treating this progression?
   a. Epinephrine 1:10,000 0.3 mg IM
   b. Epinephrine 1:1,000 0.3 mg IM
   c. Epinephrine 1:10,000 0.3 mg IV
   d. None of the above

Suggested Readings

Circulation 2005 112 [Suppl I]: IV-143–145; published online before print November 28, 2005, doi:10.1161/CIRCULATIONAHA.105.166568.

US Department of Transportation, National Highway Traffic Safety Administration. *EMT-Paramedic: National Standard Curriculum.* Washington, DC: US Department of Transportation, National Highway Traffic Safety Administration; 1998.

Chapter 27
Gastroenterology

Your 81-year-old patient complains of a sudden onset of severe, constant pain in his abdomen which radiates to his lower back.

Assessment reveals:

B/P: 82/40

Pulse: 110, thready and weak

Respiratory rate: 16 regular

Femoral pulses are weak, and you palpate a pulsating mass in his abdomen.

What is the most likely cause of abdominal pain in this patient?

Acute abdominal pain is a common chief complaint in emergency care that may reflect serious illness.

GASTROINTESTINAL (GI) ANATOMY AND PHYSIOLOGY

Physiology

- The GI system provides the body with water, electrolytes, and other nutrients.
- The GI system is specialized to:
  - Ingest of food
  - Propel food through the GI tract
  - Absorb nutrients across the wall of the lumen of the GI tract

Anatomy

Oral Cavity

- Saliva secreted in response to the presence of food in the mouth
  - Contains mucus that helps bind food together into a bolus
  - Contains digestive enzyme (salivary amylase)
    - — Begins chemical breakdown of carbohydrates (starch)
  - Contains antibodies and enzymes that help prevent bacterial infection
- Ingested food is chewed by teeth for processing and is swallowed
  - Tongue pushes bolus of food into pharynx
  - Food pushed into esophagus by pharyngeal muscles
  - Epiglottis closes entrance to airway to prevent aspiration
- Muscular contractions push food through esophagus into stomach

Stomach

- Connects esophagus to duodenum (first part of small intestine)
- Storage area for food before release into small intestine
- Lined with mucous membranes (to protect stomach wall and duodenum) and gastric glands that secrete:
  - Hydrochloric acid—Kills bacteria and activates the protein-digesting enzyme pepsin
  - Intrinsic factor—Assists in absorption of vitamin B_{12}
  - Gastrin—Stimulates flow of gastric juice
  - Pepsin—Begins digestion of protein
  - Gastric lipase—Aids digestion of triglycerides
- Food mechanically broken down by churning activity of stomach muscles
- Mixes saliva, food, and gastric juice to form chyme

Small Intestine

- Mucosa produces secretions that contain mucus, electrolytes, and water
  - Lubricates and protects intestinal wall from acidic chyme and digestive enzymes
- Primary mechanical functions of small intestine
  - Mixing and propulsion of chyme
  - Absorption of fluid and nutrients
- Peristaltic contractions move chyme through small intestine toward the ileocecal sphincter, where chyme enters the cecum

Liver

- Largest internal organ, located just below the diaphragm in the upper abdominal cavity. The liver is very vascular; it receives blood supply from hepatic artery and portal vein.
- The liver plays a major role in maintaining normal blood glucose level.
- Breaks down glycogen to glucose (glycogenolysis) when blood glucose levels are low. Can also convert certain amino acids and lactic acid to glucose (gluconeogenesis).
- When blood sugar level is high, converts glucose to glycogen and triglycerides (lipogenesis) for storage.
- Lipid and protein metabolism.
- Removal of drugs and hormones.
- Storage of vitamins A, B_{12}, D, E, and K.
- Storage of minerals (iron and copper).
- Secretes bile (secretes 600–1000 mL [about 1 quart] of bile each day).
- Dilutes stomach acid and emulsifies fats.

Gallbladder

- Stores bile secreted by the liver
  - Dilutes stomach acids and emulsifies fat
- Releases bile into the small intestine when stimulated by hormones secreted by the intestinal mucosa

Pancreas

- Both an exocrine gland (secretes pancreatic juice) and an endocrine gland (secretes hormones, for example, insulin).

- Pancreatic juice is the most important enzyme that contains digestive enzymes, sodium bicarbonate, and alkaline substances to neutralize hydrochloric acid in the digestive juices entering the small intestine.
- Also contains amylase, which continues digestion initiated in the oral cavity.

Large Intestine

- Chyme remains in the large intestine for 18–24 hours, during which:
  - Water and salts are absorbed
  - Mucus is secreted
  - Chyme is converted to feces
- During movement through the large intestine, undigested material is acted on by bacteria.
- Additional nutrients may be released and absorbed.
- Vitamin K and B-complex vitamins are absorbed from the large intestine and enter the blood.
- Defecation reflex occurs from distention of the rectal wall.

ASSESSMENT OF THE PATIENT WITH ACUTE ABDOMINAL PAIN

- Perform an initial survey to ensure adequacy of airway, breathing, and circulation.
- Gather a thorough history focused on the patient's chief complaint.
- Assess and document baseline vital signs.
- Perform a systematic physical examination to help identify abdominal emergencies that may indicate the development of shock or the need for immediate transport for surgical intervention.

History

- When obtaining a history of abdominal pain, attempt to identify the location and type of pain and any associated signs and symptoms.
- Questions that might be included in the OPQRST evaluation:
  - O (Onset)
    - — Was the onset of pain sudden?
    - — What were you doing when it started?
  - P (Provocative): What makes it better or worse?
  - Q (Quality)
    - — What does the pain feel like?
    - — Is it sharp, dull, burning, tearing?
  - R (Region)
    - — Where is the pain located?
    - — Does it radiate?
  - S (Severity)
    - — Is the pain mild, moderate, or severe?
    - — What is the degree of discomfort on a scale of 1–10?
  - T (Time)
    - — When did the pain begin?
    - — How long does it last?

- Other important elements of a patient history include:
  - Any recent illness
  - Past significant medical history
  - Cardiac or respiratory disease that may manifest in abdominal pain
  - Medication use
  - Alcohol or other drug use
  - Last bowel movement
  - Previous abdominal surgeries
- Women should also be questioned regarding:
  - Menstrual activity (including regularity and last menstrual period)
  - Possibility of pregnancy

Location and Type of Abdominal Pain (Table 27-1)

- Recalling the anatomical location of GI organs and structures may provide a method to better assess a specific disorder.
- The types of abdominal pain that may result from chronic or acute episodes may be classified as visceral, somatic, or referred.

Visceral Pain

- Caused by stimulation of autonomic nerve fibers that surround a hollow viscus or by distention or stretching of hollow viscus organs or ligaments
- Usually described as cramping or gas-type pain that varies in intensity, increasing to a high degree of severity and then subsiding
- Is generally diffuse and difficult to localize
- Often centered at the umbilicus or lower in the midline
- Frequently associated with other symptoms of autonomic nerve involvement:
  - Tachycardia
  - Diaphoresis
  - Nausea
  - Vomiting
  - Common causes
  - Early appendicitis
  - Pancreatitis

TABLE 27-1: Location of Abdominal Pain and Possible Origin

RUQ	LUQ	RLQ	LLQ	Epigastric Pain	Diffuse Pain
Cholecystitis Hepatitis Pancreatitis Perforated ulcer Renal pain (right)	Pancreatitis Gastritis Renal pain (left)	Appendicitis Abdominal aortic dissection or rupture Ruptured ectopic pregnancy Ovarian cyst (right) Pelvic inflammatory disease Urinary calculus Hernia Ovarian or testicular torsion	Diverticulitis Abdominal aortic dissection or rupture Ruptured ectopic pregnancy Ovarian cyst (left) Pelvic inflammatory disease Urinary calculus Hernia Ovarian or testicular torsion	Gastritis Esophagitis Pancreatitis Cholecystitis Abdominal aortic aneurysm Myocardial ischemia	Intestinal obstruction Perforation Generalized peritonitis

- Cholecystitis
- Intestinal obstruction

Somatic Pain

- Produced by bacterial or chemical irritation of nerve fibers in the peritoneum (peritonitis).
- Is usually constant and localized to a specific area.
- Often described as sharp or stabbing.
- Patients are generally hesitant to move about and lie on their backs or sides with legs flexed to prevent additional pain from stimulation of the peritoneal area.
- Often exhibit involuntary guarding of abdomen and rebound tenderness during the physical examination.

Common causes

- Appendicitis
- Inflamed or perforated viscera
- Ulcer
- Gallbladder
- Small or large intestine

Referred Pain

- Pain in a part of the body considerably removed from the tissues that cause the pain
- Results from branches of visceral fibers that synapse in the spinal cord with the same second-order neurons that receive pain fibers from the skin
- When these pain fibers are intensely stimulated, pain sensations spread
- Patient experiences pain in areas distant from the original source
- Knowledge of referred pain is important because many visceral ailments cause no other symptoms except referred pain

Signs and symptoms

- The following signs and symptoms are the most common:
  - Nausea, vomiting, anorexia
    - Gastritis
    - Pancreatitis
    - Biliary tract disease
    - High intestinal obstruction
  - Diarrhea
    - Inflammatory process (gastroenteritis, ulcerative colitis)
  - Constipation
    - Dehydration, obstruction, medications (codeine, morphine)
  - Change in stool color
    - Biliary tract obstruction (clay-colored stools)
    - Lower intestinal bleeding (black, tarry stools)
  - Chills and fever
    - Bacterial infection
    - Pyelonephritis
    - Appendicitis
    - Cholecystitis

Vital Signs

- Vital sign assessment should be complete, including evaluation and documentation of the patient's blood pressure, pulse rate (including ECG assessment), respiratory rate and quality, skin color, moisture, temperature, and turgor.
- When possible, the presence or absence of orthostatic changes in the patient's blood pressure should be noted by way of a tilt test to measure orthostatic vital signs.
- A rise from a recumbent position to a sitting or standing position associated with a fall in systolic pressure (after 1 minute) of 10–15 mmHg and/or a concurrent rise in pulse rate (after 1 minute) of 10–15 beats/min indicate a significant volume depletion and a decrease in perfusion status.
- An assessment of blood pressure, pulses, and capillary refill in each extremity should also be performed as a consideration for aortic dissection.

Physical Examination

Inspection

- Note the position in which the patient is lying.
- Many patients with abdominal pain lie on their side with their knees flexed and pulled in toward their chest.
- Other visual clues that may indicate abdominal pain are:
  - Skin color
  - Facial expressions such as grimacing
  - Presence or absence of voluntary movement
- Remove the patient's clothing and inspect the abdominal wall for:
  - Bruises
  - Scars
  - Ascites
  - Abdominal distention
  - Abdominal masses

Auscultation

- Auscultation to confirm the presence or absence of bowel sounds is usually reserved for assessment in the emergency department.
- If auscultation is performed:
  - Evaluate all four quadrants for approximately 2 minutes per quadrant.
  - Bowel sounds increased in number, duration, or intensity indicate the possibility of gastroenteritis or intestinal obstruction.
  - Bowel sounds that are markedly decreased in number and intensity or are absent may indicate peritonitis or ileus.

Palpation

- Begin gentle palpation of the abdomen away from the painful area.
- Note the presence of:
  - Rigidity or spasm
  - Tenderness or masses
- Note patient's facial expressions, which may provide clues about the severity of the pain.
- Note if the abdomen is soft or rigid.

Percussion

- If time permits, a general assessment of tympany and dullness by percussion may be performed to detect the presence of fluid, air, or solid masses in the abdomen.
- A systematic approach should be used, moving either from side to side or in a clockwise direction noting:
  - Tenderness
  - Abdominal skin temperature and color
- Tympany is the major sound that should be noted during percussion due to the normal presence of air in the stomach and intestines.
- Dullness should be heard over organs and solid masses.

MANAGEMENT OF ACUTE ABDOMINAL PAIN

- Patients with acute abdominal pain cannot be definitively managed in the prehospital setting.
- Most patients require extensive evaluation in the emergency department, including laboratory analysis, radiological imaging, fluid and medication therapy, and possible surgical intervention.
- Role of paramedic is to:
  - Support patient's airway and ventilatory status.
  - Perform and document an initial patient assessment, including a thorough history.
  - Monitor vital signs and cardiac rhythm.
  - Initiate intravenous therapy for fluid replacement or fluid resuscitation.
  - Transport patient for physician evaluation.

SPECIFIC ABDOMINAL EMERGENCIES

- Abdominal emergencies can result from inflammation, infection, and obstruction.
- Some disorders may be associated with upper or lower GI bleeding.
- Disorders associated with upper GI bleeding include:
  - Lesions
  - Peptic ulceration
  - Esophagogastric varices
- Disorders associated with lower GI bleeding include:
  - Colonic lesions
  - Diverticulosis
  - Hemorrhoids
- Other disorders, such as pancreatitis and cholecystitis, are more commonly associated with acute abdominal pain in the absence of bleeding.

Gastroenteritis

- Inflammation of the stomach and intestines that accompanies numerous GI disorders.
- Symptoms include anorexia, nausea/vomiting, abdominal discomfort, or diarrhea.
- May be caused by:
  - Bacterial enterotoxins
  - Bacterial or viral invasion
  - Chemical toxins
  - Other conditions (lactose intolerance)

- Infectious forms of gastroenteritis are often transmitted through the fecal-oral route, and by ingestion of infected food or nonpotable water.
- Likely to affect travelers in endemic areas and populations in disaster areas where water supplies are contaminated.
  - Native populations in endemic areas are generally resistant.
- Onset of gastroenteritis may be slow, but more often is abrupt and violent, with rapid loss of fluids and electrolytes from persistent vomiting and diarrhea.
- Hypokalemia and hyponatremia, acidosis, or alkalosis may develop.

Management

- Primarily supportive
- Bed rest, sedation, intravenous fluid replacement, and medications to control vomiting and diarrhea
  - Some forms of gastroenteritis may be managed with antibiotic therapy
- EMS personnel working in disaster areas should observe the following guidelines:
  - Avoid patient contact if ill
  - Know the source of water supplies or drink hot beverages brisk-boiled or disinfected
  - Avoid habits that facilitate fecal-oral/mucous membrane transmission
  - Observe body substance isolation (BSI) precautions and effective hand-washing procedures

Gastritis

- Acute or chronic inflammation of the gastric mucosa that commonly results from:
  - Hyperacidity
  - Alcohol or drug ingestion (e.g., aspirin, nonsteroidal anti-inflammatory drugs [NSAIDs], corticosteroids)
  - Bile reflux
  - *Helicobacter pylori* infection

Signs and Symptoms

- Epigastric pain
- Nausea/vomiting (which may be severe)
- Mucosal bleeding (erosive gastritis)
- Epigastric tenderness on palpation
- The patient with gastritis may be hypovolemic from prolonged bleeding with or without melena (abnormal maroon-colored or dark tarry stools containing digested blood)

Management

- Diet regulation
- Medications (antibiotics and antacids)
- Fluid replacement or fluid resuscitation if hypovolemia or dehydration occurs

Colitis

- An inflammatory condition of the large intestine characterized by severe diarrhea and ulceration of the mucosa of the intestine (ulcerative colitis)
- Signs and symptoms
  - Weight loss

  - Significant pain
  - Grossly bloody stools
- Affects all age groups, with the highest incidence in the third and fourth decades of life
- A family history of the disease is present in 10–15% of cases
- Cause of colitis is unknown

Management

- Usually managed with steroids, electrolytes, antibiotics, and diet regulation

Diverticulosis

- A diverticulum is a sac or pouch that develops in the wall of the colon.
  - Common development with advancing years
  - Associated with diets low in fiber
- Diverticular outpouchings (a condition known as diverticulosis) tend to develop at the weakest point in the colon wall where intraluminal vessels penetrate the circular muscular layer.
  - Often there is a small artery or arteriole at the neck of the diverticulum from which subsequent bleeding may occur.

Signs and Symptoms

- Serious complications of diverticular disease associated with perforation are:
  - Massive, bright-red rectal bleeding (which can be brisk and commonly painless)
  - Peritonitis
  - Sepsis
- Most patients with diverticula are completely asymptomatic.
  - Up to 30% of patients experience diverticulitis when one or more diverticulum becomes obstructed with fecal matter.
- Mild complications of diverticulitis include:
  - Irregular bowel habits (alternating constipation and diarrhea)
  - Fever
  - Lower left quadrant pain
- Recurrences of diverticulitis are common within the first 5 years after the onset of symptoms.

Management

- Definitive care includes diet regulation, antibiotic therapy, and sometimes surgical repair

Appendicitis

- A common abdominal emergency that occurs when the opening between the lumen of the appendix and the cecum is obstructed by fecal material (fecalith) or from inflammation from viral or bacterial infection.
- If allowed to persist, the inflamed organ eventually becomes gangrenous and ruptures within the peritoneal cavity, resulting in peritonitis and shock, or the condition may evolve into a periappendiceal abscess.

Signs and Symptoms

- Nausea/vomiting
- Chills

- Low-grade fever
- Anorexia
- Abdominal pain or cramping
  - Pain is initially periumbilical and diffuse, later becoming intense and localized to the right lower quadrant just medial to the iliac crest (McBurney's point)
  - If the appendix ruptures, the patient's pain diminishes before the development of peritoneal signs
- The goal of definitive care for appendicitis is surgical appendectomy before rupture

Peptic Ulcer Disease

- Results from a complex pathological interaction among the acidic gastric juice and proteolytic enzymes and the mucosal barrier.
- The three most common causes of peptic ulcer disease are:
  - *H. pylori* infection
  - NSAID use
  - Increased circulatory gastrin from gastrin-secreting tumors (Zollinger-Ellison syndrome)
- These factors are responsible for the formation of ulcers (an open wound or sore) usually in the stomach or duodenum. Ulcers cause disintegration and death of tissue as they erode the mucosal layers in the affected areas.
  - If left unmanaged, massive hemorrhage or perforation may result
- The patient with a peptic ulcer often uses over-the-counter antacids.

Signs and Symptoms

- Pain—Often described as a burning or gnawing discomfort in the epigastric region or left upper quadrant. Develops before meals (classically, early morning) or during stressful periods, when the production of gastric acids increases. Is usually sudden in onset, and is commonly relieved by food intake, antacids, or vomiting.
- Vomiting of blood.
- Melena (due to hemorrhagic blood passing through the GI tract).

Management

- Prehospital care includes obtaining a pertinent history, evaluating for hypotension, and providing circulatory support as needed.
- After physician evaluation, definitive care may involve antibiotics, antacids, H_2-receptor antagonists or other medications, and occasionally, diet regulation.
- Some patients require hospitalization for fluid or blood replacement or surgery if medications are not effective or blood loss is ongoing.

Bowel Obstruction

- An occlusion of the intestinal lumen that results in blockage of normal flow of intestinal contents. May be caused by:
  - Adhesions
  - Hernias
  - Fecal impaction
  - Polyps
  - Tumors
- Obstructions can be mimicked by paralytic ileus (a decrease or absence of intestinal peristalsis), which may result from many localized or systemic conditions.

- Small bowel obstruction is most often caused by adhesions or hernia.
- Large bowel obstructions commonly result from tumors or fecal impaction.

Signs and Symptoms

- Nausea/vomiting
- Abdominal pain
- Constipation
- Abdominal distention
- The speed of onset and degree of symptoms depend on the anatomical site of obstruction (small vs. large bowel).
- The most significant danger of an obstructive condition is perforation with generalized peritonitis and sepsis.
- The patient with bowel obstruction often presents with abdominal pain, and dehydration which may result from the following:
  - Vomiting
  - Decreased intestinal absorption
  - Fluid loss into the lumen and interstitium (bowel wall edema)
- As the affected portion of the bowel distends, its blood supply is decreased and the segment becomes ischemic.
  - Distention and ischemia combine to produce perforation with secondary peritonitis
- If the intestine becomes strangulated, blood or plasma may be lost from the affected intestinal segment.

Management

- Fluid replacement, antibiotics, placement of a nasogastric (NG) tube for decompression, and frequently surgery to correct the obstructing lesion

Crohn's Disease

- A chronic, inflammatory bowel disease thought to be of autoimmune etiology, usually affecting the ileum, colon, or both structures
- The diseased segments associated with Crohn's disease may be separated by normal bowel segments or skip areas
- Formation of fistulas from the diseased bowel to the anus, vagina, skin surface, or to other loops of bowel are common

Signs and Symptoms

- Frequent attacks of diarrhea
- Severe abdominal pain
- Nausea
- Fever
- Chills
- Weakness
- Anorexia
- Weight loss
- Should be suspected in any patient with chronic inflammatory colitis and a history of anorectal problems such as fistulas or abscesses
- These patients are frequently hospitalized and, once stabilized, are treated with antibiotics, diet regulation, steroids, and antimotility agents to attempt to induce remission

Pancreatitis

- Inflammation of the pancreas
- May cause severe epigastric pain

Signs and Symptoms

- Nausea/vomiting.
- Abdominal tenderness and distention.
  - Abdominal pain is often described as severe, radiating from mid-umbilicus to the patient's back and shoulders.
- In severe cases, the patient has fever, tachycardia, and signs of generalized sepsis and shock.
- Patients are often hospitalized and managed with intravenous fluids, pain medication, and placement of an NG tube if vomiting.

Esophagogastric Varices

- Esophagogastric varices are common with hepatic disease and often result from portal hypertension caused by cirrhosis of the liver.
- Obstruction to portal blood flow produced by the fibrosis in the liver increases portal pressure and dilates vessels that drain into the portal system.
- Subsequent dilation of thin-walled veins around the lower esophagus and upper end of the stomach produces esophageal varices.
- Varices are subject to rupture and life-threatening hemorrhage.
- Other causes of esophageal bleeding include:
  - Esophagitis (associated with chronic use of alcohol and NSAIDs)
  - Malignancy
  - Episodes of prolonged, violent vomiting that produce a tear or laceration in the mucosa of the upper esophagus (Mallory-Weiss syndrome)

Signs and Symptoms

- Bright-red hematemesis and vomiting (may be severe).
- If bleeding is profuse, melena may be evident, and the patient may manifest classic signs of shock.
- Variceal bleeding is usually massive and generally difficult to control.

Management

- Ensure a patent airway
- Fluid resuscitation
- Definitive care may include placement of a Sengstaken-Blakemore tube to tamponade bleeding vessels, surgical ligation of the bleeding varices, or transendoscopic injection of a sclerosing agent into the bleeding vessels
- Mortality rate for patients with variceal bleeding is about 25%

Hemorrhoids

- Swollen, distended veins (internal and/or external) in the rectoanal area
- Present in 50% of all people by age 50

Signs and Symptoms

- Most frequently present with blood streaking rather than life-threatening hemorrhage.
- Pain is infrequent unless thrombosis, ulceration, or infection is present.

- Slight bleeding is the most common symptom and usually occurs during or after defecation.
- Blood dripping into the toilet after defecation or blood-stained toilet tissue after wiping are common indications.
- Although blood loss is usually slight, recurrent episodes of bleeding may be significant enough to produce anemia.

Management

- Conservative dietary management, tissue fixation techniques, and operative hemorrhoidectomy for severe cases

Cholecystitis

- Inflammation of the gallbladder, most often associated with the presence of gallstones (75% of which are predominantly cholesterol stones).
- Very common in the United States and occurs more often in women 30–50 years of age than in men.
- On occasion, the gallstones completely obstruct the neck or cystic duct of the gallbladder.
- This is followed by a large increase in pressure within the organ.
- The increased pressure causes a sudden onset of pain (biliary colic), which radiates to the right upper quadrant or right scapula.
- Pain often occurs at night and is generally associated with recent ingestion of fried or fatty foods.
- Other associated hallmarks of cholecystitis include:
  - Previous episodes
  - Family history of gallbladder disease
  - Low-grade fever
  - Nausea/vomiting that may be bile-stained and described as bitter (variable)
  - Pain and tenderness on palpation in the right upper quadrant
- Passage of stones into the common bile duct with subsequent obstruction may cause chills, high fever, jaundice, or acute pancreatitis.

Management

- Hospitalization, intravenous therapy, antibiotics, placement of an NG tube, and possible surgical removal of the gallbladder

Acute Hepatitis

- Inflammation of the liver, associated with the sudden onset of malaise, weakness, anorexia, intermittent nausea and vomiting, and dull right-upper-quadrant pain, usually followed within 1 week by the onset of jaundice, dark urine, or both.
- Although many viruses can infect the liver, the three classes of viruses that are of main concern as causes of acute hepatitis are:
  - Hepatitis A virus (HAV)
  - Hepatitis B virus (HBV)
  - Hepatitis C virus (HCV) formerly known as non-A/non-B hepatitis virus
- All types produce similar pathological alterations in the liver and stimulate an antibody response specific to the type of virus causing the disease.

Risk Factors for Hepatitis

- Hepatitis A
  - Health-care practice without BSI precautions
  - Household or sexual contact with an infected person

- Living in an area with HAV outbreak
- Traveling to developing countries
- Engaging in sex with infected partners and/or multiple partners
- Drug use by injection

- Hepatitis B
  - Health-care practice without BSI precautions
  - Infant born to HBV-infected mother
  - Engaging in sex with infected partners and/or multiple partners
  - Drug use by injection
  - Patients receiving hemodialysis
- Hepatitis C
  - Health-care practice without BSI precautions
  - Blood transfusion recipients before July 1992
  - Engaging in sex with infected partners and/or multiple partners
  - Drug use by injection
  - Patients receiving hemodialysis

Causes

- Alcohol or other drug use
- Autoimmune disorders
- Toxic bacterial, fungal, parasitic, and viral infections
- Patients require medical evaluation to manage the course of the disease effectively

CHAPTER QUESTIONS

1. An inflammatory condition of the large intestine characterized by severe diarrhea and ulceration of the mucosa of the intestine.
   a. Ulcerative colitis
   b. Gastritis
   c. Diverticulosis
   d. Appendicitis
2. Acute or chronic inflammation of the gastric mucosa commonly results from:
   a. ulcerative colitis
   b. gastritis
   c. diverticulosis
   d. appendicitis

Suggested Reading

US Department of Transportation, National Highway Traffic Safety Administration. *EMT-Paramedic: National Standard Curriculum.* Washington, DC: US Department of Transportation, National Highway Traffic Safety Administration; 1998.

Chapter 28
Toxicology

Your patient, a local town worker, spilled Malathion over one-third of his body while filling a spray can in order to kill mosquitoes. The responding Haz-mat team followed field decontamination procedures prior to patient transport by ambulance to a hospital. The patient is exhibiting severe respiratory difficulty, salivation, lacrimation, and uncontrollable urination, and is complaining of severe abdominal cramping and diarrhea. The patient has been decontaminated and is in the cold zone awaiting your arrival.

As a member of the ambulance crew, and prior to beginning transport, what should you do?

- Our environment contains many potentially harmful substances (natural and synthetic) that can be accidentally or deliberately introduced into the body.
- These include animal and plant toxins, industrial and household chemicals, therapeutic pharmaceuticals, and drugs of abuse.
- Early identification of these agents and prevention of systemic absorption are crucial to the successful management of patients with toxicological emergencies.

POISONING FACTS

According to the National Center for Injury Prevention and Control:

- In the United States in 2003, 5543 (19.3%) of the 28,700 poisoning deaths were intentional; 5462 were suicides and 81 were homicides (CDC 2005).
- In 2004, intentional poisoning led to about 279,802 emergency department (ED) visits; 272,275 involved self-harm and 7527 were assaults (CDC 2005).
- Self-harm poisoning was the second-leading cause of ED visits for intentional injury in 2004 (CDC 2005).
- In 2003, 19,457 (67.8%) of the 28,700 poisoning deaths in the United States were unintentional, and 3700 (12.9%) were of undetermined intent (CDC 2005).
- Unintentional poisoning was second only to motor vehicle crashes as a cause of unintentional injury death that same year (CDC 2005).
- In 2004, unintentional poisoning caused about 577,886 emergency department (ED) visits (CDC 2005).
- Almost 25% of these unintentional ED visits resulted in hospitalization or transfer to another facility (CDC 2005).

POISON CONTROL CENTERS

- More than 63 poison control centers exist in the United States to help manage poisoning emergencies.
- Most are based in major medical centers or teaching hospitals.

- Each belongs to 1 of 41 American Association of Poison Control Centers—Designated regional poison control centers.
- Regional centers are staffed by medical professionals and offer 24-hour telephone access to population bases of at least 1 million.
- Each year, more than 2 million poisonings are reported to poison control centers throughout the United States.
- More than 90% of these poisonings happen in the home.
- 53% percent of poisoning victims are children younger than 6 years old.
- By helping people manage emergencies at home, these centers prevent about 50,000 hospitalizations and 400,000 visits to doctors' offices each year.
- By request, information and treatment advice are immediately provided by the poison control center through a comprehensive group of references on more than 350,000 toxic substances, including drugs (legal, illicit, foreign, and veterinary), chemicals, plants, animals, insects, fish, snakes, cosmetics, and hazardous materials.
- Each request for patient care information is followed up to determine effectiveness and confirm desired outcome.
- In addition, the centers are responsible for the following six elements of an organized poison system:
  - Treatment information and toxicological consultation with health-care providers and the public, using a toll-free number with linkage into various 911 systems
  - Professional education to train those involved in care of poisoned patients
  - Data collection on all poisonings in the region for epidemiological and evaluation purposes
  - Public education and prevention
  - Research
  - Regional emergency medical service (EMS) poison system development (e.g., patient classification criteria, triage and treatment protocols, and regional transfer agreements)

Use by EMS Agencies

- Regional poison control centers are a ready source of information for any toxicological emergency.
- Depending on local protocol, poison control centers may be contacted directly by EMS providers.
- Immediate determination of potential toxicity is based on:
  - The specific agent or agents
  - Amount ingested
  - Time of exposure
  - Weight and medical condition of the patient
  - Any treatment rendered before EMS arrival
- The poison control center can coordinate treatment by notifying the receiving hospital while the patient is en route to the emergency department.

GENERAL GUIDELINES FOR MANAGING A POISONED PATIENT

- Poisons may enter the body through:
  - Ingestion
  - Inhalation

- Injection
- Absorption
- Types of toxicological emergencies:
  - Accidental poisoning from dosage errors, idiosyncratic reactions, childhood poisoning, environmental exposure, and occupational exposure
  - Drug/alcohol abuse
  - Intentional poisoning/overdose
    - — Chemical warfare
    - — Assault/homicide
    - — Suicide attempts
- Since most poisoned patients require only supportive therapy to recover, the poisoned patient can often be appropriately managed in the prehospital setting using the following guidelines:
  - Ensure adequate airway, ventilation, and circulation
  - Obtain a thorough history and perform a focused physical examination
  - Consider hypoglycemia in an unconscious or convulsing patient
  - Administer naloxone or nalmefene to a patient with respiratory depression
  - If overdose is suspected, obtain an overdose history from the patient, family, or friends
  - Consult with medical direction or a poison control center for specific treatment to prevent further absorption of the toxin (or antidote therapy)
  - Frequently reassess the patient; monitor vital signs and electrocardiogram (ECG)
  - Safely obtain any substance or substance container of a suspected poison and transport it with the patient
  - Transport the patient for physician evaluation

POISONING BY INGESTION

- About 80% of all accidental ingestions of poisons occur in children 1–3 years of age. Most result from household products (petroleum-based agents, cleaning agents, cosmetics, medications, toxic plants, contaminated foods).
- Poisoning in adults is usually intentional, although accidental poisoning from exposure to chemicals in the workplace also occurs.
  - Deliberate poisonings are often an attempt at suicide or a result of recreational or experimental drug abuse.
    - — Intentional poisonings also may result from chemical warfare or acts of terrorism, or be a factor in assault and homicide.
- The toxic effects of ingested poisons may be immediate or delayed, depending on the substance ingested.
  - Corrosive substances such as strong acids and alkalis may produce immediate tissue damage, as evidenced by burns to the lips, tongue, throat, and upper gastrointestinal (GI) tract.
  - Medications and toxic plants usually require absorption and distribution through the blood stream to produce toxic effects.
    - — Because minimal absorption occurs in the stomach, poisons may take several hours to enter the blood stream through the small intestine.
- Early management of the ingested poisoning focuses on:
  - Removing the toxin from the stomach or binding it to prevent absorption before the poison enters the intestines.

Assessment and Management

- The primary goal of physical assessment of poisoned patients is to identify effects on the three vital organ systems—respiratory system, cardiovascular system, and central nervous system—which most likely will produce immediate morbidity and mortality.
- Five signs of major toxicity include:
  - Coma
  - Cardiac dysrhythmias
  - GI disturbances
  - Respiratory depression
  - Hypotension or hypertension

Respiratory Complications

- After ensuring scene safety, secure a patent airway and provide adequate ventilatory support. This includes providing high-concentration oxygen and possibly aggressive airway management to protect against potential airway compromise or aspiration.
- Other respiratory complications that may be associated with poisoning include:
  - Early development of noncardiogenic pulmonary edema
  - Later development of adult respiratory distress syndrome and bronchospasm, which may result from direct or indirect toxic effects

Cardiovascular Complications

- The most common complication is cardiac rhythm disturbances—Closely monitor circulatory status by ECG and take frequent blood pressure measurements.
- Tachydysrhythmias or bradydysrhythmias may indicate serious disorders such as hypoxia and acidosis.
- Other complications include hypotension (associated with decreased vascular tone) and, rarely, hypertension, which may lead to cerebral vascular hemorrhage.

Neurological Complications

- Perform and document a baseline neurological examination.
- Deviations from normal mental status may range from mild drowsiness and agitation to hallucinations, seizures, cardiopulmonary depression, and death.
- Neurological complications may result from the toxin itself (such as lead poisoning in children who have ingested paint chips) or be secondary to an underlying metabolic or perfusion problem.

History

- If possible, ascertain the following through questioning:
  - What was ingested?
    - — Obtain the poison container and remaining contents (unless it poses a threat to rescuer safety)
  - When was the substance ingested?
    - — This may affect the decision to induce emesis or to use gastric lavage, activated charcoal, or antidote administration
  - How much of the substance was ingested?
  - Was an attempt made to induce vomiting?
  - Has an antidote or activated charcoal been administered?
  - Does the patient have a psychiatric history pertinent to suicide attempts or recent episodes of depression?

Gastrointestinal Decontamination

- The goal of treating serious poisonings by ingestion is to prevent the toxic substance from reaching the small intestine (limiting its absorption). This may be accomplished through the use of activated charcoal and sometimes gastric lavage or syrup of ipecac.
- Activated charcoal:
  - An inert, nontoxic product of wood material that has been heated to extremely high temperatures.
  - Surface characteristics enable it to adsorb (collect in a condensed form) molecules of many chemical toxins while in the intestinal tract, thereby inhibiting absorption of the poison by as much as 50% and preventing systemic toxicity.
  - Is a safe and effective treatment for most toxic ingestions and is administered in nearly all cases unless strong acids, strong alkali, or ethanol is the toxicant.
  - Other agents not well adsorbed by activated charcoal include cyanide, ferrous sulfate, and methanol.
    - — If these substances have been ingested, activated charcoal should probably be withheld.

      Consult with medical direction or a poison control center
    - — May be withheld when:

      Specific oral antidotes are available
      - N-Acetylcysteine (Mucomyst) for acetaminophen overdose
      - The ingestion occurred 1 or more hours before presentation
  - Activated charcoal comes mixed in an aqueous solution with or without a cathartic (an agent that causes bowel evacuation).
    - — A cathartic (most commonly sorbitol) decreases the transit time and expels the charcoal within a short period.
  - Complications of activated charcoal therapy include poor patient acceptance and vomiting.
  - EMS personnel should protect themselves, the patient, and the immediate area from the staining properties of activated charcoal and should use personal protective measures when administering this agent.
- Gastric lavage—A method of GI decontamination that has the advantage of immediate recovery of some gastric contents (if performed within 1 hour after ingestion).
  - It also provides a method for the administration of activated charcoal
  - Is generally performed by using a large-bore orogastric tube (36–40 French in adults, 24–28 French in children)
  - Procedure for gastric lavage
    - — Place the conscious patient in a left lateral Trendelenburg ("swimmer's") position to minimize the possibility of aspiration should emesis occur

      Endotracheal intubation should precede gastric lavage in patients with a depressed level of consciousness or in those without an intact gag reflex
    - — Insert the tube through the mouth into the patient's esophagus and continue to advance the tube until it is placed in the stomach

      If any resistance to passage is noted, the procedure must cease
    - — Check tube placement before lavage by air insufflation into stomach with large syringe
    - — Aspirate gastric contents to confirm correct placement
    - — Infuse tap water or normal saline in amounts not to exceed 150–200 mL aliquots in adults, or 50–100 mL aliquots in patients younger than 5 years old

- Gastric lavage should continue until the return fluid appears clear.
- The return fluid should be approximately the same amount as the fluid administered.
- Contraindications
  - Gastric lavage is contraindicated in:
    - Patients with unprotected airway
    - Patients with altered level of consciousness
    - Patients who have ingested low-viscosity hydrocarbons or caustic agents
  - Potential complications include:
    - Agitation of the patient (produced by the procedure)
    - Inadvertent tracheal intubation
    - Esophageal perforation
    - Aspiration pneumonitis
    - Fluid and electrolyte imbalances in pediatric patients

- Syrup of Ipecac
  - Once considered the treatment of choice in preventing absorption of poisons
    - Studies have shown the agent reduces absorption by only 30%
    - Use may interfere with the efficacy of activated charcoal
  - If administered, it should be given within the first 20 minutes after ingestion of a poison and only to patients who are alert with an intact gag reflex
  - Potential complications of ipecac-induced emesis include:
    - Mallory-Weiss tear of the esophagus
    - Pneumomediastinum
    - Fatal diaphragmatic or gastric rupture
    - Aspiration pneumonitis
  - Contraindications include:
    - Altered level of consciousness
    - Ingestion of caustic substances (esophagus would be exposed to the agent twice)
    - Loss of gag reflex
    - Seizures
    - Pregnancy
    - Acute myocardial infarction
    - Ingestion of
      - Acids
      - Alkalis
      - Ammonia
      - Nontoxic agents
      - Petroleum distillates
      - Rapidly acting central nervous system (CNS) depressants (cyanide, tricyclic antidepressants)
      - Rapidly acting CNS irritants (strychnine)
      - Hydrocarbons (controversial)

Management of Specific Ingested Poisons

- Strong acids and alkalis may cause burns to the mouth, pharynx, esophagus, and sometimes the upper respiratory and GI tracts.
  - Perforation of the esophagus or stomach may result in vascular collapse, mediastinitis, or pneumoperitoneum.

- Ingestions of caustic and corrosive substances generally produce immediate damage to the mucous membrane and the intestinal tract.
- Acids generally complete their damage within 1–2 minutes after exposure.
- Alkali, particularly solid alkali, may continue to cause liquefaction of tissue and damage for minutes to hours.
- Prehospital care is usually limited to airway and ventilatory support, intravenous (IV) fluid replacement, and rapid transport.
- In some situations, medical direction may recommend attempts to dilute the acid or alkali in a conscious patient with oral administration of milk or water (200–300 mL in the adult, 15 mL/kg maximum in a child).
- Efforts to neutralize the ingested agent with other fluids, such as fruit juice, lemon juice, or vinegar, are contraindicated because of the potential for intense exothermic reactions, which may produce severe thermal burns.

Hydrocarbons

- A group of saturated and unsaturated compounds derived primarily from crude oil, coal, or plant substances.
- Mixtures vary in their viscosity, surface tension, and volatility, which, with other factors (e.g., the presence of other chemicals in the product, total amount, and route of exposure), determine the toxic effects of these agents.
- Hydrocarbons are found in many household products and in petroleum distillates, such as:
    - Cleaning and polishing agents (mineral seal oil or signal oil)
    - Spot removers
    - Paints
    - Cosmetics
    - Pesticides
    - Hobby and craft materials
    - Petroleum distillates—Turpentine, kerosene, gasoline, lighter fluids
    - Pine-oil products
- Hydrocarbon poisonings are common, accounting for 7% of all ingestions in children less than 5 years old.
- Viscosity is the most important physical characteristic in potential toxicity.
- The lower the viscosity, the higher the risk of aspiration and associated complications. An agent with low viscosity, such as gasoline or turpentine, rapidly disperses over the pharyngeal and glottic surfaces, the more volatile components becoming gas on contact with warm, mucous membranes.
- Exposure causes irritation, coughing, and possible aspiration, which may allow a toxic amount of hydrocarbons to enter the tracheobronchial tree.
- Chemical characteristics (aromatic, aliphatic, or halogenated) and the presence of toxic additives also are important in determining toxicity.
- Clinical features of hydrocarbon ingestion vary widely, depending on the type of agent involved (see Table 28-1).
- If the patient is asymptomatic on EMS arrival, the chances of serious complications are usually minimal; these patients are generally observed in the emergency department for several hours and often require no treatment.
- Any patient who chokes, coughs, cries, or has spontaneous emesis on swallowing should be assumed to have aspirated.
- Hydrocarbon ingestion may involve the patient's respiratory, GI, and neurological systems. Clinical features may be immediate or delayed in onset.

TABLE 28-1: Clinical Features of Hydrocarbon Ingestion

System	Immediate: Up to 6 Hours	Delayed: Days to Weeks
GI	Mucous membrane Hyperemia irritation Abdominal pain Nausea/vomiting Belching	Diarrhea Hepatic toxicity
Respiratory	Cough and choking Inspiratory stridor Tachypnea Cyanosis Dyspnea	Bacterial pneumonia Dyspnea Sputum production Atelectasis Pulmonary edema
Neurological	Lethargy Coma Seizures	
Systemic factors	Fever Malaise	Spontaneous hemorrhage Hemolytic and aplastic anemias

- Emergency care for symptomatic patients who have ingested hydrocarbon products includes the following:
  - Ensure a patent airway and provide adequate ventilatory and circulatory support as needed.
  - Identify the substance and contact medical direction or a poison control center, per local protocol.
  - Gastric decontamination is generally avoided in these patients to prevent potential aspiration pneumonitis.
    - It is contraindicated with ingestion of mineral seal oil, signal oil, or polishing oils because of their low viscosity and the likelihood of aspiration.
    - Medical direction may recommend gastric emptying of a petroleum product containing significant amounts (greater than 1 mL/kg) of camphor, benzene and its derivatives, organophosphates, halogenated hydrocarbons, and heavy metals such as arsenicals, lead, and mercury.

      In these situations, the chance of systemic toxicity is greater than the risk of aspiration.

      The use of activated charcoal or diluents is not effective in managing hydrocarbon ingestion.
  - Initiate IV fluid therapy.
  - Monitor cardiac rhythm.
  - Transport for physician evaluation.

Methanol (Wood Alcohol)

- A common industrial solvent obtained from distillation of wood.
- A poisonous alcohol found in a variety of products, such as gas line antifreeze, windshield washer fluid, paints, paint removers, varnishes, canned fuels such as Sterno, and many shellacs.

- Methanol is a colorless liquid that has an odor distinct from that of ethanol, the form of alcohol designed for consumption.
- Poisonings may result from intentional or accidental ingestions, absorption through the skin, or inhalation.
- Commonly used by chronic alcoholics to maintain an inebriated state.
- Accidental ingestion resulting from misuse or distribution of methanol for ethanol.
- As the alcohol is absorbed, it rapidly is converted in the liver to formaldehyde and in minutes to formic acid. The accumulation of formic acid in the blood results in a group of symptoms relating to the
  - CNS depression
  - GI tract (pain, nausea, vomiting)
  - Eyes (as little as 4 mL causing blindness)
  - Development of metabolic acidosis
    - Onset of symptoms after ingestion ranges from 40 minutes to 72 hours
- Symptoms of methanol poisoning correlate with the degree of acidosis; they include:
  - CNS depression—Lethargy, confusion, coma, seizures
  - GI tract—Nausea and vomiting, abdominal pain
  - Visual complaints—Blurred or indistinct vision, pupils that are dilated and sluggish to react to light, "spots before the eyes," "snow-filled vision," blindness
  - Metabolic acidosis—Shortness of breath, tachypnea, shock, multisystem failure, and death
- Emergency care for methanol poisoning is as follows:
  - Secure a patent airway and provide adequate ventilatory and circulatory support as needed.
  - Adequate ventilation is essential to ensure adequate oxygenation, help correct the profound metabolic acidosis, and maximize respiratory excretion.
  - An IV line should be established, and the patient should be placed on a cardiac monitor.
  - GI decontamination:
    - If the patient is seen within 1 hour after ingestion, gastric lavage is indicated.
    - The efficacy of activated charcoal in adsorbing methanol is controversial; consult with medical direction or a poison control center.
  - Correction of metabolic acidosis:
    - Attempts to correct metabolic acidosis with sodium bicarbonate administration (1 mEq/kg) may be recommended by medical direction.
    - Larger or repeated doses may be necessary.
    - Although serum formic acid may be neutralized with bicarbonate administration, hemodialysis probably will be necessary to remove toxic levels of methanol and formate.
  - Prevention of the conversion of methanol to formic acid:
    - The conversion of methanol to formic acid may be prevented by the administration of ethanol. If the patient is conscious, give 30 to 60 mL of 80-proof ethanol by mouth or gastric lavage tube.
    - Unconscious patients should have their airway protected with an endotracheal tube (ET) before gastric tube administration of ethanol.
    - Rapidly transport the patient to an appropriate medical facility for definitive treatment.

Ethylene Glycol

- A colorless, odorless, water-soluble liquid commonly used in windshield deicers, detergents, paints, radiator antifreeze, and coolants.
- Early signs and symptoms of CNS depression are usually caused by the ethanol-like effects of ethylene glycol.
- Toxicity is caused by the accumulation of intermediary metabolites, especially glycolic and oxalic acids after metabolism, which occurs primarily in the liver and kidneys.
  - Metabolic intermediaries may affect the CNS and cardiopulmonary and renal systems and result in hypocalcemia (from the precipitation of oxalic acid as calcium oxalate).
- Signs and symptoms of poisoning usually occur in three stages:
  - Stage 1: CNS effects occurring 1–12 hours after ingestion—Slurred speech, ataxia, somnolence, nausea and vomiting, focal or generalized convulsions, hallucinations, stupor, coma
  - Stage 2: Cardiopulmonary system effects occurring 12–36 hours after ingestion—Rapidly progressive tachypnea, cyanosis, pulmonary edema, cardiac failure
  - Stage 3: Renal system effects occurring 24–72 hours after ingestion—Flank pain, oliguria, crystalluria, proteinuria, anuria, hematuria, uremia
- Emergency care for ethylene glycol poisoning is similar to that used in treating methanol poisoning, and includes the following:
  - Ensure a patent airway and provide adequate ventilatory and circulatory support as needed; monitor the patient for dysrhythmias.
  - Use gastric lavage if patient presents within 1 hour after ingestion; administer activated charcoal (shown to decrease GI absorption of ethylene glycol by 50%).
  - Initiate IV therapy with a volume-expanding fluid to maintain adequate urine output.
  - Administer IV sodium bicarbonate levels to correct acidosis.
  - Administer 80-proof ethanol (30–60 mL) by mouth or gastric tube to block the conversion of ethylene glycol into toxic metabolites.
    - — Unmetabolized ethylene glycol is excreted by the lungs and kidneys
  - Rapidly transport the patient for definitive treatment, which may include hemodialysis and continued ethanol administration.
  - Anticipate orders from medical direction or a poison control center for the following:
    - — Thiamine to degrade glycolic acid to nontoxic metabolites
    - — Calcium gluconate or calcium chloride to treat hypocalcemia
    - — Diazepam (Valium) to control seizure activity

Isopropanol (Isopropyl Alcohol)

- A volatile, flammable, colorless liquid with a characteristic odor and bittersweet taste.
- Rubbing alcohol is the most common household source of this agent.
- Used in disinfectants, degreasers, cosmetics, industrial solvents, and cleaning agents.
- Common routes of toxic exposure include:
  - Intentional ingestion as a substitute for ethanol
  - Accidental ingestion
  - Inhalation of high concentrations of local vapor, as from alcohol sponging of febrile children (a harmful and inappropriate procedure)
- More toxic than ethanol but less toxic than methanol or ethylene glycol.
- A potentially lethal dose in adults is 150–240 mL.

- In children, any amount of ingestion should be considered potentially toxic.
  - After ingestion, the majority of isopropanol (80%) is metabolized to acetone.
- The rest is excreted unchanged by the kidneys.
- The acetone is excreted by the kidneys and to a lesser extent by the lungs.
  - Isopropanol poisoning affects several body systems including the CNS, GI, and renal systems.
- Signs and symptoms frequently occur within 30 minutes after ingestion and include:
  - CNS and respiratory depression
  - Abdominal pain
  - Gastritis
  - Hematemesis
  - Hypovolemia
    - Although isopropanol poisoning causes acetonemia and ketonuria, there is usually no associated metabolic acidosis unless the patient manifests hypotension
- Emergency care is primarily supportive.
  - Airway and ventilatory support to ensure adequate respiratory elimination of acetone
  - Gastric lavage (isopropanol also is secreted by the salivary glands and stomach)
  - Fluid resuscitation as needed
  - Rapid transport to an appropriate medical facility, where dialysis may be necessary

Metals

Infants and children are high-risk groups for accidental iron, lead, and mercury poisoning due to their immature immune systems or increased absorption as a function of age.

Iron poisoning

- Approximately 10% of the ingested iron (mainly ferrous sulfate) is absorbed each day from the small intestine.
- After absorption, the iron is converted, stored in iron storage protein, and transported to the liver, spleen, and bone marrow for incorporation into hemoglobin.
- When ingested iron exceeds the body's ability to store it, the free iron circulates in the blood and is deposited into other tissues.
- Accidental or intentional ingestion of iron is a common poisoning that may have lethal complications.
  - Ingested iron is corrosive to GI tract mucosa and may produce bloody vomitus, painless bloody diarrhea, and dark stools.
- Prehospital care includes supportive measures and the prevention of further absorption by GI decontamination.
  - Activated charcoal is generally not recommended, since it adsorbs iron poorly.
  - Most patients with iron poisoning survive the episode, and the long-term prognosis is favorable.

Lead poisoning

- Metallic lead has been used by humans for more than 5000 years, but was not widely recognized as a potential health hazard until 1978 when it was banned from household paints in the United States.
- Lead can be found in:
  - Homes in the city, country, or suburbs

    - Apartments, single-family homes, and both private and public housing painted before 1978
    - Soil around a home (soil contaminated from exterior paint or other sources such as past use of leaded gasoline in cars)
    - Painted windows and window sills
    - Doors and door frames
    - Stairs, railings, and banisters
    - Porches and fences
    - Paint surfaces that have been scraped, dry-sanded, or heated (lead dust)
    - Old painted toys and furniture
    - The air after vacuuming or sweeping contaminated surfaces
    - Food and liquid stored in lead crystal or lead-glazed pottery or porcelain
    - Lead smelters or other industries
    - Hobbies that use lead (e.g., making pottery or stained glass)
    - Folk remedies ("greta" or "azarcon" used to treat an upset stomach)
- Children are the most common victims of lead poisoning; an estimated 889,000 children in the United States have levels of lead in their blood stream of 10 mg/dL or greater.
- Most pediatric poisonings result from ingestion of lead-based paint chips and contaminated house dust.
- Lead toxicity in adults most commonly results from exposure by inhalation.
- If not detected early, children with high levels of lead in their bodies can suffer from:
    - Damage to the brain and nervous system
    - Behavioral and learning problems
    - Hyperactivity
    - Slowed growth
    - Hearing problems
    - Headaches
- Adults can suffer from many problems including:
    - Difficulties during pregnancy
    - Reproductive problems
    - Hypertension
    - GI disorders
    - Nerve disorders
    - Memory and concentration problems
    - Muscle and joint pain
- Most lead poisoning is slow in onset (from chronic ingestion or inhalation), eventually resulting in toxicity.
    - The metal is excreted by the body very slowly, and tends to accumulate in body tissues (primarily bone).
    - Lead causes the most significant pathophysiology in the hematopoietic, neurological, and renal systems; but it also affects the reproductive, GI, skeletal, hepatic, and cardiovascular systems.
- Signs and symptoms of chronic exposure:
    - Malaise
    - Mental disturbances
    - Incoordination
    - Abdominal pain
    - Diarrhea
    - Vomiting

- If the intoxication is acute, anemia, weakness or paralysis of the limbs, seizures, and death may result.
- Prehospital care is focused on recognizing the potential for lead poisoning and transporting the patient for physician evaluation.

Mercury poisoning

- Mercury is the only metallic element that is liquid at room temperature.
- Used in thermometers, sphygmomanometers, and dental amalgam (dental fillings).
- Various compounds of mercury are used in some paints, pesticides, cosmetics, drugs, and in certain industrial processes.
- All forms of mercury (except dental amalgam) are poisonous.
- Some are absorbed into the body more readily than others and are more dangerous.
- Liquid mercury is highly volatile and mercury vapor is readily absorbed into the body via the lungs.
- Inhalation of mercury vapor (the most common route of poisoning) may cause shortness of breath and lung damage.
- Mercury may also be absorbed through the skin (causing severe inflammation) or intestines after ingestion, resulting in nausea, vomiting, diarrhea, and abdominal pain.
- After mercury enters the body, it passes into the blood stream and later accumulates in various organs (principally the brain and kidneys), causing a wide range of symptoms that may include:
  - Malaise
  - Incoordination
  - Excitability
  - Tremors
  - Numbness in the limbs
  - Vision impairment
  - Nausea and emesis (symptoms of renal failure)
  - Mental status changes
- Prehospital care primarily is supportive.
  - Following physician evaluation, patients are managed with GI decontamination (if the ingestion was recent) and chelating agents.
  - In severe cases, hemodialysis may be indicated.

Food Poisoning

A term used for any illness of sudden onset (usually associated with stomach pain, vomiting, and diarrhea) suspected of being caused by food eaten within the previous 48 hours.

Infectious (bacterial) types

- Salmonella is one of the most common types of bacteria responsible for food poisoning—An organism found in many animals (especially poultry) as well as humans. Salmonella bacteria also may be transferred to food from the excrement of infected animals or humans and by food handling by an infected person.
- Other bacteria (strains of staphylococcal bacteria) cause formation of toxins, which may be difficult to destroy even with thorough cooking.
- Bacteria that commonly cause diarrhea are certain strains of
  - *Escherichia coli* (traveler's diarrhea)
  - *Campylobacter*
  - *Shigella*

- Botulism is a rare, but life threatening, form of food poisoning that may result from eating improperly canned or preserved food contaminated with the bacterium *Clostridium botulinum.*
  - This is found in soil and untreated water in most parts of the world and is harmlessly present in the intestinal tracts of many animals, including fish.
  - Its spore-forming properties resist boiling, salting, smoking, and some forms of pickling, allowing the bacterium to thrive in improperly preserved or canned foods.
  - Botulism is associated with severe CNS symptoms that appear in a characteristic head-to-toe progression:
    - Headache, blurred or double vision, dysphagia, respiratory paralysis, and quadriplegia
    - Death from respiratory failure occurs in about 70% of untreated cases
  - *Clostridium difficile* can produce another form of life-threatening diarrhea (pseudomembranous colitis) and is usually associated with long-term administration of certain antibiotics.

Infectious (viral) types

- Viruses that most commonly cause food poisoning are Norwalk virus, a common contaminant of shellfish, and rotavirus
- May be responsible for illness when raw or partly cooked foodstuffs have been in contact with water contaminated by human excrement

Noninfectious types

- May result from consuming mushrooms and toadstools or from eating fresh foods and vegetables accidentally contaminated with large amounts of insecticide.
- Chemical food poisoning also may result from eating food stored in a contaminated container and from improperly preparing and cooking various exotic foods.
  - Quinidine, certain antacids, some antibiotics, and stool softeners or laxatives may cause diarrhea
- Onset of signs and symptoms from food poisoning varies by cause and by how heavily the food was contaminated.
  - As a rule, symptoms usually develop
    - Within 30 minutes in the case of chemical poisoning
    - In 1–12 hours in the case of bacterial toxins
    - In 12–48 hours with viral and bacterial infections
- Use precautions to avoid contamination of self (gloves, gown if appropriate) and equipment.
- Ensure adequate airway, ventilatory, and circulatory support.
- Gather a complete history, including time and onset of symptoms, recent travel, the relation of symptoms to ingestion of a particular food, and effects on others who ate the same food.
  - In addition, information on the consistency, frequency, and odor of stool (including the presence of mucus or blood) should be obtained, and fever should be noted
  - Any patient history also should include significant past medical history, allergies, and use of medications
- Initiate IV therapy with a crystalloid solution to manage dehydration and electrolyte disturbances resulting from vomiting and diarrhea.
- Transport the patient for physician evaluation.

Plant Poisoning

Toxic plant ingestion is a frequently reported category of poisonings, second only to ingestion of cleaning substances. The majority of these exposures occur in children less than 6 years old.

- Signs and symptoms
  - Toxic manifestations of major poisonous plant ingestions are predictable and are categorized by the chemical and physical properties of the plant.
  - Anticholinergic crisis may result from ingestion of certain alkaloid components (jimsonweed and lantana), manifesting in tachycardia, dilated pupils, hot dry skin, decreased bowel sounds, altered vision, and abnormal mental status.
  - Cholinergic symptoms may result from ingestion of certain mushroom species, which is usually manifested by bradycardia, miosis, salivation, hyperactive bowel sounds, and diarrhea.
  - Nicotinic alkaloids (poison hemlock and delphinium) may initially act as stimulants but generally are soon followed by depression and weakness.
  - Most signs and symptoms appear within several hours after ingestion, but some symptoms may be delayed 1–3 days.
- Management
  - Many similar species of plants and mushrooms have widely varying potencies and combinations of toxins, and such factors as the age of the plant and soil conditions may influence the severity of toxic symptoms.
  - Management guidelines should therefore be customized to the patient's symptoms rather than to a particular type of ingestion
  - Although it is important to identify the plant if possible, the inability to do so should not delay treatment.
  - Consult with medical direction or a poison control center regarding appropriate emergency care procedures.
  - Ensure adequate airway, ventilatory, and circulatory support.
  - In patients with a depressed gag reflex, unresponsiveness, or seizures, secure the airway with an ET, and then use orogastric decontamination.
    - — Medical direction or a poison control center may recommend administration of activated charcoal in place of gastric emptying or after it
  - Initiate IV fluid therapy with a volume-expanding solution.
  - Monitor the patient's vital signs and cardiac rhythm.
  - Obtain a sample of the suspected plant or mushroom (if possible).
  - Transport the patient for physician evaluation.
  - Most patients are hospitalized for observation and treatment as indicated for the toxin involved.
    - — Dialysis has not been effective in removing most plant toxins

POISONING BY INHALATION

Accidental or intentional inhalation of poisons can lead to a life-threatening emergency. The type and location of injury caused by toxic inhalation depends on the specific action and behaviors of the chemical involved.

Physical Properties

- The concentration of a chemical in the air and the duration of exposure help determine the severity of inhalation injury.

  - At low concentrations and with brief exposure, the chemical may be removed from the air before reaching the tracheobronchial tree.
  - Large concentrations or prolonged exposure are more likely to cause contact with the lungs and damage to lung tissue.
- Solubility also influences inhalation injury.
  - Soluble chemicals such as chlorine and anhydrous ammonia can be converted to hydrochloric acid and ammonium hydroxide, respectively, when they contact moisture in the respiratory tract mucus, producing injury in the nasopharynx and conducting airways.
  - Insoluble chemicals such as phosgene and nitrogen dioxide may have little impact on the upper airways but can produce severe damage to the alveoli and respiratory bronchioles.
- Chemicals may be inhaled as gases and vapors, mists, fumes, or particles.
- Gases and vapors mix with air and distribute themselves freely throughout the lung and its airways.
- Mists are liquid droplets dispersed in air.
  - Toxic effects depend on droplet size (the larger the size, the greater the exposure).
  - Fumes contain fine particles of dust dispersed in air.
    - Large particles are likely to be trapped in the nasopharynx and conducting airways, whereas small particles (1–5 μm) are more likely to penetrate the lower airways.

Chemical Properties

- The ability of a chemical to interact with other chemicals and body tissue is called its reactivity. As a rule, highly reactive chemicals cause more severe and rapid injury than less-reactive chemicals.
- Four potential properties of chemicals that determine reactivity are:
  - Chemical pH—The likelihood for severe injury from alkaloid or acid exposure increases as the pH approaches its extremes (a pH of less than 2 for acidic substances and greater than 11.5 for alkaline substances).
  - Direct-acting potential of chemicals—Direct-acting chemicals are capable of producing injury without first being transformed or changed, such as Hydrofluoric acid, which causes severe corrosive burns on contact with mucous membranes of the upper airways.
  - Indirect-acting potential of chemicals—Indirect-acting chemicals must be transformed before they can produce injury. An example of this would be phosgene, a gas that may cause acidic burns of the alveolar membranes after conversion to hydrogen chloride (a process that may take up to several hours).
  - Allergic potential of chemicals—Some reactive chemicals bind with proteins to form structures that stimulate allergic reactions. In general, the allergic potential of a chemical is related to its reactivity.

Classifications

- Toxic gases can be classified in three categories: simple asphyxiants, chemical asphyxiants, and irritants/corrosives.
  - Simple asphyxiants (methane, propane, and inert gases) cause toxicity by displacing or lowering ambient oxygen concentration.
  - Chemical asphyxiants (carbon monoxide and cyanide) possess intrinsic systemic toxicity manifested after absorption into the circulation.
  - Irritants/corrosives (chlorine and ammonia) cause cellular destruction and inflammation as they come into contact with moisture.

Management

- The general principles of managing patients who have inhaled poisons are the same as for any other hazardous materials incident.
- Scene safety takes priority!
- Personal protective measures—Protective clothing and appropriate respiratory protective apparatus.
- Rapid removal of the patient from the poison environment.
- Surface decontamination.
- Adequate airway, ventilatory, and circulatory support.
- Initial assessment and physical examination.
- Irrigation of the eyes (as needed).
- IV line with a saline solution.
- Regular monitoring of vital signs and cardiac rhythm by ECG.
- Rapid transport to an appropriate medical facility.

Management of Specific Inhaled Poisons

Cyanide

- Refers to any of a number of highly toxic substances that contain the cyanogen chemical group.
- The agent has few applications (due to its toxicity), but is sometimes used in industry in electroplating, ore extraction, fumigation of buildings, cleaning jewelry, and as a fertilizer. It has also been used in gas chambers as a means of execution.
- Cyanide poisoning may result from:
    - Inhalation of cyanide gas (most rapid effects).
    - Ingestion of cyanide salts, nitriles, or cyanogenic glycosides (amygdalin).
    - Infusion of nitroprusside (when infused at high doses or over a prolonged period).
- Cyanide is a rapidly acting poison that combines and reacts with ferric ions (Fe^{+3}) of the respiratory enzyme cytochrome oxidase to inhibit cellular oxygenation.
- Cytotoxic hypoxia produces a rapid progression of symptoms from dyspnea to paralysis, unconsciousness, and death—Large doses are usually fatal within minutes.
- May produce a characteristic odor of bitter almonds on the patient's breath or body, although 20–40% of the population is unable to detect this odor.
- After ensuring personal safety, emergency care for a patient with cyanide poisoning begins with securing a patent airway and providing adequate ventilatory support with high-concentration oxygen.
- Oxygen competitively displaces cyanide from cytochrome oxidase and enhances the efficacy of drug administration.
- After these measures, the principal treatment of cyanide poisoning is to convert (oxidize) ferrous ions in hemoglobin (Fe^{+2}) to ferric ions (Fe^{+3}), forming methemoglobin, hemoglobin with ferrous ion in the oxidized (Fe^{+3}) state.
- Cyanide, which has a greater affinity for iron in the ferric state, is released from the cytochrome oxidase and combines with methemoglobin, thus allowing cytochrome oxidase to resume its function in normal cellular respiration.
- Cyanide antidotes are thought to be effective because they induce methemoglobin.
- Methemoglobin cannot transport oxygen and must therefore be reconverted to hemoglobin by sodium thiosulfate.
- This is accomplished in a three-step process, which includes administration of:
    - Amyl nitrite by inhalation (converting about 5% of hemoglobin to methemoglobin)
    - Sodium nitrite (300 mg IV), which results in methemoglobinemia approaching 25–30%
    - Sodium thiosulfate (12.5 mg IV)

- Prehospital care for patients with cyanide poisoning
  - Don personal protective equipment as needed to prevent rescuer contamination.
  - Remove the patient from the cyanide source.
  - Rapid decontamination and removal of any contaminated clothing are essential.
  - Ensure a patent airway and provide adequate ventilatory support.
  - Administer high-concentration oxygen.
  - If using the Pasadena cyanide antidote kit, consult with medical direction or a poison control center and follow the instructions provided by the manufacturer.
  - If an antidote kit is not available, a pearl of amyl nitrite should be crushed and held under the patient's nose for 15 of every 30 seconds, followed by continuation of supplemental oxygen.
  - If the patient's respirations are being assisted, place the crushed pearl under the intake valve of a bag-valve device.
  - Initiate IV fluid therapy with a volume-expanding solution.
  - Monitor cardiac rhythm by ECG.
  - Rapidly transport the patient for physician evaluation.

Ammonia Inhalation

- Ammonia is a toxic irritant that causes local pulmonary complications after inhalation. Exposure to ammonia vapors results in inflammation, irritation, and in severe cases, erosion of the mucosal tissue of all respiratory structures as the ammonia vapor combines with water, producing a highly caustic alkaline compound.
  - Patients usually develop coughing, choking, congestion, burning and tightness in the chest, and a feeling of suffocation.
  - These respiratory symptoms are often accompanied by burning of the eyes and lacrimation.
  - In severe cases, bronchospasm and pulmonary edema may occur.
- Besides the general management principles, emergency care may include positive-pressure ventilation and the administration of diuretics and bronchodilators.

Hydrocarbon Inhalation

- Hydrocarbons that pose the greatest risk for injury have a low viscosity, a high volatility, and a high surface tension or adhesion of molecules along a surface.
- These characteristics combine to allow hydrocarbons to enter the pulmonary tree, causing aspiration pneumonitis and the potential for systemic effects such as CNS depression and liver, kidney, or bone marrow toxicity.
- Most hydrocarbon inhalations result from "recreational use" of halogenated hydrocarbons such as carbon tetrachloride and methylene chloride or aromatic hydrocarbons such as benzene and toluene.
  - These agents may produce a state of inebriation or euphoria through "sniffing" or "huffing" (placing the solvent on a rag and inhaling the vapors through a plastic bag).
  - The onset of these effects is usually rapid (occurring within seconds) and may be followed by CNS depression, respiratory failure, or cardiac dysrhythmias.
- Other signs and symptoms of hydrocarbon inhalation include:
  - Burning sensation on swallowing
  - Nausea and vomiting
  - Abdominal cramps
  - Weakness
  - Anesthesia

- Hallucinations
- Changes in color perception
- Blindness
- Seizures
- Coma

- Emergency care is generally supportive and includes:
  - Airway, ventilatory, and circulatory support
  - IV fluid therapy
  - Vital sign and ECG monitoring
  - Rapid transport for physician evaluation

POISONING BY INJECTION

- Human poisonings from injection may result from drug abuse and from arthropod bites and stings, reptile bites, and hazardous aquatic life.
- Injected poisons are often mixtures of many different substances, which may produce several different toxic reactions.
- Be prepared to manage reactions in many organ systems simultaneously.

Arthropod Bites and Stings

- There are about 900,000 species of arthropods throughout the world. Some arthropods bite, some sting, and a few bite and sting.
- Hymenoptera (bees, wasps, and ants) and Arachnid (including spiders, scorpions, and ticks) cause the highest incidence of need for emergency care.
- Arthropod venoms are complex and diverse in their chemistry and pharmacology and may produce major toxic reactions such as anaphylaxis and upper airway obstruction in sensitized individuals.
- Reactions to venoms are classified as local, toxic, systemic, and delayed.
- Medically important venoms are mixtures of protein or polypeptide toxins, enzymes, and other compounds such as histamines, serotonin, acetylcholine, and dopamine.
- Stings are most commonly inflicted on the head and neck followed by the foot, leg, hand, and arm.
- The mouth, pharynx, and esophagus may be stung when bees or yellow jackets in soft-drink or beer containers are accidentally ingested.
- A single wasp, bee, or ant sting in an unsensitized individual usually causes instant pain followed by a wheal-and-flare reaction with variable edema.
- Large local reactions spread more than 15 cm beyond the sting site and persist for more than 24 hours.
- Anaphylaxis is the most serious complication of hymenoptera stings.
- Individuals with a history of allergic reactions to stings often wear medical alert identification and carry an emergency kit containing a preloaded syringe of epinephrine (Epi-Pen).
- The ant species of greatest concern in the United States is the imported fire ant, whose venom is primarily alkaloid.
- The fire ant is the only hymenopteran species whose venom results in necrotic activity, and sterile pustules at the sting site are not uncommon.
- Stings or bites from fire ants may produce systemic reactions and are managed like other hymenoptera stings.
- Secondary infection may occur (requiring antibiotic therapy), and extensive scarring may require skin grafts (rare).

Management

- Prehospital care for mild hymenoptera stings includes close observation for signs or symptoms of an allergic reaction.
- If an extremity is involved, immobilization and elevation can help limit the reaction's duration.
- If physician evaluation is warranted, as evidenced by signs of anaphylaxis or vigorous reaction, an antihistamine may be prescribed.
- Honey bees frequently (and other hymenoptera rarely) leave their stingers in the wound.
- If a stinger is present, it should be scraped or brushed off.
- Stingers should not be removed with forceps, because squeezing the attached venom sac may worsen the injury.
- Severe allergic reactions should be managed in the usual manner.
- Hypovolemia (if present) should be treated in the conventional manner with a volume-expanding crystalloid infusion.

Arachnid

- Spider bites.
- About 20,000 species of spiders are found in the United States and all, with the exception of two small groups (Uloboriade and Liphistiidae), have venom glands.
- Fortunately, only about 50 of these species have fangs long enough to pierce human skin or enough venom to cause significant injury.
- The two major types of reactions that occur from spider venom are neurotoxic reactions, resulting from the black widow bite, and local tissue necrosis, resulting from the bites of most other spiders.

Black Widow Spider

- The black widow is the most notorious spider in North America.
- Although there are a number of variations in the species, the typical mature female (who often devours her mate, thus the name black widow) is shiny black, with a red hourglass marking on the undersurface of the abdomen.
- The size of the female varies with age but rarely exceeds 2.5 cm overall.
- The male is about half the size of the female, brown, and nonvenomous to humans.
- The spider generally is found in undisturbed areas (under stones, logs, and clumps of vegetation) and rarely inhabits occupied dwellings.
- Most black widow bites occur in rural and suburban areas of southern and western states between April and October.
- A bite usually occurs when the spider has been disturbed.
- Generally described by patients as a slight pinprick that is initially painless.
- Physical findings are two small fang marks about 1 mm apart surrounded by a small papule.
- Multiple bites usually rule out any type of spider envenomation because spiders rarely bite more than once.
- Within 1 hour of envenomation, the neurotoxin produces characteristic muscle spasms and cramps, which may result in abdominal rigidity (in the absence of palpable tenderness) and intense pain.
- Abdominal rigidity in the absence of palpable tenderness is an important finding that helps distinguish envenomation from an acute abdominal condition.
- Associated symptoms include:
  - Paresthesia (frequently described as a burning sensation in the soles of the feet or entire body)

  - Pain in the muscles of the shoulders, back, and chest
  - Headache
  - Dizziness
  - Nausea/vomiting
  - Edema of the eyelids
  - Increased perspiration and salivation
  - Severe envenomation may cause hypertension and ECG abnormalities similar to those from digitalis

Emergency care

- Ensure adequate airway, ventilatory, and circulatory support.
- Clean the affected area with saline, cover with a sterile dressing, and intermittently apply ice.
- Obstruction tourniquets or suction devices are not helpful in delaying absorption.
- A commercially prepared antivenin is available but should be administered only in the emergency department and only after appropriate sensitivity testing.
- Moderate-to-severe symptoms require aggressive treatment.
- Per medical direction, muscle spasm, severe headache, vomiting, and paresthesia may be managed with an IV infusion of 5–10 mL of 10% calcium gluconate solution or of 5 mg of diazepam (Valium).
- Severe hypertension may be managed with antihypertensive agents.
- Transport the patient for physician evaluation.

Brown Recluse Spider

- Most prevalent in the Mississippi-Ohio-Missouri river basin and the southwestern United States.
- Prefers hot, dry, and abandoned environments, such as vacant buildings.
- Frequently found in clothing closets.
- Fawn to dark brown in color and between and 1 and 2 cm long.
- Identifying characteristics:
  - Six white eyes arranged in a semicircle on the head (vs. the usual eight eyes of most other spiders).
  - Dark, violin-shaped marking on the top of the cephalothorax (the combined head and thorax).
- Considered shy and generally does not attack unless threatened.
- Most active from April to October.
- Venom of the brown recluse manifests in a broad spectrum of reactions.
- Initially the bite causes little pain and often is overlooked by the victim.
- Some 1–2 hours later, localized pain and erythema develop.
- This is followed within 1–2 days by a blister or vesicle.
- Over the next 24–72 hours, the area often becomes larger, and necrosis may occur with the center yielding a purple or black eschar.
- The eschar eventually sloughs within 2–5 weeks, leaving an ulcer of variable size and depth.
- Systemic involvement may occur with signs and symptoms that include fever, chills, malaise, nausea and vomiting, generalized rash, and the development of hemolytic anemia, hemoglobinuria, and hypotension.
- Death occasionally occurs, usually from disturbance of the coagulation system or hepatic injury.

- Emergency care is supportive.
- Cold compresses and sterile dressings should be applied to the lesion, and the patient should be transported for physician evaluation.
- Most patients do well with outpatient management.

Scorpion Stings

- The sculptured or bark scorpion, found in the southwestern United States and Mexico, is the only species dangerous to humans.
- The scorpion is nocturnal and favors wooded areas along the edges of desert washes, where generally it clings upside down in its hideouts.
- May be found under the bark of the eucalyptus and cottonwood trees.
- Occasionally invades homes, especially adobe houses.
- The sculptured scorpion is small (2–7.5 cm) and yellow to brown; some have tail stripes.
- Most active from April to August, hibernating during winter.
- The scorpion's venom is a mixture of proteins with complex effects on cellular sodium channels.
- It acts at the presynaptic terminal of the neuromuscular junction, releasing acetylcholine, which results in depolarization of the junction.
- The venom also stimulates sympathetic nerves and is neurotoxic, causing hyperactivity and (possibly) convulsions.

Signs and symptoms of sculptured scorpion envenomation

- Hyperesthesia at the site of the sting
- Pain, tingling, and a burning sensation radiating along the nerves at the location of the bite
- SLUDGE—Salivation, lacrimation, urination, defecation, GI distress, emesis
- Initial bradycardia followed by tachycardia
- Cardiac dysrhythmias
- Muscle twitching
- Convulsions (uncommon)
- Roving eye movements (cranial nerve dysfunction)
- Temporary blindness
- The majority of scorpion envenomations, especially in adults, produce minimal pain
- Mild analgesics, cool compresses, and in-hospital observation are usually all that are required for these patients
- Prehospital care is supportive
- Airway control is the priority
- Transport for physician evaluation

Tick Bites

- Seldom require emergency care.
- Ticks can cause human disease by transmitting microorganisms or by secreting toxins or venoms.
- Hard ticks have a leathery exterior that makes them resistant to environmental stresses.
- Relatively free of natural enemies.
- Can regenerate lost parts and have been known to survive without feeding for more than 4 years.
- Local reactions to tick bites vary from the formation of a small pruritic nodule to development of extensive areas of ulceration.

- May be accompanied by fever, chills, and malaise unrelated to infection.
- Some more important diseases for which ticks are vectors include Rocky Mountain spotted fever, Lyme disease, and tick paralysis.

Rocky Mountain spotted fever

- An infectious disease transmitted from rabbits and other small mammals to humans by the bites of the wood tick and dog tick.
- Occurs more commonly on the Atlantic seaboard.
- Accounts for more than 40 deaths in the United States each year.
- Signs and symptoms usually develop within 5–7 days of the tick bite and include headache, high fever, and loss of appetite.
- Usually within 2–3 days after the onset of symptoms, small pink spots appear on the wrists and ankles.
- The rash eventually spreads over the entire body, and the spots darken and enlarge and become petechial.
- In mild cases, recovery occurs within 20 days.
- Mortality rate, if untreated, is between 8% and 25%.

Lyme disease

- Most commonly reported tick-borne disease in United States.
- Caused by a spirochete transmitted by the bite of an *Ixodes* tick known to infect deer and dogs.
- The course of the disease follows several stages.
- Initially, a red dot appears at the site of the bite, gradually expanding into a reddened annular rash (often with central clearing).
- Second stage that may follow in 4–6 weeks is manifested by cardiac abnormalities (including arteriovenous [AV] blocks) and neurological deficits (including cranial nerve palsies).
- Later, the third stage may develop with arthritis as the primary symptom.
- Unless the disease is diagnosed and treated, symptoms may continue for several years, gradually declining in severity.

Tick paralysis

- Results from a prolonged bite by a female wood tick.
- Occurs sporadically during the spring and summer months and is caused by a neurotoxin secreted from the tick's salivary glands during a blood meal.
- Tick paralysis develops in humans within 6 days after the tick attaches to the host.
- Initially, the patient presents with restlessness and complains of paresthesia in the hands and feet.
- Over the next 24–48 hours, an ascending, symmetrical flaccid paralysis may develop with loss of deep tendon reflexes.
- In severe cases, death may result from respiratory paralysis.
- Removal of the tick usually results in rapid improvement and complete resolution within several days.
- If undiagnosed, the disease may be fatal, particularly in young and older patients.

Management

- The principal treatment of tick bites is proper removal of the tick.
- Grasp the tick as close to the skin as possible with forceps, tweezers, or protected fingers and pull it out with steady pressure.

- Take care not to crush or squeeze the body of the tick, which can transmit disease from infective tick fluid.
- An alternative method is to tie a piece of thread or suture around the tick's body and gently pull until the tick is removed.
- After removal, the bite should be disinfected with soap and water and covered with a sterile dressing.

Reptile Bites

The two main families of venomous snakes indigenous to the United States are pit vipers and coral snakes.

Pit Vipers

- The pit viper family that inhabits the United States consists of rattlesnakes (15 species), the cottonmouth (water moccasin), the copperhead, the pigmy rattlesnake, and the massasauga.
- The majority of snakebites in the United States are caused by the rattlesnake family.
- The term "pit viper" is derived from a depression or pit in the maxillary bone of these snakes. Believed to be a heat-sensing organ that detects warm-blooded prey or enemies. The pit guides the direction of the strike and possibly determines the amount of venom released, based on the size and heat emission of the prey.
- Other identifying characteristics of the pit viper are vertical elliptical pupils and a triangular head distinct from the rest of the body.
  - The rattlesnake is further characterized by "rattles" (interlocking horny segments formed on the tail) that sometimes vibrate in direct relation to environmental temperatures
- The venom apparatus consists of a gland and a duct connected to one or more elongated hollow fangs on each side of the head.
  - The venom is composed of a variety of proteins designed to immobilize, kill, and digest prey.

Signs and symptoms of pit viper envenomation

- Mild envenomation:
  - Presence of one or more fang marks
  - Local swelling and pain
  - Lack of systemic symptoms
- Moderate envenomation:
  - Presence of one or more fang marks
  - Pain and edema beyond the site
  - Systemic signs and symptoms
    - — Weakness
    - — Diaphoresis
    - — Nausea/vomiting
    - — Paresthesias
- Severe envenomation:
  - Presence of one or more fang marks
  - Massive edema
  - Subcutaneous ecchymosis
  - Severe systemic symptoms
  - Shock

- On any given strike, the snake may release a quantity of venom varying from little or none to almost the entire content of the glands.

Coral Snakes

- The coral snake has round pupils and small, fixed fangs located near the anterior end of the maxilla. Most coral snakes have a three-color pattern with red, black, and yellow or white bands that completely encircle the body, along with a black snout.
- Many nonpoisonous snakes in the United States mimic the appearance of the coral snake.
- The coral snake is identified by the sequence of colors—Red bands bordered by yellow indicate a venomous species. "Red on yellow, kill a fellow; red on black, venom lack."
- Most coral snakes are shy and docile and seldom bite unless threatened.
- The snake's small mouth and fangs make it difficult to bite anything larger than a finger, toe, or fold of skin.
- Coral snake venom is primarily neurotoxic.
  - It has a blocking action on acetylcholine receptor sites.
    - — Generally produces little or no pain and no necrosis or edema
  - Early signs and symptoms are slurred speech, dilated pupils, and dysphagia (usually delayed several hours after the bite).
  - If untreated, the venom produces flaccid paralysis and death (within 8–24 hours) by respiratory failure, secondary to CNS inhibition.

Management of snake envenomation

- Venom has absorption, distribution, and elimination characteristics.
- Tissue damage increases as venom spreads into the lymphatics and blood.
- Emergency care is directed at retarding the systemic spread of the venom.

Prehospital management

- Stay clear of the snake's striking range (about the length of the snake), and move the patient to a safe area.
- If the snake has been destroyed before EMS arrival, it should be transported in a closed container to the emergency department with the patient.
- No attempt should be made by EMS personnel to capture or destroy the snake—To do so may result in a second envenomation.
- Provide adequate airway, ventilatory, and circulatory support to the patient as needed.
- Continually monitor vital signs and the ECG.
- Establish an IV line in an unaffected extremity with a volume-expanding fluid.
- When practical, immobilize the bitten extremity in a dependent position.
- Immobilization by splinting may delay systemic absorption and diminish local tissue necrosis.
- Keep the patient at rest.
- Prepare the patient for immediate transport to an appropriate medical facility.

Hazardous Aquatic Life

- Marine animals most likely to be involved in human poisonings in U.S. coastal waters are the coelenterates, echinoderms, and stingrays.
- Their specialized venom apparatuses are used for defense and for capturing prey.
  - Aquatic life may contain other poisonous substances as a result of toxic ingestions.
- Exposures to hazardous aquatic life result from recreational, industrial, scientific, and military oceanic activities.

Coelenterates

- A group of over 9000 species that may be encountered in the ocean.
- Those that carry venomous stinging cells (nematocysts) are known as Cnidaria.
  - The nematocyst is venom filled and contains a long, coiled, hollow, threadlike tube that serves as a tiny hypodermic needle.
    - — There are many types of nematocysts, and an individual coelenterate may have more than one type.
  - The severity of envenomation is related to the toxicity of the venom (which may contain various fractions), the number of nematocysts discharged, and the physical condition of the victim.
- Jellyfish, of which the Portuguese man-of-war is the largest and most dangerous, occur throughout the Atlantic and Pacific oceans, usually near the coastline.
  - Their nematocyst-bearing tentacles may be up to 100 ft long, and a single envenomation may involve several hundred thousand nematocysts.
  - A swimmer who comes into contact with the tentacles of the jellyfish may suffer sufficient envenomation to produce systemic signs and symptoms.
  - Nematocysts frequently remain embedded in the tissues of the victim.
    - — Detached tentacle fragments can retain their potency for months.
- Sea anemones are colorful bottom dwellers (sometimes found in tidal pools) that have a flowerlike appearance.
  - They possess slender projections used to sting and paralyze passing fish.
  - Their modifications of nematocysts are capable of producing mild-to-moderate pain in humans.
- Fire corals are not true (stony) corals but rather ocean-bottom dwellers that are widely distributed in tropical waters.
  - Often mistaken for seaweed because they are frequently found attached to rocks, shells, and corals
  - May grow to 2 m in height and have a razor-sharp exoskeleton with thousands of protruding nematocyst-bearing tentacles

Management

- Envenomation ranges in severity from irritant dermatitis to excruciating pain, respiratory depression, and life-threatening cardiovascular collapse.
  - Most often mild, characterized by stinging, paresthesias, pruritus, and reddish-brown linear wheals of "tentacle prints"
  - Systemic symptoms from severe envenomation may include nausea, vomiting, abdominal pain, headache, bronchospasm, pulmonary edema, and respiratory arrest
- Emergency care is directed at stabilizing the patient and counteracting the effects of the venom.
- Stabilize the patient.
- Provide adequate airway, ventilatory, and circulatory support as needed.
- Continually monitor the patient's vital signs and ECG and be prepared to provide aggressive airway management if systemic reactions develop.
- Counteract effects of the venom:
  - Immediately rinse the wound with seawater (wet sand or freshwater will usually cause the nematocysts to discharge their venom and are therefore contraindicated).
  - Apply copious amounts of vinegar (preferred), isopropanol, a baking soda slurry, or household ammonia to inactivate the venom in intact nematocysts.
  - A paste of unseasoned meat tenderizer may be recommended; however, application to injured skin for more than 5–10 minutes may have deleterious effects.

- Remove visible tentacle fragments with forceps.
  - Avoid self-contamination
- Apply a lather of shaving cream and gently shave the affected area to remove invisible nematocysts.
  - If shaving material is unavailable, use a knife or spatula to scrape away remaining tentacles
- Rinse again until pain is largely alleviated.
  - If necessary, consult with medical direction regarding administration of analgesics
- Transport the patient for physician evaluation.

Echinoderms

- Include sea urchins, starfish, and sea cucumbers
- Sea urchins
  - Have a globular, dome-shaped body and are found on rocky bottoms or burrowed in sand or crevices
  - Have tiny spines, some of which are venomous, and between the spines of some sea urchins are small pincerlike organs that are also thought to discharge a poisonous substance
  - Spines are extremely dangerous to handle and may break off easily in the flesh, lodging deeply and making removal difficult
- Starfish
  - Are covered with thorny spines of calcium carbonate crystals that secrete toxins
  - As the spine enters the skin, it carries venom into the wound with immediate pain, copious bleeding, and mild edema
  - Multiple puncture wounds may result in acute systemic reactions
- Sea cucumbers
  - Sausage-shaped animals found in shallow and deep water
  - Substance is secreted into the surrounding ocean, producing only a minor dermatitis or conjunctivitis in swimmers and divers

Management

- Emergency management usually involves caring for puncture wounds caused by spines and inactivating the venom.
  - Protective gloves should be worn.
- Embedded spines should be removed with forceps.
  - Be careful to avoid self-contamination.
  - Larger spines may require surgical removal by a physician.
  - Echinoderm toxins may cause immediate intense pain, swelling, redness, aching in the affected extremity, and nausea.
    - Delayed toxic effects may include respiratory distress, paresthesia of the lips and face, and in severe cases, respiratory paralysis and complete atonia.
  - Be prepared to deal with a variety of physical reactions.
- Most marine venoms lose their toxicity when exposed to changes in temperature or humidity.
  - If the patient is stable, immerse the affected area (usually the foot or hand) in extremely warm water before and during transport.
    - The water should be as hot as can be tolerated without scalding (no warmer than 45°C, 113°F).
  - As a safety precaution, it generally is recommended that both hands or feet not be immersed simultaneously to protect against thermal injury that may go unnoticed by the patient because of numbness or pain in the affected part.

Stingrays

- Responsible for about 1800 injuries each year in the United States.
- Vary in size from 2 in to 14 ft and are often found half-buried in mud or sand in shallow water.
- The venom organ of stingrays consists of two to four venomous stings on the dorsum of a whiplike tail. Envenomation generally occurs from stepping on the sand-buried ray, which causes the tail to thrust up and forward, driving the sting into the victim's leg or foot.
  - The sting (which is purely defensive) produces a large, severe laceration, which may be more than 15–20 cm long.
  - In addition to injecting venom into the wound, the entire spine tip of the venom apparatus is sometimes broken and embedded in the tissue.
- Stingray venom has local and systemic complications.
  - Locally, it produces a traumatic injury that causes immediate, intense pain; edema; variable bleeding; and necrosis.
  - Systemic manifestations include weakness, nausea, vomiting, diarrhea, vertigo, seizures, cardiac conduction abnormalities, paralysis, hypotension, and death.

Management

- Prehospital care is directed to life support, alleviation of pain, inactivation of venom, and prevention of infection.
- Ensure adequate airway, ventilatory, and circulatory support.
- Continually monitor the patient's vital signs and ECG.
- Copiously irrigate the wound with normal saline or freshwater.
- If the venom apparatus is visible, it should be removed.
- Avoid self-contamination.
- If practical, immerse the affected part in very warm water (as previously described).
- Immersion should continue until pain subsides or until the patient reaches the emergency department.
- Medical direction may recommend application of lymphatic-venous constricting bands (controversial) and administration of analgesics.
- Transport the patient for physician evaluation.

POISONING BY ABSORPTION

- Although many poisons may be absorbed through the skin, more than 75,000 cases of pesticide poisoning are reported to the American Association of Poison Control Centers (AAPCC) each year.
- Many of these poisonings result from exposure to organophosphates and carbamates that are available for commercial and public use as flea collars and home and commercial insecticides.
- Organophosphates and carbamates are among the most toxic chemicals currently used in pesticides and are well absorbed by ingestion, inhalation, and dermal routes.
  - The compounds have similar pharmacological actions, inhibiting the effects of acetylcholinesterase.
    - This enzyme degrades acetylcholine at the neuromuscular junction.
    - Organophosphates have a stronger bond to this enzyme than do carbamates.
    - Carbamate poisoning is easier to treat effectively than organophosphate intoxication.

- ◦ Acetylcholine is a cholinergic neurotransmitter for preganglionic autonomic fibers, postganglionic parasympathetic fibers, somatic nerves to skeletal muscle, and many synapses in the CNS.
  - — When acetylcholinesterase is inhibited, acetylcholine accumulates at the synapses, and a cholinergic "overdrive" occurs with resulting signs and symptoms characteristic of organophosphate and carbamate poisoning.

Signs and Symptoms

- Early signs and symptoms may be nonspecific, including headache, dizziness, weakness, and nausea.
- As overstimulation and subsequent disruption of transmission in the central and peripheral nervous systems occur, signs and symptoms begin to manifest in a spectrum of physiological and metabolic derangements.
- The rapidity and sequence in which these signs and symptoms develop depend on the particular compound and the amount and route of exposure.
- The onset of symptoms is probably quickest after inhalation and slowest (possibly delayed for several hours) after a primary skin exposure.
- A helpful mnemonic to recognize the signs of poisoning is SLUDGE (salivation, lacrimation, urination, defecation, GI cramping, and emesis).
- Signs and symptoms of organophosphate or carbamate poisoning:
  - ◦ Cardiovascular—Bradycardia, variable blood pressure (usually hypotensive)
  - ◦ Respiratory—Rhinorrhea, bronchoconstriction, wheezing, dyspnea
  - ◦ GI—Cramps, emesis, defecation, increased bowel sounds
  - ◦ Vision—Miosis, rapidly changing pupil size, lacrimation, blurred vision
  - ◦ CNS—Anxiety, dizziness, coma, convulsions, respiratory depression
  - ◦ Musculoskeletal—Fasciculations, flaccid paralysis
  - ◦ Skin—Diaphoresis
  - ◦ Other—Salivation, urination

Management

- Emergency care begins with scene safety, personal protection, and decontamination procedures; after these measures, patient care can be initiated.
- General principles of management include:
  - ◦ Respiratory support
    - — Respiratory tract symptoms are usually first to appear, and respiratory paralysis may occur suddenly without warning.

      The need for aggressive airway management and ventilatory support should be anticipated throughout the patient care encounter.
    - — Copious bronchial secretions may require suctioning.
    - — Bronchoconstriction may require positive-pressure ventilation and positive end-expiratory pressure.
  - ◦ Drug administration
    - — Is directed at inhibiting the release of acetylcholine, separating cholinesterase from the chemical compound and suppressing seizure activity (if present)
    - — Atropine

      Reverses the muscarinic effects (bradycardia, bronchoconstriction, respiratory secretions, and miosis) of moderate-to-severe poisoning

      Completely antagonizes the actions of acetylcholine, resulting in a decrease in the hyperactivity of smooth muscles and glands

      Initial dose is 2 mg IV push every 5–15 minutes as required to dry the patient's secretions and to decrease pulmonary resistance to ventilation

- Pediatric dose is 0.05 mg/kg, repeated every 15 minutes as necessary

Because potentially hypoxic patients may require large doses of atropine, ECG monitoring for signs of dysrhythmias (other than tachycardia) and provision of supplemental oxygen must be undertaken to minimize the risk of ventricular fibrillation (VF)

Atropine is the drug of choice for carbamate poisonings

— Pralidoxime (2-PAM Chloride) is the treatment of choice for organophosphate poisoning and should be used for nearly all patients with clinically significant exposures, particularly for those with muscle fasciculations and weakness

Has three desirable effects in managing organophosphate poisoning:

- The primary effect of cleaving the phosphorylation-acetyl-cholinesterase bond, thus freeing and reactivating acetylcholinesterase
- Directly reacting with and detoxifying the organophosphorus molecules
- An anticholinergic "atropine-like" effect

Initial adult dose of pralidoxime is 600 mg IM or 1–2 g IV over 15–30 minutes

- Pediatric dose is 20–50 mg/kg IV over 15–30 minutes

Subsequent doses may be repeated within 1–2 hours

— Diazepam (Valium)

May be indicated if seizures are present

- If the need for diazepam (Valium) arises before decontamination is complete, the drug should be administered IM in 2-mg increments as necessary to control seizure activity

Be alert to the possibility of respiratory and CNS depression

◦ ECG monitoring

— May reveal a variety of abnormalities, including idioventricular rhythms, multifocal premature ventricular contractions (PVCs), ventricular tachycardia (VT), torsades de pointes, VF, complete heart block, and asystole

— Dysrhythmias usually occur in two phases:

Beginning with a transient episode of intense sympathetic tone that results in sinus tachycardia

Followed by a period of extreme parasympathetic tone that may manifest as sinus bradycardia, atrioventricular (AV) block, and ST-segment and T-wave abnormalities

— Significant ventricular bradydysrhythmias that do not respond to conventional therapy may need to be treated with overdrive pacing

DRUG ABUSE

- Drug abuse refers to the use of prescription drugs for nonprescribed purposes or the use of drugs that have no prescribed medical use.
- Common drugs of abuse:
  - Narcotics
  - Sedatives-hypnotics
  - Stimulants
  - Phencyclidine (PCP)
  - Hallucinogens
  - Tricyclic antidepressants (TCAs)
  - Lithium
  - Cardiac medications

- Monoamine oxidase (MAO) inhibitors
- Nonprescription pain medicines
- Salicylates
- Acetaminophen
- Drugs abused for sexual purposes/sexual gratification
- Metals (iron, lead, and mercury)

- Emergencies resulting from drug abuse include:
  - Adverse effects caused by the drug or impurities or contaminants mixed with the drug
  - Life-threatening infections from IV or intradermal injection of drugs with unsterile equipment
  - Accidents during intoxication
  - Drug dependence or withdrawal syndrome resulting from the habit-forming potential of many drugs

Factors That Influence Drug Abuse

- No single cause or set of conditions lead to drug abuse.
- It is widespread and common among all socioeconomic, cultural, and ethnic groups.
- It is a major medical, social, and interpersonal problem that affects individuals from all backgrounds and of all ages.
- Illicit drug use in the United States—A survey conducted by Health and Human Services' Substance Abuse and Mental Health Services Administration (SAMSHA) revealed:
  - In 2004, an estimated 2.8 million persons used an illicit drug for the first time within the past 12 months. Most initiates (58.1%) were younger than age 18 when they first used, and the majority of new users (57.9% percent) were female. The average age at initiation was 20.1 years.
  - The drug category with the largest number of recent initiates was nonmedical use of pain relievers (2.4 million), followed by marijuana (2.1 million), nonmedical use of tranquilizers (1.2 million), and cocaine (1.0 million). Inhalants had the youngest average age at first use (16.0 years), followed by marijuana (18.0 years).
  - In 2004, an estimated 1.0 million persons had used cocaine for the first time.
  - In 2004, an estimated 118,000 persons had used heroin for the first time.
  - In 2004, an estimated 934,000 persons had used hallucinogens for the first time.
  - Although there was little change between 2003 and 2004 in the number of past-year initiates of d-lysergic acid diethylamide (LSD) or Ecstasy, there were declines between 2002 and 2003. The number of past-year LSD initiates was 338,000 in 2002, 200,000 in 2003, and 235,000 in 2004. Ecstasy initiation was 1.2 million in 2002, 642,000 in 2003, and 607,000 in 2004. Most (57.7 percent) of the recent Ecstasy initiates in 2004 were aged 18 or older at the time they first used Ecstasy. The average age at initiation of Ecstasy was 19.5 years.
  - In 2004, an estimated 857,000 persons had used inhalants for the first time.
  - In 2004, an estimated 2.8 million persons had used psychotherapeutics nonmedically for the first time within the past year.
  - In 2004, the number of new nonmedical users of OxyContin was 615,000, with an average age at first use of 24.5 years.
  - The number of recent new users of methamphetamine nonmedically was 318,000 in 2004. Between 2002 and 2004, the number of methamphetamine initiates remained level at around 300,000 per year.
  - In 2004, an estimated 4.4 million persons had used alcohol for the first time.

- In 2004, the average age of first alcohol use among recent initiates was 17.5 years.
- Because of the widespread use and misuse of drugs, maintain a high degree of suspicion and consider the possibility for a drug-related problem in any patient who has seizures, behavioral changes, stupor, or coma.
- Considerations of the visibility, accessibility, and careful handling of all medications carried on an EMS vehicle should be a part of EMS policy and procedure.

Toxic Effects of Drugs

- EMS personnel frequently encounter people suffering from the toxic effects of drugs as the result of:
  - An overdose
  - A potential suicide
  - Polydrug administration
  - An accident (accidental ingestion, miscalculation, changes in drug strength)
- Common drugs of abuse (along with their names and uses) vary widely in different geographical areas and frequently change over time.

General Management Principles

- Ensure scene safety and be prepared for unpredictable patient behavior.
  - Consider the need for law enforcement assistance
- Ensure adequate airway, ventilatory, and circulatory support as needed.
- Obtain a history of the event (including the self-administration of other drugs that may have been taken by another route) and any significant past medical or psychiatric history.
- Identify the substance and consult with medical direction or a poison control center.
- Perform a thorough focused physical examination. Continually monitor the patient's vital functions and ECG.
- Initiate IV therapy:
  - Draw a blood sample for laboratory analysis and administer appropriate pharmacological antidotes such as naloxone if a narcotic overdose is suspected.
  - Personal protective measures should be given special attention because many of these patients are at high risk of harboring infectious disease.
  - Prevent further absorption of an orally administered drug by GI decontamination or the administration of activated charcoal (per protocol).
  - Rapidly transport the patient for physician evaluation.

Narcotic/Opiate Overdose

- Heroin accounts for about 90% of the narcotic abuse in the United States.
  - Pure heroin is a bitter-tasting white powder that is usually adulterated or "cut" for street distribution with various agents such as lactose, sucrose, baking soda, powdered milk, starch, magnesium silicate (talc), procaine, quinine, and recently with scopolamine.
  - A typical "bag" is the single-dose unit of heroin and may weigh 100 mg, of which on average only 5% is pure.
- Other narcotic/opiate drugs include morphine, hydromorphone, methadone, meperidine (Demerol), codeine, oxycodone, propoxyphene, and "designer opiates" that have been chemically modified such as alpha methyl fentanyl ("China white").
- Depending on the narcotic preparation, these drugs may be taken orally, injected intradermally ("skin popping") or intravenously ("mainlining"), taken intranasally ("snorted"), or smoked.

- All narcotics and opiates are CNS depressants and can cause life-threatening respiratory depression. In severe intoxication, hypotension, profound shock, and pulmonary edema may be present.
- Signs and symptoms of narcotic/opiate overdose include:
  - Euphoria
  - Arousable somnolence ("nodding")
  - Nausea
  - Pinpoint pupils
  - Coma
  - Seizures
- Antidote therapy:
  - Naloxone is a pure narcotic antagonist effective for nearly all narcotic and narcotic-like substances.
  - The drug reverses the triad of symptoms of narcotic/opiate overdose (respiratory depression, coma, and miosis) and should be administered when narcotic/opiate intoxication is suspected or when a coma of unknown origin is present.
  - Be prepared to restrain the patient, whose behavior may be unpredictable when the effects of the drug are reversed.
  - Medical direction may recommend that naloxone administration be titrated to keep the patient responsive and free from respiratory depression but somewhat docile during transport.
  - Some narcotics and opiates have a longer duration than naloxone (Narcan).
    - — The patient must be closely monitored during antidote therapy.
    - — Repeated doses of naloxone (Narcan) may be necessary.
  - Naloxone can precipitate withdrawal syndrome in narcotic/opiate-dependent patients.
    - — Narcotic/opiate withdrawal is seldom life threatening and can usually be managed by symptomatic and supportive care.
  - Signs and symptoms of narcotic/opiate withdrawal include gooseflesh, tachycardia, diaphoresis, irritability, insomnia, abdominal cramps, tremors, nausea/vomiting, anorexia, cold sweats or chills, fever, diarrhea, and general malaise.

Sedative-Hypnotic Overdose

- Sedative-hypnotic agents include benzodiazepines and barbiturates.
  - Are usually taken orally but may be diluted and injected IV
  - Use with alcohol markedly increases their effects
  - Are commonly known as downers
- Benzodiazepines:
  - Among the best-known and most widely prescribed drugs used to control symptoms of anxiety, stress, and insomnia.
    - — Are sometimes used to manage alcohol withdrawal and control seizure disorders
    - — Promote sleep and relieve anxiety by depressing brain function
  - Frequently abused for their sedative effects.
  - Individually, these drugs are relatively nontoxic, but they may accentuate the effects of other sedative-hypnotic agents.
  - Common benzodiazepines are diazepam (Valium) and chlordiazepoxide (Librium).
- Barbiturates:
  - General CNS depressants that inhibit impulse conduction in the ascending reticular activating system.
  - Were once widely used to treat anxiety and insomnia.

  - Addictive properties and potential for abuse have led to their replacement by benzodiazepines and other nonbarbiturate drugs.
  - Barbiturates that commonly are abused include phenobarbital (Luminal), amobarbital, and secobarbital.
- Signs and symptoms of sedative-hypnotic overdose chiefly are related to the CNS and cardiovascular system.
  - Adverse effects include excessive drowsiness, staggering gait, and in some cases, paradoxical excitability.
  - In cases of severe toxicity, the patient may become comatose, with respiratory depression, hypotension, and shock.
  - Pupils may be constricted but often become fixed and dilated even in the absence of significant brain damage.
  - Airway control and ventilatory management are the essential points in treating significant sedative-hypnotic overdose.
    - Flumazenil (Romazicon), a benzodiazepine antagonist, is useful in reversing the effects of these agents, but not for barbiturates.

Stimulant Overdose

- Amphetamines
  - Frequently used to produce general mood elevation, improve task performance, suppress appetite, and prevent sleepiness.
  - Structurally, amphetamines are similar to endogenous catecholamines (epinephrine and norepinephrine) but differ in their more pronounced effects on the CNS.
  - Adverse effects include tachycardia, increased blood pressure, tachypnea, agitation, dilated pupils, tremors, and disorganized behavior.
  - In severe intoxication, the patient may exhibit psychosis and paranoia and experience hallucinations.
  - Sudden withdrawal or cessation of amphetamine use may result in a "crash" stage in which the patient becomes depressed, suicidal, incoherent, or near coma.
  - Amphetamines commonly are known as speed or uppers.
- Cocaine
  - One of the most popular illegal drugs in the United States.
  - Most commonly used as a fine, white crystalline powder.
  - Street forms are usually adulterated and vary in purity from 25% to 90%; doses vary from near 0–200 mg.
  - This form of cocaine generally is taken intranasally by snorting a "line" containing 10–35 mg of the drug (depending on purity).
  - After absorption through the mucous membranes, the effects of the drug begin within minutes.
  - Peak effects occur 15–60 minutes after use, with a half-life of 1–2½ hours.
  - Cocaine is also used parenterally by the subcutaneous (SC), IM, and IV routes.
  - The IV route provides immediate absorption and intense stimulation (peak occurs within 5 minutes and half-life of about 50 minutes).
  - Freebase or "crack" cocaine is a more potent formulation of the drug that is prepared by mixing powdered street cocaine with an alkaline solution and then adding a solvent such as ether.
  - The combination separates into two layers, the top layer containing the dissolved cocaine.
  - Evaporation of the solvent results in pure cocaine crystals, which are smoked and absorbed via the pulmonary route.

  - Cocaine in this form is called rock or crack because of the popping sound produced when the crystals are heated.
  - Freebase cocaine is generally combined with marijuana or tobacco and smoked in a pipe or a cigarette.
  - Equal to IV use in intensity and pleasure.
  - Cocaine is a major CNS stimulant that causes profound sympathetic discharge.
  - Increased levels of circulating catecholamines result in excitement, euphoria, talkativeness, and agitation.
  - Effects of the drug can precipitate significant cardiovascular and neurological complications such as cardiac dysrhythmias, myocardial infarction, seizures, intracranial hemorrhage, hyperthermia, and psychiatric disturbances.
  - Overdose can occur with any form of the drug and any route of administration.
  - Prehospital management may be complex.
  - Toxicity may range from minor symptoms to life-threatening overdose.
  - Emergency care may require a full spectrum of basic and advanced life-support measures including:
    - — Aggressive airway management, ventilatory and circulatory support
    - — Pharmacological therapy
    - — Rapid transport to an appropriate medical facility

Phencyclidine (PCP) Overdose

- PCP is a dissociative analgesic (originally used as a veterinary tranquilizer) with sympathomimetic and CNS stimulant and depressant properties.
  - It is a potent psychoactive drug illegally sold in tablet or powder form to be taken orally, intranasally, or with other drugs to be smoked (a "Sherman").
    - — Rarely taken IV
  - Most tablets contain about 5 mg of PCP.
    - — As a rule, PCP in its powder form is relatively pure (50–100% PCP)
- Chronic use results in permanent memory impairment and loss of higher brain functions.
- Pharmacological effects are dose related.
- Low-dose toxicity.
  - In low doses (less than 10 mg), PCP intoxication produces an unpredictable state that can resemble drunkenness; the user may have a sense of euphoria or confusion, disorientation, agitation, or sudden rage.
  - An intoxicated patient often has a blank stare and a stumbling gait and is in a dissociative state.
  - Pupils are generally reactive.
  - The patient may experience flushing, diaphoresis, facial grimacing, hypersalivation, and vomiting.
  - Nystagmus with a burstlike quality is characteristic of low-dose PCP use.
  - In this range of toxicity, death is usually related to behavioral disturbances resulting from spatial disorientation, drug-induced immobility, and insensitivity to pain.
  - Low-dose toxicity is best managed by keeping sensory stimulation to a minimum (verbal and physical stimulation exacerbate clinical symptoms).
    - — Violent and combative patients require protection from self-injury; provide safeguards for EMS crew and bystanders.
    - — Closely monitor vital signs and level of consciousness.
    - — Increasing motor activity and muscle rigidity often precede seizures.

- High-dose toxicity (more than 10 mg):
  - Patients may be in a coma, which may last from hours to several days, and thus often are unresponsive to painful stimuli.
  - Respiratory depression, hypertension, and tachycardia also may be present, depending on the dosage.
  - In severe cases, a hypertensive crisis causing cardiac failure, hypertensive encephalopathy, seizures, and intracerebral hemorrhage may result.
  - Prehospital care is directed at managing life-threatening complications and rapidly transporting the patient for physician evaluation.
- Phencyclidine psychosis:
  - A true psychiatric emergency that may mimic schizophrenia.
  - Usually of acute onset and may not become apparent until several days after ingestion.
    - Can occur after a single low-dose exposure to PCP and may last from several days to weeks.
  - Clinical syndromes range from a catatonic and unresponsive state to bizarre and violent behavior.
  - The patient frequently appears agitated and suspicious and often experiences auditory hallucinations and paranoia.
  - Appropriate management usually requires involuntary hospitalization, control of violent behavior, and administration of antipsychotic agents.
  - When dealing with these patients in the prehospital setting, personal safety is of paramount importance.
    - Law enforcement should be summoned for assistance.

Hallucinogen Overdose

- Hallucinogens are substances that cause perceptual distortions.
- The most common hallucinogens in use today are PCP and lysergic acid diethylamide (LSD).
- Other hallucinogens include:
  - Mescaline, found in the buttons of peyote cactus, which can be used legally in some religious settings
  - Psilocybin mushrooms, found in the United States and Mexico
  - Marijuana, the active agent of the plant *Cannabis sativa*
  - Morning glory plant
  - Nutmeg
  - Mace
  - Some amphetamines, such as MDMA ("Ecstasy") and MDEA ("Eve")
- Depending on the agent, the effects of hallucinogens may range from minor visual illusions and classic anticholinergic syndromes resembling tricyclic antidepressant (TCA) toxicity to more serious complications (associated with LSD use) such as permanent psychosis, flashbacks, and respiratory and CNS depression.
- Prehospital management is usually limited to supportive care, minimal sensory stimulation, calming measures, and transportation to a medical facility.
- After arrival at the emergency department, these patients are generally observed in a quiet environment.
- Pharmacological agents may be administered to counteract the anticholinergic effects of the drug.

Tricyclic Antidepressant (TCA) Overdose

- TCAs are commonly prescribed in the treatment of depression.
- They work by blocking the uptake of norepinephrine, serotonin, or both into the presynaptic neurons, altering the sensitivity of brain tissue to the actions of these chemicals.
- TCA toxicity is thought to result from central and peripheral atropine-like anticholinergic effects and direct depressant effects on myocardial function.
- Commonly prescribed antidepressant drugs include:
  - TCAs
    - amitriptyline (Amitril)
    - imipramine (Apo-Imipramine)
    - nortriptyline (Aventyl)
  - Selective serotonin reuptake inhibitors (SSRIs)
    - fluoxetine (Prozac)
    - sertraline (Zoloft)
    - paroxetine (Paxil)
- Early symptoms of TCA overdose are dry mouth, blurred vision, confusion, inability to concentrate, and occasionally visual hallucinations.
  - More severe symptoms include delirium, depressed respirations, hypertension, hypotension, hyperthermia, hypothermia, seizures, and coma.
- Cardiac effects may range from tachycardia to bradycardia and various dysrhythmias secondary to an atrioventricular block.
  - A prolonged QRS complex, a Glasgow coma scale less than 8, or both, are characteristic findings that should alert the paramedic to a major toxicity with potentially serious complications.
  - Sudden death from cardiac arrest may occur several days after an overdose.
- There is little effective prehospital management for major toxicity of a TCA overdose.
  - Basic supportive care and rapid transport should be instituted.
  - Sodium bicarbonate, 1–2 mEq/kg given IV per medical direction, may begin to reverse cardiac toxicity.
  - Any patient with a history of TCA ingestion should receive airway, ventilatory, and circulatory support; IV access; ECG monitoring; and rapid transport for physician evaluation.
    - More definitive treatment for specific problems (e.g., seizures, ventricular dysrhythmias) is complex, using a combination of alkalinization, anticonvulsants, and physostigmine (Antilirium) when appropriate.
  - Rapid transport to the emergency department is the most appropriate course of action.

Lithium

- A mood-stabilizing drug sometimes prescribed for the treatment of bipolar disorders.
  - Because the drug has a very low toxic-to-therapeutic dose ratio, lithium overdose is common.
  - Patients who are prescribed lithium have frequent blood tests to monitor the level of lithium in the body.
- Lithium helps to prevent "mood swings" by interfering with hormonal responses to cyclic adenosine monophosphate and by augmenting the reuptake of norepinephrine (producing an antiadrenergic effect).

- As a result of these actions, lithium has multiple effects on the body that include muscle tremor, thirst, nausea, increased urination, abdominal cramping, and diarrhea.
- With toxic ingestion (a single ingestion of 20 mg/kg or more), signs and symptoms may include:
  - Muscle weakness
  - Slurred speech
  - Severe trembling
  - Blurred vision
  - Confusion
  - Seizure
  - Apnea
  - Coma
- Prehospital care for patients with suspected lithium overdose should focus on airway management, ventilatory and circulatory support, and the control of seizure activity (if present).
  - Gastric lavage may be indicated with recent lithium ingestion, but is usually performed in the emergency department.

Cardiac Medications

Cardiac drugs are a common cause of poisoning fatalities in children and adults. The drugs responsible for the majority of these fatalities are digoxin (Lanoxin), propranolol (Inderal), beta blockers, and calcium channel blockers.

Digoxin (Lanoxin)

- Exerts direct and indirect effects on SA and AV nodal fibers.
- At toxic levels, can halt impulses in the SA node, depress conduction through the AV node, and increase sensitivity of the SA and AV nodes to catecholamines.
- Also affects the Purkinje fibers by decreasing the resting potential and action potential duration, and by enhanced automaticity that can lead to an increase in PVCs.
- Can produce almost any dysrhythmia or conduction block.
- Common signs and symptoms of toxicity include nausea, anorexia, fatigue, visual disturbances, and a variety of disorders of the GI, ophthalmological, and neurological systems.
- Oral overdoses generally are managed with activated charcoal (and sometimes gastric lavage), and drugs to treat life-threatening dysrhythmias.
- Severe overdoses are treated with IV digoxin-specific FAB (Digibind), a binding compound that decreases the morbidity and mortality associated with digitalis overdose.

Beta Blockers

- Are rapidly absorbed after ingestion.
- Toxicity impairs SA and AV node function, leading to bradycardias and AV blocks.
- Associated depression in ventricular conduction makes these patients susceptible to wide QRS complexes and, occasionally, ventricular dysrhythmias (rarely VT or VF).
- Other signs and symptoms include CNS and respiratory depression, hypotension, and seizures.
- Emergency care includes activated charcoal and drugs to manage hypotension and dysrhythmias.
- In-hospital care may include infusions of glucagon, various catecholamines, and possible hemodialysis.

Calcium Channel Blockers

- Toxic ingestion can lead to myocardial depression and peripheral vasodilation with negative inotropic, chronotropic, dromotropic, and vasotropic effects.
- Hypotension and bradycardia are early manifestations of toxicity.
- Overdose may result in serious dysrhythmias including AV block of all degrees, sinus arrest, AV dissociation, junctional rhythm, and asystole.
- Other signs and symptoms of toxicity include nausea and vomiting, hypotension, and CNS and respiratory depression.
- In addition to airway, ventilatory, and circulatory support, emergency care may include the use of antidysrhythmics, vasopressors, activated charcoal, and gastric lavage (for patients with acute overdoses).

MAO Inhibitors

- MAO inhibitors block or diminish the activity of monoamines (norepinephrine, dopamine, and serotonin). These CNS transmitters are widely distributed throughout the body, with the highest concentration in the brain, liver, and kidneys.
- MAO inhibitors are prescribed as antidepressants, antineoplastics, antibiotics, and antihypertensives.
  - Some MAO inhibitors (e.g., the antidepressants phenelzine and tranylcypromine) have active metabolites that include significant amounts of amphetamine and methamphetamine and therefore are sometimes abused for their effects.
- Effects of MAO inhibitor toxicity:
  - Neuromuscular system manifestations
    - — Agitation
    - — Rigidity
    - — Hyperreflexia
    - — Nystagmus
    - — Hallucinations
    - — Seizure
  - Cardiovascular system manifestations
    - — Sinus tachycardia
    - — Hypotension with vascular collapse
    - — Hypertension
    - — Bradyasystolic rhythms
- Prehospital care primarily is supportive and includes airway, ventilatory, and circulatory support; cardiac medications as needed; and rapid transport for physician evaluation.
- Activated charcoal is recommended for all patients; gastric lavage may be indicated with recent ingestion.

Nonsteroidal Anti-Inflammatory Drugs (NSAIDs)

- A group of agents that have an analgesic and antipyretic action that reduces inflammation of joints and soft tissues, such as muscles and ligaments
- Work by blocking the production of prostaglandins, chemicals that cause inflammation and trigger transmission of pain signals to the brain
- Widely used to relieve symptoms caused by types of arthritis (rheumatoid arthritis, osteoarthritis, gout), and in the treatment of back pain, menstrual pain, headaches, minor postoperative pain, and soft tissue injuries
- Common NSAIDs include difunisal (Dolobid), fenoprofen (Nalfon), ibuprofen (Advil, Motrin), and naproxen (Aleve)

Ibuprofen Overdose

- Ibuprofen (Advil, Motrin) is the most commonly overdosed ingested NSAID.
- Effects are usually reversible and seldom life threatening (although significant toxicity may result in coma, seizure, hypotension, and acute renal failure).
- Common symptoms of chronic and acute ingestion (more than 300 mg/kg) include mild GI and CNS disturbances that usually resolve within 24 hours after ingestion.
  - Less common effects include mild metabolic acidosis, muscle fasciculations, chills, hyperventilation, hypotension, and asymptomatic bradycardia.
- Emergency care for patients who have ingested toxic amounts of ibuprofen consists of gastric decontamination with activated charcoal, and careful monitoring for secondary complications, such as hypotension and dysrhythmias.

Salicylate Overdose

- Salicylates are widely available in prescription and over-the-counter products such as acetylsalicylic acid (aspirin), many cold preparations, and oil of wintergreen (methyl salicylate), as well as in combination with some analgesics such as propoxyphene and oxycodone.
- Mechanism of toxicity with salicylate poisoning is complex and includes direct CNS stimulation, interference with cellular glucose uptake, and inhibition of Krebs cycle enzymes that affect energy production and amino acid metabolism.
- The volume of distribution is dose dependent and usually small.
  - With toxic ingestion, redistribution of the drug into the CNS occurs and prolongs elimination of the drug from the body.
  - Complications that may result from chronic or acute ingestion of salicylates include CNS stimulation, GI irritation, glucose metabolism, fluid and electrolyte imbalance, neurological symptoms, and coagulation effects.
- CNS stimulation:
  - Salicylates initially produce direct stimulation of the respiratory center in the CNS, causing an increased rate and depth of respiration.
  - This early respiratory alkalosis is followed by a compensatory elimination of bicarbonate ions by the kidneys and a subsequent compensatory metabolic acidosis.
  - After this period, there is an accumulation of intermediate acids involved in energy metabolism, leading to profound metabolic acidosis.
  - Confusion, lethargy, convulsions, respiratory arrest, coma, and brain death all can occur in severe salicylate poisoning.
- GI irritation:
  - Salicylates have irritant effects on the gastric mucosa, which can lead to nausea, vomiting, and hematemesis.
- Glucose metabolism:
  - Interference with cellular glucose uptake causes accumulation of serum glucose.
  - Eventually, cellular glucose is depleted, and the patient can demonstrate tissue effects of hypoglycemia (particularly in CNS tissue).
  - Patients who die of salicylate poisoning frequently demonstrate primary CNS tissue toxicity and severe cerebral edema.
- Fluid and electrolyte imbalance:
  - Total body fluids are adversely affected by hypermetabolism.
  - Fluid and electrolyte losses occur via GI fluids, emesis, and renal clearance.
  - Acid-base disturbances may result in hypokalemia and hyperchloremia.
  - Cardiac dysrhythmias, including PVCs, VT, and VF, are possible.

- Neurological symptoms:
  - Mild neurological effects such as tinnitus and lethargy are common; severe intoxication may result in hallucination, seizure, and coma.
- Coagulation effects:
  - Salicylates alter normal platelet function and often lead to coagulation disorders when taken in toxic amounts.
    - These patients are at increased risk of significant bleeding.
  - Patients taking anticoagulants are at even greater risk for hemorrhage after salicylate ingestion.
- Prehospital care may include:
  - Administration of activated charcoal for intestinal decontamination.
  - IV glucose to manage hypoglycemia.
  - Because salicylates are weak acids excreted by the kidney, medical direction may recommend the administration of sodium bicarbonate to produce an alkaline urine.
  - Definitive care includes in-hospital intensive care observation, continued support of vital functions, and perhaps hemodialysis.

Acetaminophen Overdose

- Acetaminophen is a commonly prescribed analgesic and antipyretic agent available in many prescription and nonprescription preparations.
  - Due to widespread availability of acetaminophen, there is a high incidence of accidental and intentional poisoning.
- Acetaminophen can cause life-threatening hepatic toxicity from formation of a hepatotoxic intermediate metabolite if not managed within 16–24 hours of ingestion. Acetaminophen is also present in many drug combinations including Darvocet-N, Excedrin, and Sinutab.
- Toxic effects of acute acetaminophen ingestion (doses of 140 mg/kg or greater) can be classified in four stages.
  - The course of toxicity begins with mild symptoms that may be overlooked or masked by more dramatic effects of other agents followed by transient clinical improvement and finally peak liver abnormalities. If acetaminophen was the sole ingestant and a dangerously high dose was ingested, there may be no symptoms in the first two stages.
  - If antidote treatment is started within 16–24 hours of ingestion, complete recovery should occur.
- Emergency care includes respiratory, cardiac, and hemodynamic support in critically ill patients.
  - If ingestion is recent (within 1 hour) and the patient is alert, medical direction may recommend gastric decontamination and the administration of activated charcoal (controversial).
  - Definitive care for patients with progressive acetaminophen toxicity is in-hospital administration of the antidote, N-acetylcysteine (Mucomyst).

Drugs Abused for Sexual Purposes/Sexual Gratification

- Drugs abused for sexual purposes or for sexual gratification commonly are classified by users as "uppers," "downers," and those that have more than one primary effect ("all-arounders").
  - Uppers are CNS stimulants
  - Downers are CNS depressants

- The third category encompasses drugs such as anesthetics and mood-altering agents that are generally taken alone or in combination to produce one or more of the following effects:
  - A sense of euphoria
  - Excitation ("rush")
  - Relaxation ("blissed out")
  - Loss of inhibition
- Uppers
  - Ecstasy
  - Speed/Meth/Crystal
  - Coke/Crack
  - Anabolic steroids
- Downers
  - Alcohol
  - Heroin
  - Benzodiazepines (diazepam/temazepam/rohypnol)
  - Gamma hydroxybutyrate (GHB)
- All-arounders
  - Ketamine
  - Cannabis/skunk
  - Poppers (alkyl nitrates)
  - LSD
- Each of these drugs has different chemical structures, mechanisms of action, and side effects.
- Signs and symptoms of abuse can range from mild nausea and vomiting to life-threatening respiratory depression, coma, and death.
- Emergency care is supportive and includes airway, ventilatory, and circulatory support, and rapid transport for physician evaluation.
- As with all other cases of patients who use mood-altering agents, personal safety is important.

Alcohol and Related Illness Continue to Be a Major Problem in the United States

- Alcohol is a key factor in:
  - 40% of vehicle fatalities
  - 68% of manslaughters
  - 62% of assaults
  - 54% of murder attempts
  - 48% of robberies
- The economic cost of alcohol and other drug-related crime is $61.8 billion annually and is rising.

ALCOHOL DEPENDENCE

- A disorder characterized by chronic, excessive consumption of alcohol that results in injury to health or in inadequate social function and the development of withdrawal symptoms when the patient stops drinking suddenly.
  - Alcohol dependence should be considered a chronic, progressive, potentially fatal disease characterized by remissions, relapses, and cures.

- There is no single cause of alcohol dependence, but three causative factors are thought to interact in the development of the illness: personality, environment (widespread social acceptance and availability), and the addictive nature of the drug.
    - It is generally believed that any person, regardless of environment, genetic background, or personality traits can become dependent when the drug is consumed for long periods.
- The development of alcohol dependence can be divided into four main stages, which merge imperceptibly.
    - In the first stage, tolerance of the drug develops in the heavy social drinker, allowing the individual to consume larger quantities of alcohol before experiencing its ill effects.
    - On entering stage two, the drinker experiences memory lapses relating to events during the drinking episodes.
    - The third stage is characterized by lack of control over alcohol; the drinker can no longer be certain of discontinuing alcohol consumption at will.
    - The final stage begins with prolonged binges of intoxication with associated mental and physical complications.
    - Some drinkers halt their consumption temporarily or permanently during one of the first three stages.

Ethanol

- The active ingredient in all alcoholic beverages is ethanol, a colorless, flammable liquid produced from the fermentation of carbohydrates by yeast.
- All alcoholic drinks are rated based on their ethanol percentage.
    - The alcohol content of beer and wine is measured as a percentage by weight or volume.
    - In the United States, beer contains 2.3–5.1% alcohol by volume.
    - Wines vary in content up to 14–16%.
- Distilled liquors are subjected to a rating process called proof.

Metabolism

- A total of 80–90% of ingested alcohol is absorbed within 30 minutes (20% in the stomach, the remainder in the small intestine).
- Once absorbed, the drug is rapidly distributed throughout the vascular space and reaches virtually every organ system.
- About 3–5% of alcohol is excreted unchanged via the lungs and kidneys.
- The rest is metabolized in the liver to carbon dioxide and water.
- Alcohol generally is metabolized at a constant rate of about 20 mg/dL per hour (in nonalcoholics), regardless of its concentration.
- The rate of metabolism may be increased in alcoholics.

Blood alcohol content

- The alcohol content of blood is measured in terms of weight (milligrams) of alcohol per given volume of blood (deciliter).
- The time it takes for the alcohol concentration to peak in the blood depends on:
    - The rate at which the alcohol is consumed.
    - The amount of food present in the stomach before drinking.
    - Physical characteristics of the drinker.
- Although blood alcohol content is widely used to evaluate the CNS status of an intoxicated person, there is marked individual variation in blood alcohol content and degree of intoxication.
- In many states the legal limit of intoxication is 100 mg/dL (equivalent to 0.10%).

MEDICAL CONSEQUENCES OF CHRONIC ALCOHOL INGESTION

Because alcohol affects nearly every organ system, people who consume large quantities of alcohol are susceptible to numerous physical and mental disorders.

Neurological Disorders

- Alcohol is a potent CNS depressant.
- When consumed in moderate amounts, the drug reduces anxiety and tension and provides most drinkers with a feeling of relaxation and confidence.
- Clinical manifestations of alcohol are dose dependent and progress predictably as the level of consumption increases and blood alcohol content rises.
- Initial feelings of well-being give way to impaired judgement and discrimination, prolonged reflexes, and incoordination and drowsiness, which may ultimately progress to stupor and coma.
- Long-term neurological effects of chronic alcohol abuse are similar to those of the aging process and include:
  - Short-term memory deficit
  - Problems with coordination
  - Difficulty with concentration and abstraction

Nutritional Deficiencies

- Alcohol may temporarily satisfy the body's caloric requirements and also decrease a drinker's appetite through an irritant effect on the stomach.
- While providing satiation, alcohol does not have essential vitamins, proteins, or fats.
- Alcohol-dependent persons have a potential for decreased dietary intake and malabsorption, leading to multiple vitamin and mineral deficiencies.
- Clinical manifestations associated with these deficiencies include:
  - Altered immunity
  - Anorexia
  - Cardiac dysrhythmias
  - Coma
  - Irritability and disorientation
  - Muscle cramps
  - Paresthesias
  - Poor wound healing
  - Seizures
  - Tremor and ataxia

Wernicke-Korsakoff Syndrome

- A disease that results from chronic thiamine (vitamin B1) deficiency combined with an inability to use thiamine from a heritable disorder or from a reduction in intestinal absorption and metabolism of thiamine by alcohol
- Affects the brain and nervous system by disrupting central and peripheral nerve function
- May consist of two stages: Wernicke's encephalopathy, Korsakoff's psychosis, or a combination of the two
  - Wernicke's encephalopathy usually develops suddenly with the clinical manifestations of ataxia, ocular changes (nystagmus), disturbances of speech and gait, signs of neuropathy (paresthesias, impaired reflexes), stupor, or coma (rare).

    - Since the body uses up thiamine stores to metabolize sugar, the syndrome may be precipitated in the malnourished patient by the IV administration of glucose or glucose-containing fluids.
    - IV administration of thiamine should precede the IV administration of glucose in patients with altered mental status or coma of unknown origin.
    - After receiving thiamine, patients with Wernicke's encephalopathy usually become more alert and attentive, but gait and mental difficulties often persist for days or months; fewer than half the affected patients recover completely.
  - Korsakoff's psychosis is a mental disorder often found with Wernicke's encephalopathy.
    - Signs include apathy, poor retentive memory, retrograde amnesia, confabulation (invention of stories to make up for gaps in memory), and dementia
    - Is usually considered irreversible, leaving the patient permanently handicapped by memory loss and in need of continual supervision

Fluid and Electrolyte Imbalances

- Urinary output increases (over and above that expected from the amount of fluid ingested) after alcohol consumption.
- The diuresis results from an inhibition of antidiuretic hormone secretion, which can lead to dehydration as well as electrolyte imbalances.

GI Disorders

Effects of alcohol on the GI system can produce several types of alcohol-related illnesses and diseases.

GI Hemorrhage

Primary causes of GI hemorrhage in patients who drink alcohol are gastritis, ulcer formation, esophageal tear (Mallory-Weiss syndrome), and variceal hemorrhage.

Gastritis

- Results from the toxic effects of ethanol on the gastric mucosa, which leads to diffuse or localized areas of erosion.
- In the chronic form of gastritis, blood may continually ooze from the mucosal lining and ulcers may develop.
- An esophageal tear of the gastroesophageal junction, stomach, or esophagus can occur from severe or protracted vomiting or retching.
- The injury results when gastric contents are forced against an unrelaxed gastroesophageal junction, which produces a sudden increase in pressure and a mucosal tear with subsequent bleeding.
- Bleeding can be exacerbated by clotting abnormalities, which are common in patients with alcoholic liver disease.

Varices

- Varices are a result of portal hypertension caused by cirrhosis.
  - Any of these thin-walled, blood-engorged veins are subject to rupture and hemorrhage, although the most common site is the varices of the esophagus.
  - Bleeding esophageal varices remain one of the most difficult conditions to treat.
  - Severe hematemesis requires aggressive supportive care through large-bore IV lines and fluid resuscitation.

Cirrhosis

- Cirrhosis of the liver is caused by chronic damage to liver cells that results in inflammation and eventually necrosis.
- Bands of fibrosis (scar tissue) develop and break up the normal structure of the liver.
  - The distortion and fibrosis of the liver lead to portal hypertension, with the resultant complications of ascites, splenomegaly, and bleeding esophageal and gastric varices.
- Cirrhosis may also lead to hepatic encephalopathy caused by the accumulation of toxic metabolic waste products, which would normally be detoxified by a healthy liver and which have an adverse effect on the brain.

Acute or Chronic Pancreatitis

- Alcohol is the most common cause of acute and chronic pancreatitis, although the exact mechanism by which alcohol produces pancreatic inflammation is not clear.
  - It may be caused at least in part by activation of pancreatic proenzymes, obstruction of pancreatic ducts, and stimulation of enzymatic secretion.
  - There may also be a direct toxic effect, as has been demonstrated for the liver.
- Chronic pancreatitis usually produces the same symptoms as the acute form.
  - Pain may last from several hours to several days and the attacks may become more frequent as the condition progresses.
  - Other effects of chronic pancreatitis include malabsorption (a result of a deficiency of pancreatic enzymes), electrolyte imbalances such as hypocalcemia, and diabetes mellitus (caused by insufficient insulin production).
- Complications of pancreatitis, hemorrhagic pancreatitis, sepsis, and pancreatic abscess are associated with high mortality.

Cardiac and Skeletal Muscle Myopathy

- Is thought to result from a direct toxic effect of alcohol or its metabolites.
- Pathological changes associated with these alcoholic muscle syndromes include intracellular edema, formation of lipid droplets, excessive cellular glycogen, and deranged sarcoplasmic reticula and mitochondria.
- In heart muscle, these changes result in a decreased force of contraction (negative inotropic effect), dysrhythmias, and a tendency to develop congestive heart failure.
- In skeletal muscle, the major symptoms are weakness and muscle wasting.
- The clinical prevalence of cardiac and skeletal myopathy has been estimated at between 50–60% of all chronic alcoholics.

Immune Suppression

- Long-term alcohol abuse renders the immune system less effective by suppressing bone marrow production of white blood cells; red blood cells and platelet production are also often decreased.
- Alcohol has direct, specific effects on lung tissue, which impairs macrophage mobilization and mucociliary function.
  - As a result, the body's ability to fight pulmonary infection is altered, making the alcoholic more susceptible to viral and bacterial pneumonia, which may occur secondary to aspiration during alcoholic stupor or for other reasons.
  - Although the exact mechanism is unknown, there is an increased incidence of cancer in alcoholic patients, which may also be related to immune suppression.

Trauma

- Alcohol suppresses 11 of the 12 blood-clotting factors produced in the liver. This blood-clotting deficiency makes alcoholics susceptible to bruising and internal hemorrhage and adds to the frequency of subdural bleeding, even after relatively minor head trauma.
- There also is evidence that alcohol causes increased myocardial irritability and a decrease in tidal and minute volume, which may alter the trauma patient's ability to compensate for the metabolic acidosis seen in shock.

ALCOHOL EMERGENCIES

Several other conditions caused by consumption or abstinence from alcohol may require emergency care.

Acute Alcohol Intoxication

- Alcohol ingestion can cause acute poisoning if consumed in sufficiently large amounts over a relatively short period.
- Clinical features are similar to those induced by sedative-hypnotic agents and can be correlated to a degree with blood alcohol content.
- At toxic levels, hypoventilation (including respiratory arrest), hypotension, and hypothermia may develop.
- The patient with signs and symptoms of acute alcohol intoxication should be carefully considered for occult trauma and coexisting medical conditions such as:
  - Hypoglycemia
  - Cardiac myopathy and dysrhythmias
  - GI bleeding
  - Polydrug abuse (particularly barbiturates or tranquilizers)
  - Ethylene glycol or methanol ingestion

Management

- A mildly intoxicated patient should be transported for physician evaluation.
- Usually, the patient will be observed in the emergency department until he or she is sober.
- Carefully monitor vital signs and level of consciousness en route to the hospital.
- A thorough physical examination is warranted to rule out illness or injury masked by alcohol ingestion.
- Treatment of the acutely intoxicated patient is directed at protecting the patient from further injury and maintaining vital functions.
- If the patient is conscious and agitated, it may be necessary to use restraints to protect the patient and various health-care providers from bodily harm.
- If physical restraint becomes necessary, summon police.
- After scene safety has been established, initial assessment and resuscitation should include the following:
  - Rapidly evaluate airway patency with spinal precautions and ventilatory and hemodynamic status while obtaining a patient history.
  - The patient's account of the history of the event may be unreliable as a result of alcohol ingestion.
  - Initiate IV therapy.
  - Draw blood samples for laboratory analysis. Per protocol, administer thiamine, 50% dextrose (if hypoglycemia is likely or confirmed), and naloxone (Narcan), if opiate overdose is suspected.

- Continually monitor the patient's airway and provide adequate ventilatory and circulatory support as needed.
- Be prepared to provide suction and aggressive airway management.
- Monitor ECG for dysrhythmias.
- Rapidly transport the patient for physician evaluation.

Alcohol Withdrawal Syndrome

- A period of relative or absolute abstinence from alcohol may cause withdrawal in an alcoholic.
- Severity of syndromes depends on:
  - Magnitude of blood alcohol content (serum ethanol level)
  - Length of time the level was maintained
  - Abruptness of cessation
  - Tissue tolerance to alcohol
  - General physical and psychological condition of the patient
- Although the pathophysiological mechanism of alcohol withdrawal remains largely undefined, it is thought to result from CNS hyperexcitability (as the CNS depressant is removed) and from biochemical changes such as respiratory alkalosis and hypomagnesemia.
- Alcohol withdrawal syndromes can be divided into four general categories—Minor reactions, hallucinations, alcohol withdrawal seizures, and delirium tremens.

Minor Reactions

- Begin about 6–8 hours after cessation or reduction of alcohol intake.
- Symptoms peak within 24–36 hours and may persist for 10–14 days.
- When alcohol withdrawal is confined to minor reactions, the prognosis for full recovery is excellent with appropriate management.
- Minor reactions include:
  - Sudden and unexpected startle
  - Flushed face and diaphoresis
  - Anorexia
  - Nausea and vomiting
  - Insomnia
  - General muscle weakness
  - Slight disorientation
  - Generalized tremor (worsened by agitation)
  - Mild tachycardia, hypertension, hyperreflexia

Hallucinations

- Usually occur 24–36 hours after cessation of alcohol.
- Disorders of perception are common and may vary from auditory and visual illusions to frank hallucinations, which can produce agitation, fear, and panic
- The patient may show signs of suicidal and homicidal tendencies and minor reactions may be more pronounced.
- Prognosis is the same as for minor reactions with appropriate management.

Alcohol Withdrawal Seizures (or Rum Fits)

- Usually occur 7–48 hours after ethanol cessation, with a peak incidence between 13 and 24 hours.
- Seizures may occur singly or in groups of two to six.

- Are most often grand mal and of short duration (status seizures are rare).
- Are associated with varying degrees of tremor, anorexia, hallucinations, and autonomic hyperactivity.
- This category of withdrawal may be self-limiting or may progress to delirium tremens with or without a lucid interval.
- Because of the drug tolerance level of alcoholic patients, seizure activity may require IV administration of large doses of diazepam (Valium), 5 mg every 5 minutes up to 30 mg.
  - Diazepam (Valium) may synergistically interact with any ethanol still in the patient's system, so vital signs, respirations, and mental status should be closely monitored.

Delirium Tremens (DTs)

- The most dramatic and serious form of alcohol withdrawal.
- Affects about 5% of all alcoholics hospitalized for withdrawal.
- Usually occurs 72–96 hours after cessation of alcohol but may be delayed up to 14 days.
- Characterized by psychomotor, speech, and autonomic hyperactivity; profound confusion; disorientation; delusion; vivid hallucinations; tremor; agitation; and insomnia.
- Autonomic hyperactivity is the most distinguishing feature of DTs.
  - It is characterized by tachycardia, fever, hypertension, dilated pupils, and profuse diaphoresis.
  - In severe cases, cardiovascular collapse may be present.
- DTs is a true medical emergency, with a mortality rate as high as 15%.
  - Associated alcohol-related illnesses such as pneumonia, pancreatitis, and hepatitis are frequent contributing causes of death.

Management

- Prehospital care is primarily supportive.
- Ensure scene safety.
- Monitor the patient's airway, ventilatory, and circulatory status.
- Initiate IV therapy with saline solution for rehydration.
- Pharmacological therapy may be indicated for an altered level of consciousness, dysrhythmias, or seizure activity.
- Provide calm reassurance and frequent reorientation.
- Transport for physician evaluation.

Disulfiram-Ethanol Reaction

- Disulfiram (tetraethylthiuram disulfide or Antabuse) is a medication prescribed to some alcoholic patients to help them abstain.
  - The drug works by inhibiting ethanol metabolism and by allowing the accumulation of the metabolite acetaldehyde.
  - Acetaldehyde produces ill effects on the GI, cardiovascular, and autonomic nervous systems and is the metabolic product thought to be responsible for the common "hangover."
- Patients who take disulfiram and then ingest ethanol experience an unpleasant and potentially life-threatening physiological response.

- The reaction begins 15–30 minutes after ingestion of 2–5 alcoholic drinks and continues for 1–2 hours.
  - Causes the patient to experience vertigo, headache, vomiting, flushing (which may give the skin a "lobster-red" appearance), dyspnea, diaphoresis, abdominal pain, and sometimes chest pain.
  - More serious reactions include hypotension, shock, and dysrhythmias.
  - Sudden death, myocardial and cerebral infarction, and cerebral hemorrhage have been reported after as little as one drink of ethanol in patients taking disulfiram.

Management

- Provide airway, ventilatory, and circulatory support.
- Administer IV fluids to treat hypotension.
- Provide pharmacological therapy as needed to manage dysrhythmias.
- Rapidly transport the patient for physician evaluation.
  - Most episodes are self-limiting
- Supportive care and in-hospital observation are usually all that are required.

GENERAL MANAGEMENT PRINCIPLES FOR TOXIC SYNDROMES

- Most poisoned patients (regardless of the toxic agent) require only supportive therapy to recover.
- General management guidelines for the poisoned patient:
  - Ensure scene and personal safety.
  - Provide adequate airway, ventilation, and circulation.
  - Obtain a thorough history and perform a focused physical examination.
  - Consider hypoglycemia in an unconscious or convulsing patient.
  - Administer naloxone (Narcan) or nalmefene (Revex) to a patient with respiratory depression.
  - If overdose is suspected, obtain an overdose history from the patient, family, or friends.
  - Consult with medical direction or a poison control center for specific treatment to prevent further absorption of the toxin (or antidote therapy).
  - Frequently monitor vital signs and ECG.
  - Safely obtain any substance or substance container of a suspected poison and transport it with the patient.
  - Transport the patient for physician evaluation.
- Grouping toxicologically similar agents and physical findings into toxic syndromes, however, can give the paramedic important clues to narrow a differential diagnosis and to more easily remember assessment and management strategies.

Cholinergic ("Wet" Patient Presentation)

- Common signs—Confusion, CNS depression, weakness, SLUDGE (salivation, lacrimation, urination, defecation, GI upset, emesis), bradycardia, wheezing, bronchoconstriction, myosis, coma, convulsion, diaphoresis, seizures
- Causative agents—Organophosphate and carbamate insecticides, nerve agents, some mushrooms
- Specific treatment—Atropine, pralidoxime (2-PAM Chloride), diazepam (Valium), activated charcoal

Anticholinergic ("Dry" Patient Presentation)

- Common signs—Delirium, tachycardia, dry, flushed skin, dilated pupils, seizures and dysrhythmias (in severe cases)
- Causative agents—Antihistamines, antiparkinson medications, atropine, antipsychotic agents, antidepressants, skeletal muscle relaxants, many plants (e.g., jimsonweed and *Amanita muscaria*)
- Specific treatment—Diazepam (Valium), activated charcoal, rarely physostigmine (Antilirium)

Hallucinogen

- Common signs—Visual illusions, delusions, bizarre behavior, flashbacks, respiratory and CNS depression
- Causative agents—LSD, PCP, mescaline, some mushrooms, marijuana, jimsonweed, nutmeg, mace, some amphetamines
- Specific treatment—Minimal sensory stimulation and calming measures

Opioids

- Common signs—Euphoria, hypotension, respiratory depression/arrest, nausea, pinpoint pupils, seizures, coma
- Causative agents—Heroin, morphine, codeine, meperidine (Demerol), propoxyphene (Darvon), fentanyl
- Specific treatment—Naloxone (Narcan), nalmefene (Revex)

Sympathomimetic

- Common signs—Delusions, paranoia, tachycardia or bradycardia, hypertension, diaphoresis; seizures, hypotension, and dysrhythmias in severe cases
- Causative agents—Cocaine, amphetamine, methamphetamine, over-the-counter decongestants
- Specific treatment—Minimal sensory stimulation and calming measures

? CHAPTER QUESTIONS

1. The primary goal of inducing vomiting in a patient who ingested a poison is to prevent the toxic substance from reaching the:
   a. small intestine
   b. stomach
   c. kidneys
   d. large intestine
2. Patients who have ingested a caustic substance commonly present with all of the following except:
   a. shortness of breath
   b. oropharyngeal burn
   c. diarrhea
   d. severe throat and thoracic pain

3. Treatment of cyanide poisoning includes:
   a. administration of vitamin B1
   b. administration of naloxone
   c. administration of sodium thiosulfate
   d. administration of potassium thiocyanate
4. The initial treatment for cyanide poisoning is:
   a. amyl nitrite
   b. narcan 2–8 mg
   c. sodium thiosulfate
   d. ventilatory support with high flow O_2

Suggested Reading

US Department of Transportation, National Highway Traffic Safety Administration. *EMT-Paramedic: National Standard Curriculum.* Washington, DC: US Department of Transportation, National Highway Traffic Safety Administration; 1998.

Chapter 29
Hematology

You are treating a 12-year-old male, who fell off his skateboard and is complaining of abdominal pain and uncontrollable bleeding from an abrasion to his left elbow. The patient, who should not be riding a skateboard, states, he has "hemophilia." He states he currently takes desmopressin. The patient's mother is enroute to the scene and has authorized any needed treatment. Vital signs have been taken and are as follows:

B/P: 108/72

Heart rate: 110 regular/strong

Respiratory rate: 18 regular

Skin: Cool and moist

Cardiac monitor: Sinus tachycardia with no ectopic focus

Your partner attempts to control external bleeding and you establish a normal saline IV, large bore (16-gauge) and begin a fluid bolus. The patient denies neck or back pain, and states he was never unconscious prior to or after the fall. Treatment continues. What are some concerns regarding this patient and his medical history?

BLOOD AND BLOOD COMPONENTS

- Blood consists of cells and formed elements, surrounded by plasma.
- About 95% of formed elements consist of red blood cells (RBCs) (erythrocytes).
- The remaining 5% consists of white blood cells (leukocytes) and cell fragments (platelets).
- The continuous movement of blood keeps the formed elements dispersed throughout the plasma, where they are available to carry out their chief functions.
  - Delivery of substances needed for cellular metabolism in the tissues
  - Defense against invading microorganisms and injury
  - Acid-base balance
- All types of blood cells are formed within the red bone marrow (present in all tissues at birth).
- In the adult, the red bone marrow is primarily found in membranous bone.
  - Vertebrae
  - Pelvis
  - Sternum
  - Ribs
- Yellow marrow produces some white blood cells (WBCs) but is composed mainly of connective tissue and fat.
- Other blood-forming organs:
  - Lymph nodes produce lymphocytes and antibodies.

- The spleen produces lymphocytes, plasma cells, and antibodies (and stores large quantities of blood).
- The liver (a blood-forming organ only during intrauterine life) plays an important role in the coagulation process.

Plasma

- The clear portion of blood, which contains approximately 92% water
- Contains three important proteins
  - Albumin
    - The most plentiful protein
    - Similar to egg white; gives blood its gummy texture
    - These large proteins keep the water concentration of blood low, so that water diffuses readily from tissues into the blood
  - Globulins (alpha, beta, and gamma)—Transport other proteins and provide immunity to disease
  - Fibrinogen—Responsible for blood clotting
- Functions of plasma proteins:
  - Maintaining blood pH (acting as either an acid or a base)
  - Transporting fat-soluble vitamins, hormones, and carbohydrates
  - Allowing the body to digest them temporarily for food
- Plasma also contains salts, metals, and inorganic compounds

Red Blood Cells

- Most abundant cells in the body.
- Primarily responsible for tissue oxygenation.
- Appear as small rounded disks with nearly hollowed-out centers.
- Consist mainly of water and the protein hemoglobin.
- RBC production continues throughout life to replace blood cells that grow old and die, are killed by disease, or are lost through bleeding.
- After RBC production in the bone marrow, the new cell divides until there are 16 red blood cells.
- The cells produce hemoglobin protein until the concentration of the protein becomes 95% of the dry weight of the cell, at which time the cell expels its nucleus, giving the cell its characteristic "pinched" look.
- The new shape of the RBC increases the cell's surface area—and thus its oxygen-carrying potential.
- RBCs have a life span of about 120 days.
  - Characteristics of aging RBCs:
    - Weakened internal chemical machinery
    - Loss of elasticity
    - Become trapped in small blood vessels in the bone marrow, liver, and spleen
  - RBCs are then destroyed by specialized white blood cells (macrophages).
- Each RBC contains about 270 million hemoglobin molecules.
  - Each hemoglobin molecule carries four oxygen molecules
  - Hemoglobin (Hgb) is reported in grams per 100 mL of blood.
    - Normal hemoglobin for men is 13.5–18 g/100 mL.
    - In women a normal hemoglobin is 12–16 g/100 mL.
- The number of RBCs is about 4.5–5 million cells/cubic millimeter.

- Hematocrit (Hct) is the fraction of the total volume of blood that consists of red blood cells, normally about 45%.
  - For example, a value of 46% implies that there are 46 mL of RBCs in 100 mL of blood.
  - The normal hematocrit for men is 40–54%; for women, 38–47%.
- Reticulocyte count provides information about the rate of RBC production.
  - A reticulocyte count of less than 0.5% of the RBC count usually indicates a slowdown during RBC formation.
  - A reticulocyte count greater than 1.5% usually indicates an acceleration of RBC formation.

White Blood Cells

- WBCs arise from the bone marrow and are released into the bloodstream.
- Function of the WBCs includes destroying foreign substances, and clearing the blood stream of debris.
- Leukocyte production increases in response to infection, causing an elevated WBC count in the blood.
- The bone marrow and lymph glands continually produce and maintain a reserve of WBCs.
  - There are not many WBCs in the healthy bloodstream.
- The normal WBC count is about 5000–10,000 cells/cubic millimeter.
  - Monocytes make up about 5% of the total WBC count and will increase with chronic infections.
  - Lymphocytes account for about 27.5% of the total.
  - Neutrophils make up about 65% of the total.
  - Eosinophils and basophils together comprise about 2.5% of the total WBC count.
- Because WBCs are somewhat specific for various illnesses, a rise in their numbers can aid in the diagnosis of some diseases.
- Leukocyte disorders:
  - Leukemia—An increased number of WBCs in the tissues and/or in the blood.
  - Leukocytosis—An abnormal increase in the number of circulating WBCs.
    - — Types of leukocytosis include basophilia, eosinophilia, and neutrophilia.
  - Leukopenia—An abnormal decrease in the number of WBCs.
- The inflammatory process:
  - Inflammation is characterized by redness, heat, swelling, and pain.
  - When tissues are injured or irritated, injured cells release histamine and other substances.
    - — Blood vessels in the injured tissue dilate.
      Dilated blood vessels bring more blood to the area.
      Increased blood flow causes redness and heat.
    - — Increased blood flow also carries neutrophils and monocytes (phagocytic cells) to the site of injury.
  - Histamine and other substances cause the walls of the blood vessels to leak.
    - — Fluid and dissolved substances leak out of the blood vessels into the tissue spaces.
      Results in swelling.
    - — The fluid that collects in the tissues contains fibrinogen (a clotting factor).
      Fibrinogen creates fibrin threads within the tissue spaces.
      Fibroblasts (cells that form connective tissue) may also invade the injured area and help restrict the area of inflammation.
      - Prevents the spread of infection throughout the body

  - Fluid and irritating chemicals accumulate at the injured site, stimulating pain receptors.

Immunity

- Natural (native)—Present at birth and is not produced by the immune response.
- Acquired:
  - Gained after birth from exposure to a specific antigenic agent or pathogen
  - Includes that resulting from inoculation (immunization) against certain infectious diseases
  - Further classification
    - Humoral immunity—Associated with the production of antibodies that combine with and eliminate foreign material
    - Cell-mediated immunity
      - Body's best defense against viruses, fungi, parasites, and some bacteria
      - Responsible for the body rejecting transplanted organs
      - Characterized by the formation of a population of lymphocytes that attack and destroy foreign material
  - Alterations in immunologic response
    - Deficiencies in immunity and inflammation refer to the failure of mechanisms of self-defense to function at their normal capacity
    - Possible sources of the deficiency
      - Congenital (caused by an anomaly present at birth)
      - Acquired
        - Far more common than congenital forms
        - Types of acquired immune deficiencies
          - Nutritional deficiencies (e.g., severe deficits in calorie or protein intake)
          - Iatrogenic deficiencies (caused by some form of medical treatment)
          - Deficiencies caused by trauma (e.g., bacterial infection, burns)
          - Deficiencies caused by stress (depressed immune function)
          - Acquired immunodeficiency syndrome (AIDS)
        - Causes of acquired immune deficiencies
          - Infection (such as the human immunodeficiency virus, or HIV)
          - Cancer
          - Immunosuppressive drugs
          - Aging
- Whether congenital or acquired, the cause of the deficiency is usually the disruption of lymphocyte function.

Platelets

- Platelets (thrombocytes) are small, sticky cells that play an important role in blood clotting.
- When a blood vessel is cut, platelets travel to the site and swell into odd, irregular shapes and adhere to the damaged vessel wall.
  - Platelets "plug" the leak and allow other cells to stick to them and form a clot.
  - If the damage to the vessel is too great, however, the platelets will chemically signal the complex clotting process, the clotting cascade.
  - Platelets repair millions of ruptured capillaries on a daily basis, often making the rest of the clotting cascade unnecessary.

- Clotting time is normally about 7–10 minutes.
  - If this time is prolonged, the patient will have a bleeding tendency.
  - If the clotting time is less than normal, the patient will have a tendency to develop intravascular clots.
- Prothrombin time (PT time) is the time it takes plasma to clot (normally about 12–13 seconds). A patient who is taking anticoagulants will normally have frequent lab tests to measure prothrombin time.

Blood Groups

- When combined with foreign plasma, red blood cells may clump together (agglutinate).
- Two distinct agglutinins (substances on red blood cells acting as antigens) are responsible for this clumping.
- Based on possible combinations of antigens, four types of human blood have been identified—A, B, AB, and O.
  - Type A blood has anti-B antibodies in the plasma and will clump type B blood.
  - Type B blood has anti-A antibodies and will clump type A blood.
  - Type AB blood has neither antibody and can receive any of the four types of blood (universal recipient).
  - Type O blood has both anti-A and anti-B antibodies, so it cannot receive any type of blood other than type O.
  - Type O blood has neither antigen, however, and can therefore be given to patients with any blood type.
  - Type O blood is called the universal donor.

Rh Factor

- The term *Rh factor* refers to the presence or absence of the Rh antigen on the surface of red blood cells.
- A person with the factor is Rh-positive; a person without it is Rh-negative.
- Antibodies to the Rh factor are acquired through exposure to Rh-positive blood.

Hemostasis

- Hemostasis is the process that stops bleeding after injury and involves the interaction of plasma and tissue factors with the platelets and vessels.
- Ensures that leaky vessels are sealed within minutes of injury.
- The smooth muscle in the wall of the injured blood vessel constricts in response to injury (vascular spasm).
  - Decreases the amount of blood flowing through the vessel
- If the innermost lining of a blood vessel is injured, the blood contacts the underlying collagen fibers.
  - As platelets contact collagen, they swell, become sticky, and secrete chemicals that activate surrounding platelets.
  - The process causes platelets to stick to one another, creating a "platelet plug" in the injured vessel.
    - Platelets stick to the injury site with the help of von Willebrand factor.
    - If the opening in the vessel wall is small, the plug may be sufficient to stop blood loss completely.
    - For larger wounds, a blood clot is necessary to arrest the flow of blood.
- At the same time, the actual process of clotting is set off by two mechanisms.
  - An extrinsic system, triggered by tissue factors released when a tissue is damaged

- An intrinsic system, activated by contact between clotting factor XII and the collagen fibers
  - Both systems can activate, either individually or in combination, plasma factor X that, with other factors, converts prothrombin to thrombin.
  - This in turn converts fibrinogen to fibrin.
  - Fibrin forms a netlike structure at the site of injury.
  - RBCs and platelets become trapped within the net, forming a blood clot.
- Possible causes of an abnormal reduction in the blood's ability to clot, resulting in a tendency to hemorrhage, are:
  - Congenital lack of a clotting factor (lack of factor VIII leading to hemophilia A)
  - Acquired deficiency of a factor (liver damage, vitamin K deficiency)
  - Too few or diseased thrombocytes (thrombocytopenia)
  - Certain vascular diseases
  - Excessive fibrinolysis
  - Increased consumption of a particular factor

SPECIFIC BLOOD DISORDERS

Anemia

- Is a condition in which the concentration of hemoglobin or erythrocytes in the blood is below normal.
- Precipitating causes of anemia include chronic or acute blood loss, decreased production of erythrocytes, or an increased destruction of erythrocytes.
- Two common forms of anemia:
  - Iron-deficiency anemia
  - Hemolytic anemia

Iron-Deficiency Anemia

- Iron is the critical part of a hemoglobin molecule's ability to bind oxygen.
- The lack of iron in iron-deficiency anemia prevents the bone marrow from making sufficient hemoglobin for the red blood cells.
- The cells produced are small and pale centered, and have a reduced oxygen-carrying capacity.
- Causes include:
  - Insufficient intake of iron
  - GI disorders (e.g., ulcer disease)
  - External and/or internal bleeding
  - Prolonged aspirin or nonsteroidal anti-inflammatory drug (NSAID) therapy
  - Gastrectomy (surgical removal of part or all of the stomach)
- Signs and symptoms:
  - Those related to the underlying cause (e.g., bleeding)
  - Those common to all forms of anemia
- Management:
  - Correction of the underlying cause
  - Supplemental iron tablets or injections

Hemolytic Anemia

- Caused by the premature destruction of RBCs in the blood (hemolysis)
- May result from an inherited disorder inside the red cell or from a disorder outside the cell

- Usually acquired later in life
- Inherited disorders
  - Hemolysis can occur from abnormal rigidity of the cell membrane.
  - This rigidity causes the cell to become trapped at an early stage of its life span in the smaller blood vessels (usually of the spleen), where it is destroyed by macrophages.
- Causes of hemolytic anemia:
  - Genetic defect in the hemoglobin within the cell (e.g., sickle cell anemia, thalassemia)
  - Defect in one of the cell's enzymes, which help protect the cell from chemical damage during infectious illness
    - A deficiency of a certain enzyme—glucose-6-phosphate dehydrogenase—is common in African Americans
- Acquired disorders
  - Acquired hemolytic anemia results from one of three conditions:
    - Disorders in which normal RBCs are disrupted because of mechanical forces (e.g., abnormal blood vessel linings, blood clots)
    - Autoimmune disorders—Conditions in which antibodies are produced by the immune system and directed against RBCs (e.g., incompatible blood transfusion)
    - Conditions that cause hemolytic anemia when RBCs are destroyed by microorganisms in the blood (e.g., malaria)
- Signs and symptoms of hemolytic anemia
  - Jaundice
  - Those common to all forms of anemia
- Management of hemolytic anemia
  - Splenectomy
  - Immunosuppressant drugs
  - Avoidance of drugs or foods that precipitate hemolysis
  - Antimalarial drugs
  - Blood transfusions

Signs and Symptoms of Anemia

- All forms of anemia share certain signs and symptoms
  - Fatigue and headaches
  - Possibly a sore mouth or tongue
  - Brittle nails
  - In severe cases, breathlessness and chest pain
- Other specific complaints of patients with anemia
  - Fatigue
  - Lethargy
  - Fever
  - Cutaneous bleeding
  - Bleeding from mucous membranes

Diagnosis

- Patient's signs and symptoms
- Patient history
- Examining the patient's blood through blood tests and bone marrow biopsy
  - Iron-deficiency anemia will usually reveal RBCs that are smaller than normal.
  - Hemolytic anemia will show red blood cells that are immature and abnormally shaped.

Management

- Directed at correcting, modifying, or diminishing the mechanism or process that is leading to defective red cell production or reduced red cell survival

Leukemia

- Refers to any of several types of cancer in which there is usually a disorganized proliferation of WBCs in the bone marrow. The production of leukemic cells crowds and impairs the normal production of RBCs, platelets, and WBCs.
- More common in men than in women; more common in Caucasians than African Americans.
- About 30,000 cases diagnosed in the United States each year.
- Exact cause(s) of leukemia is not known. Genetics may play a role.
- Some patients with a certain form of leukemia have an abnormal chromosome called the Philadelphia chromosome in their blood cells. Philadelphia chromosome is an acquired abnormality; it is neither inherited nor passed on to children.
- Abnormal chromosomes associated with congenital disorders, such as Down syndrome, and HIV-type viruses have been associated with a rare form of this disease.
- Other factors that may play a role in the development of leukemia:
  - Exposure to radiation
  - Viral infections
  - Immune defects
  - Various chemicals in the home and work environments
- Classifications:
  - Acute or chronic
    - — Acute leukemia—Cancer cells start multiplying before they develop beyond their immature stage
    - — Chronic leukemia—Progresses more slowly, with cancer cells developing to full maturity
  - Further classification according to the type of WBC involved
    - — Acute lymphoblastic leukemia

      Affects mostly young children

      Sometimes called childhood leukemia
    - — Acute myeloblastic leukemia

      Usually affects middle-age adults

      One of the most intractable (unmanageable) blood cancers
    - — In both acute lymphoblastic and acute myeloblastic leukemias, abnormal WBCs are produced in such large amounts that they eventually accumulate in the body's vital organs (liver, spleen, lymph, and brain), impeding their function and leading to death
- The proliferation of leukemic cells, or the resulting inadequate production of other normal blood cells, makes the patient highly susceptible to serious infections, anemia, and bleeding episodes.

Signs and Symptoms

- Fatigue, bone pain, diaphoresis
- Elevated body temperature
- Sternal tenderness
- Heat intolerance
- Abdominal fullness
- Bleeding

- Frequent bruising
- Headache
- Weight loss
- Night sweats
- Enlarged lymph nodes
- Enlargement of the liver, spleen, and testes

Diagnosis

- Confirmed by bone marrow biopsy
- Severity of the leukemia is assessed by the degree of liver and spleen enlargement, anemia, and lack of platelets in the blood

Management

- Acute leukemia
  - Transfusion of blood and platelets
  - Antibiotic therapy
  - Use of anticancer drugs and sometimes radiation to destroy leukemic cells
  - In some cases, bone marrow transplantation (BMT)
- Chronic leukemia
  - May be effectively managed with medication
  - Many patients require no management in early stages

Lymphomas

- Refers to a varied group of diseases that range from slowly growing chronic disorders to rapidly evolving acute conditions.
- Hodgkin's disease represents one type; all others, despite their diversity, are commonly called non-Hodgkin's lymphomas.

Hodgkin's Lymphoma

- Hodgkin's disease is a malignant disorder of lymphoid tissue (found mainly in the lymph nodes and spleen) in which there is a proliferation of constituent cells and a resultant enlargement of lymph nodes. Left unchecked, these cancer cells multiply and eventually displace healthy lymphocytes, suppressing the immune system.
- Signs and Symptoms
  - Swollen lymph nodes in the neck, armpits, or groin
  - Fatigue
  - Chills
  - Night sweats
  - Severe itching
  - Persistent cough
  - Weight loss
  - Shortness of breath
  - Chest discomfort
- Hodgkin's disease is a relatively rare cancer of unknown etiology that may have a heritable component. More common in men than in women, with peak incidences in people in their 20s and between 55 and 70 years of age.
- Diagnosis:
  - Confirmed by identification of Reed-Sternberg cells in lymph nodes or organs affected by the cancer

- Management:
  - Depends on the level of lymph node and organ system involvement (the stage of the disease)
  - May consist of radiation and chemotherapy with anticancer drugs

Non-Hodgkin's Lymphoma

- Non-Hodgkin's lymphomas vary in their malignancy according the nature and activity of the abnormal cells.
- At least 10 types of non-Hodgkin's lymphoma have been identified.
- Each type is ranked as low-, intermediate-, or high-grade (according to how aggressively the disease behaves). Low-grade diseases usually progress slowly and tend not to spread beyond the lymphatic system. High-grade diseases may spread to distant organs within a few months.
- Signs and Symptoms
  - Painless swelling of one or more groups of lymph nodes
  - Enlargement of the liver and spleen
  - Fever
  - Abdominal pain
  - GI bleeding (in rare cases)
- Largely unknown, one form, Burkitt's lymphoma, is strongly associated with infection by Epstein-Barr virus, commonly found in Africa
- Other types have been linked to infection by HIV-type viruses and other conditions that affect the immune system (e.g., organ transplantation, radiation and chemotherapy, lupus, and rheumatoid arthritis)
- Management
  - Radiation therapy
  - Anticancer drugs
  - Sometimes, bone marrow transplantation

Polycythemia

- A rare disorder characterized by overabundant production of RBCs, WBCs, and platelets
- May be a natural response to hypoxia (secondary polycythemia) or may occur for unknown reasons (primary polycythemia)

Secondary Polycythemia

- In people who live in or visit areas of high altitude, may be naturally present because of reduced air pressure and low oxygen
  - When oxygen supply to the blood is reduced, kidneys produce the hormone erythropoietin, which stimulates RBC production in the bone marrow to compensate for the reduced oxygen supply.
  - The result is an increase in the oxygen-carrying efficiency of the blood.
  - Upon returning to sea level, the person's RBC numbers return to normal.

Primary Polycythemia (Polycythemia Vera)

- A rare disorder of the bone marrow in which the increased production of RBCs causes the blood to thicken.
- This condition primarily develops in people over 50 years of age and can lead to a number of physiological problems.
  - Headache
  - Dizziness
  - Blurred vision

  - Generalized itching
  - Red hands and feet; red-purple complexion
  - Hypertension
  - Splenomegaly
- Other complications that may be associated with primary polycythemia:
  - Platelet disorders (causing a tendency to bleed or to form clots)
  - Stroke
  - Development of other bone marrow diseases (e.g., leukemia)

Management

- May consist of phlebotomy (the slow removal of blood through a vein)
- Anticancer drug therapy to control the overproduction of RBCs in the marrow

Disseminated Intravascular Coagulopathy (DIC)

- A complication of severe injury, trauma, or disease
- A relatively common abnormal clotting disorder
- Most often seen in the critical care setting
- Disrupts the fine balance between procoagulants and inhibitors, thrombus formation, and lysis
- Those associated with hypotension and hypoperfusion
- Occurs in two phases
  - The first phase is characterized by free thrombin in the blood, fibrin deposits, and aggregation of platelets.
  - The second phase is characterized by hemorrhage caused by depletion of clotting factors.
- The clinical consequences of these processes predispose the patient to multiple-system organ failure from bleeding and coagulation disorders
- Causes
  - A loss of platelets and clotting factors
  - Fibrinolysis
  - Fibrin degradation interference
  - Small vessel obstruction, tissue ischemia, RBC injury, and anemia from fibrin deposits

Signs and Symptoms

- Dyspnea
- Bleeding

Management

- Once DIC is confirmed though laboratory tests, management is aimed at reversing the underlying illness or injury that triggered the event.
- To control the depletion of clotting factors, initial care may include the replacement of platelets, coagulation factors, and blood, while attempts are made to manage the primary process.

Hemophilia

- Hemophilia (meaning "love of blood") is an inherited bleeding disorder.
- Hemophilia A is caused by a deficiency of a particular blood protein called factor VIII, which is essential to the process of blood clotting.
- Hemophilia B is a less common form of hemophilia caused by a deficiency of factor IX.
  - Called "Christmas disease"—Named for a man first diagnosed with the disease in 1952.

- Clotting Factors
  - Fibrinogen
  - Prothrombin
  - Thromboplastin
  - Calcium
  - Proaccelerin
  - None in use
  - Serum prothrombin conversion accelerator (SPCA)
  - Antihemophilic globulin (AHG)
  - Antihemophilic factor (AHF)
  - Plasma thromboplastin component (PTC)
  - Christmas factor
  - Stuart factor
  - Plasma thromboplastin antecedent (PTA)
  - Hageman factor
  - Fibrin-stabilizing factor
- Bleeding from hemophilia may occur spontaneously, after even minor injury.
- Hemorrhage can occur anywhere in the body, but bleeding into joints, deep muscles, the urinary tract, and intracranial sites are the most common sites.
- Hemophilia is controlled by infusions of concentrates of factor VIII, which may be self-administered by the patient.
- Serious or unusual bleeding episodes, however, often require hospitalization.
- Hemophiliacs are cautioned to avoid activities that might expose them to increased risk of injury. Most hemophiliacs are knowledgeable about their disease and seek emergency care only for complicated problems and trauma-related difficulties.

Sickle Cell Disease

- Also known as sickle cell anemia. A debilitating and unpredictable recessive genetic illness that affects persons of African descent (and less commonly, persons of Mediterranean origin).
  - It is estimated that 1 in 12 African Americans suffers from sickle cell disease.
  - Another 1 in 12 African Americans has sickle cell trait.
- Pathophysiology:
  - Sickle cell anemia produces an abnormal type of hemoglobin called hemoglobin S, which has an inferior oxygen-carrying capacity.
  - The deficiency of oxygen causes hemoglobin S to crystallize, distorting the red blood cells into a sickle shape.
  - The sickle-shaped cells are fragile and easily destroyed.
    - — These cells also are unable to pass easily through tiny blood vessels, so they block flow to various organs and tissues, causing a vaso-occlusive sickle cell crisis (that can be life threatening).
    - — As fewer and fewer RBCs pass through congested vessels, tissues and joints become starved for oxygen and other nutrients, causing excruciating pain.
  - Sickle cell crisis:
    - — Can occur in any part of the body
    - — Can vary in intensity from person to person, and from one crisis to the next Over time, the crises can destroy the spleen, kidneys, gallbladder, and other organs
  - Sickle cell crisis may occur for no apparent reason or be triggered by certain conditions:
    - — Dehydration

— Infection
— Stress
— Trauma
— Exposure to extremes in temperature
— Lack of oxygen
— Strenuous physical activity

Signs and symptoms

- Episodes of severe pain ("crisis")
- Fatigue
- Pallor
- Delayed growth, development, and sexual maturation in children
- Priapism in adolescent and adult males
- Increased weakness
- Aching
- Chest pain
- Sudden, severe abdominal pain
- Bony deformities
- Icteric (jaundice) sclera
- Fever
- Arthralgia (joint pain)

Management

- At present, no cure exists for sickle cell disease.
- Because of the eventual damage that occurs to the spleen, these patients are at increased risk for septicemia if infected by certain types of bacteria.
- When in crisis, these patients require prompt management.
  - Oxygen
  - IV therapy to manage dehydration
  - Antibiotics to manage infection
  - Analgesics to manage pain
  - In severe cases, a blood transfusion may be indicated to effect a temporary replacement of hemoglobin S

Multiple Myeloma

- A malignant neoplasm of the bone marrow.
  - The tumor, composed of plasma cells, destroys bone tissue (especially in flat bones).
  - Causes pain, fractures, hypercalcemia, and skeletal deformities.
- In myeloma, the neoplastic cells produce large amounts of protein (M-protein) that affect the viscosity of the blood.
  - Masses of coagulated protein may accumulate within the patient's tissues and impair function.
  - Some patients with this disease die of kidney failure from the accumulation of proteins that infiltrate the kidneys and block the renal tubules.
- Other disorders associated with multiple myeloma:
  - Weakness
  - Skeletal pain

    - Hemorrhage
    - Hematuria
    - Lethargy
    - Weight loss
    - Frequent fractures
    - Proteinuria
    - Anemia
    - Pulmonary complications (secondary to rib fracture)
    - Recurrent infections from suppression of the immune system (from unknown factors secreted from the malignant plasma cells)
- Rare before the age of 40; occurrence increases with age.
- More common in men than in women and may have a heritable component.
- Multiple myeloma is diagnosed through x-ray, blood studies, and tumor biopsy.
- Treatment may consist of chemotherapy with anticancer drugs, radiation, plasma exchange, and bone marrow transplant.

General Assessment and Management of Patients with Hematologic Disorders

- Most patients with hematologic disorders are knowledgeable about their disease.
- Often, they will have summoned emergency medical service (EMS) to help manage a change in their condition or to arrange for transport to an emergency department for physician evaluation.
- Situations that may initiate a call for emergency care will vary by patient and disease.
- Common chief complaints can be classified by body system.
    - Central nervous system
        - Altered level of consciousness
        - Increased weakness
    - Integumentary system
        - Prolonged bleeding
        - Bruising
        - Itching
        - Pallor
        - Jaundice
    - Visual disturbances
    - Epistaxis
    - Gastrointestinal system
        - Bleeding or infected gums
        - Ulceration
        - Melena
        - Liver disease
        - Pain
    - Skeletal system
        - Bone or joint pain
        - Fracture
    - Cardiorespiratory system
        - Dyspnea
        - Chest pain

- Hemoptysis
- Tachycardia
- ◦ Genitourinary system
  - Hematuria
  - Amenorrhea
  - Infections

Emergency Management

- Often, emergency care will primarily be supportive.
- Ensure adequate airway, ventilatory, and circulatory support.
- Vital signs and a detailed physical examination will help determine the appropriateness of emergency transport. Calming measures and emotional support are particularly important, as some of these patients will be seriously ill.
- Other prehospital care measures:
  - ◦ IV fluid replacement
  - ◦ Use of antidysrhythmics
  - ◦ Administration of analgesics for pain management

CHAPTER QUESTIONS

1. Which organelle contains the genetic material of the cell?
   a. Mitochondria
   b. Nucleus
   c. Endoplasmic reticulum
   d. Ribosome's
2. The role of the mitochondria in cellular function is to produce ATP (energy).
   a. True
   b. False

Suggested Reading

US Department of Transportation, National Highway Traffic Safety Administration. *EMT-Paramedic: National Standard Curriculum*. Washington, DC: US Department of Transportation, National Highway Traffic Safety Administration; 1998.

Chapter 30
Infectious and Communicable Diseases

You suspect your 3-year-old conscious patient has meningitis. Examination reveals cool clammy skin, nonlabored respirations of 32/minute, pulse rate of 132, and blood pressure of 60/40. The patient has been complaining of a sore neck and you note on examination nuchal rigidity. Your management should include high flow oxygen and what other modalities?

- Infectious and communicable disease emergencies are common in the prehospital setting and can pose a significant health risk to the paramedic.
- Infectious disease refers to any illness caused by a specific microorganism.
- Communicable disease is an infectious disease that can be transmitted from one person to another.

PUBLIC HEALTH PRINCIPLES RELATIVE TO INFECTIOUS DISEASES

- Infectious (communicable) diseases affect entire populations of humans.
- It is important to consider the demographic characteristics of the population (location, age, socioeconomic considerations) and the relationships between populations when considering the dynamics of infectious diseases.
- Factors affecting the life cycle of an infectious agent include:
  - Population and ability to move internationally
  - Age distributions
  - Socioeconomic considerations
  - Population settling and migrating dictated by religion
  - Genetic factors
  - Efficacy of therapeutic interventions once infection has been established.
  - A disease cluster is a discrete population infected in a defined span of time in defined geographical areas. It is, by its nature, regional but may lead to an international infection.
  - When dealing with infectious disease, consider the needs of the patient, the potential, consequences on public health, and the patient's person-to-person contacts with family members and friends.
  - When a disease "outbreak" occurs, local, state, private, and federal health agencies and organizations become involved in prevention and management.

Private Sector

- Regional and national health-care providers.
- Laboratories (hospital and private).
- Local and national health maintenance organizations.
- Infection control/disease specialists.
  - Influences protocols and guidelines for dealing with disease surveillance/response to outbreaks
  - Local (municipal/city/county public health agencies)
    - — First line of defense in disease surveillance
    - — First line of defense in disease outbreaks

State Health Agencies

- Regulate and enforce federal guidelines
- Obliged by statute or law to meet or exceed federal guidelines and recommendations

Federal and National Organizations

- U.S. Congress—Plays a role in national health policy through public laws and drafting of the federal budget
- U.S. Department of Labor (OSHA rules and guidelines)
- U.S. Department of Health and Human Services (CDC, NIOSH guidelines)
- U.S. Department of Defense and Federal Emergency Management Agency (FEMA guidelines)
- National Fire Protection Association (NFPA standards), U.S. Fire Protection Administration (USFPA), and International Association of Firefighters (IAFF)

Agency Responsibility Relative to Infectious Agent Eposure

National concerns regarding communicable disease and infection control have resulted in the development of public law, standards, guidelines, and recommendations to protect health-care providers and emergency responders from infectious diseases.

Components of a Health-Care Agency Exposure Control Plan

Health Maintenance and Surveillance

- Appointment of a Designated Officer (DO) to serve as a liaison between the agency and community health agencies involved in monitoring/response to communicable diseases
- Identification of job classifications, and in some cases, specific tasks where the possibility exists for exposure to bloodborne pathogens
- Schedule of when and how the provisions of bloodborne pathogen standards will be implemented
- Personal protective equipment (PPE)
- Body substance isolation (BSI)
- Procedures for evaluating exposure and post exposure counseling (per Ryan White Act)
- Interfacing with and notification of local health authorities and state and federal agencies
- Vehicular and equipment disinfection

- Education for employees regarding disinfection agents
- After-action analysis of agency response
- Correct disposal of needles and sharps in appropriate containers
- Correct handling of body-fluid tinged linens and supplies used in patient care
- Identification of agency and/or contracted personnel for counseling, authorization of acute medical care, and documentation

Guidelines, Recommendations, Standards, and Laws

- OSHA requirements to protect against infection:
  - PPE available to all employees considered to be at high risk for exposure to infectious diseases
  - All employees offered preexposure prophylaxis to hepatitis by inoculation with hepatitis vaccines
- CDC and NFPA have established similar guidelines, recommendations, and standards regarding the protection of health-care workers and emergency providers from bloodborne pathogens, including regular testing for tuberculosis and vaccination for measles in nonimmune individuals.
- The Ryan White Comprehensive AIDS Resources Emergency Act of 1990 (PL 101-381) lists notification requirements for emergency responders, to be advised if they have been exposed to infectious diseases.
- Also requires that employers name a DO to coordinate communications between the hospital and emergency response organization in case of an exposure.
- Notification must occur as soon as practical but no later than 48 hours after determination of the disease has been made.

Body Substance Isolation

- In 1987, the CDC published recommendations for prevention of HIV transmission in health-care settings, which recommended body fluid precautions (Universal Precautions recommended by the CDC in 1983) be extended and consistently used for all patients regardless of their bloodborne infection status. Since then, the FDA has worked with the CDC to clarify application of universal precautions.
- Body fluids to which universal precautions apply:
  - Blood and other body fluids containing visible blood
  - Semen and vaginal secretions
  - Human tissue
  - Human fluids (CSF, synovial fluid, pleural fluid, peritoneal fluid, pericardial fluid, amniotic fluid)
- Body fluids to which universal precautions do not apply (in the absence of blood):
  - Feces
  - Nasal secretions
  - Sputum
  - Sweat
  - Tears
  - Urine
  - Vomitus
- Precautions for other body fluids in special settings:
  - Human breast milk in mothers infected with HBV
  - Saliva in some persons infected with HBV or HIV
- BSI is based upon the premise that all exposures to body fluids, under any circumstances, are potentially infectious.

PATHOPHYSIOLOGY OF INFECTIOUS DISEASE

- Infectious (communicable) disease ranks as the fifth most common cause of death in the United States.
- The manifestation of clinical disease is dependent on several factors:
  - Virulence (degree of pathogenicity)
  - Number of infectious agents (dose)
  - Resistance (immune status) of the host
  - Correct mode of entry
- All of these factors rely on an intact "chain of elements" necessary to produce an infectious disease.
  - The pathogenic agent
  - A reservoir
  - A portal of exit from the reservoir
  - An environment conducive to transmission of the pathogenic agent
  - A portal of entry into the new host
  - Susceptibility of the new host to the infectious disease
  - Exposure, even in the presence of all necessary elements, does not mean a person will become infected with the disease

Pathogenic Agent

- Organisms that can create pathological processes in the human host.
- Some pathogens (such as certain bacteria) are metabolically equipped so that they can survive outside a host, whereas others (such as viruses) can survive only in the human cell.

Infectious Agents and Their Properties

- Most bacteria are susceptible to certain drugs (antibiotics) that kill them or inhibit their growth.
- Viruses, however, are more difficult to treat because they reside in cells for most of their life cycle and become intricately enmeshed in the host cell's deoxyribonucleic acid (DNA).
- Factors affecting any pathogen's ability to create a pathological process:
  - Ability to invade and reproduce within a host and the mode in which it does so
  - Speed of reproduction, ability to produce a toxin, and the extent of tissue damage that it causes
  - Potency
  - Ability to induce an immune response in the host

Bacteria

- Procaryotic (nuclear material not contained within a distinctive envelope)
- Self-reproducing without a host cell
- Signs and symptoms depend on the cells and tissues affected
- Produce toxins (often more lethal than the bacterium itself)
  - Endotoxins (chemicals, usually proteins, that are integral parts of a bacterium's outer membrane and steadily shed from living bacteria)
  - Exotoxins (proteins released by bacteria that can cause disease symptoms by acting as neurotoxins or enterotoxins)
- Lysis of bacteria may release endotoxins
- Can cause localized or systemic infection

Viruses

- Eukaryotic (nuclear material contained within a distinct envelope)
- Must invade host cells to reproduce
- Cannot survive outside a host cell
- May contain other microorganisms

Fungi

- Has protective capsules that surround the cell wall to protect the fungi from phagocytes

Protozoa

- Single-celled microorganisms
- More complex than bacteria
- Helminths (worms, including tapeworms, roundworms)
- Pathogenic parasites
- Not necessarily microorganisms

Reservoir

- The environment (reservoir) in which a pathogen lives and reproduces may be a human or other animal host, an arthropod, a plant, soil, water, food, or some other organic substance, or a combination of these reservoirs.
- When infected, the human host may exhibit signs of clinical illness or be an asymptomatic carrier, transmitting the pathogen to others.
- The life cycle of the infectious agent depends on several factors:
  - The demographics of the host
  - Genetic factors
  - The efficacy of therapeutic interventions once infection has been established

Portal of Exit

- The mechanism or method by which a pathogenic agent leaves one host to invade another involves a "portal of exit."
- The portal of exit from the human host depends on the agent and may be single or multiple. They include:
  - Genitourinary (GU) tract
  - Intestinal tract
  - Oral cavity
  - Respiratory tract
  - Open lesion
  - Any wound through which blood escapes
- The period in which an actively infectious pathogen can escape to produce disease in another organism coincides with the period of communicability, which varies with each disease.

Transmission

- Determined by the portal of exit, which may be direct or indirect.
- Direct transmission—Occurs when there is physical contact between the source and the victim. Examples include:
  - Oral transmission
  - Transmission by airborne mucus droplets

- ◦ Transmission by fecal contamination
- ◦ Transmission by sexual contact
- Indirect transmission—The organism survives on animate or inanimate objects for a period without a human host. Diseases can be indirectly transmitted by air, food, water, soil, or biological matter.

Portal of Entry

- Refers to the means by which the pathogenic agent enters a new host.
- Entry may be by ingestion, inhalation, percutaneous injection, crossing of a mucous membrane, or crossing of the placenta.
- The duration of exposure to the pathogen and the number of organisms required to initiate the infectious process vary with the disease and host susceptibility. Exposure to an infectious agent does not always produce infection.

Host Susceptibility

- Host susceptibility is influenced by a person's immune response, and by several other factors:
  - Human characteristics
    - — Age
    - — Gender
    - — Ethnic group
    - — Heredity
    - — General health status
    - — Nutrition
    - — Hormonal balance
    - — Presence of concurrent disease
    - — History of previous disease
    - — Immune status
    - — Prior exposure to disease (conferring resistance)
    - — Effective immunization against disease (conferring host immunity)
  - Geographical and environmental conditions
  - Cultural behaviors
  - Eating habits
  - Personal hygiene
  - Sexual behaviors

PHYSIOLOGY OF THE HUMAN RESPONSE TO INFECTION

- The human body is constantly exposed to pathogens capable of producing illness; yet most people do not succumb to infectious disease. This protection is provided by external and internal barriers that serve as lines of defense against infection.

External Barriers

- The first line of defense against infection is the surface of the body exposed to the environment. This surface, inhabited by an indigenous flora (agents that could produce disease if allowed access to the interior of the body), includes the skin and the mucous membranes of the digestive, respiratory, and GU tract that forms a continuous closed barrier between the internal organs and the environment.

- Flora—Normal microbial floras inhabit nearly the whole body surface. Indigenous flora competes with pathogens for space and nutrients and maintains a pH optimal for their own growth, which can be incompatible with what is needed for many pathogens to survive.
- Some floras also secrete germicidal substances and are thought to stimulate the immune system.
- Although resident (normal) flora play an important role in defense, some can be pathogenic under certain conditions and can be responsible for infection when the skin or mucous membranes are interrupted or when flora is displaced from their natural habitat to another area of the body.

Skin

- Intact skin defends against infection by preventing penetration and by maintaining an acidic pH that inhibits growth of pathogenic bacteria.
- Microbes are also sloughed from the skin surface with dead skin cells, and oil and sweat wash microorganisms from the skin's pores.

Gastrointestinal (GI) System

- Resident bacterial flora in the GI system provide competition between colonies of microorganisms for nutrients and space and help to prevent proliferation of pathogenic organisms.
- Stomach acid may destroy some microorganisms or deactivate their toxic products.
- The digestive system also eliminates pathogens through feces.

Upper Respiratory Tract

- The sticky membranes of the upper respiratory tract protect against pathogens by trapping large particles, which may be swallowed or expelled by coughing or sneezing.
- Coarse nasal hairs and cilia also trap and filter foreign substances in inspired air, preventing pathogens from reaching the lower respiratory tract.
- Lymph tissues of the tonsils and adenoids also permit a rapid local immunological response to pathogens that may enter the respiratory tract.

Genitourinary Tract

- The natural process of urination and the bacteriostatic properties of urine help prevent the establishment of microorganisms in the GU tract.
- Antibacterial substances in prostatic fluid and the presence of vaginal flora also help to prevent GU system infection.

Internal Barriers

- Protect against pathogenic agents when the external lines of defense are breached. Internal barriers include the inflammatory response and the immune response, which share many of the same processes and cellular components.

Inflammatory Response

- Inflammation (a local reaction to cellular injury).
- May be initiated by microbial infection.
- When invasion occurs, this line of defense is activated to prevent further invasion of the pathogen by isolating, destroying, or neutralizing the microorganism.

- The inflammatory response is generally protective and beneficial but may initiate destruction of the body's own tissue if the response is sustained or directed toward the host's own antigens.
- The inflammatory response may be divided into three separate stages—Cellular response to injury, vascular response to injury, and phagocytosis.

Cellular response to injury

- Metabolic changes occur with any type of cell injury.
- The most common primary effect on the cell's aerobic respiration and oxidative phosphorylation leads to decreased energy reserves.
- Sodium-potassium pump can no longer function effectively, and the cell swells from the accumulation of sodium ions.
- Swelling, along with increased acidosis, leads to further impairment of enzyme function and further deterioration in the integrity of the membranes.
- Eventually, the membranes of the cellular organelles begin to leak, and release of hydrolytic enzymes by the lysosomes contributes further to cellular destruction and autolysis.
- As the cellular contents are dissolved by enzymes, the inflammatory response is stimulated in surrounding tissues.

Vascular response to injury

- After cellular injury, localized hyperemia develops as the surrounding arterioles, venules, and capillaries dilate.
- The associated increase in filtration pressure and capillary permeability causes fluid to leak from the vessels into the interstitial space, producing edema.
- Leukocytes (particularly neutrophils and monocytes) begin to collect along the vascular endothelium, and as a result of release of chemotactic factors, eventually migrate to injured tissue.

Phagocytosis

- The process by which leukocytes engulf, digest, and destroy pathogens.
- Circulating macrophages are also responsible for clearing the injured area of dead cells and other debris.
- Intracellular phagocytosis (ingestion of bacteria and dead cell fragments) occurs at the site of tissue invasion and may extend into the general circulation if the infection becomes systemic—stimulating the release of chemicals that induce lysis of the leukocytes.

Immune Response

- The first two lines of defense against infection respond to all infectious agents—using the identical nonspecific mechanism—but the immune response is specific to individual pathogens.

Characteristics of the Immune System

- Possesses "self-nonself" recognition and therefore normally responds only to foreign antigens.
- Produces antibodies that are antigen-specific and can produce new antibodies in response to new antigens.
- Some of the antibody-producing lymphocytes become "memory cells" that allow a more rapid response to subsequent invasions by the same antigen.

- Self-regulated to activate only when there is an invading pathogen.
- Ability to activate or deactivate the immune response prevents the destruction of healthy tissues.
- When this regulatory function goes awry, autoimmune disease (rheumatoid arthritis, active glomerulonephritis, and systemic lupus erythematosus) can occur.
- May require extrinsic regulation with certain medications in patients with transplanted organs or severe autoimmune diseases.
- The immunological response to an invading pathogen depends somewhat on the size and antigenic properties of the pathogen.
- Often, peripheral phagocytic cells encounter a pathogen first, but circulating B and T lymphocytes also play a reconnaissance role.
- The B lymphocyte's role is to produce antibody (humoral immunity), which coats the pathogen and makes phagocytosis easier.
- Antibody can also fix complement, a protein cascade that often results in the death of the organism and in the production of chemotactic factors.
- The T lymphocyte not only processes antigen for the B lymphocyte but also has a subpopulation of "killer cells," which are a major component of cell-mediated immunity.
- Sensitized T cells develop into distinct subsets, each with a specific set of functions that coordinate the activity of other components of the immune system.
- Killer T cells (like B cells) are sensitized and stimulated to multiply by the presence of antigens present on abnormal body cells.
- Unlike B cells, killer T cells do not produce antibodies
- Helper T cells "turn on" the activities of killer (cytotoxic) cells and control other aspects of the immune response.
- Suppressor T cells "turn off" the action of the helper and killer T cells, preventing them from causing harmful immune reactions.
- Inflammatory T cells stimulate allergic reactions, anaphylaxis, and autoimmune reactions.

The Reticuloendothelial System (RES)

- Works with the lymphatic system to dispose of debris that results from the immune system's attack on invading organisms.
- The RES is composed of immune cells in the spleen, lymph nodes, liver, bone marrow, lungs, and intestines.
- These structures serve as sites where mature B and T cells are stored until the immune system is activated.

STAGES OF INFECTIOUS DISEASE (TABLE 30-1)

- The progression from exposure to an infectious agent to the onset of clinical disease follows specific stages.
- The duration of each stage and the potential outcomes vary, depending on the infectious agent and individual host factors.

Latent Period

- Begins with pathogenic invasion of the body and ends when the agent can be "shed" or communicated. During the latent period, the infectious agent cannot be transmitted to another host or cause clinically significant symptoms.

TABLE 30-1: Stages of Infectious Disease

Stage of Disease	Begins	Ends
Latent period	With invasion	When the agent can be shed
Incubation period	With invasion	When the disease process begins
Communicability period	When the latent period ends	Continues as long as the agent is present and can spread to others
Disease period	Follows incubation period	Of variable duration

Incubation Period

- Period during which the organism reproduces. Begins with invasion of the agent and ends when the disease process begins.
- The interval between exposure to an infectious agent and the first appearance of symptoms associated with the infection.

Communicability Period

- Begins when the latent period ends and continues as long as the agent is present and can spread to other hosts.
- Clinically significant symptoms from the infection may manifest during this period.
- This stage is variable and is often the major determining factor in ease of transmission.
- The communicable period and the method of transmission can be altered in some diseases (tuberculosis, syphilis, gonorrhea), depending on the stage of the disease and the primary site of infection.

Disease Period

- Follows the incubation period and is of variable disease-specific duration.
- This stage may be subclinical or produce overt symptoms, which can arise directly from the invading organism or from the host's physiological responses.
- During this period, the pathological process may resolve completely, or the organism may become incorporated and dormant inside certain cells.
- The infection is then considered to be in a latent stage.
- A number of viruses, including HIV and hepatitis, can lead to latent infection.

HIV

- HIV is present in blood and serum-derived body fluids (semen, vaginal, or cervical secretions) in individuals infected with the virus.
- The disease is directly transmitted person-to-person by several routes:
  - Through anal or vaginal intercourse
  - Across the placenta
  - By contact with infected blood or body fluids on mucous membranes or open wounds
- HIV may be indirectly transmitted by several methods:
  - Transfusion with contaminated blood or blood products
  - Transplanted tissues and organs
  - Use of contaminated needles or syringes

- Occurrence is highest in persons with certain risk factors.
  - High-risk sexual behavior
  - IV drug abuse
  - Transfusion recipient between 1978 and 1985
  - Hemophilia or other coagulation disorders requiring blood products
  - Infant born of HIV-positive mother
- Other factors that may affect susceptibility to HIV include coexisting sexually transmitted diseases (especially with ulceration) and penile foreskin.
- Race and gender do not appear to be risk factors for the disease.

Pathophysiology

- HIV results from one of two retroviruses—A group of viruses that convert genetic ribonucleic acid (RNA) to DNA after entering the host cell (referred to as HIV-1 and HIV-2).
- Once inside the cell, the cell's genetic material is altered into a hybrid that is part virus, part cell. The virus essentially commandeers the cell's machinery to make more virus particles.
- When sufficient quantities of the virus are produced, the host cell ruptures, destroying the cell and releasing the virus into the blood to seek new target cells.
- The cell receptor sought by HIV is called CD4+ T lymphocyte (a type of lymphocyte used to diagnose AIDS).
- It is found on the surface of T-4 lymphocytes (T helper cells, T-4 cells), certain nerve cells, and monocytes and macrophages that probably carry the virus to other parts of the body.
- Even though the body develops antigen-specific antibodies to HIV, they are not protective.
- Secondary complications are generally related to opportunistic infections that arise as the immune system deteriorates.
  - Pulmonary tuberculosis
  - Recurrent pneumonia
  - *Pneumocystis carinii* pneumonia
  - Kaposi's sarcoma
  - Wasting syndrome
  - HIV dementia
  - Sensory neuropathy
  - Toxoplasmosis of the central nervous system (CNS)

Classification and Categories

- The average time from HIV transmission to serious complications in the absence of treatment is about 10 years, although there is considerable variation.
- HIV can be categorized by CD4+ T cell counts.
- Category 1—Greater than or equal to 500 cells per mL.
- Category 2—200–499 per microliter (FL).
- Category 3—Less than 200 per FL.
- After viral transmission of HIV (which occurs almost always through sexual intercourse or exposure to contaminated blood), the progression of the disease in adolescents and adults can be divided into three clinical categories.

Category A

- Acute retroviral infection
- This syndrome generally occurs 2–4 weeks after exposure
- Clinical features are those of an infectious mononucleosis-like illness with fever, adenopathy, and sore throat
- The febrile illness is self-limited, usually lasting 1–2 weeks
- During this stage, there is a transient decrease in CD4+ T cell counts

Seroconversion

- The serological response with antigen-specific antibodies to HIV generally takes place between 6 and 12 weeks after transmission
- Accompanied by a return of CD4+ T lymphocyte counts to normal levels
- Asymptomatic infection
- The person with HIV infection may have persistent generalized lymphadenopathy (enlarged lymph nodes involving two noncontiguous sites other than inguinal nodes) and a gradual decline in the CD4+ T lymphocyte count

Category B

- Early symptomatic HIV infection
- Usual CD4+ T-cell count in this group is 100–300 per FL
- Common complications at this stage include localized *Candida* infections (thrush, *Candida esophagitis*, *Candida vaginitis*), oral lesions, shingles, pelvic inflammatory disease, peripheral neuropathy, and constitutional symptoms such as fever or diarrhea lasting more than 1 month

Category C

- Late symptomatic HIV infection
- Represents all AIDS-defining diagnoses found primarily with CD4+ T-lymphocyte counts of 0–200 per FL, including severe opportunistic infections; bacterial pneumonia (*Pneumocystis carinii* pneumonia); pulmonary tuberculosis; debilitating diarrhea; tumors in any body system, including Kaposi's sarcoma; HIV-associated dementia; and neurological manifestations

Advanced HIV Infection

- Applies to individuals with CD4+ T-lymphocyte counts of 0–50 per FL.
- This group of patients has a limited life expectancy, and most die from AIDS-related complications.

Personal Protection

- Strict compliance with universal precautions is the only known prophylactic measure that health-care workers can take to protect themselves against HIV infection. The chance of emergency medical service (EMS) personnel acquiring this disease by exposure to infected blood appears to be low (0.2–0.44%).
- HBV poses a much greater occupational hazard.
- Factors that increase the risk to health-care workers include exposure involving a large quantity of blood—when a device is visibly contaminated with blood; when care of the patient involves placing a needle in a vein or artery; and in deep injuries. Needle size and type (hollow bore vs. suture) and depth of penetration influence volume transferred to skin of a health-care worker.
- Exposure that involves a source patient with a terminal illness, possibly reflecting a higher dose of HIV in the late course of AIDS.

Post Exposure Prophylaxis

- If a known or possible exposure occurs, immediately notify the Designated Officer (per protocol) so that elective postexposure prophylaxis (PEP) can begin.
- Information about primary HIV infection indicates that systemic infection does not occur immediately, leaving a brief "window of opportunity" during which postexposure antiretroviral intervention may modify viral replication.
- Several antiretroviral agents from at least three classes of drugs are available for the treatment of HIV disease.
  - Nucleoside analogue reverse transcriptase inhibitors (NRTIs)
  - Nonnuceloside reverse transcriptase inhibitors (NNRTIs)
  - Protease inhibitors (PIs)
- Among these drugs, ZDV (an NRTI) is the only agent shown to prevent HIV transmission in humans.
- Following PEP, testing for HIV is again performed 2–3 weeks after the exposure and again at 6 weeks, 3 months, 6 months, and 1 year.

Psychological Reactions to HIV Infection

- HIV infection is almost invariably a progressive disease with morbid late consequences.
- During the infection, HIV-infected persons are likely to feel and express anger about many aspects of their illness, including pain, dying prematurely and without dignity, and the social rejection and prejudice that they may experience.
- An important aspect of patient care is to help these patients feel that they can obtain acceptance and compassion from health-care workers.
- Although no immunization exists for HIV infection, new developments in treatment are evolving rapidly.
- Despite current limitations, progression of the illness can be delayed with drug therapy and other strategies, permitting access to new therapeutic options in the future.

HEPATITIS

- Hepatitis is a viral disease that produces pathological alterations in the liver.
- The three main classes of hepatitis viruses are hepatitis A (HAV), or viral hepatitis; hepatitis B (HBV), or serum hepatitis; and hepatitis C (HCV), or non-A/non-B hepatitis.
- Hepatitis non-ABC is a fourth class of hepatitis caused by infection from the hepatitis D virus and the newer hepatitis viruses (E and G).
- The routes of transmission of these viruses are similar to those for HBV and often are mistaken for HBV infection.

Hepatitis Facts

Hepatitis A Virus

- HAV is the most common type of viral hepatitis in the United States.
- Acquired by the ingestion of HAV-contaminated food or drink or by the fecal-oral route. The virus localizes in the liver, reproduces, enters the bile, and is carried to the intestinal tract, where it is shed in the feces.
- Fecal shedding usually occurs before the onset of clinical symptoms.
- Antibodies (anti-HAV) develop during acute disease and later during convalescence.
- Once infected with the virus, the person is immune to HAV for life.

- HAV is the only hepatitis virus that does not lead to chronic liver disease or a chronic carrier state.
- Many HAV infections are subclinical and often present with influenza-like symptoms. About 1 in 100 patients with HAV suffer from a fulminant infection that may require a liver transplant.
- Immune globulin (IG) can provide a temporary immunity to the virus for 2–3 months if given before exposure to HAV or within 2 weeks after contact.
- Hepatitis A vaccines have been approved for persons 2 years of age and older who meet certain criteria:
  - Persons who have close physical contact with people who live in areas with poor sanitary conditions, or who are traveling or working in developing countries
  - Men who have sex with other men
  - Users of illicit drugs
  - Children in populations that have repeated epidemics of hepatitis A (Alaskan Natives, American Indians, Pacific Islanders, and certain closed religious communities)
  - Persons who have chronic liver disease or clotting factor disorders
- Each year an estimated 180,000 HAV infections occur in the United States.
- Hepatitis A is the cause of 30 days of missed work and about $2600 in lost wages each year per case.
- Medical care alone for hepatitis A can cost $2800 for each hospitalized case.
- About 100 Americans die each year from hepatitis A.
- The annual cost associated with hepatitis A is estimated at $200 million in the United States.

Hepatitis B Virus

- Infectious HBV particles are found in blood, in secretions containing serum (oozing, cutaneous lesions), and in secretions derived from serum (saliva, semen, vaginal secretions).
- Like other viral types of hepatitis, HBV affects the liver and causes similar signs and symptoms.
- May produce chronic infection that can lead to cirrhosis and other complications.
- Other complications associated with HBV include coagulation defects, impaired protein production, impaired bilirubin elimination, pancreatitis, and hepatic cancer.
- Exposure generally occurs in one of five ways.
  - Direct percutaneous inoculation of infectious serum or plasma by needle or transfusion of infected blood or blood products
  - Indirect percutaneous introduction of infective serum or plasma through skin cuts or abrasions, tattoo/body piercing, etc.
  - Absorption of infective serum or plasma through mucosal surfaces (such as those of the eyes or mouth), across the placenta, or through contamination from the mother's infective blood at birth
  - Absorption of infective secretions (such as saliva or semen) through mucosal surfaces, as might occur during vaginal, anal, or oral sexual contact, but never by fecal transmission
  - Transfer of infective serum or plasma via inanimate environmental surfaces
- The exposure risk for health-care providers to HBV-positive patients is estimated to be between 2 and 40%, making HBV a serious concern to all health-care workers.
- Blood is the most important potential source of HBV in the workplace.
- Risk of infection is directly proportional to certain factors.
  - Probability that the blood contains hepatitis B virus
  - Immunity status of the recipient

- An estimated 200,000 Americans are infected with HBV each year.
- About 12 million Americans are chronically infected with hepatitis B.
- Approximately 70% of new cases occur among people between the ages of 15 and 39.
- Every year 5000 Americans die from cirrhosis and 1000 die from liver cancer caused by HBV infections.
- HBV affects 22,000 pregnant women in the United States who can transmit it to their newborns.
- HBV can live on a dry surface for at least 7 days.
- Hepatitis B vaccine can provide immunity in over 95% of young healthy adults.
- HBV is 100 times more infectious than HIV.

Hepatitis C Virus

- HCV is a bloodborne virus that causes a disease similar to HBV.
- The virus was associated with receipt of contaminated blood during transfusion before 1992 (accounting for more than 90% of posttransfusion hepatitis in the United States).
- It is estimated that about 4 million Americans are infected with the virus.
- Of health-care workers who become infected, 85% become chronic carriers.
- About one-half to two-thirds of those infected with HCV develop chronic hepatitis; one in five suffers severe liver disease such as cirrhosis and liver cancer.
- There is no available HCV vaccine.
- Transmission of HCV occurs in the same manner as other forms of hepatitis, but the virus is not easily spread through sexual contact.
- Signs and symptoms of the disease, when they occur, are similar to those of other types of hepatitis.
- The majority of persons infected with HCV are asymptomatic.
- About 36,000 Americans contract HCV each year.
- An estimated 3.9 million Americans, nearly 2% of the population, are chronically infected with HCV.
- An estimated 300,000 Americans contracted HCV from blood transfusions given before 1992.
- More than 80% of patients infected with HCV will remain chronically infected.
- Each year, 8000–10,000 people in the United States die of HCV-related cirrhosis or liver cancer.
- Almost one-third of all liver transplants are performed for HCV-related chronic liver disease.
- A conservative estimate of the cost of HCV infections and related chronic liver disease is about $600 million per year.

Efficacy of transmission

- HBV vaccination is available to provide protection for 18 years in those who respond to the inoculation.
- Generally requires three IM (deltoid) doses over 6 months.
- For optimal protection against HBV infection, the vaccination series should be completed before an exposure occurs.
- HBV vaccinations currently available include Recombivax HB and Engerix-B.
- Postexposure prophylaxis.
- May be indicated if a nonvaccinated person or an individual who has not completed the vaccination schedule is exposed to HBV.

- Before treatment, a blood test is usually performed to determine immunity to HBV.
- If the candidate is seronegative, he or she generally receives the HBV vaccine and hepatitis B immune globulin, an antibody used in postexposure patients to provide passive immunity to HBV.

Signs and Symptoms

- Infection with any of the causative viruses may be symptomless or may cause a typical hepatitis with an abrupt onset of flulike illness followed by jaundice, dark urine, or both.
- Within 2–3 months after infection, the patient will generally develop nonspecific symptoms such as anorexia, nausea and vomiting, fever, joint pain, and generalized rashes.
- About 1% of patients hospitalized with HBV develop full-blown liver crisis and die.

Patient Management and Protective Measures

- Out-of-hospital care primarily is supportive for maintenance of circulatory status and prevention of shock.
- All health-care workers involved in the patient's care must observe personal protective measures, including effective hand washing and proper care in the use of diagnostic and therapeutic equipment (high-level disinfection of laryngoscope blades and the appropriate disposal of sharps).

TUBERCULOSIS

- About 8 million new cases of tuberculosis (TB) occur each year in the world, and 3 million people die of the disease. Although reports of TB in the United States declined continually after the turn of the century, this trend reversed in 1985.
- The rate of TB for patients with HIV is 40 times the rate for people who are not HIV-infected.

Pathophysiology

- TB is a chronic pulmonary disease acquired by inhalation of a dried-droplet nucleus containing tubercle bacilli (*Mycobacterium tuberculosis*, *M. bovis*, or a variety of atypical mycobacteria).
- Infection is transmitted primarily from infected persons who are coughing or sneezing the bacteria into the air or from contact with sputum that contains virulent TB bacilli.
- The pathology of TB is related to the production of inflammatory lesions throughout the body and to the ability of the TB bacillus to break through the body's natural defenses leading to the formation of caseating granulomas (necrotic inflammatory cells) and TB cavities, which may cause chronic and debilitating lung disease.
- Susceptibility to mycobacterial infection generally is highest in children under 3 years of age, in adults older than 65, and in chronically ill, malnourished, and immunosuppressed or immunocompromised individuals.
- The infection may remain dormant for an indefinite length of time (often not causing disease) or may lead to active disease that is contagious.
- TB is characterized by stages of early infection (frequently asymptomatic), latency, and a potential for recurrent postprimary disease.
- Signs and symptoms include cough, fever, night sweats, weight loss, fatigue, and hemoptysis.

- Associated complications by organ system:
  - Cardiovascular
    - Pericardial effusions
  - Lymphadenopathy (cervical lymph nodes usually involved)
  - Skeletal
    - Intervertebral disk deterioration
    - Chronic arthritis of one joint is common
  - CNS
    - Subacute meningitis
    - Brain granulomas
- Systemic miliary TB (extensive dissemination by the blood stream of tubercle bacilli)

TB Testing

- Although signs and symptoms of initial infection may be minimal, early infection can be detected with the Mantoux tuberculin skin test (purified protein derivative [PPD]).
- A positive reaction to PPD test indicates past infection and the presence of antibodies.
- Patients who test positive generally will have a chest x-ray examination and an acid-fast bacilli (AFB) sputum culture obtained before management.
- All persons with TB infection should be offered counseling and HIV-antibody testing, because medical management may be altered in the presence of HIV infection.
- TB reporting is required by law in every state.

Patient Care and Protective Measures

- Prehospital care for patients with infectious TB primarily is supportive.
- As with any other infectious disease, universal precautions (including respiratory barriers for patient and paramedic) should be taken during the patient care encounter.
- Paramedics should be alert to those populations that have significant prevalence of active TB in their jurisdictions (as reported by local public health authorities) and use particulate filter respirators approved by the National Institute of Occupational Safety and Health (NIOSH).
- Other methods that may help prevent exposure to droplet nuclei during patent transport:
  - Enhancing ventilation by opening windows on both sides of the ambulance
  - Operating the vehicle's air-conditioning system on a non-recirculating cycle
  - Placing a mask on the patient

Management of TB

- TB is usually curable if effective management is instituted without delay.
- Because of the increase in multidrug-resistant TB, most persons with TB are started on a lengthy four-drug regimen of isoniazid (INH), rifampin (RIF), pyrazinamide (PZA), and ethambutol (EMB) or streptomycin (SM) until the drug susceptibility results are known.
- Patients given preventive therapy should be monitored for drug side effects, especially signs and symptoms of hepatitis.

- Positive-to-negative sputum conversion and results of culture are usually available within 3–8 weeks after initiation of therapy.
- Prophylactic INH.
  - Recommended routinely for persons less than 35 years of age who are PPD skin-test positive.
  - Not routinely recommended for persons younger than 35 years old because of hepatic complications, except under certain circumstances.
    - — Recent infection as evidenced by PPD skin test conversion
    - — Close or household contact with a known case of infectious TB
    - — Abnormal chest x-ray examination
    - — Prolonged therapy with immunosuppressant drugs
    - — HIV or other immunosuppressive disease
  - Patients receiving INH should avoid alcohol.
  - Side effects include paresthesias, seizures (toxic reaction), orthostatic hypotension, nausea and vomiting, hepatitis, and hypersensitivity to the drug.

MENINGOCOCCAL MENINGITIS

- Meningococcal meningitis (also known as spinal meningitis) refers to inflammation of the membranes that surround the spinal cord and brain.
- Can be caused by a variety of different bacteria, viruses, and other microorganisms. A major cause of bacterial meningitis is *Neisseria meningitidis*, which, like *M. tuberculosis*, is spread by airborne pathogens.
- The usual mode of transmission is prolonged, direct contact with upper respiratory secretions (discharge from the nose and throat) from an infected person or carrier. Once inhaled, the bacteria invade the respiratory passages and travel by way of blood to the brain and spinal cord. As the infecting agent spreads to additional organs, it causes toxic manifestations in the involved organ system.

Other Infectious Agents Known to Cause Meningitis

Other common pathogens that cause meningitis include *Streptococcus pneumoniae* and *Haemophilus influenzae* type b (Hib), and some viruses.

S. Pneumoniae

- Second most common cause of bacterial meningitis in adults
- Most common cause of pneumonia in adults
- Most common cause of otitis media (middle ear infection) in children
- Spread by droplets, prolonged personal contact, or contact with linen soiled with respiratory discharges
- Episodic contact rarely results in infection

H. Influenzae

- Same mode of transmission as *N. meningitidis.*
- Before the introduction of vaccines for children in 1981, *H. influenzae* was the leading cause of bacterial meningitis in children aged 6 months to 3 years.
- Also implicated in conditions such as pediatric epiglottitis, septic arthritis, and generalized sepsis.
- Although bacterial meningitis can be treated effectively with antibiotics, 50% of all infected children with the disease specific to *H. influenzae* will have long-term neurological sequelae.

Viral Meningitis (Aseptic Meningitis)

- A syndrome generally associated with an existing systemic viral disease (mumps).
- Toxic and meningeal symptoms are similar to those of bacterial meningitis but are usually less severe.
- In most cases, viral meningitis is self-limited with complete recovery.
- The patient may experience muscle weakness and malaise during prolonged convalescence.
- Viral meningitis is not considered communicable.

Signs and Symptoms

- In infants, signs of meningeal irritation may be absent or include only irritability, poor feeding or vomiting, a high-pitched cry, and fullness of the fontanelle. Maternal antibodies protect neonates to 6 months of age.
- In older infants and children, signs of meningitis may include the presence of malaise, low-grade fever, projectile vomiting, petechial rash, headache, and stiff neck from meningeal irritation (nuchal rigidity).
- Diagnostic signs of meningitis in older children:
  - Brudzinski's sign—Involuntary flexion of the arm, hip, and knee when the neck is passively flexed.
  - Kerning's sign—Loss of the ability of a seated or supine patient to completely extend the leg when the thigh is flexed on the abdomen.
    - The patient, however, can usually extend the leg completely when the thigh is not flexed on the abdomen.
- Extensive meningeal involvement in a toxic or debilitated patient may be accompanied by acute adrenal insufficiency, convulsions, coma, and disseminated intravascular coagulation (Waterhouse-Friderichsen syndrome), associated with hemorrhage into the adrenal glands causing adrenal insufficiency. Death can ensue in 6–8 hours.
- Other conditions and long-term complications associated with severe cases of meningitis include blindness and deafness (from cranial nerve damage), arthritis, myocarditis, and pericarditis. Death can follow overwhelming infection.

Immunization and Control Measures

- Vaccines against Hib and some strains of *N. meningitidis* and many types of *S. pneumoniae* are available.
- The vaccines against Hib are very safe and highly effective.
- By 6 months of age, most infants will have received at least three doses of an Hib vaccine; a fourth dose ("booster") is recommended between 12 and 18 months of age.
- Vaccine against some strains of *N. meningitidis* is not routinely used in the United States, and is not effective in children under 18 months of age.
- The vaccine is sometimes used to control outbreaks of some types of meningococcal meningitis.
- Vaccines to prevent meningitis due to *S. pneumoniae* can prevent other forms of infection caused by the bacterium.
- This vaccine is not effective in children under 2 years of age but is recommended for all persons over age 65 (and younger persons with certain chronic medical problems).

Patient Management and Protective Measures

- Patient management will be primarily supportive—ensuring adequate airway, ventilatory, and circulatory support.

- Use protective measures when caring for patients who have signs and symptoms suggesting meningitis.
- The use of universal and BSI precautions (with surgical masks applied to the patient) are indicated during care and transport.
- Post-EMS exposure activities should be addressed as part of an agency Exposure Control Plan.
- Early diagnosis and management of bacterial meningitis are very important.
- Diagnosis is usually confirmed by identifying the type of bacteria responsible from a sample of spinal fluid obtained through a spinal tap (lumbar puncture).
- The disease is then managed with a number of effective antibiotics.
- Effective prophylactic drug treatments for those who may have intimate contact with the patient (e.g., family members) also are available.

PNEUMONIA

- Pneumonia is an acute inflammatory process of the respiratory bronchioles and alveoli.
- Routes of transmission include droplet spread and direct and indirect contact with respiratory secretions.
- Etiological agents responsible for this disease may be bacterial *(S. pneumoniae, M. pneumoniae, S. aureus, H. influenzae, Klebsiella pneumoniae, Moraxella catarrhalis, Legionella*), viral, or fungal.
- These organisms may affect several body systems, including the respiratory system (pneumonia); the CNS (meningitis); and the ears, nose, and throat (otitis, pharyngitis media).

Signs and Symptoms

- Sudden onset of chills, high-grade fever, chest pain with respirations, dyspnea
- Tachypnea and chest retractions (an ominous sign in children)
- Congestion from the development of purulent alveolar exudates in one or more lobes
- A productive cough with yellow-green phlegm

Susceptibility and Resistance

- Susceptibility is increased by processes that adversely affect the status of respiratory tissues:
  - Pulmonary edema
  - Influenza
  - Exposure to inhaled toxins
  - Chronic lung disease
  - Aspiration of any form (postalcohol ingestion, near-drowning, regurgitation due to gastric distention from gag-valve mask ventilation)
- Extremes of age also appear to increase susceptibility to the disease:
- Older adults
- Infants with low birth weight and/or malnourishment
- Other risk factors for pneumonia:
  - Sickle cell disease
  - Cardiovascular disease
  - Asplenia (congenital absence or surgical removal of a spleen)

    ◦ Diabetes
    ◦ Chronic renal failure (or other kidney disease)
    ◦ HIV infection
    ◦ Organ transplantation
    ◦ Multiple myeloma, lymphoma, Hodgkin's disease

Patient Management and Protective Measures

- Airway support
- Oxygen
- Ventilatory assistance (as needed)
- IV fluids
- Cardiac monitoring
- Transport for physician evaluation
- Patients with bacterial pneumonia are usually managed with bed rest, analgesics, decongestants, expectorants, and antibiotic therapy.
- Patient isolation generally is not warranted except in clinical facilities where a patient with a resistant strain of pneumonia may be in contact with other patients who have increased susceptibility to infection.
- Protective measures against the disease for health-care workers includes BSI precautions and effective hand washing.
- Immunizations exist for some causes of pneumonia but generally are not recommended for persons who come in contact with patients who have the disease.

TETANUS

- Tetanus is a serious, sometimes fatal, disease of the CNS caused by infection of a wound with spores of the bacterium *Clostridium tetani.*
- Tetanus spores live mainly in soil and manure, but are also found in the human intestine and elsewhere. If the spores enter tissue, they multiply and produce a toxin that acts on the nerves controlling muscular activity.
- Dead or necrotic tissue is a favorable environment for *C. tetani.*
- Only about 100 cases of tetanus are reported annually in the United States.
- The relatively low number of tetanus cases in the United States is a result of immunizing the general population with tetanus vaccines.

Signs and Symptoms

- Trismus (stiffness of the jaw; also known as "lockjaw")
- Muscular tetany (muscle spasms and twitching)
- Painful muscular contractions in the neck, moving to the trunk
- Abdominal rigidity (often the first sign in pediatric patients)
- Painful spasms (contortions) of the face
- Respiratory failure

Patient Management and Protective Measures

- The goal of prehospital care for a patient with tetanus is to support vital functions, which may include aggressive airway management (intubation, surgical/needle cricothyrotomy).
- Muscle spasms should be managed to maintain patient comfort with diazepam (Valium) or paralytic agents (per medical direction).

- Other drugs that may be indicated to manage a patient with tetanus include IV fluids, magnesium sulfate, narcotics, and antidysrhythmics.
- After physician evaluation and stabilization, care for patients with tetanus will include administration of antitoxin (tetanus immunoglobulin [TIG]) to provide postexposure passive immunity, treatment to eliminate the toxin, active immunization with tetanus toxoid, and wound care. Given prompt treatment, most patients recover completely.

Immunization

- Immunization against tetanus begins during childhood by way of DPT vaccination—A combined immunization against diphtheria (laryngitis, pharyngitis with discharge), pertussis (whooping cough), and tetanus.
- Initial immunization is followed by a booster before entry into elementary school and every 10 years thereafter, conferring effective active immunity.

RABIES

- An acute viral infection of the nervous system. The disease primarily affects animals but can be transmitted from an infected animal to a human through virus-laden saliva.
- In the United States, wildlife rabies is common in skunks, raccoons, bats, foxes, dogs, wolves, jackals, mongoose, and coyotes. Hawaii is the only area in the United States that is rabies free.
- Humans are highly susceptible to the rabies virus after being exposed to saliva from a bite or scratch of an infected animal. The severity of infection is governed by several factors:
  - Severity of the wound
  - Richness of nerve supply close to the wound
  - Distance from the wound to the CNS
  - Amount and strain of the virus
  - Degree of protective clothing

Signs and Symptoms

- The incubation period between bite and appearance of symptoms varies from 9 days to 7 years.
- Initial symptoms include:
  - Low-grade fever
  - Headache
  - Loss of appetite
  - Hyperactivity
  - Disorientation
  - In some cases, seizures
- Often the patient will have intense thirst, but attempts to drink will induce violent and painful spasms in the throat (thus the name "hydrophobia").
- As the disease progresses, eye and facial muscles may become paralyzed. Without medical intervention, the disease lasts 2–6 days, often resulting in death from respiratory failure.

Patient Management and Protective Measures

- After evaluation by a physician, signs and symptoms of the disease are treated with respiratory and cardiovascular support (as needed) and the administration of sedatives and analgesics.

- Thorough debridement of the wound without sutures (if possible) is indicated so that free bleeding and drainage occur.
- Passive immunization may be given with human rabies immune globulin, and a rabies vaccine—human diploid cell rabies vaccine (HDCV), rabies vaccine (DEV)—is given by a course of injections lasting several weeks.
- Injections are no longer administered in the stomach.
- Tetanus prophylaxis and antibiotics may be indicated.
- Most human cases of rabies are the result of bites from a rabid dog.
- The possibility of rabies, however, must be considered with all mammal bites.
- Scene safety and use of BSI precautions during wound management are important.
- Contact law enforcement personnel and animal-control authorities to assist in scene control.
- Immunization of contacts with open wounds or exposure of mucous membranes to saliva should receive treatment.
- Immunization should also be directed toward persons with high probability of contact with animal reservoirs.
- If an animal is suspected of being rabid, it will be destroyed and its brain examined for the presence of rabies inclusion bodies. In the absence of these inclusion bodies, the patient's rabies treatment will be stopped.

HANTAVIRUS

- Hantavirus was previously known to be associated with hemorrhagic fever in renal syndrome that occurs in Asia.
- Hantaviruses are also associated with a syndrome of severe respiratory distress and shock occurring in persons in several areas of the United States.
- The virus is carried by rodents and transmitted via inhalation of aerosols of material contaminated with rodent urine and feces.
- Hantavirus can cause significant disease in humans. Patients are typically healthy adults who experience an onset of fever and malaise, followed in several days by respiratory distress. The severity of the illness is determined by the strain of the virus. Other signs and symptoms may include fever, chills, headache, GI upset, and capillary hemorrhage.
- With severe infection, oliguria, kidney failure, and hypotension ensue.
- Death typically occurs from depressed cardiac output and eventual cardiovascular collapse.
- Management primarily is supportive and should be guided by medical direction.
- These viruses are very infectious; BSI precautions are indicated.

VIRAL DISEASES OF CHILDHOOD

- Childhood infectious diseases include rubella (German measles), rubeola (red measles or hard measles), mumps (parotitis), chicken pox (varicella), and pertussis (whooping cough).
- These infectious diseases are preventable with immunization for chicken pox and with the triple-immunization measles, mumps, and rubella (MMR) vaccine.
- With widespread immunization of children, the incidence of these childhood infectious diseases has decreased.
- Immunization provides long-lasting immunity and is known to be 98–99% effective against these diseases.

Rubella

- A mild, febrile, and highly communicable viral disease (caused by the rubella virus) characterized by a diffuse punctate macular rash.
- Usually transmitted by direct contact with nasopharyngeal secretions or droplet spray from an infected person.
- May also be transmitted transplacentally (producing active infection in the fetus) and by contact with articles contaminated with blood, urine, or feces.
- After inoculation, the virus invades the lymph system.
- From there, it enters the blood and produces an immune response; subsequent rash spreads from forehead to face to torso to extremities (lasting 3 days).
- Maximal communicability appears to be during the first few days before and 5–7 days after the onset of rash.
- Complications from the disease are rare, although young females sometimes develop a self-limiting arthritis.
- Congenital rubella syndrome (CRS) is a serious manifestation that affects about 90% of infants born to women who were infected with rubella during the first trimester of pregnancy.
- The disease is associated with multiple congenital anomalies, mental retardation, deafness, and an increased risk of death from congenital heart disease and sepsis during the first 6 months of life.
- The CDC recommends that all health-care providers receive immunization (if they are not immune from previous rubella infection) to reduce the risk of exposure to themselves and those they treat.
- As a precaution, pregnant EMS providers should not be exposed to these patients.

Rubeola

- Rubeola (caused by the measles virus) is an acute, highly communicable viral disease characterized by fever, conjunctivitis, cough, bronchitis, and a blotchy red rash. The virus is found in the blood, urine, and pharyngeal secretions.
- The disease is usually transmitted directly or indirectly through contact with infected respiratory secretions.
- After exposure, the virus invades the respiratory epithelium and spreads via the lymph system.
- Rubeola may predispose to secondary bacterial complications such as otitis media, pneumonia, and myocarditis.
- The most serious life-threatening complication is subacute sclerosing panencephalitis (a slowly progressing neurological disease marked by deterioration of mental capacity and muscle coordination).
- Early (prodromal) symptoms that mark the onset of disease include high fever, nasal discharge, conjunctivitis, photophobia, and cough.
- A day or two before the rash, patients with rubeola usually have white spots on the internal cheek (Koplik's spots).
- Dermal rash begins a few days after respiratory tract involvement.
- Rash is red and maculopapular and spreads from the forehead to the face, neck, torso, and eventually to feet by the third day.
- Uncomplicated cases of rubeola usually last 6 days.
- Immunity acquired after illness is lifelong.

Mumps

- Mumps is an acute, communicable systemic viral disease characterized by localized unilateral or bilateral edema of one or more of the salivary glands (usually the parotid), with occasional involvement of other glands.
- Virus is transmitted through direct contact with the saliva droplets of an infected person.
- Virus invades and multiplies in the parotid gland or epithelium of the upper respiratory passages.
- From there, it enters the blood and localizes in glandular or nervous tissue.
- Parotid gland, testes, and pancreas are most frequently involved.
- When mumps occurs past the age of puberty, it may cause a painful inflammation of the testicle (orchitis) and testicular atrophy; however, sterility is rare.
- The intensity of symptoms in mumps is variable; 30% of infections are asymptomatic.
- Immunity after clinical and subclinical disease is lifelong.
- Placental transfer of antibodies sometimes occurs.

Chicken Pox

- Chicken pox (caused by the varicella-zoster virus) is a common childhood disease caused by a member of the herpesvirus family and transmitted by direct and indirect contact with droplets (mainly airborne) from respiratory passages of an infected person. Exposure to linen tainted with vesicle or mucous membrane discharges of infected persons has been implicated.
- Chicken pox is highly communicable and is characterized by a sudden onset of low-grade fever, mild malaise, and a skin eruption that is maculopapular for a few hours and vesicular for 3–4 days, leaving a granular scab.
- Initially the skin lesions appear on the trunk and usually move to the extremities. The crops of skin eruptions (each associated with itching) generally are more abundant on covered areas of the body; the scalp, conjunctivae, and upper respiratory tract may be affected. The appearance of crops of vesicles (fresh vesicles appearing while other lesions are scabbed) differentiates chicken pox from smallpox, which has vesicles of the same age.
- Treatment is symptomatic, and the disease is self-limited.
- Complications are rare but may include secondary bacterial infections, aseptic meningitis, mononucleosis, and Reye's syndrome.
- After recovery, the virus is believed to remain in the body in an asymptomatic latent stage (possibly localized in the dorsal root ganglia).
- The virus may reactivate during periods of stress or immunosuppression, producing an illness known as shingles.
- The vesicles associated with shingles are restricted to the skin area supplied by the sensory nerves of a single group or associated groups of dorsal root ganglia.
  - Unlike chicken pox, shingles is not transmitted through respiratory droplets but can cause chicken pox in susceptible individuals who are in contact with skin lesions.
  - Antiviral drugs exist that shorten the duration of symptoms and pain in the older patient.
- EMS workers who have not had chicken pox should consider receiving the chicken pox vaccine.
- Data indicates that adult antibody production occurs in 82% of patients after one dose, and 92% of patients after two doses.
  - About 5% of patients who receive the vaccine develop a rash, and some develop frank chicken pox, which is very debilitating in adults.

- Varicella zoster immune globulin (VZIG) is recommended for pregnant women with significant exposure to chicken pox (without history of previous exposure) to protect the fetus.

Pertussis

- Pertussis (caused by *Bordetella pertussis* bacterium) is an infectious disease that mainly affects infants and young children.
- Spread by direct contact by discharges from mucous membranes contained in airborne droplets.
- Leads to inflammation of the entire respiratory tract and causes an insidious onset of cough that becomes paroxysmal in 1–2 weeks, lasting 1–2 months.
- Coughing episodes are violent (sometimes without an intervening inhalation), causing the high-pitched inspiratory "whoop" and ending with expulsion of clear mucus and vomiting.
- The "whoop" is often not present in children less than 6 months of age.
- The communicability for pertussis is thought to be greatest before the onset of paroxysmal coughing (thus the need for BSI and surgical mask protection for paramedic and patient).
- Erythromycin is known to decrease the period of communicability but can reduce symptoms only if given during the incubation period (before the onset of paroxysmal cough).
- Infection with pertussis generally confers immunity; however, subsequent attacks after immunization in older children and adults indicate that immunity may wane over time.

OTHER VIRAL DISEASES

Influenza

- Influenza primarily is a respiratory infection spread by influenza viruses A, B, and C. Popularly known as "the flu."
- Spread by virus-infected droplets coughed or sneezed into the air.
- Usually occurs in small outbreaks or every few years in epidemics.
- Resistance is normally conferred after recovery.
- Persons infected with certain strains of influenza type A or B acquire immunity to that strain.
- Type A and B viruses, however, occasionally alter to produce new strains, leading to new infection.
- Type B virus is relatively stable but occasionally alters to overcome resistance and may lead to small outbreaks of infection.
- Type A virus is highly unstable and has caused flu epidemics throughout the world.
- These variants are named for geographical site and year of isolation (e.g., the Spanish flu in 1918, Asian flu in 1957, and the Hong Kong flu in 1968) and the culture number (e.g., A/Japan/305/57).
- Type C virus stimulates antibodies that provide immunity for life.
- Signs and symptoms typically include chills, fever, headache, muscular aches, loss of appetite, and fatigue.
- These are followed by upper respiratory infection and cough (which is often severe and protracted), lasting 2–7 days.
- Patient management primarily is supportive, and mild cases of viral infection generally are not treated.

- Severe cases (particularly in older adults and those with lung or heart disease) may result in secondary bacterial infection (e.g., *S. pneumoniae*), and can be fatal.
- Anti-influenza vaccines (containing killed strains of type A and B viruses currently in circulation) may help prevent infection.
- Immunity is short-lived; the vaccine must be repeated each year just before the start of "flu season" (November to March in the United States).
- Amantadine (Symmetrel, Symadine), rimantadine (Flumadine), or zanamivir (Relenza) may be given to institutionalized patients to protect against influenza A.
- Despite advances in prevention and management, influenza and its complications are fatal to about 20,000 people in the United States each year.

Mononucleosis

- Mononucleosis (often referred to as "mono") is caused either by the Epstein-Barr virus (EBV) or cytomegalovirus (CMV), both members of the herpesvirus family.
- A very common illness that is spread person to person through the oropharyngeal route and saliva (thus the name "kissing disease").
- Blood transfusions also can be a mode of transmission, but resultant clinical disease is rare.
- Most people with a healthy immune system are able to ward off the infection, even after significant exposure.
- Transmission from care providers to young children is common.
- Signs and symptoms of mononucleosis generally appear gradually.
    - Characterized by fever (which may last for weeks), sore throat, oropharyngeal discharges, lymphadenopathy (especially posterior cervical), and splenomegaly with abdominal tenderness
    - About 10% of people also will develop a generalized rash or darkened areas in the mouth that resemble bruises
- Recovery usually occurs in a few weeks, but some people take months to regain their former level of energy.
- The patient may remain a carrier for several months after symptoms disappear.
- Immunization for mononucleosis is not available.

SEXUALLY TRANSMITTED DISEASES

- Sexually transmitted diseases (STDs) are a group of disease syndromes that can be spread sexually, whether or not the disease has genital pathological manifestations.
- More than 20 etiological agents have been identified as belonging to this group of diseases (including HBV and HIV infections).
- Other common STDs include syphilis, gonorrhea, chlamydia, and herpesvirus infections.
- A number of pathogenic agents are responsible for the host of STDs, including bacteria, viruses, protozoa, fungi, and ectoparasites.
- Many of these pathogens can produce multiple disease syndromes, and patients with STD syndromes frequently have multiple STDs.
- These infections usually result in a short-lived cellular immune response and a longer-lasting humoral antibody response, neither of which protects against future exposures.

Syphilis

- A systemic disease.
- Characteristics include a primary lesion, a secondary eruption involving skin and mucous membranes.

- Long periods of latency
- Late seriously disabling lesions of the skin, bone, viscera, CNS, and cardiovascular system
- Caused by penetration of *Treponema pallidum* into intact mucous membranes or abraded skin.
- Common modes of transmission include direct contact with exudate from lesions on skin and mucous membranes, blood transfusions/needle sticks (rare), and congenital transmission.
- After penetration, the organisms travel (within hours) to lymph nodes, where they are disseminated throughout the body.
- After initial infection, syphilis follows well-defined stages of disease.
- Syphilis is treatable with antibiotic therapy.
- No immunization is available.

Primary Stage

- Within 10–90 days after exposure, a primary lesion or chancre develops at the site of initial invasion.
- The surface of the chancre is usually crusted or ulcerated and varies in size from 1–2 cm in diameter.
- The lesion is usually single and painless, and it generally heals spontaneously within 1–5 weeks.
- During this stage, syphilis is highly communicable.

Secondary Stage

- The secondary stage begins about 2–10 weeks after the appearance of the primary lesion and lasts 2–6 weeks.
- This stage is heralded by systemic symptoms, including headache, malaise, anorexia, fever, sore throat, lymphadenopathy, and bald spots in the area of infection.
- In addition, the patient may develop a rash, which is usually bilaterally symmetrical and frequently involves the palms and soles.
- Painless, wartlike regions (condyloma latum) that are extremely infectious also may be found in moist, warm sites.
- The CNS, eyes, bones, joints, or kidneys may be affected in this stage of the illness.

Latency

- A period of latency (ranging from 1 to 40 years or more) follows the secondary stage in untreated persons.
- During latency, there may be recurrent episodes of secondary-stage symptoms (in about 25% of cases) with subclinical infection.
- About 33% of these patients will progress to tertiary syphilis; the rest will remain asymptomatic.
- Tertiary syphilis—Infectious involvement of the skin, CNS, and cardiovascular systems.

Gonorrhea

- Caused by the sexually transmitted bacterium *Neisseria gonorrhoeae*, which is communicated by a purulent exudate from mucous membranes of an infected person. Other modes of transmission include maternal infection during pregnancy and transmission of the pathogen during birth.
- The disease occurs in both men and women but differs in course, severity, and ease of recognition.

- Immunization is not available.
- Affected areas of the male anatomy are the urethra, Littre's gland, Cowper's gland, prostate gland, seminal vesicles, and epididymis.
- Several days after exposure, there is usually a sudden onset of dysuria, urgency, and frequency.
- The associated discharge rapidly becomes purulent and profuse.
- Direct spread of the infection may result in prostatitis, epididymitis, and seminal vesiculitis.
- Primary gonorrheal infections may also affect the pharynx, conjunctivae, and anus.
- Affected areas of the female anatomy are the Bartholin glands, Skene glands, urethra, cervix, and fallopian tubes.
- Contiguous spread of the disease may lead to endometritis, salpingitis, parametritis (pelvic inflammatory disease), and the formation of tubo-ovarian abscesses.
- Complete or partial occlusion of the fallopian tubes may result in sterility and increased risk for ectopic pregnancy.
- Between 1% and 3% of gonococcal infections become disseminated in the blood.
- This extension of the disease may produce septicemia, arthritis, endocarditis, meningitis, and skin lesions.
- In the bacteremic stage, the patient may complain of fever, chills, and malaise.
- Erythematous lesions are common, especially on the extremities, and may occur in groups or singly.

Chlamydia

- *Chlamydia trachomatis* is a major cause of sexually transmitted nonspecific urethritis (NSU) or nongonococcal genital infection.
- The disease is prevalent worldwide, is the most common sexually transmitted disease in the United States (an estimated 25% of men are carriers), and is the world's leading cause of preventable blindness.
- Signs and symptoms of the disease are similar to gonorrhea, making differentiation difficult.
- No immunization is available.
- In men, NSU may cause a penile discharge and complications such as swelling of the testes, which if untreated may lead to infertility.
- In women, NSU is usually symptomless but may cause a vaginal discharge or pain with urination, salpingitis, and cervicitis.
- Transmission occurs from direct contact with exudates, either sexually or during birth.
- Infections are treated with antibiotics.

Herpesvirus Infections

- Herpes simplex virus (HSV), which is associated with STD
- Cytomegalovirus, which is associated with mononucleosis, hepatitis, and severe systemic disease in the immunosuppressed host
- Epstein-Barr virus, which causes mononucleosis
- Varicella-zoster virus, which causes chicken pox and shingles

Herpes Simplex Virus

- Two antigenically distinct HSV agents responsible for STDs.
  - Herpes simplex virus type 1 (HSV-1)
    - Most often associated with herpes above the waist

  - Herpes simplex virus type 2 (HSV-2)
    - — Generally associated with genital herpes
- Immunization is not available for either virus.
- Herpesvirus infections are common in the United States, producing 300,000–500,000 new infections each year.
- The mode of transmission for HSV is strictly by skin-to-skin contact with an infected area of the body.
- The virus enters through a break in the skin or through mucous membranes.
- Sexual contact is not required for transmission.
- The virus may also be spread to other external body sites by autoinoculation (e.g., lip to finger to genitalia).
- Initial HSV-1 transmission usually occurs by age 4 and is manifested by gingivostomatitis ("cold sores" or "fever blisters").
- Initial HSV-2 transmission generally occurs during sexual activity and is manifested by painful vesicular lesions in the genital area.
- Once the virus is present in tissue, HSV produces an acute infection with self-limited tissue destruction.
- This "primary infection" produces a vesicular lesion (blister) that heals spontaneously without residual scarring.
- After the primary infection, the HSV enters the nervous system (nearest the site of initial infection) and travels along sensory nerve pathways to a sensory nerve ganglion, where it remains in a latent stage until it is reactivated.
- When triggered by another infectious disease, menstruation, emotional stress, trauma, or immunosuppression, the virus reaches the epidermis by way of peripheral nerves.
- Reproduces a recurrent infectious disease state that usually lasts 4–10 days—Lesions generally occur in the area of initial inoculation.
- The disease is manifested by clusters of painful vesicles that become pustular and dry, leaving shallow, painful ulcers.
- HSV can remain dormant indefinitely—It is unknown why many infected people never exhibit the disease, whereas others experience a lifetime of periodic outbreaks.
- Acyclovir (Zovirax) may shorten the disease episode and is useful as a prophylactic agent in instances of frequent recurrence.

LICE AND SCABIES

Lice and scabies are potential health hazards for all emergency care providers. Both are medically important as potential vectors of communicable skin disease and systemic illness, as well as dermatitis and discomfort.

Lice

- Lice are small, wingless insects that are ectoparasites of birds and mammals, and most are host-specific.
- Two of the species are human parasites.
  - *Phthirus pubis*, the pubic or crab louse
  - *Pediculus humanus*, with two varieties, *P. humanus capitis*, the head louse, *and P. humanus corporis*, the body louse (involved in outbreaks of epidemic typhus and trench fever in World War I)

- There is a three-stage life cycle for lice.
  - Eggs hatch in 7–10 days
  - Nymph stage lasts 7–13 days
  - Egg-to-egg cycle lasts about 3 weeks
- Lice subsist on blood from the host and have mouths modified for piercing and sucking.
- During biting and feeding, secretions from the louse cause a small, red macule and pruritus.
- Long periods of infestation may bring a decrease in pruritus and often impart a thick, dry, scaly appearance to the skin. In severe cases, oozing and crusting may be present.
- If sensitization to lice saliva and feces occurs, inflammation may develop.
- Secondary infection may result from scratching of lesions.
- Lice spread through close personal contact and sharing of clothing and bedding.
- Pubic lice have a distinctive appearance, suggestive of a miniature crab.
- Grayish-blue spots may be observed on the abdomen and thighs of infested patients.
- The eggs (nits or ova) often are evident on the shaft of pubic hairs and sometimes in eyelashes, eyebrows, and axillary hairs.
- Pubic lice are usually acquired during sexual activity or from unchanged bedding where egg-infested pubic hairs have been shed.
- Primary bite lesions are seldom evident, but the patient normally complains of intense pruritus and pubic scratching.
- Head lice have an elongated body with a head that is narrower than the thorax.
- Each louse has three pairs of legs that possess delicate hooks at the distal extremities.
- The white ova of head lice (usually one nit to a shaft) are easily mistaken for dandruff, but the nits cannot be brushed out.
- These parasites most frequently affect children.
- Body lice are larger than head lice and concentrate about the waist, shoulders, axillae, and neck.
- Body lice and their nits are usually found in seams and on fibers of clothing.
- The lesions from their bites begin as small, noninflammatory red spots that quickly become papular wheals that resemble linear scratch marks (parallel scratch marks on the shoulders are a common finding).
- Head lice and body lice interbreed.
- The management of all types of lice is aimed at eradicating the parasites and nits and at preventing reinfestation.
- Patients are usually advised to wash all clothing, bedding, and personal articles thoroughly in hot water and to wash the infected body area with gamma benzene hexachloride shampoo (Kwell), crotamiton (Eurax), Rid, or Nix.
- Overtreatment should be avoided out of concern for toxicity.

Scabies

- The human scabies mite *(Sarcoptes scabiei var. hominis)* is a parasite that completes its entire life cycle in and on the epidermis of its host.
- Infestation resembles that of lice, but scabies bites generally are concentrated around the hands and feet, especially between the webs of the fingers and toes.
- Other common areas of infestation include the face and scalp of children, the nipples in females, and the penis in males.
- The scabies mite is usually passed by intimate contact or from infested bedding, furniture, and clothing.

- Scabies infestation is often manifested by severe nocturnal pruritus (although it takes 4–6 weeks for sensitization to develop and itching to begin).
- The adult female mite is responsible for symptoms.
- After impregnation, she burrows into the epidermis to lay her eggs and remains in the burrow for a life span of about 1 month.
- Vesicles and papules form at the surface, but they often are disguised by the results of scratching. In severe cases, oozing, crusting, and secondary infection may result.
- Susceptibility is general, but people with a previous exposure usually develop less mites on successive exposures, and experience symptoms earlier (usually in 1–4 days).
- Treatment is similar to that prescribed for lice infestation.
- Symptoms may persist for over a month until the mite and mite products are shed with the epidermis.
- Mites are communicable until all mites and eggs are destroyed.
- Reinfestation is common.
  - If itching has not been abated within several weeks, the patient should be reexamined.
- Antibiotic therapy may be required to treat secondary infection.
- Immunization is not available.

Protective Measures Against Lice and Scabies

- Observe BSI guidelines; bag linen separately.
- Spray the patient compartment of the ambulance with an effective insecticide.
- Most commercial sprays contain effective pyrethrins, Malathion, or carbamates.
- Spray floor, gurney, and immediate areas where the patient's head was positioned (lice do not jump great distances).
- Remove all insecticide residues with appropriate solution.
- Wear gloves during all steps and practice effective hand washing when finished.
- Personal treatment:
  - Use appropriate body/hair pedulicide; repeat in 7–10 days
  - Launder personal clothing in hot cycles of washer and dryer (of questionable benefit)

REPORTING AN EXPOSURE TO AN INFECTIOUS/COMMUNICABLE DISEASE

- All suspected exposures to an infectious or communicable disease must be reported to the Designated Officer.
- An exposure incident (significant exposure) is contact with any specific eye, mouth, other mucous membrane, nonintact skin, parenteral contact with blood, blood products, bloody body fluids, or other potentially infectious materials.
- Reporting a possible exposure is important for several reasons.
  - It permits immediate medical follow-up, permitting identification of infection and immediate intervention.
  - It enables the Designated Officer to evaluate the circumstances surrounding the incident and to implement engineering or procedural changes to avoid a future exposure.
  - It facilitates follow-up testing of the source individual if permission for testing can be obtained.
- The Ryan White Act stipulates that an employer will designate a person or officer within the organization to whom exposed employees will report.
- That officer will then initiate those elements of the Exposure Control Plan to comply with standards and guidelines relative to the exposure, and follow any local reporting requirements.

Medical Evaluation and Follow-Up

- Employers must, by law, provide free medical evaluation and treatment to exposed employees.
- Counseling about the risks, signs and symptoms, probability of developing clinical disease, and how to prevent future further spread of the potential infection.
- Appropriate treatment in line with current U.S. Public Health Service recommendations.
- A discussion of medications offered, including side effects and contraindications.
- Evaluation of any reported illness to determine whether the symptoms could be related to HIV or hepatitis.
- Steps involved:
    - Blood tests of exposed employees are always contingent upon employee agreement.
    - The employee has the option of providing blood samples, but can refuse permission for HIV testing at the time the sample is drawn.
    - The employer must maintain the blood samples for 90 days in case the employee changes his or her mind about testing should HIV- or hepatitis-like symptoms develop.
    - A health-care provider, acting as an agent of the employer, must provide certain services.
    - Counsel the employee based on test results.
    - Provide informed consent about prophylaxis to therapeutic regimens.
    - Implement those regimens with the approval of the employee.
- Vaccines also should be made available to the employee and all employees who have occupational exposure to blood and other potentially infectious materials.

The Written Report and Confidentiality

- The health-care provider will provide a written report to the Designated Officer of the employer.
- This report will identify only whether vaccination was recommended to the exposed employee and whether or not the employee received vaccination.
- The written report must also note that the employee was informed of the results of the evaluation and told of any medical conditions resulting from the occupational exposure that may require further evaluation or treatment.
- A copy of this report must be provided to the employee and to the Designated Officer for the agency's files.
- All other elements of the employee's medical record are confidential and cannot be supplied to the employer.
- The employee must give written consent for anyone to see the records.
- The records must be maintained for the duration of employment, plus 30 years, to comply with OSHA standards on access to employee exposure and medical records.

The Paramedic's Role in Preventing Disease Transmission

- Paramedics deal with infectious disease emergencies and must be vigilant about consequences to themselves, patients, and coworkers.
- Part of this professional responsibility in preventing the spread of disease is to know when *not* to go to work.
    - When you have a fever
    - When you have diarrhea
    - When you have a draining wound or any type of wet lesion
    - When you are jaundiced
    - When you have been told you have mononucleosis
    - When you have been treated with a medication and/or shampoo for lice or scabies

  - Until you have been taking antibiotics for at least 24 hours for a strep throat
  - When you have a cold (unless you wear a surgical mask to protect your patients)
- The health-care worker should also ensure that personal immunization status is current for MMR, hepatitis, DPT, polio, chicken pox, and influenza.

Other Considerations in Disease Prevention

- When providing emergency care duties, always approach the scene with caution and be aware that an uncontrolled scene increases the likelihood for transmission of body fluids.
- BSI guidelines should be observed at all times.
  - Wear gloves
  - Don protective eyewear, face shield, and gown (if splash or spray is possible)
  - Wear an appropriate particulate mask when airborne disease is suspected
- BSI guidelines are based upon the premise that all body fluids, in any situation, may be infectious.
- As a rule, the paramedic should consider any patient who presents with cough, headache, general weakness, recent weight loss, nuchal rigidity, or high fever to have an infectious process.
- Regardless of the patient's infectious status, however, the paramedic should follow certain guidelines:
  - Provide the same level of care to all patients
  - Disinfect equipment and the patient compartment with appropriate disinfectant solution
  - Practice effective hand-washing procedures
  - Report any infectious exposure to the agency's Designated Officer

CHAPTER QUESTIONS

1. A common childhood disease that is caused by the varicella-zoster virus is called?
   a. Mumps
   b. Chicken pox
   c. Measles
   d. Rubella
2. *Bordetella pertussis* bacterium is an infectious disease that mainly affects infants and young children. This bacterial infection is named:
   a. pertussis
   b. measles
   c. rubella
   d. chicken pox

Suggested Reading

US Department of Transportation, National Highway Traffic Safety Administration. *EMT-Paramedic: National Standard Curriculum.* Washington, DC: US Department of Transportation, National Highway Traffic Safety Administration; 1998.

Chapter 31

Behavioral and Psychiatric Disorders

A 45-year-old female is anxious and says she feels like she is going crazy. The patient has a past medical history of anxiety and is in good physical health. During initial contact with the patient, what should your first step be?

Behavioral and psychiatric emergencies require a different approach than your typical medical or trauma calls.

- Most behavioral emergencies require only excellent communication skills and supportive measures to prevent the escalation of a crisis.
- The paramedic's primary role will often be to provide understanding, compassion, and direction for someone with temporary turmoil.
- Emergency medical service (EMS) personnel must be oriented to helping and protecting these patients until they are able to gain self-control or until other therapeutic skills can be applied.
- Mental illness accounts for 4 of the 10 leading causes of disability in established market economies worldwide.
- The cost of mental illness in the United States (including days lost from work) exceeds 148 billion dollars each year.
- It has been estimated that as much as 20% of the U.S. population has some form of mental health problems and that one person out of very seven will require treatment for an emotional disturbance at some point during their lives.
- Mental health problems incapacitate more people in the United States than all other health problems combined.

UNDERSTANDING BEHAVIORAL EMERGENCIES

- Although there is no clear agreement or ideal model for "normal" behavior, it is generally considered to be adaptive behavior accepted by society, which can vary by culture and ethnic group.
- The concept of abnormal (maladaptive) behavior is also defined by society when behavior does one of the following:
    - Deviates from society's norms and expectations
    - Interferes with well-being and ability to function
    - Is harmful to the individual or group
- A behavioral emergency can be defined as a change in mood or behavior that cannot be tolerated by the involved person or others and that requires immediate attention.

- Behavioral emergencies may range from disordered and disturbed patients who are dangerous to themselves and others to less intense situations in which the patient has a transient inability to cope with stress or anxiety.
- Most behavioral emergencies result from the following:
  - Biological/organic causes
  - Psychosocial causes
  - Sociocultural causes
- Common misconceptions about mental illness:
  - Abnormal behavior is always bizarre
  - All patients with mental illness are unstable and dangerous
  - Mental disorders are incurable
  - Having a mental disorder is cause for embarrassment and shame

Terms and Definitions

- Affect—An outward manifestation of a person's feelings or emotions
- Anger—A feeling of displeasure resulting from injury, mistreatment, or opposition
- Anxiety—A state or feeling of apprehension, uneasiness, agitation, uncertainty, and fear resulting from the anticipation of some threat or danger
- Confusion—A state of disorder or failure to distinguish between things
- Depression—A mood disturbance characterized by feelings of sadness, despair, and discouragement
- Fear—A feeling of anxiety and agitation caused by the presence or nearness of danger or pain
- Mental status—The degree of competence shown by a person in intellectual, emotional, psychological, and personality function
- Open-ended question—Question that encourages a person to answer in detail
- Posture—The position or carriage of the body

Biological/Organic Causes

- Physical or biochemical disturbances (which may have an inherited component) can result in significant changes in behavior.
- Instances of organic causes of behavioral emergencies include the following:
  - Substance abuse
    - Alcohol
    - Barbiturates
    - Sedative hypnotics
    - Amphetamines and other stimulants
    - Hallucinogens
  - Trauma
    - Concussion
    - Intracranial hematoma (especially subdural hematoma)
- Illness
  - Endocrine disorders
    - Diabetes
    - Thyroid disease
    - Parathyroid disease
    - Adrenal hormone imbalance

- ◦ Metabolic disorders
  - — Glucose, sodium, calcium, or magnesium imbalance
  - — Acid-base imbalance
  - — Acute hypoxia
  - — Renal failure
  - — Hepatic failure
- ◦ Cardiovascular disorders
  - — Cardiac dysrhythmias
  - — Hypotension
  - — Transient ischemic attack
  - — Cerebrovascular accident (CVA)
  - — Hypertensive encephalopathy
  - — Infectious diseases
    - Encephalitis
    - Meningitis
    - Brain abscess
    - Severe systemic infection
- ◦ Tumors
  - — Central nervous system (CNS) tumors or metastases
- ◦ Dementia
  - — Dementia of the Alzheimer's type
  - — Other dementia
- ◦ Drug reactions from:
  - — Beta-blockers
  - — Antihypertensives
  - — Cardiac drugs
  - — Bronchodilators
  - — Beta-agonists
  - — Anticonvulsants

- It is important to consider the possibility of organic causes in all behavioral emergencies.

Psychosocial Causes

- Psychosocial mental illness may have many causes, but it is often the result of one of the following:
  - ◦ Childhood trauma
  - ◦ Parental deprivation
  - ◦ Dysfunctional family structure
- Most mental conditions are characterized by one of the following:
  - ◦ Neurosis—A restricted ability to achieve optimal functioning in social life
  - ◦ Psychosis—Maladaptive behavior that involves major distortions of reality
- Behavioral changes associated with these illnesses manifest in a wide range of psychological and physiological responses, including the following:
  - ◦ Depression
  - ◦ Withdrawal
  - ◦ Catatonic state
  - ◦ Violence or homicidal acts

  - Suicidal acts
  - Paranoid reactions
  - Phobias
  - Disorientation or disorganization

Sociocultural Causes

- Most people maintain a delicate balance among emotions, thoughts, and actions. When this equilibrium shifts rapidly, the person may experience emotional turmoil that results in crisis.
- Changes in behavior caused by interpersonal or situational stress are frequently linked to a specific incident or series of incidents.

Assessment and Management of Behavioral Emergencies

- Evaluate the scene for possible danger. Most EMS services operate under protocol that includes law enforcement response for any behavioral emergency. If a dangerous situation is suspected, do not approach the patient until police are present and the potential for danger is controlled.
- Four general principles must be remembered when dealing with behavioral emergencies:
  - Ensure scene safety
  - Contain the crisis
  - Render appropriate emergency medical care
  - Transport the patient to an appropriate health-care facility

Assessment

- Patient assessment should begin by gathering the information necessary for immediate management of life-threatening conditions.
- Survey the scene for evidence of the following:
  - Violence
  - Substance abuse
  - Suicide attempt
- Gather information from the following people:
  - The patient
  - The patient's family
  - Bystanders
  - First responders
- Limit the number of people around the patient; isolate the patient if necessary.
- Stay alert to signs of possible danger (patient rage or hostility).
- During the patient assessment, attempt to gather the following data:
  - Patient's mental state (i.e., alertness, orientation, and ability to communicate)
  - Patient's name and age
  - Significant past medical history
  - Medications that have been taken
  - Past psychiatric problems
  - Precipitating situation or problem

Interview Techniques

- After any life-threatening illness or injury has been managed, alert and communicative patients should be interviewed.
- Do not ask for more information than is necessary; however, limited and supportive interviews help strengthen rapport with a patient and can help establish and maintain a relationship during the patient encounter.
- Effective interviewing techniques include the following:
  - Active listening
  - Being supportive and empathetic
  - Limiting interruptions
  - Respecting the patient's personal space by limiting physical touch
- Assessment findings that are important to note during the interview include the following:
  - Physical/somatic complaints
  - Intellectual functioning
  - Thought content
  - Language
  - Mood
  - Appearance
  - Psychomotor activity
  - Difficult patient interviews
  - Some patients with behavioral or psychiatric disorders will be difficult to interview
- A patient may refuse to talk to the paramedic, especially if the family requested EMS assistance without the patient's consent.
- The patient may be extremely talkative and have a disorganized speech pattern.
- The patient may be confrontational.
- If the patient refuses to be interviewed, the following techniques may be employed:
  - Speaking to the patient in a quiet voice
  - Avoiding questions that may be interpreted by the patient as an "interrogation"
  - Allowing extra time for the patient to respond
- Patients who are too talkative will need to be focused on the interview; try the following techniques:
  - Calling out the patient's name
  - Raising your hand to get the patient's attention
- If a patient is confrontational, the following situations may arise:
  - Additional manpower may be required at the scene to ensure scene safety
  - Restraint may be required

Other Patient Care Measures

- After the initial assessment and history taking, the remainder of the examination is determined by the patient's overall condition and the nature of the psychiatric problem.
- Benefits of a thorough physical examination must be weighed against the risks involved in an encounter that the patient may construe as a physical violation.
- If there is reason to suspect an organic cause and the patient demonstrates no apprehension or disapproval, perform the examination.
  - If this is not possible, prehospital management may be limited to maintaining an effective rapport with the patient during transfer to the hospital

- Elements of the physical examination that may be associated with a behavioral emergency include the following:
  - Abnormal pupillary size and reactivity, which indicates toxic ingestion or an intracranial process
  - Odor of alcohol on breath
  - Needle tracks on the extremities
  - Unilateral weakness or loss of sensation

SPECIFIC BEHAVIORAL/PSYCHIATRIC DISORDERS

- More than 250 psychiatric conditions have been identified by mental health workers. Prehospital care for most behavioral emergencies is primarily supportive and includes the following:
  - Protecting the patient and others from harm; restraints may be necessary
  - Assessing and managing coexisting emergency medical problems
  - Transporting the patient for physician evaluation

Cognitive Disorders

- Cognitive disorders may have an organic etiology or be the result of a physical or chemical injury.
- All cognitive disorders result in a disturbance of cognitive functioning, which may manifest as delirium or dementia.
- Delirium is an abrupt disorientation of time and place, usually with illusions and hallucinations.
- Symptoms vary according to personality, environment, and the severity of illness.
- Common signs and symptoms include the following:
  - Inattention
  - Memory impairment
  - Disorientation
  - Clouding of consciousness
  - Vivid visual hallucinations
- Treatment
  - Treatment is aimed at correcting the underlying physical disorder to reduce anxiety
  - Sedatives may be required to manage the patient
- The exact occurrence rate of delirium is unknown, because it often is overlooked. Some groups are more susceptible to delirium than others, including the following:
  - The elderly
  - Children
  - Patients with burns
  - Patients who have had major heart surgery
  - Patients with previous brain damage
  - Patients with AIDS
- Dementia is a clinical state characterized by loss of function in multiple cognitive domains. It involves a slow, progressive loss of awareness for time and place, usually with an inability to learn new things or remember recent events.
- Although about 75 different types of dementia have been identified, the majority of cases result from one of the following:
  - Cerebrovascular disease, including stroke
  - Alzheimer's disease (an irreversible, gradual loss of brain cells and shrinkage of brain tissue)

- Dementia is a major health problem in the United States because of long life spans; it affects some 10% of people more than 65 years old and 20% of people more than 75 years old.
- The personal habits of patients with dementia often deteriorate.
  - Speech may become incoherent
  - Many of these patients may revert to a "second childhood" and require total care of their feeding, toilet, and physical activities
- Treatment of certain illnesses may be effective in arresting the mental decline associated with this disease.

Schizophrenia

- Schizophrenia is composed of a group of disorders. It is characterized by recurrent episodes of psychotic behavior that may include abnormalities of the following:
  - Thought processes
  - Thought content (delusions)
  - Perception (auditory hallucinations are particularly common)
  - Judgement
- There often is a family history of schizophrenia, and the disorder usually becomes apparent during adolescence or early adulthood.

Facts about Schizophrenia

- More than 2 million adult Americans are affected by schizophrenia.
- In men, schizophrenia usually appears in the late teens or early twenties.
- In women, schizophrenia usually appears in the twenties or early thirties.
- Schizophrenia affects men and women with equal frequency.
- Most people with schizophrenia suffer chronically throughout their lives.
- One of every 10 people with schizophrenia eventually commits suicide.
- Schizophrenia costs the nation more than 32 billion dollars annually.
- Many schizophrenic patients function quite well with medication therapy.
- Others function poorly between frank psychotic episodes, which are often due to medication noncompliance.
- Most require lifelong management with antipsychotic drugs and agents that block the action of the brain chemical dopamine.
- Compliance with drug therapy is usually effective in suppressing obvious symptoms of the disease. Drug therapy may result in side effects, especially dyskinesia (abnormal muscular movements) and tremor.
- The management of paranoid reactions associated with schizophrenia should include the following:
  - Clearly identifying yourself as a paramedic and expressing your intent to provide help
  - Exhibiting an attitude that is friendly but also somewhat distant and neutral
    - Kindness and warmth may be interpreted by the patient as an attempt to gain his or her confidence for ulterior motives
  - Never responding to the patient's anger
  - Not speaking with family members or bystanders in hushed or secretive tones
  - Using tact and firmness in persuading the patient to be transported to the hospital
  - Remembering that paranoid reactions can lead to violent behavior
    - Precautions regarding personal safety must be a priority

Anxiety Disorders

A certain amount of anxiety is useful and necessary in adapting constructively to stress. A patient who suffers from an anxiety disorder displays a persistent fearful feeling that cannot be consciously related to reality.

Facts about Anxiety Disorders

- More than 16 million adults in the United States who are between the ages of 18 and 54 suffer from anxiety disorders.
- Anxiety disorders are frequently complicated by depression, eating disorders, or substance abuse.
- Anxiety disorders cost the nation more than $46 billion annually.
- This type of illness may be disabling, because the patient withdraws from daily activities in a usually unsuccessful attempt to avoid the episodes of intense activity.
- Severe anxiety disorders may manifest as panic disorders ("panic attacks").

Facts about Panic Disorders

- Panic disorders affect about 2.4 million people in the United States each year.
- Panic disorders typically strike in young adulthood; about half of the people who develop the condition do so before age 24.
- Women are twice as likely as men to develop panic disorders.
- People with panic disorders also may suffer from depression and substance abuse.
- About 30% of people with panic disorders abuse alcohol.
- About 17% abuse recreational drugs.
- About a third of people with panic disorders develop agoraphobia.
- Signs and symptoms of panic disorder:
    - Hyperventilation
    - Feeling of breathlessness or smothering
    - Blurred vision
    - Perioral and hand and foot paresthesias
    - Fear of losing control
    - Fear of dying
    - Somatic complaints
    - Chest discomfort
    - Palpitations or tachycardia
    - Dyspnea
    - Choking
    - Faintness
    - Syncope
    - Vertigo
    - Trembling and sweating
    - Urinary frequency and diarrhea
- Patient management primarily is supportive.
- Assure these patients that, although they may feel like they are dying, they are not, and let them know that effective treatment is available.
- Panic attacks may mimic many medical emergencies, including myocardial infarction.
- Any patient who exhibits the signs and symptoms described should be thoroughly assessed and transported for physician evaluation.
- Sedation may be required.
- Patients with anxiety disorders should not be left alone.

Phobia

- Phobia is a type of anxiety disorder. Phobic patients transfer anxiety to a situation or object as an irrational, intense fear of that situation or object.
  - Fear of heights
  - Fear of closed spaces
  - Fear of water
  - Fear of other people
- As the object or situation comes closer to the person, the anxiety increases, and this anxiety may escalate into a panic attack.
- These patients generally recognize that their fear is unreasonable, but they feel that they cannot do anything to prevent it.
- Sometimes the phobia did not initiate the EMS response, but it can become a secondary complication during emergency care.

Patient management

- Explain each step of the care being provided.
- Explain all maneuvers or procedures.
- A careful rehearsal with the patient, explaining exactly what will happen and how care will be accomplished, is important.
- Show patience and understanding of the phobia and assure the patient that no forceful steps will be taken to place the patient in an uncomfortable situation.

Posttraumatic Syndrome (Posttraumatic Stress Disorder)

- Posttraumatic syndrome is an anxiety reaction to a severe psychosocial event.
- These events are often life threatening and associated with repetitive, intrusive memories.
- Manifestations of this condition may include the following:
  - Depression
  - Sleep disturbances
  - Nightmares
  - Survivor guilt
- The syndrome is frequently complicated by substance abuse.

Facts about posttraumatic syndrome

- About 5.2 million people in the United States have posttraumatic syndrome during a given year.
- Posttraumatic syndrome can develop at any age, even during childhood.
- Posttraumatic syndrome is more common in women than in men.
- About 30% of men and women who spent time in war zones develop this disorder.
- Posttraumatic syndrome frequently occurs after violent personal assaults, such as rape, mugging, or domestic violence; terrorism; natural or human-caused disasters; and accidents.
- Depression, alcohol or other substance abuse, or another anxiety disorder often accompanies posttraumatic syndrome.

Mood Disorders

The term mood disorder is used to describe the illnesses of depression and bipolar disorder. Both conditions are associated with an increased risk for suicide.

Depression

- Depression is an impairment of normal functioning.
- It is one of the most prevalent major psychiatric conditions, and it affects 10–15% of the general population.

Facts about depression

- More than 19 million adults in the United States suffer from a major depressive illness each year. Many will be unnecessarily incapacitated for weeks or months because their illness is untreated.
- Twice as many women (12%) as men (7%) are affected by depressive illness each year.
- Depression is a frequent and serious complication of heart attack, stroke, diabetes, and cancer.
- Depression increases the risk of heart attack.
- Depression costs in the United States are more than $30 billion per year in direct and indirect costs.
- Major depression is the leading cause of disability worldwide.
- Major depression is characterized as episodic (usually lasting longer than 1 month), with periods of remission. It is known to have a gradual or rapid onset and, occasionally, a clustering of episodes.
- Patients with depression may show feelings of hopelessness, extreme isolation, tenseness, and irritability.
- In severe cases, depression may be followed by the following:
  - Anhedonia (an inability to feel pleasure or happiness from experiences that ordinarily are pleasurable)
  - Insomnia or hypersomnia
  - Weight loss from decreased appetite or weight gain
  - Decreased libido
  - Deep feelings of worthlessness and guilt
- Depression is associated with an increased risk for suicide.
- Care is directed at quietly talking to the patient about things that appear to be of interest to him or her and at attempting to gain responsiveness.
- Depression may be treated with antidepressant drug therapy, counseling, psychotherapy, and, sometimes, electroconvulsive therapy (ECT).

Bipolar Disorder

- Bipolar disorder is a biphasic emotional disorder in which depressive and manic episodes alternate.
- Mania is characterized by the following:
  - Excessive elation
  - Talkativeness
  - Flight of ideas
  - Motor activity
  - Irritability
  - Accelerated speech
  - Delusions that involve personal grandeur
- Bipolar disorders sometimes begin gradually, but they also may occur abruptly and be precipitated by a single event.
  - The manic phase can be very brief or last weeks to months
- The most frequent age for initial manic episodes is between 20 and 35 years, with initial attacks of depression occurring about 10 years later.

Facts about bipolar disorder

- More than 23 million American ages 18 and over (about 1% of the U.S. population) suffer from bipolar disorder.
- As many as 20% of people with bipolar disorder die by suicide.
- Men and women are equally likely to develop bipolar disorder.
- Prehospital care should focus on the following:
  - Calm, firm emotional support.
  - Transport for physician evaluation.
  - If this is the patient's first manic episode, consider the possibility of drug abuse.
  - Sensory stimulation should be kept to a minimum.
  - If the patient's condition permits, EMS transport should proceed without audible or visual warning devices.

Suicide and Suicide Threats

- A threat of suicide is an indication that a patient has a serious crisis that requires immediate intervention.
- In many cases, suicide attempts are a cry for help or a form of direct or indirect communication, such as "I don't want to live" or "I am angry with you."
- Other suicide attempts are an effort by the patient to manipulate relationships so that he or she will be surrounded by individuals ready and willing to provide advice and support.
- When assessing the risk of suicide, consider these facts:
  - Suicide is the third leading cause of death in people between the ages of 15 and 25 years and the fourth leading cause of death in people between the ages of 25 and 45 years.
  - The highest suicide rates in the United States are found among white men more than 85 years old.
  - Women attempt suicide more often than men.
  - Men successfully commit suicide more often than women.
  - Men use more violent means (e.g., guns, knives) than do women (e.g., pills, razor blades).
  - About 60% of people who successfully commit suicide have a history of a previous attempt.
  - The more specific and detailed the suicide plan, the greater the suicide potential.
- Other factors associated with suicide threats include the following:
  - Recent death of a loved one or loss of a significant relationship
  - Financial setback or job loss
  - Chronic or debilitating illness
  - Social isolation
  - Alcohol or other drug abuse
  - Depression
  - Schizophrenia
- Patient management
  - If a suicide attempt is suspected, it generally is recommended that this suspicion be discussed with the patient.
    - Questions such as "Do you have thoughts about killing yourself or others?" or "Have you ever tried to kill yourself?" are appropriate.
    - Many depressed patients are willing to discuss their suicidal (or homicidal) thoughts.

- Try to ascertain the following:
  - If the patient has a plan (i.e., how and when the suicide will be performed).
  - If the plan is intended to be successful.
  - If the patient has the available means or a method to follow through with the plan.
- When responding to a suicide attempt, request police protection before approaching the scene.
- After scene safety is ensured and access to the patient is gained, the scene should be evaluated for the presence of dangerous objects.
- The priority in patient management is medical care.
- Unconscious patients should be managed with airway, ventilatory, and circulatory support and rapid transport.
- If the patient is conscious, attempt to develop a rapport within a relatively short period.
- Conduct a brief interview to assess the situation and to determine the need and direction for further action.
- The following five steps are helpful in reducing the potential for suicide:
  - Provide support and honest assurance about the patient's well-being.
  - Provide for physical safety and emotional security.

    Establish protective limits and measures to prevent the person from injuring himself or herself or others; this conveys to patients that you will help them control their behavior until they can gain self-control.
  - Listen to the person, even if his or her talk seems bizarre, inappropriate, or unrealistic.

    Do not feel that you must answer every statement or give advice or opinions.

    During the interview, acknowledge the patient's feelings.

    Do not argue with the patient's wish to die.

    Explain alternatives to suicide that the patient may not have considered.
  - Determine the patient's support system or significant others when possible.

    People that know the patient may be better able to communicate with and calm him or her.
  - Encourage and reassure the patient through the crisis.

- Transport the patient to an appropriate facility for emergency intervention.

Substance-Related Disorders

- Psychiatric illness and behavioral problems are often a result of drug dependence, drug abuse, and intoxication from use or misuse of the following:
  - Narcotics and opiates
  - Sedative-hypnotics
  - Stimulants (cocaine)
  - Phencyclidine (PCP)
  - Hallucinogens
  - Tricyclic antidepressants
  - Drugs abused for sexual purposes or sexual gratification
  - Alcohol

Somatoform Disorders

- Somatoform disorders are a group of conditions in which there are physical symptoms for which no physical cause can be found and for which there is definite or strong evidence that the underlying cause is psychological.

- Two of the most common disorders in this group are the following:
  - Somatization disorder
  - Conversion disorder
- Both disorders are associated with anxiety, depression, and threats of suicide.
- Treatment for both disorders often requires psychotherapy.

Somatization Disorder

- Somatization disorder is a condition in which the individual has complaints (lasting several years) of various physical problems for which no physical cause can be found.
- This condition is more common in women than in men.
- It sometimes results in unnecessary surgery and other treatments.
- Symptoms most commonly complained of are as follows:
  - Neurological symptoms
  - Double vision
  - Seizure
  - Weakness
  - Gynecological symptoms
  - Painful menstruation
  - Painful intercourse
  - Gastrointestinal symptoms
  - Abdominal pain
  - Nausea

Facts about somatization disorders

- The lifetime prevalence rate for somatization disorders is 0.2–2.0% of the United States population.
- Somatization disorders are rare in men.
- Somatization disorders tend to run in families and occur in 10–20% of the primary female relatives of patients with somatization disorders.
- Most somatization disorders begin in adolescence or early adulthood and are chronic in nature.
- Symptoms sometimes increase and decrease in severity over time, but usually there are few symptom-free episodes.
- Anxiety and depression often accompany the disorder.
- Suicide threats are common in these patients, but suicide is rarely actually attempted or accomplished.

Conversion Disorder

- Conversion disorder is a mental illness in which painful emotions are repressed and unconsciously converted into physical symptoms.
- There may be a loss of sensory skills, motor skills, or special senses.
- The person suddenly cannot speak, hear, see, or feel.
- An arm or leg is paralyzed.
- In many cases, the areas of the body that are affected do not correspond to the actual arrangement of neural pathways.
- Symptoms also may come and go or appear at different times and in different areas of the body.

Facts about conversion disorder

- True conversion disorder is rare in the United States.
- The disorder is seen more commonly in lower socioeconomic groups and may be more common in military personnel who are exposed to combat situations.
- Conversion disorder may present at any age, but it is rare before the age of 10 years or after the age of 35 years.
- In pediatric patients, the incidence of conversion disorder is increased after physical or sexual abuse.
- The incidence also increases in those children whose parents are either seriously ill or that have chronic pain.
- About 64% of adult patients with conversion disorder have evidence of organic brain disorder.

Management

- Treat symptoms of somatoform disorders as if they are real, because differentiating them from an organic ailment may be difficult.
- It is important to recognize that these patients are not "faking"; they believe their illness or loss of function to be real.
- These patients require physician evaluation.

Factitious Disorders

- Factitious disorders are a group of disorders in which symptoms mimic a true illness but have actually been invented and are under the control of the patient and used as a means of receiving attention.
- The most common disorder in this group is Munchausen's syndrome.
- With this syndrome, the patient makes habitual pleas for treatment and hospitalization for a symptomatic but imaginary acute illness.
- Munchausen's syndrome by proxy is a psychological disorder in which people injure or induce illness in others (usually children) to gain sympathy.
- Factitious disorders include the following:
  - Bereavement
  - Cushing syndrome
  - Dental problems
  - HIV infection
  - Hypoglycemia
  - Munchausen's syndrome
  - Stroke
- Symptoms (which are often dramatic, but plausible) usually resolve with treatment, after which the person seeks further treatment for another imaginary disease.
- Once the factitious disorder is diagnosed, treatment is aimed at protecting these people from unnecessary surgeries and treatments.

Dissociative Disorders

- Dissociative disorders are a group of psychological illnesses in which a particular mental function is separated (dissociated) from the mind as a whole.
- Dissociative disorders include the following:
  - Dissociative amnesia—A disorder characterized by a blocking out of critical personal information, usually of a traumatic or stressful nature.
    - Unlike other types of amnesia, dissociative amnesia does not result from other medical trauma.

  - Dissociative fugue—A rare disorder in which an individual suddenly and unexpectedly takes physical leave of his or her surroundings.
  - Dissociative identity disorder—A disorder also known as multiple personality disorder.
  - Depersonalization disorder—A condition marked by a feeling of detachment or distance from one's own experience, body, or self.
- Dissociative disorders are usually associated with emotional conflicts that are so repressed that a split personality occurs, resulting in an altered state of consciousness or confusion in identity.
- They may also be caused by an inability to cope with a severe stress or conflict, where dissociation occurs suddenly after a catastrophic event (e.g., the traumatic death of a child or spouse).
- With dissociative disorders, a person often is unable to remember his or her name or personal history but can still speak, read, and learn new material.
- Treatment for this condition may include anitianxiety medications, hypnosis, and psychotherapy.

Eating Disorders

- The two most common eating disorders, which are considered forms of psychiatric illness, are the following:
  - Anorexia nervosa
  - Bulimia nervosa
- Both disorders can result in starvation and can be fatal.
  - They are best managed with supervision and regulation of eating habits, psychotherapy, and, sometimes, antidepressants.
  - Most patients with these disorders require hospitalization.

Facts about Eating Disorders

- More than 5 million Americans suffer from eating disorders.
- Anorexia, bulimia, and binge-eating disorders are diseases that affect the mind and body simultaneously.
- Three percent of adolescent and adult women and 1% of men have eating disorders.
- A young woman with anorexia is 12 times more likely to die than a woman of the same age without anorexia.
- Fifteen percent of young women have substantially disordered eating attitudes and behaviors.

Anorexia Nervosa

- Anorexia nervosa is an eating disorder characterized by intense fear of being obese, severe weight loss, and, eventually, amenorrhea.
- The patient with this condition often feels intensely hungry but denies the existence of hunger pains.
- Signs and symptoms:
  - Weight loss
  - Obsession with exercise
  - Fatigue
  - Binge eating
  - Induced vomiting and use of laxatives to promote weight loss
- Anorexia nervosa is primarily seen in adolescents and predominantly in females.
- It is also usually associated with emotional stress or conflict.
- Frequently it is difficult to identify an exact underlying cause of this condition.

Bulimia Nervosa

- Bulimia nervosa (sometimes considered a variant of anorexia) is an insatiable craving for food that often results in episodes of binge eating followed by purging (through self-induced vomiting or use of laxatives), depression, and self-deprivation.
- Bulimia is most common in adolescent girls and young women.
- Anorexic and bulimic patients are often highly distressed about their compulsive behavior, and, as a result, may become depressed and suicidal.
- Anorexia and bulimia can lead to serious dehydration, starvation, and electrolyte imbalances that may cause critical illness or death.

Impulse Control Disorders

- Impulse control disorders are a group of psychiatric disorders characterized by the inability to resist an impulse or temptation to do some act that is unlawful, socially unacceptable, or self-harmful.
- Examples include the following:
  - Pathological gambling
  - Kleptomania (an impulse to steal)
  - Pyromania (an impulse to set fires)
- These disorders are often difficult to treat.
- Imprisonment of patients with these conditions is not unusual.
- Obsessive-compulsive disorder (OCD):
  - OCD is a psychiatric disorder in which the person feels stress or anxiety about thoughts or rituals over which he or she has little control.
  - Facts about obsessive-compulsive disorder.
    - — About 3.3 million adults in the United States have OCD during any given year.
    - — OCD affects both men and women with equal frequency.
    - — The nation's social and economic loss due to OCD totals more than 8 billion dollars each year.
  - OCD can take many forms, including the following:
    - — Frequent hand washing or showering
    - — Thoughts or mental images of an upsetting nature (e.g., violence, vulgarities, harm to self or others)
    - — Obsessions about special numbers, colors, single words, phrases, or even melodies
  - It is common for a person with OCD to have clinical depression, panic attacks, or both.
  - Although most adults realize in part that these obsessions and compulsions are senseless, they have great difficulty stopping them.
    - — Children with OCD may not realize that their behavior is unusual.
  - People with OCD often cleverly hide their condition from family, friends, and coworkers.
  - Medications (e.g., antidepressants) and behavior therapies give many patients significant relief from OCD.

Personality Disorders

- Personality disorders are a large group of conditions characterized by a general failure to learn from experience or adapt appropriately to changes; they often result in personal distress and impairment of social functioning.
- These disorders (which may have an environmental or heritable component) often produce behavior that is especially obvious during times of stress.

- Symptoms are generally first recognized in adolescence and continue throughout life.
  - Depression and anxiety are common in this group
- Maladaptive behavior patterns associated with these conditions impair a person's ability to function in society and severely limit adapting potential.
- Examples of personality disorders include the following:
  - Eccentric behavior
  - Paranoia
  - Narcissism (intense self-love)
  - Obsessive-compulsive behavior
- Treatment of these conditions involves behavior modification techniques, counseling, and individual psychotherapy.

SPECIAL BEHAVIORAL PROBLEMS

Assessing the Potentially Violent Patient

- Only a small proportion of people with mental health problems are potentially violent; nonetheless, assessment and management of the potentially violent patient should be part of an EMS protocol.
- Factors that may help determine the potential for a violent episode:
  - Past history—Has the patient exhibited hostile, aggressive, or violent behavior in the past?
  - Posture—Is the patient sitting or standing? Does the patient appear to be tense or rigid?
  - Vocal activity—Loud, obscene, and erratic speech indicates emotional distress.
  - Physical activity—Is the patient pacing, agitating, or displaying protection of physical boundaries?
- If any signs of potentially violent behavior are present, attempt to reduce the impact of the stress, but avoid confrontation and prepare a way to cope with the crisis that reduces the potential for a life-threatening incident or psychologically damaging consequences.
- Controlling violent situations:
  - Severely disturbed patients who pose a threat to themselves or others may need to be restrained, transported, and hospitalized against their will.
  - Each state has a statute covering the criteria for involuntary commitment; be familiar with all applicable laws in your state of employment.
  - The premise on which most state laws are based suggests that one person may restrain another to protect life or prevent injury.
  - When a psychiatric patient refuses care in the prehospital setting, EMS personnel should consult with medical direction.
  - The decision to restrain, treat, or release the patient is the decision of medical direction.
  - If violent behavior must be contained, "reasonable force" to restrain the patient should be carried out in as humanely a way as possible.
  - In most cases where restraint is deemed necessary, the restraint duty should be given to law enforcement personnel.
  - As in all other aspects of health care, details of the incident should be carefully recorded for future reference.
  - When dealing with a patient who may require restraint, be sure to do the following:
    - — Ensure a safe environment
    - — Gather a pertinent medical and psychiatric history
    - — Attempt to gain the patient's cooperation
    - — Be confident but not confrontational

Restraint Guidelines

- If the patient is homicidal, do not attempt restraint without law enforcement assistance.
- If the patient is armed, move everyone out of range, retreat from the scene, and wait for law enforcement personnel to arrive.
- Remember that the patient may not be responsible for his or her actions.
- Plan your restraining action to include a backup plan in case the initial action fails.
- Be sure that adequate help is available.
- Be sure that a minimum of four capable individuals are available to help restrain an adult patient.
- Remember that the potential for personal injury and legal liability is always present.
  - The dignity of the patient should be respected as much as possible during the restraining process.
- Restraint methods:
  - Begin with a gentle, nonthreatening, low-profile approach and progress to more direct intervention as needed.
  - Always explain the options of physical restraint to the patient before applying force.
  - If the patient is still unwilling to cooperate, he or she should be advised that restraint is necessary to protect against injury and to ensure the safety of others.
  - Before approaching the violent patient, be aware of the patient's surroundings.
    - — Note seemingly harmless items including ashtrays, lighted cigarettes, hot coffee, letter openers, soda bottles, cans, and furniture.
  - Do not attempt to enter the patient's physical space (usually considered one arm's length) until the other members involved in the restraint action are ready to proceed.
    - — Consider the patient's muscle groups and potential range of motion before initiating restraint procedures.
    - — Plan to position the patient in a way that limits the effectiveness of his or her strength and range of motion.
    - — Each member of the restraint team should be assigned a specific body part or responsibility before actual restraint activity.
  - Be familiar with the restraint devices available, and improvise if the need arises.
    - — The preferred method of restraint is to use commercially manufactured wrist/waist/ankle padded leather or Velcro straps or full-jacket restraints.
    - — Effective restraints may also be improvised using common materials such as the following:

      Small towels that can be wrapped around the patient's wrists and ankles and secured with tape to the stretcher

      Cravats

      Webbed straps ordinarily used to secure patients to spine boards

      Roller bandages

      Blanket roll
    - — Whatever the types of restraint used, they should be strong enough to produce the desired effect without compromising the patient's circulatory or respiratory status.
- Sequence of restraint actions:
  - Offer the patient one final opportunity to cooperate.
  - If there is no response, a minimum of two rescuers should move swiftly toward the patient and position themselves close to and slightly behind the patient.
    - — Each rescuer should then position an inside leg in front of the patient's leg to force the patient into a prone position if needed.

  - — Swift movement by two or more rescuers minimizes the patient's ability to focus on restraint actions and decreases the accuracy of kicks or blows.
  - — During the restraint procedure, the patient should be continually reassured by a rescuer that is not involved in the physical maneuver.
- ◦ If the patient calms and agrees to be transported without restraints, the paramedic positions the patient supine on a stretcher (if not contraindicated by mechanism of injury or medical condition) and secures the patient with straps to limit range of motion.
  - — If the patient becomes dangerous on the way to the hospital, restraints should be employed.
- ◦ Once applied, restraints should not be removed until the patient is delivered to the emergency department or until there are adequate resources to control the situation.
  - — Restrained limbs should be checked periodically for adequacy of circulation and the presence of soft tissue injury.
  - — If a change in the restraints is required, adequate assistance must be available and only one limb should be repositioned at a time.
- ◦ The patient's respiratory and circulatory status should frequently be assessed (and documented) to ensure that the restraint action has not compromised vital functions.
- ◦ Restraint procedures should be thoroughly documented on the prehospital care report.
  - — Attempts at negotiations and the sequence of patient behavior that led to the need for restraint should be clearly described.
  - — Documentation also should verify that circulatory evaluation and continued monitoring of the patient were performed after restraint.
  - — Again, physical restraint is recommended only when all verbal and nonverbal techniques have been exhausted and only when an individual presents a danger to self or others.

Personal Safety

- Although personal safety should be considered during any emergency response, behavioral emergencies are more likely to require that the paramedic protect himself or herself and the crew from hostile injury.
- The following methods to avoid personal injury should be considered:
  - ◦ When possible, remain at a safe distance from the patient.
  - ◦ Do not allow the patient to block your exit.
  - ◦ Keep large furniture between you and the patient.
  - ◦ Do not allow a single paramedic to remain alone with the patient.
  - ◦ Do not make threatening statements.
  - ◦ Use folded blankets or cushions to absorb the impact of thrown objects.
  - ◦ Be familiar with the various training programs have been developed to provide safety and security to the rescuer and to the violent patient.
- Nonviolent personal protection maneuvers should be learned and practiced under the supervision of someone trained in these procedures.

Behavioral Problems in Children

- Young children who are victims of an emotional crisis need to be managed with techniques that differ from those used to care for older children and adults.
- The following suggestions may be helpful when dealing with children:
  - ◦ Gain the child's trust and try to convince the child that you are a friend who can help.
  - ◦ Make it clear to the child that you are strong enough to be in control but that you will not hurt him or her.

    - Keep the interview questions brief; the child's attention span may be extremely short.
    - Never lie; be honest.
    - Use all available resources to communicate (e.g., draw pictures, tell stories).
    - Involve parents or caregivers in the interview or examination (if appropriate).
    - Take any threat of violence seriously.
- If the child's behavior or physical condition makes restraint necessary, use only reasonable force (with sufficient help) to ensure the patient's safety and the safety of the EMS crew.
- If calming measures fail to work, wrapping the child in a full body blanket and securing the child and blanket to the stretcher with straps often is sufficient during transport for physician evaluation.
    - Monitor the child's airway and circulation and ensure that they are not compromised.
    - Documentation should be thorough and complete.

CHAPTER QUESTIONS

1. A 65-year-old male is anxious and says he feels like he is going crazy. The patient has no past medical history of mental illness and is in good physical health. During initial contact with the patient, your first step should be to:
   a. place patient in soft restraints and transport
   b. reassure the patient that it was a good idea to call for help
   c. advise the patient to seek drug counseling services
   d. perform a detailed exam
2. Which one of the following is least characteristic in a person with a suicide plan?
   a. Excessive grieving over death of a spouse
   b. Giving one's possessions away
   c. Obsessing about death and dying
   d. Exhibiting transient personality disorders
3. You are called to assist a 30-year-old female in crisis who just lost her job. She has a history of chronic emotional instability and poly substance drug abuse. Your patient tells you she feels helpless and worthless. You are concerned about her risk for suicide because of all of the following EXCEPT for her:
   a. gender
   b. history of drug abuse
   c. age
   d. history of emotional instability

Suggested Reading

US Department of Transportation, National Highway Traffic Safety Administration. *EMT-Paramedic: National Standard Curriculum*. Washington, DC: US Department of Transportation, National Highway Traffic Safety Administration; 1998.

Chapter 32
Gynecology

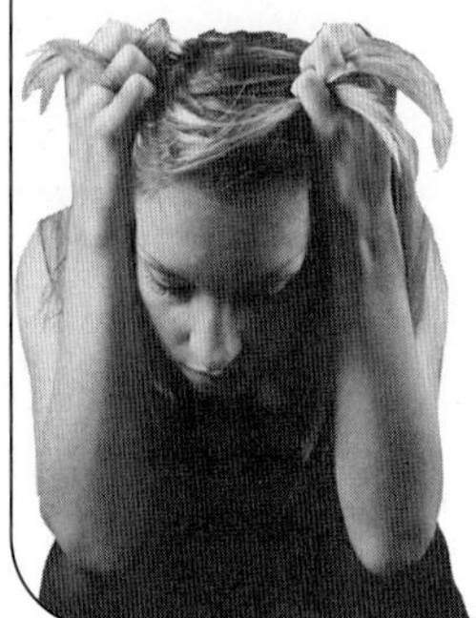

You are treating a conscious and alert 32-year-old female patient that presents with vaginal bleeding, abdominal pain, cool and clammy skin, tachycardia, and hypotension. The patient states the pain has been increasing in intensity throughout the day and is now unbearable. She denies any recent history of trauma and states she may be pregnant! Her last menstrual cycle was 2 months ago.

You suspect an ectopic pregnancy. What would your primary management include?

A number of disorders can occur in the female reproductive system, some of which lead to gynecological emergencies.

FEMALE REPRODUCTIVE SYSTEM (FIGURE 32-1)

- Components of the female anatomy:
  - Ovaries
  - Uterine (fallopian) tubes
  - Uterus
  - Vagina
  - External genital organs
  - Mammary glands
- Purpose of female organs is to produce oocytes, and to receive spermatozoa for fertilization, conception, gestation, and birth.

Ovaries

- The two small ovaries are attached to the posterior of the broad ligament (mesovarium).
- Other ligaments associated with the ovaries are the suspensory ligaments and the ovarian ligaments.
- Ovarian arteries, veins, and nerves traverse the suspensory ligament and enter the ovary through the mesovarium.
- Each ovary consists of a dense outer portion (cortex) and a looser inner portion (medulla).
- Ovarian follicles (each of which contains an oocyte) are distributed throughout the cortex.

Uterine Tubes

- Uterine tubes are ducts for the ovaries and open directly into the peritoneal cavity to receive the oocyte.

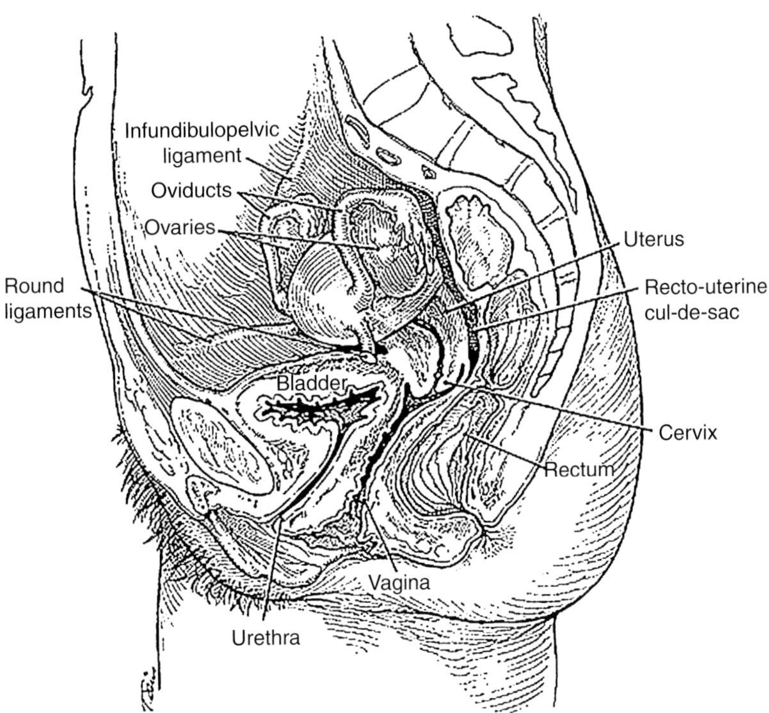

Figure 32-1 Female reproductive system. (*Used with permission from Cunningham FG, Leveno KL, Bloom SL, et al (eds). Williams Obstetrics. 22nd Edition. New York: McGraw-Hill, p. 19.*)

Uterus

- The uterus is the size and shape of a medium-sized pear.
- The fundus (the larger, rounded portion of the uterus) is directed superiorly, and the cervix, inferiorly.
- The main portion of the uterus is positioned between the fundus and the cervix.
- Ligaments that hold the uterus in place are as follows:
  - Broad ligament
  - Round ligaments
  - Uterosacral ligaments

Vagina

- The vagina functions to receive the penis during intercourse.
- It also provides a passageway for menstrual flow and childbirth.
- The vaginal orifice is covered by a thin mucous membrane (hymen).

External Genitalia (Vulva)

- The external genitalia of the female consists of the vestibule and surrounding structures and is bordered by a pair of skin folds (labia minora)

Clitoris

- The clitoris is a small erectile structure located in the anterior margin of the vestibule.
- The two labia minora unite over the clitoris to form a fold of skin (prepuce).

Labia Majora

- The labia majora are the two prominent folds of skin lateral to the labia minora.
- They unite anteriorly over the pubic symphysis to form the mons pubis.

Perineum

- The perineum is divided into triangles by perineal muscles.
- The urogenital triangle contains the external genitalia.
- The posterior anal triangle contains the anal opening.
- The clinical perineum is the region between the vagina and the anus; this area sometimes tears during childbirth.

Mammary Glands

- Mammary glands are the organs of milk production located within the breasts.
- The breasts of both males and females have a raised nipple surrounded by a circular pigmented areola.
- The nipples are sensitive to tactile stimulation.
- They may become erect in response to sexual arousal.
- Female breasts enlarge during puberty under the influence of estrogen and progesterone.
- Each adult female mammary gland consists of 15–20 glandular lobes that are covered by adipose tissue.
- Each lobe possesses a single lactiferous duct that divides to form smaller ducts, each of which supplies a lobule.
- These ducts expand at their ends to form secretory sacs called alveoli, which secrete milk during nursing.

MENSTRUATION AND OVULATION

Menstruation

- Menstruation is the normal periodic discharge of blood, mucus, and cellular debris from the uterine mucosa. The normal menstrual cycle is about 28 days.
- Menstruation occurs at more or less regular intervals from puberty to menopause (except during pregnancy and lactation).
- The average menstrual flow of 25–60 mL usually lasts 4–6 days and is fairly constant for each individual from cycle to cycle.
- The onset of menses (menarche) generally begins between the ages of 12 and 13 years and ends permanently (menopause) at an average age of 47 years; however, there is wide variation for both menarche and menopause.
- Depending on the individual, normal menopause may occur as early as age 35 or as late as age 60.

Follicle and Oocyte Development

- By the fourth month of prenatal life, the ovaries contain about 5 million cells from which oocytes (immature ova) develop.
- At birth, a female infant is carrying about 2 million primary oocytes; this number declines to about 300,000–400,000 at puberty.
- Of these primary oocytes, only about 400 are eventually released from the ovary.
- Oocytes are surrounded by a layer of cells (granulosa cells), and the entire structure is known as a primary follicle.

- The menstrual cycle is associated with hormonal changes that stimulate some primary follicles to continue development and become secondary follicles.
- The secondary follicle continues to enlarge and forms a lump on the surface of the ovary.
- The fully mature follicle is known as the vesicular or Graafian follicle.

Ovulation

- Cellular secretions of the graafian follicle cause it to swell more rapidly than can be accommodated by follicular growth.
- The follicle expands and ruptures, thereby forcing a small amount of blood and follicular fluid out of the vesicle.
- Shortly after this initial burst of fluid, an oocyte escapes from the follicle.
- The release of this secondary oocyte is called *ovulation.*
- After ovulation, the follicle is transformed into a yellow glandular structure called the *corpus luteum.*
- Cells of the corpus luteum secrete large amounts of progesterone and smaller amounts of estrogen.
- If pregnancy occurs, the fertilized oocyte (zygote) begins releasing a hormonelike substance (chorionic gonadotropin) that keeps the corpus luteum from degenerating.
- As a result, blood levels of estrogen and progesterone do not decrease, and the menstrual period does not occur.
- In the absence of pregnancy, the corpus luteum degenerates, and the secondary oocyte passes out of the system with the menstrual flow.

Hormonal Control of Ovulation and Menses

- Ovulation and menses are controlled by hormones released from the following organs:
  - The hypothalamus
  - The anterior pituitary
- Follicle-stimulating hormone (FSH) stimulates development of the follicle, including the cells that produce estrogen.
  - Before ovulation, these cells release estrogen and cause a surge in the pituitary production of luteinizing hormone (LH).
- LH initiates the ovarian cycle (leading to ovulation), which in turn regulates the uterine cycle.
- Under the influence of the ovarian hormones, the lining of the uterus (endometrium) goes through two phases of development—The proliferative phase and the secretory phase.
  - The proliferative phase is initiated and maintained by the increasing amounts of estrogen produced by the maturing follicle.
    — Estrogen stimulates the endometrium to grow and increase in thickness, which prepares the uterus for the implantation of a fertilized ovum.
  - The secretory phase begins after ovulation and is under the combined influence of estrogen and progesterone.
  - During this phase, tortuous secretory glands and spiral vessels develop to prepare the endometrium for implantation of the fertilized ovum.
  - Within 7 days after ovulation (about day 21 of the menstrual cycle), the endometrium is ready to receive the developing embryo if fertilization has occurred.
- In the absence of fertilization, the ovum can survive only 6–24 hours, after which the hormone levels drop and the endometrium is shed as menstrual flow. This process normally occurs on day 28 of the menstrual cycle (about 14 days after ovulation). The oocyte can be fertilized for up to 24 hours after ovulation.

SPECIFIC GYNECOLOGICAL EMERGENCIES

Nontraumatic Abdominal Pain

- Besides gastrointestinal causes of abdominal pain, acute or chronic infection involving the patient's uterus, ovaries, fallopian tubes, and adjacent structures may be a source of severe abdominal pain.
- The scope of abdominal pain associated with the female reproductive system may range from benign episodes of difficult menstruation to a potentially life-threatening hemorrhage from a ruptured ovarian cyst or ectopic pregnancy.

Pelvic Inflammatory Disease

- Pelvic inflammatory disease (PID) affects about 1 million women annually and is responsible for more than 250,000 hospitalizations each year.
- It results from infection of one or more of the following:
  - Cervix
  - Uterus
  - Fallopian tubes
  - Ovaries and their supporting structures
- PID is usually caused by sexually transmitted bacteria, most commonly *Neisseria gonorrhoeae* and *Chlamydia trachomatis.*
- Staphylococci, streptococci, and other pathogens may also cause PID, but these organisms are usually transmitted by doctor's instruments during medical procedures.
- This condition is characterized by ascending infection of the vaginal area:
  - The cervix (cervicitis)
  - The uterus proper (endometritis)
  - The fallopian tubes (salpingitis)
  - The supporting structures around the uterus and the fallopian tubes (parametritis)

Signs and symptoms of PID

- Diffuse lower abdominal pain
- Low-grade fever (variable)
- Vaginal discharge
- Dyspareunia (pain with intercourse)
- PID frequently follows onset of menstrual bleeding by 7–10 days
- It may also be accompanied by pain during ambulation ("PID shuffle")
- Consequences of PID include the following:
  - Secondary infertility
  - Ectopic pregnancies
  - Tubo-ovarian abscesses
  - Surgical removal of reproductive organs (in severe cases)
- Definitive treatment usually consists of antibiotic therapy

Ruptured Ovarian Cyst

- A ruptured ovarian cyst is a gynecological emergency that can result in significant internal hemorrhage.
- An ovarian cyst is a thin-walled, fluid-filled sac on the surface of the ovary.

- Abdominal pain caused by an ovarian cyst may result from the following:
  - Rapid expansion
  - Torsion that produces ischemia
  - Acute rupture
- Corpus luteum cyst is the type of cyst most prone to rupture.
  - It forms because of hemorrhage in a mature corpus luteum
  - Most ruptures occur approximately 1 week before menstrual bleeding is due to begin
    - — Corpus luteum develops after ovulation
- Some patients may present with vaginal bleeding or report a late or missed period at the time of rupture.

Signs and symptoms

- Localized, unilateral abdominal pain
- Generalized signs of peritonitis
- Onset of pain is often associated with one of the following:
  - Minimal abdominal trauma
  - Sexual intercourse
  - Exercise

Cystitis

- Cystitis is an inflammation of the inner lining of the bladder. And is usually caused by a bacterial infection.
- Although both sexes can develop infection, cystitis in women is more common because the urethra is shorter, making it easier for infectious agents from the vagina or rectum to pass from the mucous membrane around the urethral opening and into the bladder.
- Signs and symptoms:
  - Frequent urge to pass urine, but only a small amount of urine passed each time (primary symptom)
  - Painful (burning) urination
  - Fever
  - Chills
  - Lower abdominal pain
  - The urine may occasionally be foul smelling or contain blood
- Prompt treatment of cystitis with antibiotics usually settles the infection within 24 hours.

Dysmenorrhea and Mittelschmerz

- Many women experience dysmenorrhea (painful menstruation)

Signs and symptoms

- Painful menses.
- Headache.
- Faintness.
- Dizziness.
- Nausea.
- Diarrhea.
- Backache.
- Leg pain.

- In severe cases, chills, headache, diarrhea, nausea, vomiting, and syncope can occur.
- The condition is more common in unmarried women and in women who have not borne children.
- Abdominal pain is associated with this condition and thought to be related to the following:
    - Muscular contraction of the myometrium (the muscular layer of the uterus) mediated by local prostaglandins
    - Infection
    - Inflammation
    - Presence of intrauterine contraceptive device
- Mittelschmerz (German for "middle pain"):
    - Mittelschmerz may occur during the menstrual cycle due to rupture of the graafian follicle and bleeding from the ovary
    - It is characterized by right- or left-lower-quadrant abdominal pain that occurs in the normal midcycle of a menstrual period (after ovulation)
    - It usually lasts about 24–36 hours
    - Hormones produced by the ovary may also result in slight endometrial bleeding and low-grade fever
- Dysmenorrhea and mittelschmerz are not life threatening.
    - Physician evaluation is required to rule out more serious causes of menstrual pain

Endometritis

- It is an inflammation of the uterine lining.
- It usually occurs as the result of infection. It most often occurs after childbirth or abortion as a result of retained placental tissue.
    - The condition is also a feature of PID and other sexually transmitted infections.
- It may affect the uterus and fallopian tubes.
    - If untreated, endometritis may result in sterility, sepsis, and death.
- Signs and symptoms:
    - Fever
    - Purulent vaginal discharge
    - Lower abdominal pain
- Treatment includes removal of any foreign tissue and antibiotic therapy.

Endometriosis

- Endometriosis is an abnormal gynecological condition characterized by ectopic growth and functioning of endometrial tissue.
- It is thought to result from fragments of endometrium being regurgitated backward during menstruation through the fallopian tubes into the peritoneal cavity, where they attach and grow as small cystic structures.
- The endometrial tissue of endometriosis functions cyclically and undergoes periodic menstrual breakdown that results in bleeding within the cysts, stretching of the walls of the cysts, and pain.
- It is more common in women who defer pregnancy.
    - The average age of women found to have endometriosis is 37 years.

Signs and symptoms

- Pain (particularly dysmenorrhea)
- Painful defecation

- Suprapubic soreness
  - Premenstrual vaginal staining of blood
  - Infertility
- After physician evaluation, treatment of endometriosis may consist of medication with analgesics or hormones and sometimes surgery

Ectopic Pregnancy

- Ectopic pregnancy is a pregnancy that develops outside of the uterus (most commonly in a fallopian tube but sometimes in an ovary or rarely in the abdominal cavity or cervix).
- Most ectopic pregnancies are discovered during the first 2 months of pregnancy, often before the woman realizes she is pregnant.

Signs and symptoms

- Severe abdominal pain.
- Vaginal "spotting."
- If rupture occurs, internal hemorrhage, sepsis, and shock may develop.
- This condition is treated with surgery to remove the developing fetus, the placenta, and any damaged tissue at the site of the pregnancy.
- Ectopic pregnancy is common (occurs in 19.7 out of every 1000 pregnancies).
- It should be considered in any female of reproductive age with abdominal pain.
- Vaginal bleeding is due to the loss of blood from the uterus, cervix, or vagina.
- The most common source of nontraumatic vaginal bleeding is menstruation, which rarely results in a request for emergency care.
- Possible causes of serious nonmenstrual bleeding include the following:
  - Spontaneous abortion
  - Disorders of the placenta
  - Hormonal imbalances (especially menopause)
  - Lesions
  - PID
  - Onset of labor

Traumatic Abdominal Pain

- Traumatic abdominal pain in the female patient is usually associated with vaginal bleeding or sexual assault.
- Vaginal bleeding:
  - Traumatic causes of vaginal bleeding include the following:
    - Straddle injuries
    - Blows to the perineum
    - Blunt force to the lower abdomen
  - Other causes include the following:
    - Foreign bodies inserted into the vagina
    - Injury during intercourse
    - Abortion attempts
    - Soft tissue injures that result from sexual assault
  - Complications of vaginal bleeding that result from trauma may cause organ rupture of any or all of the pelvic organs.
    - This can lead to life-threatening hypovolemia and shock
  - Treatment is consistent with severe internal injuries and often requires surgical repair.

GENERAL PRINCIPLES OF ASSESSMENT AND MANAGEMENT

- Precise diagnosis of lower abdominal pain in the female is difficult because many gynecological conditions produce common clinical characteristics.
- Ruptured ectopic pregnancy, ruptured ovarian cyst, and PID can have identical presentations.
- The goal of prehospital care is to quickly identify conditions that require aggressive therapy and rapid transport for surgical intervention.
- Prehospital care includes the following:
  - Obtaining a history of the present illness, including a thorough gynecological history
  - Providing airway, ventilatory, and circulatory support as needed
  - Transporting the patient for physician evaluation

History of Present Illness and Obstetric History

- A history of the present illness should be obtained to better understand the patient's chief complaint.
- Associated symptoms that may be important include the following:
  - Fever
  - Diaphoresis
  - Syncope
  - Diarrhea
  - Constipation
  - Abdominal cramping
- Besides gathering information appropriate for all patients, the interview should be expanded to include a thorough obstetric history.
- The obstetric history includes:
  - Pregnancy
    - — Total number of pregnancies (gravida)
    - — Number of pregnancies carried to term (para)
    - — Previous Cesarean deliveries
  - Last menstrual period
    - — Date
    - — Duration
    - — Normalcy
    - — Bleeding between periods
    - — Regularity
    - — Possibility of pregnancy
    - — Missed or late period
  - Breast tenderness
  - Urinary frequency
  - Morning sickness (nausea and/or vomiting)
  - Unprotected sexual activity
  - History of previous gynecological problems
    - — Infections
    - — Bleeding
    - — Dyspareunia
    - — Miscarriage

    — Abortion
    — Ectopic pregnancy
  - Present blood loss
    — Color
    — Amount (number of pads soaked per hour)
    — Duration
  - Vaginal discharge
    — Color
    — Amount
    — Odor
  - Use and type of contraceptive
    — Birth control pills
    — Intrauterine device
    — Spermicide
    — Condoms
    — Withdrawal/rhythm method
    — Tubal ligation
    — Contraceptive systems (Norplant, Depo-Provera)
  - History of trauma to the reproductive system
  - Degree of emotional distress

Physical Examination

- The physical examination should be conducted with a comforting and professional attitude.
- Attempts should be made to protect the patient's modesty, to maintain privacy, and to be considerate of reasons for the patient's discomfort.
- When evaluating the potential for serious blood loss, assess the patient's skin and mucous membranes for color, cyanosis, or pallor.
- Vital sign assessment should include orthostatic measurements.
- If indicated, the vaginal area should be inspected for bleeding or discharge, and the following should be noted:
  - Color
  - Amount
  - Presence of clots or tissue
- The abdomen should be auscultated (if time permits) and palpated to assess for the following:
  - Masses
  - Areas of tenderness
  - Guarding
  - Distention
  - Rebound tenderness

Patient Management

- Patient management includes support of the patient's vital functions.
- High-concentration oxygen should be administered during transport.
- Intravenous (IV) access is usually not necessary unless the patient is demonstrating signs of impending shock or has excessive vaginal bleeding.

- Many patients will prefer to be transported in a left-lateral, recumbent, knee-chest position or in a hips-raised, knees-bent position for comfort.
- During transport, monitor the patient for the onset of serious bleeding.
  - If this occurs or if the patient's condition begins to deteriorate, establish one or two large-bore IV lines with normal saline solution or lactated Ringer's solution
  - Monitor ECG and pulse oximetry
  - Drug therapy (such as, analgesics) may mask important symptoms and generally should not be administered before physician evaluation

SEXUAL ASSAULT

Characteristics of Sexual Assault

- Sexual assault is a crime of violence with serious physical and psychological implications. Men and women of all ages may be victims of sexual assault, but it most often affects women and young girls. It is estimated that one in three women will be raped during their lifetime and that only 16% of these crimes will be reported.
- The paramedic is often the first to encounter victims of sexual assault.
- The emergency medical service (EMS) worker must use tact, kindness, and sensitivity during patient care.
- Treat all life-threatening injuries in the usual manner. If possible, move the patient to a private area for physical examination and history taking.
- If possible, allow the patient to be examined and interviewed by a crew member of the same gender.

History Taking

- Avoid detailed questions about the incident. Limit questions to those necessary to provide emergency care. Allow the patient to speak openly about the event. Record all information accurately and thoroughly.

Assessment

- Identify physical trauma outside the pelvic area that needs immediate attention.
- Common injuries include the following:
  - Facial fractures
  - Human bites of the hands and breasts
  - Long bone fractures
  - Broken ribs
  - Abdominal trauma
- Examine the genitalia only if severe injury is present or suspected.
- If possible, explain all procedures to the patient before the examination takes place.
- Document all findings and observations, including the following:
  - Patient's emotional state
  - Condition of the victim's clothing
  - Obvious injuries
  - Any care rendered
- Maintain a nonjudgmental and professional attitude.

Management

- After managing a life-threatening injury, emotional support is the most important patient care procedure that can be offered to a victim of sexual abuse.
- Provide a safe environment for the patient.

- Respond appropriately to the victim's physical and emotional needs.
- Be aware of the need to preserve evidence from the crime scene.
- Special considerations include the following:
  - Handle the victim's clothing as little as possible.
  - Do not clean wounds unless absolutely necessary.
  - Do not allow the patient to drink or to brush teeth.
  - Do not use plastic bags for bloodstained articles.
  - Bag each item of clothing separately using a paper bag.
  - Ask the victim not to change clothes or bathe.
  - Disturb the crime scene as little as possible.

CHAPTER QUESTIONS

1. When examining the victim of sexual assault, the paramedic should:
   a. avoid examining the genitalia due the emotional state of the victim
   b. examine the genitalia if severe injury is present or suspected
   c. question the victim in detail about the incident in order to determine the need for an examination of the genitalia
   d. complete a thorough examination of the genitalia to collect evidence
2. Of the following, the most important aspect in the management of the sexually abused female patient is:
   a. offering psychological and emotional support
   b. assisting the patient if she wants to wash up before transport
   c. careful vaginal examination
   d. thoroughly questioning the victim about the incident

Suggested Reading

US Department of Transportation, National Highway Traffic Safety Administration. *EMT-Paramedic: National Standard Curriculum.* Washington, DC: US Department of Transportation, National Highway Traffic Safety Administration; 1998.

Chapter 33
Obstetrics

You are caring for an 18-year-old primigravida patient who is in her 30th week. She complains of being dizzy with a severe headache. Her pulse is 90, respirations 16, and blood pressure 168/128. While your partner is taking off a ring which appears to be impairing her circulation in her finger, she becomes unresponsive and exhibits tonic-clonic activity.

Which IV medication should be included in your management of this patient?

- Childbirth is common in the prehospital setting.
- Most often, emergency medical service (EMS) personnel only assist in this natural process and provide appropriate care for the mother and newborn.
- Obstetrical emergencies can develop suddenly and become life threatening.
- The paramedic must be prepared to recognize and manage these events and sometimes assist in abnormal deliveries.

NORMAL EVENTS OF PREGNANCY

- Fertilization occurs in a fallopian tube when the head of a sperm penetrates a mature ovum. After penetration, the nuclei of the sperm and ovum fuse, and the newly fertilized ovum becomes a zygote.
- The zygote undergoes repeated cell divisions as it passes down the fallopian tube.
- After a few days of rapid cell division, a ball of cells called a morula is formed and develops into a blastocyst, and implantation in the uterus occurs.
- Implantation begins within 7 days after fertilization and is completed when the trophoblast cells make contact with maternal circulation (about day 12).

SPECIALIZED STRUCTURES OF PREGNANCY

Placenta

- For about 14 days after ovulation, the trophoblast cells continue to develop and form the placenta. The placenta is a disclike organ composed of interlocking fetal and maternal tissues.
- The placenta serves as the organ of exchange between the mother and fetus and is responsible for the following five functions:
  - Transfer of gases
    - The diffusion of oxygen and carbon dioxide through the placental membrane is similar to that which occurs through the pulmonary membranes.
    - Dissolved oxygen in maternal blood passes through the placenta into fetal blood because of the pressure gradient between the blood of the mother and fetus.

    — Conversely, as fetal PCO_2 accumulates, a low-pressure gradient of carbon dioxide develops across the placental membrane, and diffusion of carbon dioxide from fetal blood to maternal blood occurs.
- ◦ Transport of nutrients
    — Other metabolic substrates needed by the fetus diffuse into fetal blood in the same manner as oxygen.
    — Other substrates transported by way of diffusion include fatty acids, potassium, sodium, and chloride.
    — Some nutrients are also actively absorbed by the placenta from maternal blood.
- ◦ Excretion of wastes
    — Waste products such as urea, uric acid, and creatinine diffuse from fetal blood into maternal blood where they are excreted along with the waste products of the mother.
    — This transfer of wastes from fetus to mother occurs in the same manner as does carbon dioxide.
- ◦ Hormone production
    — The placenta becomes a temporary endocrine gland (secreting sufficient quantities of estrogen and progesterone), so that by the third month of fetal development, the corpus luteum is no longer needed to sustain the pregnancy.
    — Estrogen, progesterone, and other hormones maintain the uterine lining, prevent the occurrence of menses, and stimulate changes in the mother's breasts, vagina, and cervix that prepare her body for delivery and motherhood.
- ◦ Formation of a barrier
    — The placenta provides a barrier against some harmful substances and chemicals in the mother's circulation.
    — The placental barrier is incomplete and nonselective and therefore does not provide total protection to the fetus.
    — Among the drugs easily transported across the placenta are steroids, narcotics, anesthetics, and some antibiotics.

Umbilical Cord

- Blood flows from the fetus to the placenta by way of two umbilical arteries carrying deoxygenated blood; oxygenated blood returns to the fetus by one umbilical vein.
- The blood remains in a closed system independent of and separated from the maternal circulation.
- Other structures unique to fetal circulation are the ductus venosus, foramen ovale, and ductus arteriosum.
- The ductus venosus is a continuation of the umbilical cord and serves as a shunt to allow most blood returning from the placenta to bypass the immature liver of the embryo and empty directly into the inferior vena cava.
- The foramen ovale and ductus arteriosum allow blood to bypass the nonfunctional lungs, which remain collapsed until birth.
- The foramen ovale shunts blood from the right atrium directly into the left atrium, and the ductus arteriosum connects the aorta and pulmonary artery.
- Thus, well-oxygenated blood from the placenta enters the left side of the heart rather than the right side and is pumped by the left ventricle into the vessels of the head and forelimbs.
- The blood entering the right atrium from the superior vena cava is directed downward through the tricuspid valve into the right ventricle.

- Most of this blood is deoxygenated blood from the head region of the fetus and is pumped by the right ventricle into the pulmonary artery. From there it passes through the ductus arteriosum into the descending aorta and through the two umbilical arteries into the placenta for oxygenation.
- At birth, the various arteriovenous (AV) shunts close.

Amniotic Sac and Amniotic Fluid

- The amniotic sac is a fluid-filled cavity that surrounds and protects the embryo.
- Amniotic fluid originates from several fetal sources, including fetal urine and secretions from the respiratory tract, skin, and amniotic membranes.
  - The fluid accumulates rapidly and amounts to about 175–225 mL by the fifteenth week of pregnancy and about 1 L at birth.
- The rupture of the amniotic membranes produces a watery discharge at the time of delivery.

FETAL GROWTH AND DEVELOPMENT

- During the first 8 weeks of pregnancy, the developing ovum is known as an embryo, and after that until birth, it is called a fetus.
- The period during which intrauterine fetal development takes place (gestation) usually averages 40 weeks from time of fertilization to delivery.
- The progress of gestation is usually considered in terms of 90-day periods or trimesters.
- Since conception occurs about 14 days after the first day of the last menstrual period, fetal development and the estimated date of confinement (delivery date) can be calculated with some reliability.

Adjustments of the Infant to Extrauterine Life

- Birth results in the infant's loss of the placental connection with the mother and therefore loss of metabolic support. This requires circulatory adjustments that permit adequate blood flow through the lungs.
- After a normal delivery by the mother who has not been depressed with anesthetics, an infant ordinarily begins to breathe with a normal respiratory rhythm immediately or with minimal stimulation.
- At birth the walls of the alveoli are held together by the surface tension of the viscid fluid that fills them.
  - More than 25 mmHg of negative pressure is required to oppose the effects of this surface tension, allowing the alveoli to open for the first time.
- The initial respirations of the newborn can create as much as 50 mmHg of negative pressure in the intrapleural space.
- These powerful first breaths open the alveoli and allow further respirations to occur with much less effort.
- Immature liver and nonfunctional lungs of the developing fetus are bypassed by the ductus venous, ductus arteriosum, and foramen ovale.
  - When blood flow through the placenta ceases at birth, there is a resultant increase in systemic vascular resistance and in aortic, left ventricular, and left arterial pressures.
    - Pulmonary vascular resistance also decreases greatly because of expansion of the lungs, which reduces the pulmonary arterial, right ventricular, and right atrial pressures.
  - Because of these changes in pressure gradients, the AV shunts close normally within a few hours after birth and are eventually occluded by growth of fibrous tissue.

Obstetrical Terminology

- Gravida—Refers to the number of current and past pregnancies
- Para—Refers only the number of past pregnancies that have remained viable to delivery
- Antepartum—The maternal period before delivery
- Gestation—Period of intrauterine fetal development
- Grand multipara—A woman who has had seven deliveries or more
- Multigravida—A woman who has had two or more pregnancies
- Multipara—A woman who has had two or more deliveries
- Natal—Connected with birth
- Nullipara—A woman who has never delivered
- Perinatal—Occurring at or near the time of birth
- Postpartum—The maternal period after delivery
- Prenatal—Existing or occurring before birth
- Primigravida—A woman who is pregnant for the first time
- Primipara—A woman who has given birth only once
- Term—A pregnancy that has reached 40 weeks' gestation

Assessment of the Patient—Maternal Changes During Pregnancy

- Besides cessation of menstruation and the obvious enlargement of the uterus, the pregnant woman undergoes many other physiological changes.
- These changes affect the genital tract, breasts, gastrointestinal (GI) system, cardiovascular system, respiratory system, and metabolism.

Genital Tract

Uterus

- Uterine size increases from 70 g (nongravid) to 1000 g by term.
- By the second month, the uterus triples in size and weight.
- By the third month, the uterus occupies the entire pelvic cavity and may be palpated suprapubically.
- By the fourth month, the uterus becomes an abdominal organ, and the top of the uterus (fundus) reaches the level of the umbilicus.
- In the last trimester, the uterine fundus recedes a little when the fetus descends into the pelvis.

Cervix

- Increased uterine blood and lymphatic flow cause pelvic congestion and edema, resulting in softening and bluish discoloration of the cervix (Chadwick's sign).

Vagina

- The vagina develops a characteristic violet color from increased vascularity.
- The vaginal walls prepare for labor, and the vaginal mucosa increases in thickness.
- Vaginal secretions increase, and the pH decreases to about 3.5 because of increased production of lactic acid from glycogen in the vaginal epithelium.

Bladder

- Frequency of urination occurs from pressure of the expanding uterus on the bladder.

Breasts

- The breasts become tender in the early weeks of pregnancy.
- By the second month, the breasts increase in size from hypertrophy of the mammary alveoli.
- The nipples become larger, more deeply pigmented, and more erectile early in pregnancy.
- As breast glands proliferate, they begin to secrete a clear fluid by the tenth week after conception.

GI System

- Morning sickness and nausea may occur anytime (usually beginning by the sixth and tapering off by the fourteenth week). The cause is thought to be related to the high serum levels of chorionic gonadotropin in early pregnancy.
- The patient's stomach and intestines are displaced upward and laterally by the enlarging uterus. This may cause indigestion and can increase the risk for aspiration in unconscious patients.
- The liver is displaced backward, upward, and to the right.
- The tone and motility of the GI tract decrease, leading to prolonged gastric emptying and relaxation of the pyloric sphincter; heartburn and constipation are common.

Cardiovascular System

- The heart is displaced to the left and upward by elevation of the diaphragm.
  - Flat or negative T waves may be present in lead III on the electrocardiogram (ECG).
- Cardiac output rises 30% by the thirty-fourth week.
- The pulse rate may increase 15–20 beats/min above baseline late in the third trimester (variable).
- Pulmonic systolic and apical systolic murmurs are common because lowered blood viscosity and increased flow lead to turbulence in the great vessels.

Circulation

- Total blood volume is increased by 30%, and plasma volume is increased by 50%.
- Blood pressure decreases 10–15 mmHg during the second trimester because of the reduction in peripheral resistance but gradually increases to prepregnancy levels toward term.
- The enlarged uterus interferes with venous return from the legs.
- Hemorrhoids, slight edema of the ankles, and varicose veins may be present.
- The supine position may cause the uterus to compress the inferior vena cava, producing decreased cardiac filling and decreased cardiac output (supine hypotension syndrome).
  - The patient may become faint and hypotensive while lying on her back after the first or second trimester.
- Increased plasma volume results in a drop in hemoglobin and hematocrit concentrations.
- The leukocyte count is elevated.
- Fibrinogen levels increase 50% because of the influence of estrogen and progesterone.

Respiratory System

- Tidal volume and minute ventilation increase by 30–40% in late pregnancy.
- Functional residual capacity decreases about 25%.
- The respiratory rate may be normal or increased because of elevation of the diaphragm by the uterus.

- PCO_2 is normally decreased due to increased respiratory rate (30 torr vs. 40 torr, which provides a gradient for fetal carbon dioxide) and may cause dizziness and a sensation of shortness of breath.

Metabolism

- The mother experiences a normal weight gain of 9.1 kg (20 lb).
- Increased water retention produces increased intracapillary hydrostatic pressure, which favors filtration from the vascular bed and resultant edema.
- Metabolic rate increases, as does caloric demand (especially for protein).
- Glucose escapes into urine because of increased glomerular filtration.
- Maternal gestational diabetes mellitus (GDM) may result from an impaired ability to metabolize carbohydrates, which is usually caused by a deficiency of insulin.
- Fetal demands for calcium and iron may deplete maternal stores if not supplemented through diet.

History

- When obtaining a history from an obstetrical patient, the paramedic should first gather information on the chief complaint, which may not be related to the pregnancy.
- After ruling out any life-threatening illness or injury, interview the patient to obtain relevant data, including:
  - Obstetrical history
    - Length of gestation
    - Parity and gravidity
    - Previous cesarean delivery
    - Maternal lifestyle (alcohol or other drug use, smoking history)
    - Infectious disease status
    - History of previous gynecological or obstetrical complications
  - Presence of pain
    - Onset (gradual or sudden)
    - Character
    - Duration and evolution over time
    - Location and radiation
  - Presence, quantity, and character of vaginal bleeding
  - Presence of abnormal vaginal discharge
  - Presence of "show" (expulsion of the mucous plug in early labor) or rupture of membranes
  - Current general health and prenatal care (none, physician, nurse midwife)
  - Allergies, medications taken (especially the use of narcotics in the last 4 hours)
  - Maternal urge to bear down or sensation of imminent bowel movement, suggesting imminent delivery

Physical Examination

- The patient's chief complaint determines the extent of the physical examination.
  - The objective in examining an obstetrical patient is to rapidly identify acute surgical or life-threatening conditions or imminent delivery and take appropriate management steps.
- Evaluate the patient's general appearance and skin color.
  - If she is markedly pale, suspect hemorrhage.
  - Sunken cheeks, cracked lips, or hollow eyes with a history of vomiting suggests dehydration.

- Assess vital signs and frequently reassess them throughout the patient encounter.
  - Orthostatic vital signs may be useful in eliciting the early presence of significant bleeding or fluid loss.
  - Remember that normal physiological changes in the pregnant patient can produce variations in vital signs.
    - — Mild tachycardia
    - — A slight fall in systolic and diastolic blood pressure
    - — An increase in respiratory rate
- Examine the abdomen for previous scars and any gross deformity, such as that caused by a hernia or marked abdominal distention.
  - Gentle palpation may reveal the presence of:
    - — Masses
    - — Enlarged organs
    - — Intestinal distention
    - — Distended bladder
  - Peritoneal irritation may be discernible during the physical examination.
    - — Diagnosed by the presence of tenderness, guarding, or rebound tenderness
  - If the patient is obviously pregnant, evaluation of uterine size and fetal monitoring may be indicated.
- Evaluation of uterine size:
  - The uterine contour is usually irregular between weeks 8 and 10.
    - — Early uterine enlargement may not be symmetrical
    - — The uterus may be deviated to one side
  - At 12–16 weeks' gestation, the uterus is above the symphysis pubis.
  - At 24 weeks, at the level of the umbilicus.
  - At term, near the xiphoid process.
- Fetal monitoring:
  - Fetal heart sounds may be auscultated between 16 and 40 weeks by use of a stethoscope, fetoscope, or Doppler.
  - Benefits of fetal monitoring include:
    - — Detecting the presence or absence of fetal circulation
    - — Providing baseline measurements for use in evaluating fetal or maternal distress
  - When auscultating the fetal heart rate, position the high-intensity diaphragm of the stethoscope (the bell of the fetoscope or the microphone of the Doppler) firmly on the mother's abdominal wall.
    - — Move the diaphragm in a circular pattern about 6–8 in. in diameter around the woman's umbilicus until the fetal heart tones can be heard.
    - — Once found, the fetal heart rate should be measured in beats per minute.
  - The normal fetal heart rate is 120–160 beats/min.
    - — A persistent fetal heart rate above 160 (fetal tachycardia) or below 120 beats/min (fetal bradycardia) is an early sign of fetal distress and fetal or maternal hypoxia.
    - — Intermittent, short-term acceleration or deceleration of the fetal heart rate is usually normal and can occur anytime.
    - — Short-term periodic changes in fetal heart rate are common during fetal sleep, fetal movement, and contractions associated with labor and delivery.

General Management of the Obstetrical Patient

- If birth is not imminent, prehospital care for the healthy patient will often be limited to basic treatment modalities (airway, ventilatory, and circulatory support) and transport for physician evaluation.
- In the absence of distress or injury, the patient should be transported in a position of comfort (usually left lateral recumbent).
- ECG monitoring, high-concentration oxygen administration, and fetal monitoring may be indicated for some patients, based on patient assessment and vital sign determinations.
- Medical direction may recommend that IV access be established in some patients.
- Medications are usually deemed inappropriate because they may mask symptoms of a deteriorating condition.

COMPLICATIONS OF PREGNANCY

Trauma in Pregnancy

- Poor fetal outcome has been correlated with increasing severity of maternal injury. When the mother sustains life-threatening injuries, 40.6% of fetuses die compared to only 1.6% in non-life-threatening cases.
- Anatomical and physiological changes associated with pregnancy can alter the patient's response to injury, requiring modified assessment, treatment, and transportation strategies.
- Causes of maternal injury in decreasing order of frequency are:
  - Vehicular crashes
  - Falls
  - Penetrating objects
- These injuries can result in trauma to the gravid uterus and to the maternal bladder, liver, and spleen. In addition, an injury that results in a pelvic fracture can produce massive hemorrhage and damage to the fetal skull.
- During pregnancy, the fetus is well protected within the uterus.
  - Amniotic fluid surrounds the fetus and serves as an excellent shock absorber.
  - Experiencing physical trauma is extremely rare for a fetus except from direct penetrating wounds or extensive blunt trauma to the maternal abdomen.
- The greatest risk of fetal death is from fetal distress and intrauterine demise caused by trauma to the mother or her death.
  - When dealing with a pregnant trauma patient, promptly assess and intervene on behalf of the mother.
- Severe abdominal injury may result in:
  - Premature separation of the placenta
  - Premature labor or abortion
  - Rupture of the uterus
  - Fetal death
- Causes of fetal death from maternal trauma include:
  - Death of the mother
  - Separation of the placenta
  - Maternal shock
  - Uterine rupture
  - Fetal head injury

Assessment and Management

- Priorities in assessing and managing a pregnant trauma patient are the same as for a nongravid patient.
  - Adequate airway, ventilatory, and circulatory support with spinal precautions
  - Hemorrhage control
  - Rapid assessment, stabilization, and rapid transport to a medical facility
- Resuscitating the mother is the key to survival of both mother and fetus.
  - During the initial stages of assessment and management, efforts should be directed toward the mother's status.
- Perform a thorough physical examination.
  - Injuries that would contribute to hypovolemia or hypoxia must be detected, identified, and treated early.
  - With the normal increase in maternal blood volume, the mother can tolerate more blood loss before demonstrating signs and symptoms of hypoperfusion.
    - A 30–35% reduction in blood volume can produce minimal changes in blood pressure but will reduce uterine blood flow by 10–20%.
  - Fetal monitoring is the best available indicator of fetal well-being after trauma.
    - Accelerations of fetal heart rate above baseline are associated with fetal movement and contractions but also may be an early sign of fetal distress.

      Decreased fetal movement and increased fetal heart rate can suggest maternal shock.
    - Decelerations of fetal heart rate below the baseline are associated with a decrease in cardiac output and the presence of hypoxia.
    - A hypoxic fetus in metabolic acidosis cannot accelerate heart rate and thus becomes bradycardic (a heart rate of less than 120 beats/min).
    - Sustained fetal bradycardia (lasting 10 minutes or more) may be a response to increased parasympathetic tone and can be tolerated for only a short time before the fetus becomes acidotic.
    - Fetal bradycardia is usually a late occurrence from maternal hypoxia and decreased maternal circulating volume.
- Include oxygenation, volume replacement, and hemorrhage control.
  - Labor also is a complication of trauma in pregnancy, so be prepared to manage imminent delivery or spontaneous abortion.
- If cardiac arrest occurs, begin CPR in the usual fashion.
  - Aggressive resuscitation is justified in patients near term to allow for emergency cesarean delivery at the emergency department.
  - Fetal survival is good if the interval between maternal death and delivery is less than 5 minutes and poor if longer than 20–25 minutes.
  - Advance notice to the receiving emergency department of impending emergency cesarean delivery is paramount.
- Oxygenation:
  - Adequate airway maintenance and oxygenation are essential to prevent fetal hypoxemia.
  - Oxygen requirements are 10–20% greater than in the nongravid patient.
    - Fetal hypoxia may occur with even small changes in maternal oxygenation.
    - Administer high-concentration oxygen.
  - If available, pulse oximetry should be used to monitor oxygen saturation.
- Volume replacement:
  - Signs and symptoms of hypovolemia may not be present until a blood loss is large.
  - Blood is preferentially shunted from the uterus to preserve maternal blood pressure.

- Bleeding also may occur inside the uterus.
- Crystalloid fluid replacement is initiated, even in normotensive patients.
- Pneumatic antishock garment application is controversial.
  - If applied, only the leg compartments are inflated.

    Use of the abdominal compartment may increase blood loss from disrupted vasculature of the pelvis.

    Abdominal compartment inflation may rarely be indicated when maternal and fetal deaths are imminent (by order of medical direction).
- Vasopressors generally are not recommended because they decrease uterine blood flow and fetal oxygen delivery.

- Hemorrhage control:
  - Control external hemorrhage.
  - Vaginal bleeding may suggest placental separation or uterine rupture.
  - A vaginal examination should be avoided, as it may increase bleeding and precipitate delivery, especially if unsuspected placenta previa is present.
  - Note and document the amount and color of vaginal bleeding.
  - Collect any expelled tissue and transport it with the patient to the hospital.
- Transportation strategies:
  - After 3–4 months' gestation, pregnant patients should not be transported in a supine position because of the potential for supine hypotension.
  - If spinal injury is not suspected, the patient should be transported in a left lateral recumbent position.
  - If spinal injury is suspected, the paramedic should prepare the patient for transport in the following manner:
    - Fully immobilize the patient on a long spine board
    - After immobilization, carefully tilt the board on its left side by log-rolling the secured patient 10–15°.
    - Place a blanket, pillow, or towel under the right side of the board to move the uterus to the left side.

Medical Conditions and Disease Processes

- Medical conditions and disease processes that may be masked or aggravated by pregnancy include:
  - Acute appendicitis
  - Acute cholecystitis
  - Hypertension
  - Diabetes
  - Infection
  - Neuromuscular disorders
  - Cardiovascular disease
- Preeclampsia and eclampsia are two hypertensive disorders specific to pregnancy.
- Preeclampsia is a disease of unknown origin that primarily affects previously healthy, normotensive primigravidae.
- Occurs after the twentieth week of gestation, often near term.
- The pathophysiology of preeclampsia (which is not reversed until after delivery) is characterized by:
  - Vasospasm
  - Endothelial cell injury

    - Increased capillary permeability
    - Activation of the clotting cascade
- Signs and symptoms of preeclampsia result from hypoperfusion to the tissue or organs involved.
    - Cerebrum
        - Headache
        - Hyperreflexia
        - Dizziness
        - Confusion
        - Seizures
        - Coma
    - Retina
        - Blurred vision
        - Diplopia
    - GI system
        - Nausea/vomiting
        - Right-upper-quadrant or epigastric pain and tenderness
    - Renal system
        - Proteinuria
        - Azotemia
        - Oliguria
        - Anuria
        - Hematuria
        - Hemoglobinuria
    - Vasculature or endothelium
        - Hypertension
        - Edema
        - Activation of the clotting cascade
    - Placenta
        - Abruptio placentae
        - Fetal distress
- Eclampsia is characterized by the same signs and symptoms plus seizures or coma.
- The criteria for diagnosis of preeclampsia are based on the presence of the "classic triad."
    - Hypertension (blood pressure greater than 140/90 mmHg, an acute rise of 20 mmHg in systolic pressure, or a rise of 10 mmHg in diastolic pressure over prepregnancy levels)
    - Proteinuria
    - Excessive weight gain with edema
- Besides nulliparity, factors predisposing to preeclampsia include:
    - Advanced maternal age
    - Chronic hypertension
    - Chronic renal disease
    - Vascular disease
    - Multiple gestation
- Preeclampsia is a clinical diagnosis that may be confirmed by postpartum renal biopsy.
    - When the disease is suspected, most patients are hospitalized or confined to bed rest at home until delivery

Management

- Not all hypertensive patients have preeclampsia, and not all preeclamptic patients have hypertension. Because of the potentially devastating course of the illness, the disease should always be considered when hypertension is present in late pregnancy.
- If preeclampsia or eclampsia is suspected, prehospital care is directed at preventing or controlling seizures and treating hypertension.
- Seizure activity in eclampsia is similar to generalized grand mal seizures of other etiologies and is characterized by tonic-clonic activity.
  - The seizure often begins around the mouth as facial twitching
  - Labor can begin spontaneously and progress rapidly
- The procedure for managing severe preeclampsia is:
  - Place the patient in a left lateral recumbent position to maintain or improve utero-placental blood flow and to minimize risk of insult to the fetus.
  - Handle the patient gently and minimize sensory stimulation (darken the ambulance) to avoid precipitating seizures.
  - Administer high-concentration oxygen and assist respirations as needed.
  - Initiate IV therapy per protocol.
  - Anticipate seizures at any moment and be prepared to provide airway, ventilatory, and circulatory support.
- Be prepared to administer the following medications per medical direction and local protocol:
  - Magnesium sulfate 10%
    - Have antidote (calcium gluconate) nearby to treat respiratory depression
  - Diazepam (Valium)
  - Hydralazine (Apresoline) to treat hypertension
    - May precipitate a fall in blood pressure
    - May jeopardize fetal circulation
    - Closely monitor vital signs
  - Gently transport patient to appropriate medical facility

Vaginal Bleeding

May result during pregnancy from abortion (miscarriage), ectopic pregnancy, abruptio placentae, placenta previa, uterine rupture, or postpartum hemorrhage. Patients who have vaginal bleeding develop varying degrees of blood loss; some require aggressive resuscitation.

Abortion

The termination of pregnancy from any cause before the twentieth week of gestation (after which it is known as a preterm birth). The most frequent cause of vaginal bleeding in pregnant women and occurs in about 1 in 10 pregnancies.

Classifications of Abortion

- Complete abortion—An abortion in which the patient has passed all of the products of conception.
- Criminal abortion—An intentional ending of any pregnancy under any condition not allowed by law.
- Incomplete abortion—An abortion in which the patient has passed some but not all of the products of conception.
- Induced abortion—An abortion in which the pregnancy is intentionally terminated.

- Missed abortion—The retention of the fetus in utero for 4 or more weeks after fetal death.
- Spontaneous abortion—An abortion that usually occurs before the twelfth week of gestation.
  - Lay term is *miscarriage*
  - Predisposing factors include:
    - Acute or chronic illness in the mother
    - Abnormalities in the fetus
    - Abnormal attachment of the placenta
    - Often, the cause is unknown
- Therapeutic abortion—A pregnancy legally terminated for reasons of maternal well-being.
- Threatened abortion—An abortion in which a patient has some uterine bleeding with an intrauterine pregnancy in which the internal cervical os is closed.
  - May stabilize and end in normal delivery or progress to an incomplete or complete abortion
- Most abortions occur in the first trimester, usually before the tenth week.
- The patient is often anxious and apprehensive and complains of vaginal bleeding, which may be slight or profuse.
  - The patient may have suprapubic pain referred to the lower back and described as "cramplike" and similar to the pain of labor or menstruation
- When obtaining a history, determine:
  - The time of onset of pain and bleeding
  - Amount of blood loss
  - If the patient passed any tissue with the blood

Management

- Assessment of all first-trimester emergencies should include close observation for signs of significant blood loss and hypovolemia.
- Measure and frequently monitor vital signs (including orthostatic vital signs) during transport.
- Depending on the patient's hemodynamic status, IV fluid therapy may be indicated.
- Provide oxygen, emotional support, and transport for physician evaluation.

Ectopic Pregnancy

- Occurs when a fertilized ovum implants anywhere other than the endometrium of the uterine cavity.
- Ectopic gestation occurs in 1 of every 200 pregnancies.
  - It is the leading cause of first-trimester death and accounts for more than 11% of all maternal deaths in the United States.
  - Death from ectopic pregnancy is usually the result of hemorrhage.
- Although ectopic pregnancy has many causes, most involve factors that delay or prevent passage of the fertilized ovum to its normal site of implantation.
- Predisposing factors include:
  - Pelvic inflammatory disease (PID)
  - Adhesions from previous surgery
  - Tubal ligation
  - Previous ectopic pregnancy
  - Possibly the presence of intrauterine contraceptive devices (IUCDs)

- Signs and symptoms are often difficult to distinguish from those of a ruptured ovarian cyst, PID, appendicitis, or abortion (thus the name "the great imitator").
- The classic triad of symptoms includes:
  - Abdominal pain
  - Vaginal bleeding
  - Amenorrhea
    - — Vaginal bleeding may be absent, spotty, or minimal, and amenorrhea may be replaced by oligomenorrhea (scanty flow)
- Other symptoms include:
  - Signs of early pregnancy
  - Referred pain to the shoulder
  - Nausea/vomiting
  - Syncope
  - Classic signs of shock

Management

- A true emergency that requires initial resuscitation measures and rapid transport for surgical intervention.
- Manage the patient like any other with hemorrhagic shock—Airway, ventilatory, and circulatory support and aggressive IV fluid resuscitation.

Third-Trimester Bleeding

Abruptio Placentae

- A partial or complete detachment of a normally implanted placenta at more than 20 weeks' gestation.
- Predisposing factors to abruptio placentae include maternal hypertension, preeclampsia, multiparity, trauma, and previous abruption.
- The common presentation of abruptio placentae is sudden, third-trimester vaginal bleeding and pain.
  - Vaginal bleeding may be minimal and often is out of proportion to the degree of shock, since much of the hemorrhage may be concealed.
  - The more extensive the abruption, the greater the uterine irritability, resulting in a tender abdomen and rigid uterus.
  - Contractions may be present.
  - In its severe form, fetal heart sounds are absent because fetal death is likely.

Placenta Previa

- Placental implantation in the lower uterine segment encroaching on or covering the cervical os.
- Characterized by painless, bright red bleeding without uterine contraction.
  - Bleeding may occur in repetitive episodes and be slight to moderate, becoming more profuse if active labor ensues.
- Fetal heart rate is often diminished because of placental insufficiency and hypoxia.
- Associated with:
  - Increasing maternal age
  - Multiparity
  - Previous cesarean section
  - Previous placenta previa episodes
- Bleeding is frequently precipitated by recent sexual intercourse.

Uterine Rupture

- A spontaneous or traumatic rupture of the uterine wall.
- May result from:
  - Reopening of a previous uterine scar (e.g., a previous cesarean section)
  - Prolonged or obstructed labor
  - Direct trauma
- Characterized by sudden abdominal pain described as steady and "tearing."
  - Active labor
  - Early signs of shock (complaints of weakness, dizziness, anxiety)
  - Vaginal bleeding, which may not be visible
- On examination, the abdomen is usually rigid with diffuse pain.
  - Fetal parts may easily be palpated through the abdominal wall.
  - A previous cesarean scar may be a good indication of the rupture.

Management of Third-Trimester Bleeding

- Prehospital management of a patient with third-trimester bleeding is aimed at preventing shock.
- No attempt should be made to examine the patient vaginally.
- Doing so may increase hemorrhage and precipitate labor.
- Emergency care measures should include the following:
  - Provide adequate airway, ventilatory, and circulatory support as needed (with spinal precautions if indicated)
  - Place patient in left lateral recumbent position
  - Begin transport immediately
  - Initiate IV therapy with volume-expanding fluid
  - Apply a fresh perineal pad and note the time of application to assess bleeding during transport
  - Check fundal height and document it for baseline measurement
  - Closely monitor the patient's vital signs en route to the hospital

Labor and Delivery

- Parturition is the process by which the infant is born.
- Near the end of pregnancy, the uterus becomes progressively more irritable and exhibits occasional contractions, which become stronger and more frequent until parturition is initiated.
- During and because of these contractions, the cervix begins to dilate.
- As uterine contractions increase, complete cervical dilation occurs to about 10 cm.
- The amniotic sac ruptures, and the fetus, and shortly after that the placenta, is expelled from the uterus through the vaginal canal.

Stages of Labor

- Labor follows several distinct stages.
- The length of these stages varies, depending on whether the mother is nullipara or multipara.
- The stages of labor should be used only as a guideline in estimating labor progression in the average pregnancy.
  - Stage I (Dilation Stage)—The onset of regular contractions. Average time: 12.5 hours.

  - Stage II (Expulsion Stage)—The full dilation of cervix to delivery. Average time: 80 minutes in primipara, of the newborn 30 minutes in multipara.
  - Stage III (Placental Stage)—Immediately follows delivery of the placenta. Average time: Usually occurs 5–20 minutes after delivery of the baby.
- About 2–3 weeks before the onset of active labor, while the cervix undergoes the process of softening, effacement (thinning), and dilation, the uterus begins to become a contractile organ.
- Contractions, which before 30 weeks' gestation were uncoordinated and of low intensity, begin to steadily increase in intensity and duration (Braxton-Hicks contractions).
- The patient may not notice the contractions or perceive them as a slight uterine hardening.
- The contractions eventually strengthen and increase in frequency and duration, heralding the onset of clinical labor.
- Labor begins with a prodromal stage that marks the infant's descent into the birth canal.
- Characterized by a relief of pressure in the upper abdomen and a simultaneous increase in pressure in the pelvis.
- During this stage, a mucous plug (sometimes mixed with blood, thus the name bloody show) is expelled from the dilating cervix and discharged from the vagina.
- The prodromal stage may go unnoticed by the mother.
- The first stage of labor begins with the onset of regular contractions and ends with complete dilation of the cervix.
- Uterine contractions generally occur at 5- to 15-minute intervals.
- Characterized by cramplike abdominal pain that radiates to the small of the back.
- As the uterus contracts, the cervix becomes soft and thinned (effaced), and the less muscular segment of the uterus is pulled upward over the presenting part.
- Usually lasts 8–12 hours in the nulliparous mother and about 6–8 hours in the multiparous mother.
- In most pregnancies, the amniotic sac ruptures (rupture of membranes) toward the end of this stage.
- The second stage of labor is measured from full dilation of the cervix to delivery of the infant.
- The fetal head enters the birth canal, and the mother's pain and contractions become more intense and frequent (usually 2–3 minutes apart).
- Often, the mother becomes diaphoretic and tachycardiac.
  - Generally experiences an urge to bear down with each contraction
  - May express the need to have a bowel movement (a normal sensation caused by pressure of the fetal head against the mother' rectum)
- The presenting part of the fetus (usually the head) emerges from the vaginal opening.
  - This process, known as crowning, indicates that delivery is imminent
- Usually lasts 1–2 hours in the nullipara mother and 30 minutes or less in a woman who is multipara.
- The third stage of labor begins with delivery of the infant and ends when the placenta has been expelled and the uterus has contracted.
- The length of this stage varies from 5 to 60 minutes, regardless of parity.

Signs and Symptoms of Imminent Delivery

- The following signs and symptoms indicate that delivery is imminent and that preparations for childbirth should be made at the scene:

- ◦ Regular contractions lasting 45–60 seconds at 1- to 2-minute intervals.
  - — Intervals are measured from the beginning of one contraction to the beginning of the next. If contractions are more than 5 minutes apart, there generally is time to transport the mother to a receiving hospital.
- ◦ The mother has an urge to bear down or has a sensation of a bowel movement.
- ◦ There is a large amount of bloody show.
- ◦ Crowning occurs.
- ◦ The mother believes delivery is imminent.
  - — If any of these signs and symptoms is present, prepare for delivery.
  - — Except for cord presentation, the delay or restraint of delivery should not be attempted in any fashion.
  - — If complications are anticipated or an abnormal delivery occurs, medical direction may recommend expedited transport of the patient to a medical facility.

- Preparing for delivery.
  - ◦ Attempt to provide an area of privacy.
  - ◦ Position the mother on a bed, stretcher, or table that has a surface long enough to project beyond the mother's vagina.
  - ◦ The delivery area should be as clean as possible and covered with absorbent material to guard against staining and contamination by blood and fecal material.
  - ◦ Place the mother on her back with her knees flexed and widely separated (or in another position preferred by the mother), and drape the vaginal area appropriately.
- If delivery occurs in an automobile, instruct the mother to lie on her back across the seat with one leg flexed on the seat and the other leg resting on the floorboard.
- If a pillow or blanket is available, place it beneath the mother's buttocks to facilitate delivery of the infant's head.
- Evaluate the mother's vital signs for baseline measurements and monitor fetal heart rate for signs of distress.
- Per protocol and medical direction, consider maternal oxygen administration and IV access for volume expansion or postdelivery administration of oxytocin (Pitocin) if needed.
- Coach the mother to bear down and push during contractions and to rest between contractions to conserve strength.
- If the mother finds it difficult to refrain from pushing, encourage her to breathe deeply or "pant" through her mouth between contractions to prevent glottic closure.

Prehospital delivery equipment (OB kit) generally includes the following:

- Surgical scissors (used to cut the umbilical cord)
- Cord clamps or umbilical tape
- Towels (for drying the infant)
- Surgical masks
- 4 × 4 gauze sponges
- Sanitary napkins (for absorption of vaginal drainage after delivery)
- Bulb syringe/DeLee suction kit (used to suction the infant's mouth and nose)
- Baby blanket/baby stocking cap
- Plastic bag (for placental transport)
- Neonatal resuscitation equipment
- IV fluid supplies
- Assisting with delivery
  - ◦ In most cases, the paramedic only assists in the natural events of childbirth.

- The primary responsibilities of the EMS crew are to:
  - Prevent an uncontrolled delivery.
  - Protect the infant from cold and stress after the birth.
- Steps in assisting the mother with a normal delivery:
  - Don sterile gloves and other personal protective equipment.
  - When crowning occurs, apply gentle palm pressure to the infant's head to prevent an explosive delivery and tearing of the perineum. If membranes are still intact, tear the sac with finger pressure to allow escape of amniotic fluid.
  - After delivery of the head, examine the infant's neck for a looped umbilical cord (nuchal cord).
    - If the cord is looped around the neck, gently slip it over the infant's head.
  - Suction the infant's mouth and nose with a bulb syringe to clear the airway.
    - Perform suction after the head appears but before the next contraction, which delivers the shoulders and chest.
  - Support the infant's head as it rotates for shoulder presentation.
  - With gentle pressure, guide the infant's head downward to deliver the anterior shoulder and then upward to release the posterior shoulder.
    - The remainder of the infant is delivered quickly by smooth uterine contraction.
  - Be careful to grasp and support the infant as it emerges.
    - Use care because the baby is very slippery.
    - Hold the infant firmly with its head dependent to facilitate drainage of secretions.
    - Maintain the infant's position at or slightly above the level of the mother's vagina to prevent overtransfusion or undertransfusion of blood from the umbilical cord.
  - Clear the infant's airway of any secretions with sterile gauze and repeat suction of the infant's nose and mouth.
  - Dry the infant with sterile towels and cover the infant (especially the head) to reduce heat loss.
  - Note and record the baby's gender and time of birth.

Evaluating the Infant

- After delivery, dry and cover the infant to prevent heat loss, position on the side or with padding under back and clear the airway, and provide tactile stimulation to initiate respirations.
- Continue to suction as necessary.
- If there is no need for resuscitation, use the Apgar score at 1 minute and 5 minutes to evaluate the infant.
- Criteria for computing the Apgar score include:
  - Appearance (color)
  - Pulse (heart rate)
  - Grimace (reflex irritability to stimulation)
  - Activity (muscle tone)
  - Respiratory effort
- Each criterion is rated on a basis of 0–2, and the numbers are then added for a total Apgar score:
  - 10 indicates that the infant is in the best possible condition
  - 7–9 indicates the infant is slightly depressed (near normal)
  - 4–6 indicates the infant is moderately depressed
  - 0–3 indicates the infant is severely depressed

- Most newborns have an Apgar score of 8–10 at 1 minute after birth.
- Neonates with an Apgar score of less than 6 generally require resuscitation; however, the Apgar score should not be used to determine the need for resuscitation.

Cutting the Umbilical Cord

- After delivery and evaluation of the infant, the umbilical cord should be clamped (or tied with umbilical tape) and cut.
- Clamp the cord about 4–6 in. away from the infant in two places.
- Cut between the two clamps with sterile scissors or a scalpel.
- Examine the cut ends of the cord to ensure there is no bleeding.
- If the cut end attached to the infant is bleeding, clamp the cord proximal to the previous clamp and reassess for bleeding.
- Do not remove the first clamp.
- Handle the cord carefully at all times; it tears easily.

Delivery of the Placenta

- The placenta normally delivers within 20 minutes of the infant.
- Do not delay transport for placental delivery.
- Placental delivery is characterized by episodes of contractions.
- A palpable rise of the uterus within the abdomen.
- Lengthening of the umbilical cord protruding from the vagina.
- A sudden gush of vaginal blood.
- As the placenta delivers, advise the mother to bear down with contractions.
- Hold the placenta with both hands and gently twist it as it delivers to facilitate complete separation from the uterine wall.
- When expelled, place the placenta in a plastic bag or other container and transport it with the mother and infant to the receiving hospital, where it will be examined for abnormality and completeness.
- After placental delivery, evaluate the perineum for tears.
- If present, the tears should be managed by applying sanitary napkins to the area and maintaining direct pressure.
- Closely monitor the mother for signs of hemorrhage or shock.
- Initiate fundal massage to promote uterine contraction.
- Oxytocin (Pitocin) may be prescribed by medical direction to manage postpartum hemorrhage.

Postpartum Hemorrhage

- More than 500 mL of blood loss after delivery of the newborn.
- Frequently occurs within the first few hours after delivery but can be delayed up to 24 hours.
- Occurs in about 5% of all deliveries and often results from ineffective or incomplete contraction of the interlacing uterine muscle fibers.
- Other causes of postpartum hemorrhage include retained pieces of placenta or membranes in the uterus, and/or vaginal or cervical tears incurred during delivery (rare).
- Risk factors associated with this condition include:
  - Uterine atony (lack of tone) from prolonged or tumultuous labor
  - Grand multiparity
  - Twin pregnancy

- Placenta previa
- A full bladder

Management

- Control external hemorrhage. Manage external bleeding from perineal tears with firm pressure.
- Uterine massage:
  - Palpate the uterus for firmness or loss of tone.
  - If the uterus does not feel firm, apply fundal pressure by supporting the lower uterine segment with the edge of one hand just above the symphysis and massaging the fundus with the other hand.
  - Continue massaging until the uterus feels firm.
  - Reevaluate the patient every 10 minutes.
    - — Note the location of the fundus in relation to the level of the umbilicus, the degree of firmness, and vaginal flow
- Encourage the infant to breast-feed.
  - If the mother and baby are stable, place the newborn to her breast and encourage the infant to breast-feed.
  - Stimulation of the breasts may promote uterine contraction.
- Administer oxytocin (Pitocin).
  - Per medical direction and after ensuring that a second fetus is not present in the uterus, add 20 units of oxytocin (Pitocin) to 1000 mL lactated Ringer's solution and infuse at 20–30 drops/min via microdrip tubing (titrated to the severity of hemorrhage and uterine response or as ordered by medical direction).
- Continue with fluid resuscitation as indicated by the patient's hemodynamic status.
- Do not attempt a vaginal examination or vaginal packing to control hemorrhage.
- Rapidly transport the patient for physician evaluation.

DELIVERY COMPLICATIONS

Factors Associated with High Risk of Abnormal Delivery

- Maternal age—Very young or very old
- Absence of prenatal care
- Maternal lifestyle—Alcohol, tobacco, or drug usage
- Preexisting maternal illness including diabetes, chronic hypertension, or Rh sensitization
- Previous obstetrical history
  - Premature delivery or miscarriage
  - Perinatal loss
  - Previous malformed neonate
  - Previous multiple births
  - Previous cesarean delivery
- Intrapartum disorders
  - Preeclampsia
  - Prolonged rupture of membranes
  - Prolonged labor
  - Abnormal presentation

  - Abruptio placentae
  - Placenta previa

Fetal Factors

- Lack of fetal well-being
  - History of decreased fetal movement
  - History of heart rate abnormalities
  - Evidence of fetal distress
- Fetal immaturity—Prematurity as established by dates, ultrasound, uterine size, amniocentesis
- Fetal growth—History of poor intrauterine growth or postdate delivery
- Specific fetal malformation detected by ultrasound—Diaphragmatic hernia or omphalocele

Cephalopelvic Disproportion

- Produces a difficult labor because of the presence of a small pelvis, an oversized fetus, or fetal abnormalities (hydrocephalus, conjoined twins, fetal tumors).
- The mother is often primigravida and experiencing strong, frequent contractions for a prolonged period.
- Definitive care is cesarean delivery because uterine rupture and fetal demise are possible.
- Prehospital care is limited to maternal oxygen administration, IV access for fluid resuscitation if needed, and rapid transport to the receiving hospital.

Abnormal Presentations

Most infants are born head first (cephalic or vertex presentation); on rare occasions, a presentation is abnormal.

Breech Presentation

- In breech presentation, the largest part of the fetus (the head) is delivered last.
- Occurs in 3–4% of deliveries at term and is more frequent with multiple births and when labor occurs before 32 weeks' gestation.

Management

- An infant in a breech presentation is best delivered in a hospital where emergency cesarean section is a possible alternative to vaginal delivery.
- When necessary to assist in a breech delivery, the EMS crew should:
  - Prepare the mother for delivery in the usual manner.
  - Provide supplemental oxygen and IV access and continuously monitor the fetal heart rate.
  - Allow the fetus to deliver spontaneously up to the level of the umbilicus.
    - If the fetus is in a front presentation, gently extract the legs downward after the buttocks are delivered.
  - After the infant's legs are clear, support the baby's body with the palm of the hand and volar surface of the arm.
  - After the umbilicus is visualized, gently extract a 4- to 6-inch loop of umbilical cord to allow delivery without excessive traction on the cord.
    - Gently rotate the fetus to align the shoulders in an anterior-posterior position.
    - Continue with gentle traction until the axilla is visible.

- ◦ Gently guide the infant upward to allow delivery of the posterior shoulder.
- ◦ Gently guide the infant downward to deliver the anterior shoulder.
- ◦ During a breech delivery, avoid having the fetal face or abdomen toward the maternal symphysis.
- ◦ Be aware that after shoulder delivery, the head is often delivered without difficulty.
- ◦ Be careful to avoid excessive head and spine manipulation or traction.
- ◦ If the head does not deliver immediately, take action to prevent suffocation of the infant.
- ◦ Place a gloved hand in the vagina with the palm toward the baby's face.
- ◦ With index and middle fingers, a V should be formed on either side of the baby's nose.
- ◦ The vaginal wall should then be gently pushed away from the baby's face until the head is delivered.
- ◦ If the head does not deliver within 3 minutes, the baby's airway should be maintained with the V formation, and the mother should be rapidly transported to the receiving hospital.

Shoulder Dystocia

- Occurs when the fetal shoulders impact against the maternal symphysis pubis, blocking shoulder delivery.
  - ◦ The head delivers normally but then pulls back tightly against the maternal perineum.
- The incidence of shoulder dystocia is small but increases significantly with increasing birth weight (up to 10% incidence with birth weights of 10 or more pounds).
- Complications include:
  - ◦ Brachial plexus damage
  - ◦ Fractured clavicle
  - ◦ Fetal anoxia from cord compression

Management

- Delivery entails dislodging one shoulder and rotating the fetal shoulder girdle into the wider oblique pelvic diameter.
  - ◦ Because of the potential for cord compression, the anterior shoulder should be delivered immediately after the head (before suctioning of the nares and mouth).
- Many maneuvers can assist in delivery; the following steps are a reasonable field approach to this problem:
  - ◦ Position the mother on her left side in a dorsal-knee-chest position to increase the diameter of the pelvis.
  - ◦ Attempt to guide the infant's head downward to allow the anterior shoulder to slip under the symphysis pubis.
    - — Avoid excessive force or manipulation.
  - ◦ Gently rotate the fetal shoulder girdle into the wider oblique pelvic diameter.
    - — The posterior shoulder usually delivers without resistance.
  - ◦ Medical direction may recommend attempting delivery of the posterior shoulder first.
    - — This may be accomplished by rotating the posterior shoulder downward and into the left posterior quadrant.
    - — The anterior shoulder usually follows.
  - ◦ After delivery, continue with resuscitative measures as needed.

Shoulder Presentation (Transverse Presentation)

- Results when the long axis of the fetus lies perpendicular to that of the mother
- Usually results in the fetal shoulder lying over the pelvic inlet, thus the name
- The fetal arm or hand may be the presenting part
- Occurs in only 0.3% of deliveries but may occur in 10% of second twins

Management

- Spontaneous delivery of a shoulder presentation is not possible.
- Give the mother adequate oxygen, ventilatory, and circulatory support, and rapid transport to the receiving hospital.
- Cesarean section is required whether the fetus is viable or nonviable.

Cord Presentation (Prolapsed Cord)

- Occurs when the cord slips down into the vagina or presents externally after the amniotic membranes have ruptured.
  - The cord is compressed against the presenting part, diminishing fetal oxygenation from the placenta
- Prolapsed cord occurs in about 1 in every 200 pregnancies and should be suspected when fetal distress is present.
- Predisposing factors include:
  - Breech presentation
  - Premature rupture of membranes
  - Large fetus
  - Multiple gestation
  - A long cord
  - Preterm labor

Management

- Fetal asphyxia may rapidly ensue if circulation through the cord is not reestablished and maintained until delivery.
- If the umbilical cord can be seen or felt in the vagina, take the following steps:
  - Position the mother with hips elevated as much as possible.
    - — Trendelenburg or knee-chest position may relieve pressure on the cord
  - Administer oxygen to the mother.
  - Instruct the mother to "pant" with each contraction to prevent bearing down.
  - If assistance is available, apply moist sterile dressings to the exposed cord to minimize temperature changes that may cause umbilical artery spasm.
  - With a gloved hand, gently push the baby back into the vagina and elevate the presenting part to relieve pressure on the cord.
    - — The cord may spontaneously retract, but no attempt should be made to reposition the cord
  - Maintain this hand position during rapid transport to the receiving hospital.
  - Definitive treatment is cesarean section.
- Other abnormal presentations:
  - Occiput posterior presentation, in which the infant's head is delivered face up instead of face down, and face or brow presentation.
    - — Result in increased perinatal morbidity and mortality because of difficult labor and delivery and associated abnormalities
    - — May require cesarean section

- Goals of prehospital management:
  - Early recognition of potential complications
  - Maternal support and reassurance
  - Rapid transport for definitive care

Premature Birth

- A premature infant is one born before 37 weeks' gestation.
- Low birth weight (less than 2.5 kg [5.5 lb]) has also been used to determine prematurity, although the conditions are not synonymous.
  - Premature deliveries occur in 6–9% of all pregnancies.
- After a preterm labor, the newborn is at increased risk for hypothermia, because of a large surface/mass ratio, and for cardiorespiratory distress because the cardiovascular system is premature.
  - These infants require special care and observation.
- After delivery, prehospital management for a premature infant includes the following:
  - Keep the infant warm—Dry the infant, wrap it in a warm blanket, place it on the mother's abdomen, and cover both mother and infant.
  - Frequently suction the infant's mouth and nares.
  - Carefully monitor the cut end of the umbilical cord for oozing.
  - Administer humidified free-flow oxygen through a makeshift oxygen tent.
    - — Aim oxygen flow toward the top of tent; do not allow it to flow directly into the baby's face.
  - Protect the infant from contamination.
    - — Don mask and gown and minimize family member and bystander contact with the baby.
  - Gently transport the mother and infant to the receiving hospital.

Multiple Gestations

- A pregnancy with more than one fetus.
  - Twins occur in 1 of every 80–90 births, and triplets occur in 1 of 8000 births
- Multiple gestation places additional stress on the maternal system and is accompanied by an increased complication rate.
- Associated complications include:
  - Premature labor and delivery (30–50% of twin deliveries are premature)
  - Premature rupture of membranes
  - Abruptio placentae
  - Postpartum hemorrhage
  - Abnormal presentation
- Delivery procedure:
  - First-twin delivery is identical to single delivery with the same presentation.
    - — Up to 50% of second-twin deliveries are in nonvertex presentation.
  - After delivery of the first twin, clamp (or tie) and cut the umbilical cord in the usual fashion.
  - Within 5–10 minutes after delivery of the first twin, uterine contractions begin again.
    - — Delivery of the second twin usually occurs within 30–45 minutes.
    - — As a rule, both twins are born before placental delivery.
  - Infants in multiple births are often smaller than infants of term births.
    - — Pay special attention to keeping these infants warm, well oxygenated, and free from unnecessary contamination.

- ◦ Postpartum hemorrhage may be more severe after multiple births, requiring fluid resuscitation, uterine massage, and even oxytocin infusion.

Precipitous Delivery

- A rapid, spontaneous delivery, with less than 3 hours from onset of labor to birth.
- Results from overactive uterine contractions and little maternal soft tissue or bony resistance.
- May be associated with soft tissue injury and uterine rupture (rare) and has an increased perinatal mortality rate secondary to trauma and hypoxia.
  - ◦ Primary danger to the fetus is from cerebral trauma or tearing of the umbilical cord
- If a precipitous delivery is anticipated, attempt to prevent an explosive delivery by providing gentle counterpressure to the infant's head.
  - ◦ No attempt should be made to detain fetal head descent.
- After the delivery, keep the infant dry and warm to prevent heat loss, and examine the mother for perineal tears that often accompany a rapid birth.

Uterine Inversion

- An infrequent but serious complication of childbirth, occurring in about 1 in 2100 deliveries.
- It essentially is a turning "inside out" of the uterus.
- May occur spontaneously after a contraction or with increased abdominal pressure caused by coughing or sneezing.
  - ◦ It is thought, however, to be more often iatrogenic (caused by medical personnel or a medical procedure) secondary to excessive cord traction and fundal pressure, particularly when fundal implantation of the placenta has occurred.
  - ◦ Is considered incomplete if the uterine fundus does not extend beyond the cervix and complete if the entire uterus protrudes through the cervical ring.

Signs and Symptoms

- Postpartum hemorrhage (which can be profuse)
- Sudden and severe lower abdominal pain
- Hypovolemic shock may develop rapidly

Management

- Prehospital care for uterine inversion includes airway, ventilatory, and circulatory support and rapid transport for physician evaluation.
- Medical direction may recommend that manual replacement of the uterus be attempted, if the cervix has not yet constricted.
- Place the patient supine.
- Do not attempt to remove the placenta, which will increase hemorrhage.
- Apply pressure with the fingertips and palm of a gloved hand and push the fundus upward and through the cervical canal.
- If this is ineffective, cover all protruding tissues with moist sterile dressings and rapidly transport.

Pulmonary Embolism

- The development of pulmonary embolism during pregnancy, labor, or the postpartum period is one of the most common causes of maternal death.
- The embolus is frequently the result of a blood clot in the pelvic circulation (venous thromboembolism) and is more commonly associated with cesarean section than vaginal delivery.

- The patient often has classic signs and symptoms including:
  - Sudden dyspnea
  - Sharp, focal chest pain
  - Tachycardia
  - Tachypnea
  - Occasionally hypotension
- If the embolism occurs in the prehospital setting, emergency care for the patient is directed at airway, ventilatory, and circulatory support; ECG monitoring; and rapid transport for physician evaluation.

Fetal Membrane Disorders

Premature Rupture of Membranes

- A rupture of the amniotic sac before the onset of labor, regardless of gestational age.
- Signs and symptoms include a history of a "trickle" or sudden gush of fluid from the vagina.
- Transport the patient for physician evaluation.
- In-hospital delivery preparations will be made if the patient enters the advanced stages of labor or if an infection of fetal membranes (chorioamnionitis) is diagnosed.
- Chorioamnionitis is associated with premature rupture of membranes of greater than 24-hours duration or with prolonged labor.
- The infection generally is accompanied by maternal fever, chills, and uterine pain and is treated with antibiotics.
- Definitive treatment for the maternal infection is delivery of the fetus.

Amniotic Fluid Embolism

- May occur when amniotic fluid gains access to maternal circulation during labor or delivery or immediately after delivery.
- Probable routes of entry include lacerations of:
  - Endocervical veins during cervical dilation
  - Lower uterine segment or placental site
  - Uterine veins at sites of uterine trauma
- Particulate matter in the amniotic fluid (meconium, lanugo hairs, fetal squamous cells) forms an embolus and obstructs the pulmonary vasculature.
- Most commonly seen in multiparous women late in the first stage of labor.
- Other conditions that can increase the incidence of this complication are:
  - Placenta previa
  - Abruptio placentae
  - Intrauterine fetal death
- Signs and symptoms are the same as those described for pulmonary embolism and may include cardiopulmonary arrest.
- Manage the patient with airway, ventilatory, and circulatory support; fluid resuscitation; and rapid transport.

Meconium Staining

- Presence of fetal stool in amniotic fluid
- Between 8% and 30% of deliveries
- Increased perinatal mortality
- Meconium in amniotic fluid could be aspirated

Assessment

- Color varies from yellow, light green, or dark green ("pea soup")
- The thicker and darker the fluid, the higher the risk of morbidity

Management

- Prepare for intubation
- Clear airway/thoroughly suction
- Mouth, pharynx, nose
- Direct visualization and suction of hypopharynx
- Intubate
- Suction proximal end of endotracheal tube

CHAPTER QUESTIONS

1. Infants of diabetic mothers tend to be:
   a. small
   b. hypoglycemic
   c. large
   d. hyperglycemic
2. Blood pressure above 140/90 in the third trimester may indicate:
   a. the onset of labor
   b. abruptio placenta
   c. placenta previa
   d. preeclampsia
3. In all ectopic pregnancies, the fertilized ovum is implanted:
   a. outside the uterus
   b. on the corpus luteum
   c. on the outer edge of an ovary
   d. in the fallopian tubes

Suggested Reading

US Department of Transportation, National Highway Traffic Safety Administration. *EMT-Paramedic: National Standard Curriculum*. Washington, DC: US Department of Transportation, National Highway Traffic Safety Administration; 1998.

Section 6

Special Considerations

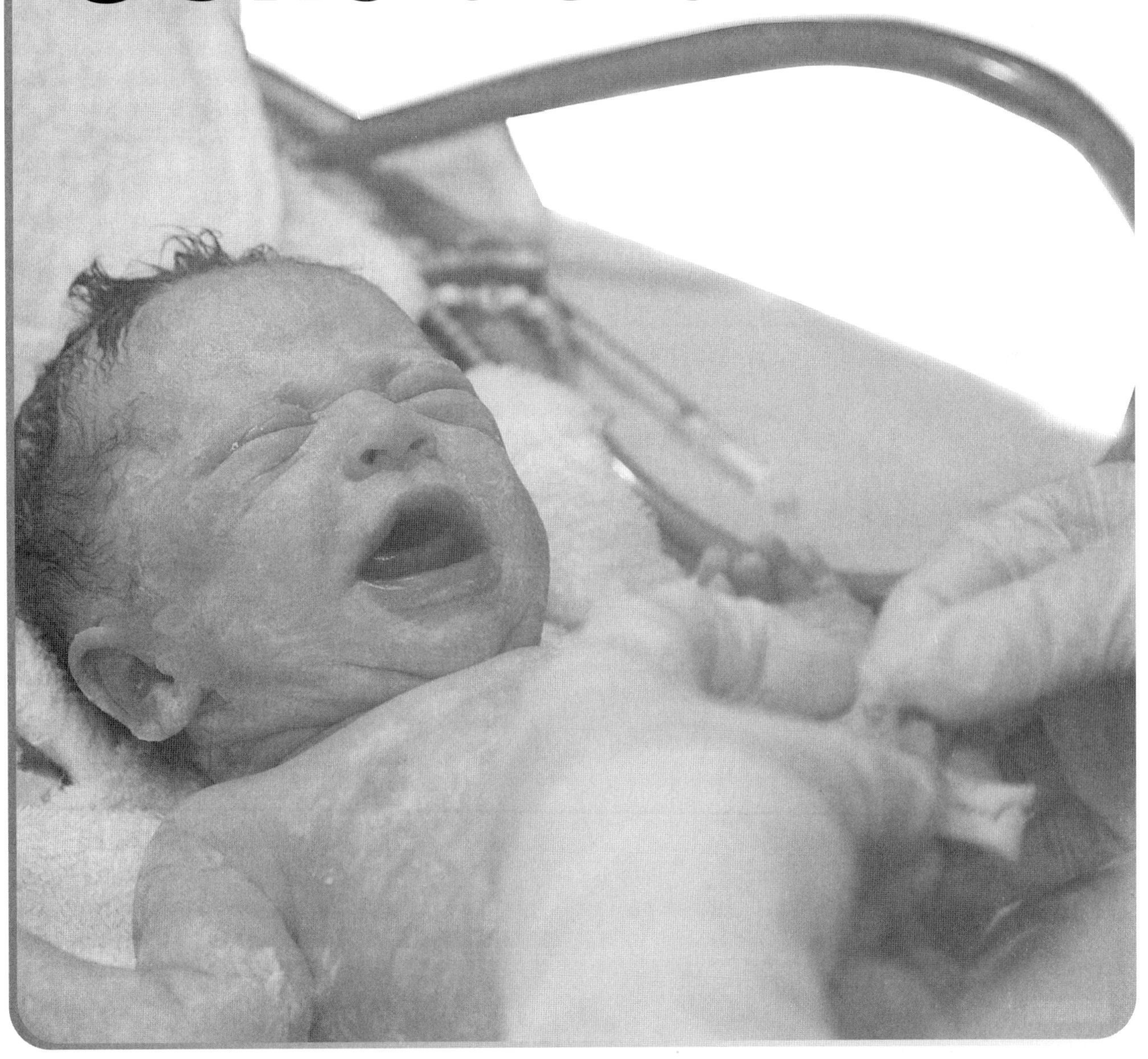

- Most will have a large trunk, short extremities, and skin that may appear translucent.
- Resuscitation should be attempted if the infant has any signs of life.
- Transportation to a facility with special services for low-birth-weight newborns is indicated.
- Healthy premature infants weighing greater than 1700 g (3.5 lb) have a survivability and outcome about that of full-term infants.

Low Birth Weight

- The average term newborn weighs about 3600 g (7.5 lb).
- Birth weight depends on many factors including the size and racial origin of the parents. Small parents tend to have small babies; Asian babies tend to be smaller than Caucasian babies.
- Newborn boys usually weigh about 8 ounces more than baby girls.
- Antepartum (before labor and delivery) and intrapartum (during labor and delivery) risk factors can affect the need for resuscitation.

Antepartum Risk Factors

- Multiple gestation
- Inadequate prenatal care
- Mother's age (less than age 16 or older than age 35)
- History of perinatal morbidity or mortality
- Postterm gestation
- Drugs/medications
- Toxemia, hypertension, diabetes

Intrapartum Risk Factors

- Premature labor.
- Meconium-stained amniotic fluid.
- Rupture of membranes greater than 24 hours before delivery.
- Use of narcotics within 4 hours of delivery.
- Abnormal presentation.
- Prolonged labor or precipitous delivery.
- Prolapsed cord.
- Bleeding.
- The paramedic should prepare equipment and drugs that may be required for neonatal resuscitation for any of the risk factors listed above.
- Medical direction should also be advised of the situation so that the appropriate destination hospital can be determined.

Congenital Anomalies

The presence of some congenital anomalies may also be a factor in the need for neonatal resuscitation. Some more common congenital anomalies include choanal atresia, cleft lip, cleft palate, diaphragmatic hernia, and Pierre Robin syndrome.

Choanal Atresia

- A bony or membranous occlusion that blocks the passageway between the nose and pharynx. Can result in serious ventilation problems in the neonate.

Chapter 34
Neonatology

You are sitting awaiting an assignment in your response area when over the radio you hear a basic life support (BLS) unit requesting advanced life support (ALS) for a female in labor. As you arrive at the scene, one of the emergency medical technician's (EMTs) meets you in the lobby and states the patient is 25 weeks pregnant and is a current crack cocaine user, the baby is crowning, and there is meconium staining present in the amniotic fluid. As you enter, the female patient has just completed delivery of a distressed neonate. The meconium, which resembles "pea soup," is observed in the amniotic fluid.

After suctioning the mouth and nose with a bulb syringe, what should your immediate next step be?

Approximately 6% of infants born in United States hospitals require resuscitation immediately after birth. This figure is thought to be much higher in the prehospital setting.

TERMINOLOGY

- Newborn refers to a recently born infant in the first few hours of life.
- Neonate refers to infants in the first 28 days of life.
- The premature infant refers to a baby born before 37 weeks' gestation.

RISK FACTORS ASSOCIATED WITH THE NEED FOR RESUSCITATION

- Most term newborns require no resuscitation beyond maintenance of temperature, suctioning of the airway, and mild stimulation.
- The incidence of complications, however, increases as birth weight decreases.
- In fact, resuscitation is required for about 80% of the 30,000 babies who weigh less than 1500 g (3.12 lb) at birth.
- Causes of low birth weight include:
  - Premature births
  - Undernourishment in the uterus
  - Maternal factors, such as:
    - — Preeclampsia
    - — Cigarette smoking during pregnancy
- The weight of these newborns is often between 0.6 and 2.2 kg or 1.5 and 5 lb.
- Premature infants have an increased risk for respiratory depression, hypothermia, and/or head and brain injury.

Cleft Lip

- One or more fissures that originate in the embryo. A vertical, usually off-center split in the upper lip that may extend up to the nose.

Cleft Palate

- A fissure in the roof of the mouth that runs along its midline that may extend through both the hard and soft palates into the nasal cavities.

Diaphragmatic Hernia

- Protrusion of a part of the stomach through an opening in the diaphragm.
- In some cases the intestines may herniate into the chest, displacing the heart and resulting in severe respiratory distress.
- Occurs in 1 in 2200 live births.
- Most commonly (90%) on the left side.
- Survival for infants who require mechanical ventilation in the first 18–24 hours of life is approximately 50%.
- If no respiratory distress within the first 24 hours of life, survival approaches 100%.

Risk factors

- Bag and mask ventilation can worsen condition

Pathophysiology

- Abdominal contents are displaced into the thorax
- Heart may be displaced

Assessment findings

- Little to severe distress
- May have cyanosis unresponsive to ventilations
- Scaphoid (flat) abdomen
- Bowel sounds heard in chest
- Heart sounds displaced to right

Management considerations

- Airway and ventilation
- Ensure adequate oxygen
- Place an orogastric tube and apply low, intermittent suction
- Endotracheal intubation may be necessary
- Circulation
- Monitor heart rate continuously
- Surgical repair required
- Transport consideration
- Identify facility to handle high-risk newborn

Pierre Robin Syndrome

- A multitude of anomalies including:
  - A small mandible
  - Cleft lip

  - Cleft palate
  - Other craniofacial abnormalities
  - Defects of the eyes and ears

PHYSIOLOGICAL CHANGES AT BIRTH

- At birth, newborns make three major physiological adaptations necessary for survival:
  - Emptying of fluids from their lungs and beginning ventilation
  - The changing of their circulatory pattern
  - Maintaining body temperature
- During vaginal delivery, the newborn's chest is usually compressed, which forces fluid from the lungs into the mouth and nose. The chest wall recoils, air is drawn into the lungs, and the newborn takes the first breath in response to chemical changes and changes in temperature.
- When the cord is cut and placental circulation shuts down, the circulatory system must become an independently functioning unit. This involves the immediate and permanent closure of the pathways that allowed the fetus to receive oxygen without the use of lungs.
- As the lungs expand with initial breaths, the resistance to blood flow in the lungs decreases, and the newborn's blood begins to be oxygenated.
- Newborns are very sensitive to hypoxia, and permanent brain damage will occur from prolonged hypoxemia.
- Causes of hypoxia include the following:
  - Compression of the cord
  - Difficult labor and delivery
  - Maternal hemorrhage
  - Airway obstruction
  - Hypothermia
  - Newborn blood loss
  - Immature lungs in the premature newborn
- Newborns are at great risk for rapidly developing hypothermia because of the following:
  - They have a larger body surface area
  - Decreased tissue insulation
  - Immature temperature regulatory mechanisms
- Newborns attempt to conserve body heat through vasoconstriction and increasing their metabolism, placing them at risk for the following:
  - Hypoxemia
  - Acidosis
  - Bradycardia
  - Hypoglycemia

ASSESSMENT AND MANAGEMENT OF THE NEONATE

- Initial steps of neonatal resuscitation except for infants born through meconium are:
  - Prevent heat loss
  - Clear the airway by positioning and suctioning
  - Provide tactile stimulation and initiate breathing if necessary
- Further evaluate the infant.
- These steps enable the paramedic to immediately recognize an infant in need of resuscitation and lead to efficient and effective emergency care delivery.

Prevention of Heat Loss

- Even healthy, term newborns are limited in their ability to conserve heat when exposed to a cold environment.
- Immediately after delivery, dry the infant's head and body to prevent evaporative heat loss and metabolic problems that may be brought on by cold stress. Take care to remove any wet coverings from the infant and to cover the infant with dry wrappings. Most heat loss can be prevented by covering the newborn's head (which accounts for 20% of the newborn's body surface area).

Opening the Airway

- After the infant has been dried and covered, establish an open airway by correctly positioning the infant and suctioning the mouth and nose.
- Place the neonate on the back or side with the neck slightly extended (sniffing position); take care to prevent hyperextension, which may compromise the airway.
- After positioning, suction the mouth and nose with a bulb syringe or mechanical suction.
- Suctioning the mouth first to prevent aspiration is preferable in case the infant gasps when the nose is cleared of secretions.
- Each application of suction should last no more than 5 seconds to prevent hypoxia.
- Be careful to avoid deep or vigorous suctioning because stimulation of the posterior pharynx can produce a vagal response with resulting bradycardia, apnea, or both.
- Monitor the newborn's heart rate during suctioning.
- Allow time during suction attempts for spontaneous ventilation or assisted ventilation with 100% oxygen.
- Suctioning provides a degree of tactile stimulation that may initiate respirations.

Meconium Staining

- The presence of fetal stool in amniotic fluid (occurring either in utero or intrapartum) occurs in about 10–15% of all deliveries, becoming more common in postterm and small-for-gestational-age newborns.
- Meconium staining is associated with:
  - Increased perinatal mortality
  - Hypoxemia
  - Aspiration pneumonia
  - Pneumothorax
  - Pulmonary hypertension
- Depending on the amount of meconium particles and the amount of amniotic fluid, the staining may range from a slight yellow or light green to a thick meconium that has a "pea-soup" appearance.
- When thick meconium is present in amniotic fluid, there is a chance the particles will be aspirated into the infant's mouth and potentially into the trachea and lungs (meconium aspiration syndrome), leading to the following:
  - Atelectasis
  - Development of pneumothorax
- Death may result from hypoxia, hypercapnia, or acidosis.
- After meconium is observed in the amniotic fluid, intervention is aimed at preventing or minimizing the risk of aspiration by the newborn.
- Emergency management includes the following:
  - Prepare the necessary equipment:
    - — Intubation equipment

    - Bulb syringe and DeLee suction
    - 10-French or larger suction catheter
    - Portable suction and irrigation solution
    - Gauze pads
    - Infant bag-valve device
  - As the baby's head is delivered (and before shoulder delivery), clear the infant's airway and thoroughly suction the mouth, pharynx, and nose in that order.
  - After delivery of the infant, remove residual meconium in the hypopharynx by suction under direct visualization.
  - If the neonate is depressed or the meconium is thick or particulate, perform direct endotracheal suctioning using the endotracheal (ET) tube as a suction catheter.
  - Quickly intubate the trachea (preferably before the baby has taken its first breath).
  - Apply suction to the proximal end of the endotracheal tube while withdrawing the tube.
  - During intubation and suction, aim 100% oxygen toward the infant's face and monitor the fetal heart rate for bradycardia.
  - If bradycardia develops, ventilate the infant's lungs using a bag-valve device after suctioning to prevent persistent bradycardia and hypoxia.
  - Repeat the intubation-suction-extubation cycle until no further meconium is obtained.
    - Do not ventilate between intubations
  - After tracheal suction is complete, continue resuscitative measures as needed. If respirations are adequate, manage the infant's airway in the normal fashion.

Tactile Stimulation

- If drying and suctioning do not induce respirations, provide additional tactile stimulation. Two safe and appropriate methods are:
  - Slapping or flicking the soles of the feet
  - Rubbing the infant's back
- If the infant remains apneic after a brief period (5–10 seconds) of stimulation, immediately initiate positive-pressure ventilation with a pediatric bag-valve device and supplemental oxygen (40–60 ventilations/min).

Evaluation of the Infant (Table 34-1)

- Drying, positioning, suctioning, and stimulating are necessary in every infant at birth and are used to clear the airway and to initiate respirations.
- The next step in the resuscitation process depends on evaluation of the infant's respiratory effort, heart rate, and color.
- The following steps are suggested for monitoring and evaluating the newborn:
  - Observe and evaluate the infant's respirations:
    - If normal (crying), continue the evaluation.
    - If respirations are inadequate or gasping is present, begin positive-pressure ventilation immediately.
    - If the respiratory response is slow or shallow, a brief period of stimulation may be attempted while 100% oxygen is administered.
    - If no response is noted after 5–10 seconds of stimulation and oxygen administration, begin positive-pressure ventilation.
  - Evaluate the infant's heart rate by stethoscope, or by palpating the pulse in the umbilical cord or brachial artery.

TABLE 34-1: Apgar Score

SIGNS	0	1	2	1-MINUTE	5-MINUTE
HEART RATE	absent	<100	>100		
RESPIRATORY EFFORT	absent	slow, irregular	good, crying		
MUSCLE TONE	limp	some flexion of extremities	active motion		
REFLEX IRRITABILITY	no response	grimace	cough, sneeze		
COLOR	blue, pale	body pink, extremities blue	completely pink		
		TOTAL SCORE:			

— If it is above 100 beats/min, continue the evaluation.

— If it is less than 100 beats/min, initiate positive-pressure ventilation.

— If the heart rate is less than 60–80 beats/min and does not increase despite 30 seconds of positive-pressure ventilation, initiate chest compressions (2–$^3/_4$ in. deep) at a rate of 120/min.

◦ Evaluate the infant's color.

— If central cyanosis is present in an infant with spontaneous respirations and an adequate heart rate, administer free-flow oxygen at 5 L/min.

— A maximum oxygen concentration of about 80% can be achieved when the tube is $^1/_2$ in. from the infant's nose.

Hold the tubing steady in a cupped hand and aim it at the nares.

Waving the end of the tubing back and forth or withdrawing the tube 1 or 2 in. from the infant's face considerably decreases oxygen concentration.

RESUSCITATION OF THE DISTRESSED NEWBORN

- Risk factors associated with the need for resuscitation include the following:
  - Premature delivery
  - Maternal health problems
  - Complicated pregnancies
  - Delivery complications
- If, with continued assisted ventilations, the infant's condition continues to deteriorate or fails to improve, the infant may require ET intubation and the administration of medications.

Before considering intubation or pharmacological therapy, reevaluate two components of the resuscitation process.

- Is chest movement adequate?
  - Check for adequacy of chest expansion and auscultate for bilateral breath sounds.
  - Is the face-mask seal tight?
    - — A relatively large mask should be turned upside down for a better fit.

- Is the airway blocked from improper head position or secretions in the nose, mouth, or pharynx?
  - — Reassess head position and reexamine the airway for the presence of secretions.
- Is adequate ventilatory pressure being used?
  - — A bag-valve mask (BVM) pop-off valve may need to be disabled to allow for higher inspiratory pressures, especially for premature or meconium-aspiration delivery.
- Is air in the stomach interfering with chest expansion?
  - — Consider nasogastric or orogastric decompression per protocol.

- Is 100% oxygen being administered?
  - Is the oxygen tubing attached to the bag and to the flow meter?
  - If using a self-inflating bag, is the oxygen reservoir attached?

Routes of Drug Administration

- Drugs and fluids may be administered to the neonate via peripheral cannulation, IO, including some drugs that can be given through the ET tube.
- Another common site for vascular access in the neonate is the umbilical vein.
- The umbilical cord contains three vessels: two arteries and one vein.
- The vein in the umbilical cord has a thin wall and is larger than the arteries.
- The arteries are thick walled and usually paired.
- To gain access to the umbilical vein:
  - Set up intravenous (IV) fluid (per protocol) and tubing with a three-way stopcock
  - Select a 3.5-French or 5.0-French umbilical catheter
  - Connect the catheter to the stopcock and purge the air from the catheter
  - Cleanse the umbilical stump and surrounding skin with antibacterial solution
  - Loosely tie umbilical tape around the cord so that pressure can be applied to control bleeding
  - Hold the umbilical stump firmly, and, with a scalpel, trim the cord several centimeters above the abdomen
  - Locate the umbilical vein and insert the catheter until blood is freely obtained
    - — Do not insert the catheter more than 6–8 cm
  - Draw blood for a sample if needed
  - Start the infusion and regulate the fluid flow per medical direction
  - Secure the catheter in place with tape and cover with a sterile dressing
  - Document the procedure
- The umbilical cord also may be cannulated by using a typical IV catheter.
- Insert the catheter-over-needle through the side of the proximal end of the cord into the vein and advance it upward through the translucent wall.
- Start the infusion.
- Adjust the fluid flow per medical direction.
- Secure the catheter in place with tape.

Medications Used in Neonatal Resuscitation

- Medications most frequently used during neonatal resuscitation are:
  - Epinephrine
  - Volume expanders
  - Naloxone

POSTRESUSCITATION CARE

The three most common complications of the postresuscitation period are:

- ET migration (including dislodgement)
- Tube occlusion by mucus or meconium
- Pneumothorax

These complications should be suspected in the presence of the following:

- Decreased chest wall movement
- Diminished breath sounds
- Return of bradycardia
- Unilateral decrease in chest expansion
- Altered intensity to pitch of breath sounds
- Increased resistance to hand ventilation

Corrective management in the field for these postresuscitative complications may include the following:

- Adjustment of the ET tube
- Reintubation
- Suction

Needle decompression to manage a suspected pneumothorax must be carefully performed.

NEONATAL TRANSPORT

- During transport of the neonate; maintain body temperature, administer oxygen, and provide ventilatory support when appropriate.
- In the prehospital phase of care, transport strategies are usually limited to providing a warm ambulance, free-flow oxygen administration, and warm blankets.
- Specialized transport equipment such as isolettes and radiant heating units are often used for interhospital transfers and require special training.
- Highly trained neonatal transport teams consisting of paramedics, nurses, respiratory therapists, and physicians are part of several well-organized regional referral systems throughout the United States.

SPECIFIC SITUATIONS

Respiratory Disorders

- Respiratory insufficiency in the neonate is generally managed by:
  - Stimulation and positioning of the airway
  - Prevention of heat loss
  - Oxygenation and ventilation
  - Suction
  - Intubation with ventilatory support (if needed)
- Pharmacological therapy that may be appropriate in managing some infants with respiratory disorders (per medical direction) includes:
  - Administration of sodium bicarbonate for prolonged resuscitation
  - Dextrose if hypoglycemia is suspected or confirmed
  - Naloxone if maternal narcotic use is suspected

- Apnea (respiratory pauses that exceed 20 seconds) is a common finding in preterm infants and, if prolonged, may lead to hypoxemia and Bradycardia.
- Primary apnea is a self-limited condition (controlled by PCO_2 levels) that is common immediately after birth.
- Secondary apnea describes respirations that are absent and that do not begin again spontaneously.
- Risk factors include:
  - Prematurity
  - In newborn, prolonged or difficult labor and delivery
  - Drug exposure

Pathophysiology

- Usually due to hypoxia or hypothermia
- May be due to other causes
  - Narcotics or central nervous system (CNS) depressant
  - Airway and respiratory muscle weakness
  - Oxyhemoglobin dissociation curve shift
  - Septicemia
  - Metabolic disorder
  - CNS disorders
- Assessment findings
  - Failure to breathe spontaneously after stimulation
  - Respiratory pauses greater than 20 seconds

Management

- Airway and ventilation:
  - Stimulate the baby to breathe
    - — Flicking the soles of the feet
    - — Rubbing the back
  - Ventilate with BVM
    - — Disable pop-off valve
    - — Subsequent ventilations with minimal pressure to cause chest rise
  - Suction as needed
  - Intubation
    - — Indications

      Heart rate less that 60 beats/min with adequate BVM ventilation and chest compressions

      Prolonged positive-pressure ventilations

      Prolonged apnea

      Central cyanosis despite adequate ventilations
  - Complications
    - — Tube dislodgement
    - — Tube occlusion by mucus or meconium
    - — Pneumothorax
- Circulation:
  - Monitor heart rate continuously

- Circulatory access
  - Umbilical vein cannulation in newborn
  - Peripheral IV
  - Intraosseous
- Pharmacological:
  - Consider narcotic antagonists if narcotic administered within 4 hours of delivery
  - No narcotic antagonist should be used if mother is a drug abuser
  - Consider dextrose (D_{10}) administration if hypoglycemic
- Maintain normal body temperature.
- Many parents use apnea detection devices to monitor their child's breathing during sleep.
- Infants should be positioned on their backs while sleeping.
- Respiratory distress and cyanosis:
  - Prematurity is the single most common factor for respiratory distress and cyanosis in the neonate
    - The condition occurs most frequently in infants weighing less than 1200 g (2.5 lb) and younger than 30 weeks' gestation

      May be related to the infant's immature central respiratory control center that easily is affected by environmental or metabolic changes
- Other risk factors for respiratory distress and cyanosis include:
  - Lung or heart disease
  - Primary pulmonary hypertension
  - CNS disorders
  - Mucus obstruction of nasal passages
  - Spontaneous pneumothorax
  - Choanal atresia
  - Meconium aspiration
  - Amniotic fluid aspiration
  - Lung immaturity
  - Pneumonia
  - Shock and sepsis
  - Metabolic acidosis
  - Diaphragmatic hernia
- Can lead to cardiac arrest, requires immediate intervention to support respirations.
- Assessment findings:
  - Tachypnea
  - Paradoxical breathing
  - Intercostal retractions
  - Nasal flaring
  - Expiratory grunt
  - Central cyanosis
- Management considerations:
  - Airway and ventilation
    - Suction
    - High concentration oxygen
    - BVM
    - Consider intubation

- Circulation—Chest compressions if indicated
- Pharmacological
  - Possible sodium bicarbonate if prolonged resuscitation (per medical direction)
  - D_{10} administration if hypoglycemic
- Maintain normal body temperature

Cardiovascular Disorders

- A neonate's heart generally is healthy and strong; however, disorders in the heart's conduction system can and do occur, usually from hypoxemia and respiratory arrest. All neonates with cardiovascular disorders should be assessed for treatable causes of hypoventilation.

Bradycardia

- Bradycardia is defined as a heart rate less than 100 beats/min.
- Causes include:
  - Hypoxia (most common)
  - Increased intracranial pressure
  - Hypothyroidism
  - Acidosis
- Considered a minimal risk to life in neonates if corrected quickly.

Cardiac Arrest

- Asystole and pulseless arrest are uncommon in children and usually result from hypoxia.
- Outcome is poor if interventions are not initiated quickly
- Increased likelihood of brain and organ damage
- Risk factors include
  - Intrauterine asphyxia
  - Drugs administered to or taken by the mother
  - Congenital neuromuscular disease
  - Congenital malformations
  - Intrapartum hypoxemia
- Pathophysiology
  - Primary apnea
  - Secondary apnea
  - Bradycardia
  - Persistent fetal circulation
  - Pulmonary hypertension
- Assessment findings
  - Peripheral cyanosis
  - Inadequate respiratory effort
  - Ineffective or absent heart rate
- Prehospital emergency management:
  - Airway and ventilation
    - — Ensure adequate oxygenation and ventilation
    - — Blow-by oxygenation is required if peripheral cyanosis is present and despite adequate respiratory effort and heart rate greater than 100 beats/min
    - — Ventilations are required if respiratory effort is inadequate, ineffective, or absent or heart rate is less than 80 beats/min

    - — Ventilate at a rate of 40–60 breaths/min
    - — Administer a tidal volume sufficient to expand the chest
    - — Intubation required if BVM ventilations are ineffective, tracheal suctioning is required, or prolonged positive-pressure ventilation is necessary
    - — Chest compressions are indicated if pulse is:
      Less than 60 beats/min
      Or between 60 and 80 beats/min and not improving despite assisted ventilations with BVM
    - — Suction airway thoroughly
  - ◦ Circulation—Perform chest compressions
  - ◦ Pharmacological therapy may include:
    - — Epinephrine
    - — Normal saline or Ringer's lactate
    - — Sodium bicarbonate
    - — Naloxone
    - — Dextrose (D_{10})
  - ◦ Maintain normal body temperature
  - ◦ Rapid transport to an appropriate facility

Hypovolemia

- May result from the following:
  - ◦ Dehydration
  - ◦ Hemorrhage
  - ◦ Trauma
  - ◦ Sepsis
- May be associated with myocardial dysfunction.
- Signs and symptoms include:
  - ◦ Mottled or pale color (that persists after oxygenation)
  - ◦ Cool skin
  - ◦ Tachycardia
  - ◦ Diminished peripheral pulses
  - ◦ Delayed capillary refill despite normal ambient temperature
- Prompt and effective treatment of early signs of compensated shock may prevent the development of hypotension (decompensated shock) and associated high morbidity and mortality.
- Prehospital management:
  - ◦ Ensure an adequate airway
  - ◦ Provide ventilatory, and circulatory support (including control of external hemorrhage)
  - ◦ Provide rapid transport to an appropriate medical facility
- When signs of hypovolemia are present:
  - ◦ Administer a fluid bolus (20 mL/kg of isotonic crystalloid immediately after IV or IO access is obtained)
  - ◦ Reassess
  - ◦ If signs of shock persist, administer a second 20-mL/kg bolus
  - ◦ Additional boluses should be infused as indicated by repeated reassessments of the patient and under the guidance of medical direction

Gastrointestinal Disorders

- Occasional vomiting or diarrhea is not unusual in the neonate. Vomiting mucus (that may occasionally be blood streaked) is common in the first few hours of life.
- Five to six stools per day is considered normal, especially if the infant is breast-feeding.
- Persistent vomiting and/or diarrhea should be considered warning signs of serious illness.

Vomiting

- Persistent vomiting is a warning sign.
- Vomiting mucus, occasionally blood streaked, in the first few hours of life is not uncommon.
- Vomiting in the first 24 hours of life suggests obstruction in the upper digestive tract or increased intracranial pressure (ICP).
- Vomitus containing dark blood is usually a sign of a life-threatening illness.
- Aspiration of vomitus can cause respiratory insufficiencies or obstruction of the airway.
- Pathophysiology:
  - Vomiting of non-bile-stained fluid
  - Anatomical or functional obstruction at or above the first portion of the duodenum
  - May be indicative of gastroesophageal reflux
  - Vomiting of bile-stained fluid
  - Obstruction below the opening of the bile duct
- Assessment findings:
  - Distended stomach
  - Signs of infection
  - Increased ICP
  - Drug withdrawal (from the mother's drug use)
- Prehospital management:
  - Usually limited to maintaining a patent airway that is clear of vomit and ensuring adequate oxygenation.
  - In severe cases, medical direction may recommend that IV fluid therapy be initiated before transport to treat dehydration and any bradycardia that may develop from vagal stimulation.
  - If possible, the infant should be transported on his or her side to help prevent aspiration.

Diarrhea

- Normal—Five to six stools per day, especially if breast-feeding.
- Severe cases can cause dehydration.
- Bacterial or viral infection may be involved.
- Severe loss can cause electrolyte imbalance.
- Pathophysiology:
  - Gastroenteritis
  - Rotavirus
  - Lactose intolerance
  - Phototherapy (a treatment for hyperbilirubinemia and jaundice in the newborn)
  - Neonatal abstinence syndrome (drug withdrawal)
  - Thyrotoxicosis
  - Cystic fibrosis

- Assessment findings:
  - Loose stools
  - Decreased urinary output
  - Signs of dehydration
- Prehospital management:
  - Support the infant's vital functions
  - IV fluid therapy (per medical direction)
  - Rapid transport to the receiving hospital

Seizures

- Occur in a very small percentage of all newborns. Represent relative medical emergencies, as they are usually a sign of an underlying abnormality.
- Prolonged and frequent multiple seizures may result in metabolic changes and cardiopulmonary difficulties.

Causes

- Hypoglycemia
- Hypoxic-ischemic encephalopathy
- Intracranial hemorrhage
- Metabolic disturbances
- Meningitis or encephalopathy
- Developmental abnormalities
- Drug withdrawal

Types of Seizures

Subtle Seizures

- Involve eye deviation, blinking, sucking, swimming movements of the arms, or peddling movements of the legs
- Apnea may be present during subtle seizures

Tonic Seizures

- Tonic extension of the limbs
- Less commonly, flexion of the upper extremities and extension of the lower extremities
- More common in premature infants, especially in those with intraventricular hemorrhage

Multifocal Seizures

- Clonic activity in one extremity
- Randomly migrates to another area of the body
- Occur primarily in full-term infants

Focal Clonic Seizures

- Localized clonic jerking
- Occur in both full-term and premature infants
- Myoclonic seizures
- Flexion jerks of the upper or lower extremities
- May occur singly or in a series of repetitive jerks

Management

- Provide airway, ventilatory, and circulatory support
- Maintain the infant's body temperature
- Pharmacological therapy prescribed by medical direction may include
  - Dextrose to treat hypoglycemia
  - Anticonvulsant agents
  - Benzodiazepines (for status epilepticus)
- Seizure activity is always considered pathological
- Rapid transport for physician evaluation is indicated

Fever

- Rectal temperature: 100.4°F (38.0°C)
  - Is generally a cause for concern
  - Often a response to an acute viral or bacterial infection
- Average normal temperature: 99.5°F (37.5°C)
  - Limited ability to control body temperature
  - Dehydration may contribute to hyperthermia
- Pathophysiology
  - Rise in core temperature is associated with increased oxygen demand
  - Increased use of glucose to maintain normal body temperature
  - Anaerobic metabolism results due to a lack of glucose
- Assessment findings
  - Mental status changes (irritability/somnolence)
  - History of decreased intake
  - Feels warm or hot
  - Observe patient for rashes, petechia
  - Term newborns will produce beads of sweat on their brow but not over the rest of their body
  - Premature infants will generally have no visible sweat
- Prehospital management
  - Primarily supportive
  - As a rule, cooling procedures and the use of antipyretics will be delayed until the child has arrived in the emergency department

Hypothermia

- Body temperature drops below 35°C
- Infants may die of cold exposure at temperatures adults find comfortable
- Four methods of heat loss need to be controlled
  - Evaporation
  - Conduction
  - Convection
  - Radiation
- Pathophysiology
  - Increased surface-to-volume relation makes newborns extremely sensitive to environmental conditions, especially when they are wet after delivery
  - Can be an indicator of sepsis in the neonate
  - Increased metabolic demand can cause metabolic acidosis

- Assessment findings
  - Pale color
  - Cool to touch (especially in extremities)
  - Respiratory distress
  - Apnea
  - Bradycardia
  - Central cyanosis
  - Irritability (initially)
  - Lethargy in late stage
  - Absence of shivering (variable)
- Prehospital management
  - Provide basic and advanced cardiac life support (depending on the severity of hypothermia)
  - Rapid transport to an appropriate facility
  - Ensure the infant is dry and warm
  - Possible administration of D_{10} to treat hypoglycemia and IV therapy with warm fluids
  - Transport in a heated ambulance (24°–26.5°C [76°–80°F])

Hypoglycemia

- A blood glucose screening test less than 40 mg/dL indicates hypoglycemia.
- Blood glucose concentration should be determined on all sick infants.
- May be due to:
  - Inadequate glucose intake
  - Increased utilization of glucose
- Persistent low blood glucose levels may have catastrophic effects on the brain.
- Risk factors include:
  - Asphyxia
  - Toxemia
  - Smaller twin
  - CNS hemorrhage
  - Sepsis
- Assessment findings:
  - Twitching or seizure
  - Limpness
  - Lethargy
  - Eye-rolling
  - High-pitched crying
  - Apnea
  - Irregular respirations
  - Possible cyanosis
- Prehospital management:
  - Ensure adequate airway, ventilatory, and circulatory support
  - Maintain body temperature
  - Rapid transport
  - IV/IO administration of D_{10} (per medical direction)
  - Repeat blood glucose evaluation if the infant fails to respond to initial resuscitative measures

- All infants with an altered level of consciousness and those who are hypoglycemic and fail to respond to the administration of dextrose should be immediately transported to an appropriate medical facility.

COMMON BIRTH INJURIES

- Used to denote avoidable and unavoidable mechanical and anoxic trauma incurred by the infant during labor and delivery.
- Estimated to occur in 2–7 of every 1000 live births.
- 5–8 of every 100,000 infants die of birth trauma.
- 25 of every 100,000 die of anoxic injuries.
- Such injuries account for 2–3% of infant deaths.
- Risk factors include uncontrolled, explosive delivery.
- Injuries that sometimes occur to the infant during childbirth include:
  - Cranial injuries
    - — Molding of the head and overriding of the parietal bones
    - — Soft-tissue injuries from forceps delivery (e.g., erythema, abrasions, ecchymosis)
    - — Subconjunctival and retinal hemorrhage
    - — Subperiosteal hemorrhage
    - — Skull fracture
  - Intracranial hemorrhage (from trauma or asphyxia)
  - Spine and spinal cord injury (from strong traction or lateral pull)
  - Peripheral nerve injury
  - Liver or spleen injury
  - Adrenal hemorrhage
  - Clavicle or extremity fracture
  - Hypoxia-ischemia
- Assessment findings:
  - Will vary by the nature of the injury and may include
    - — Diffuse, sometimes ecchymotic, edematous swelling of the soft tissues of the scalp
    - — Paralysis below the level of spinal cord injury
    - — Paralysis of the upper arm with or without paralysis of the forearm
    - — Diaphragmatic paralysis
    - — Movement on only one side of the face when the newborn cries
    - — Does not move arm freely on side of fractured clavicle
    - — Lack of spontaneous movement of the affected extremity
    - — Hypoxia
    - — Shock
- Prehospital management:
  - Support vital functions
  - Rapidly transport to an appropriate medical facility for definitive care

PSYCHOLOGICAL AND EMOTIONAL SUPPORT

- It is important to be aware of the normal feelings and reactions of parents, siblings, other family members, and caregivers while providing emergency care to an ill or injured child. These events also are often highly charged and emotional for the emergency medical service (EMS) crew.

- Those at the scene should be kept abreast of all procedures being performed and of the necessity of the procedures. As a rule, emergency responders should:
  - Never discuss the infant's chances of survival with a parent or family member
  - Not give "false hope" about the infant's condition
  - Assure the family that everything that can be done for the child is being done
  - Assure the family that their baby will receive the best possible care during transport and while at the emergency department
- The receiving hospital will have appropriate support personnel available to assist family members and loved ones.

? CHAPTER QUESTIONS

1. A neonate is an infant from the time of birth to:
   a. 1 week of age
   b. 2 weeks of age
   c. 1 month of age
   d. 3 months of age
2. The term newborn or newly born infant is used to describe a neonate:
   a. until the umbilical cord is cut
   b. during the time it spends in the delivery room
   c. until it is discharged from the hospital
   d. during the first few hours of life
3. The difference between primary apnea and secondary apnea in a newborn is that:
   a. infants with primary apnea typically will respond to simple stimulation and oxygen while those in secondary apnea will not
   b. bradycardia is present in primary apnea but not in secondary apnea
   c. infants with secondary apnea typically will respond to simple stimulation and oxygen while those in primary apnea will not
   d. bradycardia is present in secondary apnea but not in primary apnea
4. A normal newborn's respiratory rate should average:
   a. 12–20 breaths per minute
   b. 20–30 breaths per minute
   c. 40–60 breaths per minute
   d. 60–80 breaths per minute
5. A newborn's heart rate should normally be:
   a. 80–100 at birth, speeding to 140–160 thereafter
   b. 150–180 at birth, slowing to 130–140 thereafter
   c. 170–190 at birth, slowing to 80–100 thereafter
   d. 60–80 at birth, speeding to 150–180 thereafter

Suggested Reading

US Department of Transportation, National Highway Traffic Safety Administration. *EMT-Paramedic: National Standard Curriculum*. Washington, DC: US Department of Transportation, National Highway Traffic Safety Administration; 1998.

Chapter 35
Pediatrics

A 4-month-old male infant presents with respiratory distress, fever, and warm mottled skin. The baby has been ill for several days with increasing irritability. He does not appear to recognize his parents and looks very ill. He is tachycardic and displays a delayed capillary refill.

What is the most likely cause of these signs and symptoms?

- Emergencies involving pediatric patients account for about 10% or less of all emergency medical service (EMS) responses. Caring for these patients presents unique challenges that relate to size, physical and intellectual maturation, and diseases specific to neonates, infants, and children.
- Paramedics play an important role in treating infants and children through both prehospital care (primary transport) and interfacility transfer (secondary transport).
- It is important to maintain and improve knowledge and clinical skills for these patients through continuing education programs and clinical application specific to this age group.

EMERGENCY MEDICAL SERVICES FOR CHILDREN

- In 1985, the Emergency Medical Services for Children (EMSC) Demonstration Program was established through grants provided by the Department of Health and Human Services, Maternal and Child Health Bureau, and the Department of Transportation, National Highway Traffic Safety Administration.
- This program was designed to enhance and expand emergency medical services for acutely ill and injured children and has defined 12 basic components of an effective EMSC system.
    - System approach
    - Education
    - Data collection
    - Quality improvement
    - Injury prevention
    - Access
    - Prehospital care
    - Emergency care
    - Definitive care
    - Rehabilitation
    - Finance
    - Ongoing health care from birth to young adulthood

- Through the funding of EMSC grants and the efforts of organizations dedicated to improving emergency care for children, specific programs targeted to prehospital care providers have been developed.
- These include continuing education programs, educational resources for instructors, equipment guidelines, protocols for prehospital management, quality improvement procedures for evaluating prehospital care for children, and designation of facilities with special capabilities for pediatric care.
- As stated in Emergency Medical Service for Children: A Report to the Nation, "The lives of many infants, children, and young adults . . . can be saved through implementation of emergency medical services for children (EMSC)."
- ". . . Outcomes for critically ill and injured children can be influenced by the provision of timely care by health care professionals who are well trained and equipped for pediatric emergency and critical care."
- Paramedics can play a significant role in the reduction of mortality and morbidity for children by becoming active participants in school, community, and parent education programs; participating in injury prevention programs; and providing thorough documentation appropriate for prehospital trauma registries, epidemiological research, and surveillance.

GROWTH AND DEVELOPMENT REVIEW (TABLE 35-1)

Children have unique characteristics in their anatomical, physiological, and psychological makeup, which change during their development.

Pediatric Age Classifications

- Newborn—First few hours of life
- Neonate—First 28 days of life
- Infant—Up to 1 year of age
- Toddler—From 1–3 years of age
- Preschooler—From 3–5 years of age
- School-age—From 6–12 years of age
- Adolescent—The period between the end of childhood (beginning of puberty) and adulthood (18 years of age)
    - Highly child-specific (male child average—13 years; female child average—11 years)
    - May also be defined as early (puberty), middle (middle school/high school), and late (high school/college age)

Anatomy and Physiology Review for Pediatric Patients

Head

- The head is proportionally larger
- Larger occipital region
- Fontanelles open in infancy
- Smaller face in comparison with size of head
- Higher proportion of blunt trauma involves the head
- Airway positioning techniques differ for pediatric patients

TABLE 35-1: Developmental Stages and Approach Strategies for Pediatric Patients

Classification	Major Fears	Characteristics of Thinking	General Approach Strategies
Infants	Separation from strangers		• Provide consistent caretakers • Decrease parent's anxiety since it is transferred to infant • Minimize separation from parents
Toddlers	Separation and loss of control	• Primitive • Inability to recognize views of others • Little concept of body integrity	• Keep explanations simple • Choose words carefully • Let toddler play with equipment (stethoscope) • Minimize separation from parents
Preschoolers	• Bodily injury and mutilation • Loss of control • The unknown and the dark • Being left alone	• Highly literal interpretation of words • Inability to abstract • Primitive ideas about their bodies (fearing that all blood will "leak out" if a bandage is removed)	• Keep explanations simple and concise • Choose words carefully • Emphasize that a procedure will help the child be more healthy • Be honest
School-age children	• Loss of control • Bodily injury and mutilation • Failure to live up to expectations of others • Death	• Vague or false ideas about physical illness, body structure, and function • Ability to listen attentively without always comprehending • Reluctance to ask questions about something they think they are expected to know • Increased awareness of significant illness, potential hazards of managements, lifelong consequences of injury, and the meaning of death	• Ask children to explain what they understand • Provide as many choices as possible to increase the child's sense of control • Assure the child that he or she has done nothing wrong and that necessary procedures are not punishment • Anticipate and answer questions regarding long-term consequences
Adolescents	• Loss of control • Altered body image • Separation from peer group	• Ability to think abstractly • Tendency toward hyperresponsiveness to pain (reactions not always in proportion to event) • Little understanding of the structure and workings of the body	• When appropriate, allow the adolescent to be a part of decision making about his or her care • Give information sensitively • Express how important compliance and cooperation are to management • Be honest about consequences • Use or teach coping mechanisms such as relaxation, deep breathing, and self-comforting talk

- Place thin layer of padding under back of seriously injured child younger than 3 years of age to obtain neutral position
- Examine fontanelle in infants, bulging fontanelle suggests increased intracranial pressure (ICP), sunken fontanelle suggests dehydration

Airway

- Pediatric airway is narrower than adult airway at all levels
- Infants are obligate nasal breathers
- Jaw is posteriorly smaller in young children
- Larynx is higher (C3–C4) and more anterior
- Cricoid ring is the narrowest part of the airway in young children
- Tracheal cartilage is softer
- Trachea is smaller in both length and diameter

Epiglottis

- Omega-shaped in infants
- Extends at a 45° angle into airway
- Epiglottic folds have softer cartilage; more floppy, especially in children
- Keep nares clear in infants under 6 months of age
- Remember that narrower upper airways are more easily obstructed
- Possible causes of obstruction include flexion, hyperextension, particulate matter, or soft tissue swelling (injury, inflammation)

Intubation Techniques/Modifications

- Use gentler touch
- Use straight blade (Miller)
- Lift epiglottis
- Use uncuffed tube up to age 8
- Ensure precise placement

Chest and Lungs

- Ribs are positioned horizontally
- Ribs are more pliable and offer less protection to organs
- Chest muscles are immature and fatigue easily
- Lung tissue is more fragile
- Mediastinum is more mobile
- Thin chest wall allows for easily transmitted breath sounds
- Infants and children are diaphragmatic breathers
- Infants and children are prone to gastric distention
- Rib fractures are less frequent but not uncommon in child abuse and trauma
- Greater energy is transmitted to underlying organs following trauma (significant internal injury can be present without external signs)
- Pulmonary contusions are more common in major trauma
- Lungs are prone to pneumothorax following barotrauma
- Mediastinum has greater shift with tension pneumothorax
- Pneumothorax or misplaced intubation may be missed because of transmitted breath sounds

Abdomen

- Immature abdominal muscles offer less protection.
- Abdominal organs are closer together.
- Liver and spleen are proportionally larger, more vascular, and are more frequently injured.
- Multiple organ injuries are common.

Extremities

- Bones are softer and more porous until adolescence.
- Injuries to growth plate may disrupt bone growth.
- Immobilize any sprain or strain since it is likely a fracture.
- Avoid piercing growth plate during intraosseous (IO) needle insertion.

Skin and Body Surface Area (BSA)

- Skin is thinner and more elastic, therefore thermal exposure results in deeper burns.
- Less subcutaneous fat.
- Larger surface area to body mass.
- Children are more easily and deeply burned.
- Children experience greater losses of fluid and heat.

Respiratory System

- Tidal volume is proportionally smaller than that of adolescents and adults.
- Metabolic oxygen requirements of infants and children are about double those of adolescents and adults.
- Children have proportionally smaller functional residual capacity—and therefore proportionally smaller oxygen reserves.
- Hypoxia develops rapidly because of increased oxygen requirements and decreased oxygen reserves.

Cardiovascular System

- Cardiac output is rate-dependent in infants and small children.
- Infants and small children have vigorous but limited cardiovascular reserve.
- Bradycardia is a response to hypoxia.
- Children can maintain blood pressure longer than adults.
- Circulating blood volume is proportionally larger than adults.
- Absolute blood volume is smaller than adults.
- Smaller volumes of fluid/blood loss can cause shock.
- Hypotension is a late sign of shock.
- A child may be in shock despite a normal blood pressure.
- Shock assessment is based upon clinical signs of tissue perfusion.
- Carefully assess for shock if tachycardia is present.
- Monitor carefully for development of hypotension.
- Intervene early to prevent decompensation.

Nervous System

- Develops throughout childhood (developing neural tissue is more fragile).
- Brain and spinal cord are less protected by skull and spinal column.
- Fontanelles are open in early months.

- Brain injuries are more devastating in young children.
- Greater force is transmitted to underlying brain of young children.
- Spinal cord injury can occur without spinal column injury.

Metabolic Differences

- Infants and children have limited glycogen and glucose stores.
- Blood glucose can drop very low in response to stressors.
- Significant volume loss can result from vomiting and diarrhea.
- Children are prone to hypothermia because of increased body surface area.
- Newborns and neonates are unable to shiver to maintain body temperature.
- Keep children warm during management and transport.
- Cover the head to minimize heat loss.
- Assess for hypoglycemia if prolonged stress state exists.

ILLNESS AND INJURY BY AGE GROUP (TABLE 35-2)

- Several childhood diseases and disabilities are predictable by age group.
- Illnesses and accidents in the seven age groups are frequently encountered by prehospital providers.

TABLE 35-2: Illness and Injury by Age Group

Neonate (first 28 days of life)	Respiratory distress, jaundice, vomiting, fever, sepsis, meningitis, physical and sexual abuse
1- to 5-month-old infant	Respiratory distress, fever, sudden infant death syndrome (SIDS), vomiting and diarrhea with dehydration, sepsis, meningitis, physical and sexual abuse
6- to 12-month-old infant	Fever or febrile seizures, vomiting and diarrhea with dehydration, bronchiolitis, croup, sepsis, meningitis, respiratory distress (bronchiolitis, foreign body aspiration, croup), physical and sexual abuse, foreign body airway obstruction, falls, injuries from motor-vehicle crashes
1- to 3-year-old child	Fever or febrile seizure, vomiting and diarrhea with dehydration, respiratory distress (asthma, bronchiolitis, foreign body aspiration, croup), sepsis, meningitis, ingestions, foreign body airway obstruction, falls, injuries from motor-vehicle crashes, physical and sexual abuse
3- to 5-year-old child	Croup, asthma, febrile seizures, sepsis, meningitis, burns, drowning, near-drowning, injuries from motor-vehicle crashes, physical and sexual abuse
6- to 12-year-old child	Drowning, near-drowning, injuries from motor-vehicle crashes, injuries from bicycle accidents, fractures, falls, sports injuries, burns, physical and sexual abuse
12- to 15-year-old adolescent	Asthma, injuries from motor-vehicle crashes, sports injuries, alcohol or other drug use, suicide gestures, physical and sexual abuse, pregnancy, physical and sexual abuse

PEDIATRIC ASSESSMENT

- Many components of the initial patient evaluation for children can be done by observing the patient and by involving the child's parent or guardian in the initial assessment.
- The parent or guardian can often help make the child more comfortable during the assessment, and can usually provide valuable information about the child's medical history and judgements about whether certain aspects of the child's behavior or response to the illness or injury seem normal or abnormal.

Scene Assessment

- Begin the physical exam with a quick scene survey.
- Note any hazards, potential hazards, visible mechanism, injury, or illness.
- The presence of pills, medicine bottles, or household chemicals may indicate a possible toxic ingestion.
- Injury and history that does not coincide with the mechanism of injury may indicate child abuse.
- Observe the relationship between the parent/guardian/caregiver and the child and determine the appropriateness of their interaction.
- Does the interaction demonstrate concern, or is it angry or indifferent?
- Make other important assessments during the scene survey:
  - Orderliness
  - Cleanliness and safety of the home
  - General appearance of other children in the family

Initial Assessment

- Begin with formulating a general impression of the patient.
- Focus on the most valuable information to ascertain whether life-threatening conditions exist.
- Pediatric Assessment Triangle can be used to assess a child. Three components of the Pediatric Assessment Triangle include:
  - Airway and Appearance
  - Breathing (work of breathing)
  - Circulation
- Using the assessment triangle or a similar method allows the paramedic to make initial triage decisions.
- If the child's condition is urgent, care should proceed with rapid assessment of airway, breathing, and circulation; management; and rapid transport.
- If the child's condition is nonurgent, care can proceed with a focused history and detailed physical examination.
- The AVPU Scale or the modified Glasgow Coma Scale (GCS) can be used to determine the child's level of consciousness, and can be used to assess for signs of inadequate oxygenation.

Airway and Breathing (Table 35-3)

- The child's airway should be patent, and breathing should proceed with adequate chest rise and fall.
- Watch for signs of respiratory distress:
  - Tachypnea
  - Use of accessory muscles

TABLE 35-3: Normal Vital Signs

Group	Breaths/min	Beats/min	Expected Mean for BP
Newborn	30–50	120–160	74–100 mmHg/50–68 mmHg
Infant	20–30	80–140	84–106 mmHg/56–70 mmHg
Toddler	20–30	80–130	98–106 mmHg/50–70 mmHg
Preschool	20–30	80–120	98–112 mmHg/64–70 mmHg
School-age	(12–20)–30	(60–80)–100	104–124 mmHg/64–80 mmHg
Adolescent	12–20	60–100	118–132 mmHg/70–82 mmHg

- ◦ Nasal flaring, grunting
- ◦ Bradypnea
- ◦ Irregular breathing pattern
- ◦ Head bobbing
- ◦ Absent breath sounds
- ◦ Abnormal breath sounds

Circulation

- Compare the strength and quality of central and peripheral pulses
- Measure blood pressure (in children over 3 years of age)
- Evaluate skin color, temperature, moisture, turgor, capillary refill
- Look for visible hemorrhage

Focused History

- When obtaining the focused history for an infant, toddler, or preschool-age patient, the paramedic will often have to elicit information from the parent, guardian, or caregiver.
- School-age and adolescent patients can provide most information.
- School-age and adolescent patients should be questioned in private (away from parents or family members) regarding sexual activity, pregnancy, alcohol or other drug use, or suspicion of child abuse.
- Content of the focused history should include chief complaint, nature of illness or injury, the length (duration) of illness or injury, last meal, presence of fever, effects on behavior, vomiting or diarrhea, frequency of urination, medications and allergies, past medical history, physician care, and chronic illnesses.

Detailed Physical Exam

- Should proceed from head-to-toe in older children.
- Should proceed from toe-to-head in younger children (under two years of age).
- Depending on the patient's condition, some or all of the following assessments may be appropriate:
  - ◦ Pupils
  - ◦ Capillary refill (most accurate in patients under 6 years of age)
  - ◦ Hydration (skin turgor, sunken or flat fontanelles in infants, presence of tears and saliva)
  - ◦ Pulse oximetry
  - ◦ Electrocardiogram (ECG) monitoring

Ongoing Assessment

- Appropriate for all patients and should be continued throughout the patient care encounter.
- Purpose—To monitor the patient for certain changes.
  - Respiratory effort
  - Skin color and temperature
  - Mental status
  - Vital signs (including pulse oximetry measurements)
- Measurement tools (blood pressure cuffs, electrodes) should be appropriate for the size of the child.

GENERAL PRINCIPLES IN PATIENT MANAGEMENT

- Principles of management depend on patient's condition
- Basic airway management
  - Manual positioning
  - Removal of foreign body airway obstruction with basic clearing methods
  - Suction
  - Oxygenation
  - Airway adjuncts (nasal and oral)
  - Ventilation with bag-valve device
- Advanced airway management
  - Removal of foreign body airway obstruction with advanced clearing methods
  - Endotracheal (ET) intubation
  - Needle cricothyroidotomy (per medical direction)
- Circulation
  - Vascular access (intravenous [IV], IO)
  - Fluid resuscitation
- Pharmacological management
  - Pain management
  - Rapid sequence intubation (per medical direction)
  - Respiratory/cardiac/endocrine/neurological medications
- Nonpharmacological management
  - Spine immobilization for trauma patients
  - Hemorrhage control
  - Bandaging and splinting
  - Fever control
- Transport considerations
  - Appropriate mode (rapid transport vs. on-scene care)
  - Appropriate facility

Psychological Support/Communication Strategies

- Begin conversations with both the child and parent.
- With younger children (1–6 years of age), focus most of your conversation with the parent.
- Offering the child a toy may provide distraction while interviewing the parent.
- Be aware you are collecting the child's history from a parent's point of view.

- Your interview can put the parent on the defensive.
- Be cautious not to be judgmental if the parents have not provided proper care or safety for the child before your arrival.
- Be observant but not confrontational.
- Make contact with the child in a gradual approach as you are interviewing the parent.
- Communicating with the child.
- Speak to children at eye level.
- Use a quiet, calm voice.
- Be aware of your nonverbal communication.
- Be knowledgeable of effective communication with children according to their age group.

Infants

- Respond best to firm, gentle handling and a quiet, calm voice.
- Older infants may have stranger-anxiety, so keep the parent within their view.

Preschoolers

- See the world only from their perspective
- Use short sentences with concrete explanations

School-Age Children

- More objective and realistic

Adolescents

- Want to be adults
- Should not be communicated with as children

SPECIFIC PATHOPHYSIOLOGY, ASSESSMENT, AND MANAGEMENT

Respiratory Compromise

- Several conditions manifest as respiratory distress in children
  - Upper and lower foreign body airway obstructions
  - Upper airway disease (croup, bacterial tracheitis, and epiglottitis)
  - Lower airway disease (asthma, bronchiolitis, and pneumonia)

Management Considerations

- Most cardiac arrests in children are secondary to respiratory insufficiency.
- Attempt to calm and reassure the child with respiratory compromise.
- Do not agitate the conscious patient (avoid IVs, blood pressure measurements, examining the patient's mouth).
- Do not lay the child down (supine).
  - Doing so may aggravate the airway condition and lead to life-threatening airway obstruction.
- When possible, allow the parent or other caregiver to remain with the child.
- Advise the receiving hospital of the patient's status as soon as possible to make arrangements for appropriate medical personnel.

Upper and Lower Foreign Body Airway Obstructions

- May cause a partial or complete airway obstruction.
- Usually occur in toddlers and preschoolers (1–4 years of age).
- Commonly result from food (hard candy, nuts, seeds, hot dogs) or small objects (coins, balloons).
- Complete airway obstruction requires immediate intervention to relieve the obstruction.
- Signs and symptoms of airway obstruction:
  - Anxiety
  - Inspiratory stridor
  - Muffled or hoarse voice
  - Drooling
  - Pain in the throat
  - Decreased breath sounds
  - Rales (crackles)
  - Rhonchi
  - Wheezing
- History of choking (observed by an adult) may exist.
- Suspect foreign body aspiration in an otherwise healthy child with sudden onset of respiratory compromise.
- If a complete airway obstruction cannot be relieved with basic and advanced methods of clearing, tracheal intubation or cricothyroidotomy may be indicated.

Croup (laryngotracheobronchitis)

- A common inflammatory respiratory illness in children.
- Viral infection of the upper airway that most frequently occurs in children between the ages of 6 months and 4 years, frequently during the late fall and early winter months.
- Responsible organism—Usually the parainfluenza virus, although respiratory syncytial virus (RSV), rubeola, and adenovirus have been implicated.
- May involve the entire respiratory tract, but symptoms are caused by inflammation in the subglottic region (at the level of the larynx extending to the cricoid cartilage).
- Child usually has a history of recent upper respiratory infection (URI) and a low-grade fever.
- Patient may present with hoarseness, inspiratory stridor (from subglottic edema), and a "barking" cough.
- Wheezing may be present if the lower airways are involved.
- Commonly, the episode occurs in the middle of the night after the child has gone to bed.
- On EMS arrival, a patient with severe croup may exhibit all the classic signs of respiratory distress.
- Child may be sitting upright and leaning forward to facilitate breathing.
- Nasal flaring, intercostal retraction, and cyanosis (a late sign of respiratory insufficiency) may be present.
- Children with severe croup are at risk of serious airway obstruction from the narrowed diameter of the trachea.
- Differentiation between croup and epiglottitis in the prehospital setting may be difficult (Table 35-4).

TABLE 35-4: Croup and Epiglottitis Symptoms

Croup	Epiglottitis
Age 6 months to 4 years	Age 3–7 years
Slow onset	Rapid onset
Patient may lie or sit upright	Patient prefers to sit upright
Barking cough	No barking cough, possible inspiratory stridor
Lack of drooling	Drooling, pain during swallowing
Low-grade fever	High fever

Prehospital Management

- Airway maintenance
- Humidified or nebulized oxygen administration
- Transport in a position of comfort
- Symptoms may improve dramatically in patients with croup after the child is exposed to cool, humidified air
- Make all efforts to keep the child comfortable and at ease

Bacterial Tracheitis

- Bacterial infection of the upper airway and subglottic trachea may follow a viral illness.
- Generally occurs in infants and toddlers (1–5 years of age), but can occur in older children.
- Signs and symptoms are those of respiratory distress or failure (depending on severity).
  - Agitation
  - High-grade fever
  - Inspiratory and expiratory stridor
  - A cough producing pus or mucus
  - Hoarseness
  - Throat pain
- Emergency care is directed at providing airway, ventilatory, and circulatory support and rapid transport for physician evaluation.
- If airway obstruction or respiratory failure or arrest develops, tracheal intubation is required with tracheal suction to remove mucus or pus.
- Bag-valve mask (BVM) ventilation may require high pressures.
- In-hospital care will include IV antibiotics specific for the causative organism after the child's airway is stabilized.

Epiglottitis

- A rapidly progressive, life-threatening bacterial infection that most often affects children between 3 and 7 years of age (but can occur at any age).
- Usually associated with *Haemophilus influenzae* type B; however, *Streptococcus, Pneumococcus*, and *Staphylococcus* organisms have also been implicated.
- The bacterial infection causes edema and swelling of the epiglottis and supraglottic structures (pharynx, aryepiglottic folds, and arytenoid cartilage).
- Epiglottitis usually begins suddenly (within 6–8 hours).
- Commonly, the child goes to bed asymptomatic and awakens complaining of a sore throat and pain on swallowing.
- The child may have a fever, a muffled voice (from edema of the mucosa covering of the vocal cords), and drooling from the presence of pooled saliva secondary to dysphagia.

The child is typically found sitting upright and leaning forward with the head hyperextended to facilitate breathing (tripod position).

- The child may have a protruding tongue or inspiratory stridor with a characteristic "rattle" and may be gasping or gulping for air.
  - Classic signs of respiratory distress are usually present
- Definitive care for epiglottitis is in-hospital intubation and parenteral antibiotic therapy.
- Children with acute epiglottitis are in danger of progressing to complete airway obstruction and respiratory arrest (absence of breathing).
- Occlusion can occur suddenly and may be precipitated by minor irritation of the throat, aggravation, and anxiety.
- Make no attempt to lay the child down or to change his or her position of comfort.
- Make no attempt to visualize the airway if the child is still ventilating adequately.
- Advise medical direction of the suspected epiglottitis so that appropriate personnel and resources can be made available.
- Administer 100% humidified oxygen by mask unless it provokes agitation.
- Do not attempt vascular access.
- Have appropriate-sized emergency airway equipment selected and immediately available.
- Transport the child to the receiving hospital in the position of comfort.
- If the patient progresses to respiratory arrest before arrival at the emergency department, field intubation must be attempted.
- The child's lungs should be hyperventilated and preoxygenated with a bag-valve device before intubation.
- After the airway has been established, IV access should be obtained if time permits.
- Be prepared for a difficult intubation since the vocal cords are likely to be obscured by the swollen supraglottic tissues.
- An uncuffed ET tube (one to two sizes smaller than normal) should be used.
- Locate the laryngeal inlet by looking for mucus bubbles appearing in the cleft between the edematous aryepiglottic folds and the swollen epiglottis.
  - Chest compressions during glottic visualization may produce a bubble at the tracheal opening
- If intubation cannot be achieved and the child cannot adequately be ventilated via bag-valve device (rare), medical direction may recommend needle cricothyroidotomy.

Asthma

- Characterized by inflammation and bronchoconstriction that results from autonomic dysfunction or sensitizing agents.
- The hallmarks of an acute exacerbation are anxiety, dyspnea, tachypnea, and audible expiratory wheeze with a prolonged expiratory phase.
- A silent chest indicates impending respiratory failure.
- Asthma is common among children more than 2 years of age and affects 5–10% of those under 10 years of age.
- An acute exacerbation may be triggered by infection, changes in temperature, physical exercise, or emotional response.

Prehospital Management

- Ventilatory assistance with humidified oxygen administration.
- Reversal of the bronchospasm.
- Rapid transport for evaluation and management.
- Severe asthma exacerbations may be life threatening and can rapidly progress to respiratory failure.

- Be prepared to initiate aggressive airway management with ventilatory and circulatory support.
- Pharmacological therapy depends on local protocol, prior medication use, and the recommendations of medical direction.
- Aerosolized bronchodilators.
- Subcutaneous epinephrine (with severe respiratory distress or failure).
- Occasionally, corticosteroids during prolonged transports.

Bronchiolitis

- A viral disease frequently caused by RSV infection of the lower airway.
- Usually affects children under 2 years of age
- Commonly occurs in the winter months, and generally is associated with an upper respiratory infection
- Presents with tachypnea and wheezing
- Resulting inflammation of the distal airway is sometimes unresponsive to therapy

Differentiation of Bronchiolitis and Asthma

- Bronchiolitis is generally benign and self-limiting, but can be life threatening.
- The infant is at greater risk for developing respiratory failure because of the relatively small diameter of the bronchioles.
- Prehospital care is aimed at providing ventilatory support with humidified oxygen and rapid transport for physician evaluation.
- A therapeutic trial of albuterol via nebulizer may greatly decrease respiratory distress.

Pneumonia

- An acute infection of the lower airway and lung that involves either the alveolar walls or the alveoli.
- Common causes are a bacterial or viral infection.
- The child may have a history of recent airway infection and present with respiratory distress or failure (depending on severity) and any of the following:
    - Anxiety
    - Decreased breath sounds
    - Rales (crackles)
    - Rhonchi (localized or diffuse)
    - Pain in the chest
    - Fever
- Most children with pneumonia have only mild disease and require no immediate stabilization or airway support.
- If respiratory distress is present, airway stabilization is the priority.
- In severe cases, pharmacological therapy with bronchodilators may be indicated, and assisted ventilations via bag-valve device or intubation of the trachea may be necessary.

Shock

- An abnormal condition characterized by inadequate delivery of oxygen and metabolic substrates to meet the normal demands of tissues.
- Shock can be classified as:
    - Noncardiogenic (resulting from hypovolemia or distributive causes)
    - Cardiogenic (resulting from cardiomyopathy or dysrhythmias)

Special Considerations for Pediatric Patients in Shock

Circulating Blood Volume

- Adult blood volumes account for 5–6% of total body weight or 70 mL/kg/body weight; pediatric blood volumes account for 7–8% of total body weight or 88 mL/kg/body weight. Although child percentages of circulating blood volumes are greater than those of the adult, the absolute blood volume in the child is much lower. A relatively small loss of blood may be devastating.
- A child with a volume deficit will maintain stable hemodynamics until all compensatory mechanisms fail. At that point, shock progresses rapidly, with catastrophic deterioration.
- Early recognition, stabilization (airway control, fluid replacement), and rapid patient transport to an appropriate medical facility is especially important when caring for the child in shock.

Body Surface Area and Hypothermia

- Children have a relatively large body surface area in proportion to body weight, and their compensatory mechanisms (e.g., shivering) are not well developed.
- Children in shock can quickly develop hypothermia from exposure and concurrent metabolic acidosis, increased vascular resistance, respiratory depression, and myocardial dysfunction. Hypothermic states can make resuscitation and medication therapy less effective.
- Maintain the patient's body temperature.
  - Cover the patient's head
  - Use towels and blankets to warm the patient
  - Warm devices for IV fluids

Cardiac Reserve

- Because of their already high metabolic needs, infants and children have less cardiac reserve than adults for stressful situations such as shock.
- It is important to reduce the energy and oxygen requirements of the child in shock as much as possible by providing ventilatory support, decreasing anxiety, and maintaining moderate ambient temperatures.

Respiratory Fatigue

- Respiratory muscle fatigue may lead to hypoventilation, hypoxemia, and respiratory failure or arrest.
- Respiratory compensation in shock is generally at a maximum until it is depleted, when deterioration can be sudden.
- Airway control and supplemental oxygen are essential in all children who are seriously ill or injured.

Vital Signs and Assessment

- Many variables must be considered when evaluating a child's vital signs.
- Blood pressure and pulse rate vary greatly with age, body temperature, and degree of agitation.
- The most effective assessment is constant monitoring of the child's mental and physical status and assessing the response to therapy.
- Nine evaluation components should be noted when assessing a child in shock:
  - Level of consciousness (anxiety, agitation, ability to make eye contact, ability to recognize family members)
  - Skin (temperature, moisture, color, turgor, capillary refill [in children under 6 years of age])

- Mucous membranes (color, moisture)
- Nail beds (capillary refill [in children under 6 years of age], color)
- Peripheral circulation (collapse, distention)
- Cardiac (ECG findings, rate, rhythm, quality of pulses, location of pulses)
- Respiration (rate, depth)
- Blood pressure (in children over 3 years of age)
- Body temperature

Hypovolemia

- Results from intravascular volume depletion (vomiting, diarrhea, burns) and blood loss (trauma, internal bleeding).

Dehydration

- Profound fluid and electrolyte imbalances can occur in children as a consequence of diarrhea, vomiting, poor fluid intake, fever, or burns (see Table 35-5).
- Below are situations in which dehydration would compromise cardiac output and systemic perfusion:
  - Child loses the fluid equivalent of 5% or more of total body weight
  - Adolescent loses 5–7% of total body weight
- If allowed to progress, dehydration can result in renal failure, shock, and death.
- Severity of the dehydration and fluid volume deficit can be estimated from a history of the child's weight loss and a physical examination.
- Physical findings depend on the type of dehydration (isotonic, hypotonic, hypertonic).
- After provision of airway and ventilatory support, the initial management of dehydration in the child is directed at restoring and maintaining intravascular volume and systemic perfusion.
- Initiate IV therapy (per medical direction) with isotonic crystalloids such as lactated Ringer's solution (LR) or normal saline (NS).
  - Administer (in less than 20 minutes) a fluid bolus of 20 mL/kg.

TABLE 35-5: Assessment of Degree of Dehydration in Isotonic Fluid Loss

Clinical Parameters of Body Weight Loss	Mild	Moderate	Severe
Infant	5% (50 mL/kg)	10% (100 mL/kg)	15% (150 mL/kg)
Adult	3% (30 mL/kg)	6% (60 mL/kg)	9% (90 mL/kg)
Skin turgor	Slightly ↓	↓↓	↓↓↓
Fontanelle	Possibly flat or depressed	Depressed	Significantly depressed
Mucous membranes	Dry	Very dry	Parched
Skin perfusion	Warm with normal color	Cool (extremities); pale	Cold (extremities)
Heart rate	Mildly tachycardic	Moderately tachycardic	Extremely tachycardic
Peripheral pulses	Normal	Diminished	Absent
Blood pressure	Normal	Normal	Reduced
Sensorium	Normal or irritable	Irritable or lethargic	Unresponsive

  - Repeat until the patient's systemic perfusion improves and an appropriate blood pressure is obtained.
  - After physician evaluation and initial shock resuscitation, the fluid administration rate and type of fluid replacement are determined by the volume and type of fluid deficit and the patient's response to therapy.

Hemorrhage

- Even a relatively small amount of blood loss can be quite serious for the pediatric patient.
- After controlling external hemorrhage (if present), securing the patient's airway, and providing high-concentration oxygen, the child's circulatory status may require support with IV therapy (per medical direction).
- Initiate IV therapy (per medical direction) with isotonic crystalloids such as LR or NS.
- Administer (in less than 20 minutes) a fluid bolus of 20 mL/kg.
- If the volume loss is in the 20% range, physiological measurements should improve after this infusion.
- If physiological parameters improve, continue IV therapy at maintenance rate during patient transport.
- If there is little response to the first bolus (slight improvement in color and capillary refill and decreased heart rate) or if the patient does not respond to the initial infusion, a second bolus of 20 mL/kg should follow immediately.

Distributive Shock (Vasogenic Shock)

- A term used to refer to septic shock, neurogenic shock, and anaphylactic shock
- Relatively uncommon in children
- Results in peripheral pooling due to loss of vasomotor tone
- Signs and symptoms—Those of compensated or decompensated shock (hypotension), depending on severity
- Characteristic findings in distributive shock

Septic Shock

- Early stages—Skin is warm
- Late stages—Skin is cool

Neurogenic Shock

- Warm skin
- Bradycardia
- Impaired neurologic function

Anaphylactic Shock

- Allergic rash, erythema
- Airway swelling, wheezes
- Angioedema
- Gastrointestinal (GI) upset
- Emergency care—Directed at ensuring the patient's vital functions through airway, ventilatory, and circulatory support and rapid transport to an appropriate medical facility
- Medical direction—May recommend IV fluid therapy and pharmacological agents to manage specific forms of distributive shock (e.g., dopamine for neurogenic shock; epinephrine for anaphylaxis)

Cardiomyopathy

- Cardiomyopathy refers to any disease of the heart muscle that causes a reduction in the force of heart contractions and a resultant decrease in the efficiency of circulation of blood throughout the lungs and to the rest of the body.
- In children, the condition is usually the result of viral infection or congenital abnormalities that affect both ventricles of the heart.
- Symptoms include fatigue, chest pain, dysrhythmias, and in severe cases, signs of heart failure and cardiogenic shock.
  - Tachycardia
  - Tachypnea
  - Crackles
  - Hypotension
  - Jugular vein distention (difficult to determine in young children)
  - Peripheral edema
- Stable patients are managed with supportive care, oxygen administration, and transport for physician evaluation.
- Children who are hypotensive and demonstrating other signs and symptoms of decompensation may require vascular access for drug administration.
- IV fluid therapy should be restricted in these patients to avoid volume overload.

Dysrhythmias

- Most children have healthy hearts; when dysrhythmias occur, they are usually the result of hypoxia or structural heart disease.
- The most common dysrhythmias are sinus tachycardia, supraventricular tachycardia (SVT), bradycardia, and asystole.
- Ventricular tachycardia (VT) and ventricular fibrillation (VF) are not common, but do occur.

Supraventricular Tachycardia

- Heart rate associated with SVT varies with age
- In infants, the heart rate is often about 240 beats/min or higher
- The rhythm is usually regular since associated AV block is rare
- P waves may not be identifiable, especially when the ventricular rate is high
- QRS duration is normal in most children
- SVT with aberrant conduction may be difficult to distinguish from VT (but this form of SVT is rare in infants and children)

Ventricular Tachycardia

- Ventricular rate is at least 120 beats/min and regular
- The QRS is wide and P waves are often not identifiable
- Differentiating SVT with aberrant conduction (rare in children) from VT may be difficult

Bradycardia

- Rate will be less than 60 beats/min
- P waves may or may not be visible
- QRS duration may be normal or prolonged
- The P wave and QRS are often unrelated

Pulseless Arrest

- Straight line appears on ECG monitor
- P waves are occasionally observed

Ventricular Fibrillation

- There will be no identifiable P, QRS, or T waves
- VF waves may be coarse or fine

Management of Pediatric Dysrhythmias

Supraventricular Tachycardia

- Usually occurs in infants with no prior history
- Stable (compensated shock)—Patient will usually remain stable during transport with oxygen
- Unstable (decompensated shock)—*Patient requires immediate management*
- Children may be able to sustain increased rates for a while, but after several hours, they will decompensate
- Signs and symptoms
    - Compensated or decompensated shock, depending on severity
    - Narrow complex tachycardia with rates of greater than 220 beats per minute (too fast to count)
    - Poor feeding
    - Hypotension
- History
- Management
    - Stable—Supportive care
    - Unstable—Adminster high flow oxygen; consider adenosine, synchronized cardioversion
- Ventricular tachycardia with a pulse
    - Stable (compensated shock)—Patient will usually not tolerate for long periods
    - Unstable (decompensated shock)—*Patient requires immediate management*

Bradydysrhythmias

- Most common dysrhythmia in children
- Usually develops because of hypoxia
- May develop because of vagal stimulation (rare)
- Assessment
    - Signs and symptoms
        - Compensated or decompensated shock, depending on severity
        - Bradycardia
        - Slow, narrow complex heart rhythm; QRS duration may be normal or prolonged
    - History
- Management
    - Stable—Supportive care
    - Unstable
        - Ventilate patient with 100% oxygen via BVM
        - Intubate if poor response to BVM ventilation
        - Perform chest compressions if oxygen does not increase heart rate
        - Medications can be given down the ET tube
          Administer epinephrine
          Administer atropine for vagally induced bradycardia

Asystole

- May be the initial cardiac arrest rhythm
- Pathophysiology
  - Bradycardias may degenerate into asystole
  - High mortality rate
- Assessment—Pulseless, apneic; cardiac monitor indicating no electrical activity
- Management
  - Confirm in two leads
  - Ventilate patient with 100% oxygen via BVM
  - Intubate patient if poor response to BVM ventilations
  - Perform chest compressions
  - Medications can be given down the ET tube
    - — Administer epinephrine

Ventricular Fibrillation/Pulseless Ventricular Tachycardia

- Incidence—Rare
- Pathophysiology
  - Possibly caused by electrocution and drug overdoses
  - High mortality rate
- Assessment
  - Pulseless, apneic; cardiac monitor indicating no organized electrical activity or rapid wide complex tachycardia
- Management
  - Unmonitored—Perform basic life support
  - Monitored—Defibrillate up to three consecutive shocks
  - Ventilate patient with 100% oxygen via BVM
  - Intubate patient if poor response to BVM ventilations
  - Perform chest compressions
  - Medications can be given down the ET tube
    - — Administer epinephrine
    - — Administer lidocaine
  - After administration of medication, allow drug to circulate for one minute before repeat defibrillation
  - Pulseless electrical activity
    - — Incidence—Look for a treatable cause
    - — Pathophysiology—Pneumothorax, cardiac tamponade, hypovolemia, hypoxia, acidosis, hypothermia, hypoglycemia
    - — Assessment
    - — Pulseless, apneic; cardiac monitor indicating organized electrical activity
  - Management
    - — Resuscitation should be directed toward relieving cause
    - — Ventilate the patient with 100% oxygen
    - — Intubate patient
    - — Perform chest compressions
    - — Medications can be given down the ET tube

      Administer epinephrine

Seizure

- An episode of sudden abnormal electrical activity in the brain that results in abnormalities in motor, sensory, or autonomic function, usually associated with abnormal behavior, alterations in level of consciousness, or both.
- Common causes of seizures in adults and children
  - Noncompliance with a drug regimen for the management of epilepsy
  - Head trauma
  - Intracranial infection
  - Metabolic disturbance
  - Poisoning
  - Fever—Most common cause of new onset of seizure in children

Febrile seizures are associated with fever but without evidence of intracranial infection or other definable cause.

- Usually occur between the ages of 6 months and 5 years of age
- Usually associated with an underlying viral infection (most frequently of the upper respiratory tract), gastroenteritis, roseola, otitis media, or another febrile illness
  - Seizures generally occur in vulnerable patients during a rapid rise in body temperature, but the intensity of the seizure is not related to the severity of the fever
- May present with generalized tonic-clonic activity or be of more subtle presentation
  - Classic febrile seizures are of short duration (usually lasting less than 5 minutes) and have an uncomplicated and short postictal period
  - Seizures that last longer than 20 minutes require extensive investigation and should never be considered benign
- Regardless of the suspected etiology, all children who have suffered a seizure should be transported for physician evaluation per protocol

Assessment and Management

- Commonly, febrile seizure will have ceased before EMS arrival and the child will often be in a postictal state.
- The first steps are airway management and ventilatory and circulatory support including airway positioning, suctioning the airway, and administering oxygen.
- Repeated assessment of the adequacy of ventilation is necessary, with special emphasis on respiratory rate and depth.
- If the airway cannot be maintained with manual maneuvers, airway adjuncts should be used.
- After initial stabilization of the patient, vital signs should be assessed and a history should be obtained.
- Obtain important elements of the history:
  - Previous seizures.
  - Number of seizures in this episode.
  - Description of seizure activity
  - Presence of vomiting during the seizure (aspiration risk)
  - Condition of child when first found
  - Recent illness
  - Potential for toxic ingestion

- ◦ Potential head injury (as primary etiology or secondary complication)
- ◦ Significant medical problems
- ◦ Recent headache or stiff neck (which may suggest meningitis)
- ◦ Medication use and compliance with anticonvulsant medication

- Closely monitor the child during transport to the emergency department and be alert for recurrent seizures.
- Medical direction may recommend that a febrile patient be given an antipyretic (if alert) to reduce the fever en route to the receiving hospital.

Status Epilepticus

Defined as a continuous seizure activity lasting 30 minutes or longer or a recurrent seizure without an intervening period of consciousness. Status epilepticus is considered a true emergency that can lead to hypotension and cardiovascular, respiratory, renal failure, and permanent brain damage.

Management

- Provide adequate airway, ventilatory, and circulatory support.
- Intubation for airway protection or mechanical ventilation is seldom necessary and should be withheld unless the child fails to respond to initial management.
- Obtain vascular access through an IV or IO route.
- Measure blood glucose level to screen for hypoglycemia.
- If the value is below 60 mg/dL (40 mg/dL in an infant), administer dextrose 10%, 25%, 50% (per medical direction).
- If seizures do not stop, consult with medical direction for IV, IO, or rectal administration of anticonvulsants (diazepam or lorazepam).
  - ◦ Diazepam (Valium)
    - — Breaks active seizures in 75–90% of cases
    - — Has a short duration of action (15 minutes) and may require repeat administration to a maximum of three doses
    - — Be prepared for unpredictable sudden respiratory depression or hypotension associated with use of this drug
    - — If IV or IO access cannot be obtained, diazepam may be administered rectally
  - ◦ Lorazepam (Ativan)
    - — An alternative to IV or IO diazepam (preferred by some physicians)
    - — May be administered IM, IV, IO, or rectally
    - — Side effects—Resemble those of diazepam in terms of cardiorespiratory and central nervous system (CNS) depression
    - — Be alert to these complications
- Attach a cardiac monitor and observe for rhythm or conduction abnormalities that may suggest hypoxia.

Hypoglycemia and Hyperglycemia

Signs and Symptoms

- Hypoglycemia and hyperglycemia should be suspected whenever a child presents with an altered level of consciousness that has no explainable cause.

Hypoglycemia

- Mild—Hunger, weakness, tachypnea, tachycardia
- Moderate—Sweating, tremors, irritability, vomiting, mood swings, blurred vision, stomach ache, headache, dizziness
- Severe—Decreased level of consciousness, seizure

Hyperglycemia

- Early—Increased thirst, increased hunger, increased urination, weight loss
- Late (dehydration/early ketoacidosis)—Weakness, abdominal pain, generalized aches, loss of appetite, nausea, vomiting, signs of dehydration (except urinary output), fruity breath odor, tachypnea, hyperventilation, tachycardia, Kussmaul respirations and coma (if untreated)

Prehospital management

- First ensure adequate airway, ventilatory, and circulatory support.
- Obtain a blood glucose measurement in any child with altered level of consciousness and no explainable cause.
- Conscious children who are mildly hypoglycemic should receive an oral glucose solution or paste.
- Unconscious children or those with moderate or severe hypoglycemia require IV/IO dextrose or IM glucagon, followed by a repeat blood glucose measurement in 10–15 minutes.
- Children who are hyperglycemic with signs of dehydration may require IV fluid therapy and in-hospital administration of insulin.
- Any child with hypoglycemia or hyperglycemia should be transported for physician evaluation.

Infection

- Children with infection may present with varied signs and symptoms, depending on the source and extent of infection.
  - Fever
  - Hypothermia (neonates)
  - Chills
  - Tachycardia
  - Cough
  - Sore throat
  - Nasal congestion
  - Malaise
  - Tachypnea
  - Cool or clammy skin
  - Respiratory distress
  - Poor feeding
  - Vomiting and/or diarrhea
  - Dehydration
  - Hypoperfusion
  - Seizure
  - Severe headache
  - Irritability
  - Lethargy

- Stiff neck
- Bulging fontanelle (in infants)

- Often, the parent or caregiver will provide a history of recent illness, such as fever, upper respiratory tract infection, or otitis media.
- Most children with infection will need only supportive care while being transported for physician evaluation.
- In severe cases, some patients may require airway, ventilatory, and circulatory support.
- If signs of decompensated shock are present, IV therapy may be warranted (per medical direction).
- Active seizure activity may require the administration of anticonvulsant agents.
- When possible, stable children should be transported in their position of comfort in the company of the parent or caregiver.

Poisoning and Toxic Exposure

- Most poisoning events in the United States involve children
- Common sources of poisoning (accidental and intentional)
  - Alcohol
  - Barbiturates
  - Sedatives
  - Anticholinergics
  - Acetaminophen
  - Aspirin
  - Corrosives
  - Digitalis, beta-blocker agents
  - Hydrocarbons
  - Narcotics
  - Organic solvents (inhaled)
  - Organophosphates

Signs and Symptoms of Accidental Poisoning

- Vary, depending on the toxic substance and the time since the child was exposed
- May include cardiac and respiratory depression, CNS stimulation or depression, GI irritation, and behavioral changes

Management

- First ensure adequate airway, ventilatory, and circulatory support.
- Contact medical direction and the poison control center to obtain directions for specific managements.
- All pills, substances, and containers associated with the poisoning event should be transported with the child to the receiving hospital.

PEDIATRIC TRAUMA

- Blunt and penetrating trauma is a predominant cause of injury and death in children. Common pediatric trauma events:
  - Falls
    - Single most common cause of injury in children
    - Serious injury or death resulting from truly accidental falls is relatively uncommon unless from a significant height

- Motor vehicle crashes
  - Leading cause of permanent brain injury
  - Leading cause of death and serious injury in children
- Pedestrian-vehicle crashes
  - Particularly lethal form of trauma in children
  - Initial injury caused by impact with vehicle (extremity or trunk)
  - Child is thrown from force of impact, causing additional injury (head, spine) upon impact with other objects (ground, another vehicle, light standard, etc.)
- Near-downing
  - Third leading cause of injury or death in children between birth and 4 years of age
  - Causes about 2000 deaths annually
  - Severe, permanent brain damage occurs in 5–20% of children hospitalized for near-drowning
- Penetrating injuries
  - A significant problem in adolescence
  - Higher incidence in inner city (mostly intentional); significant incidence in other areas (mostly unintentional)
  - Risk of death from firearm injuries increases with age
  - Stab wounds and firearm injuries account for about 10–15% of all pediatric trauma admissions
  - Visual inspection of external injuries cannot evaluate the extent of internal involvement
- Burns
  - Leading cause of accidental death in the home for children under 14 years of age
  - Burn survival depends on burn size, inhalation injury, and concomitant injuries
  - Modified "rule of nines" is used to determine percentage of surface area involved
- Child abuse
  - Includes physical abuse, sexual abuse, emotional abuse, and child neglect
  - Social phenomena such as increased poverty, domestic disturbances, younger aged parents, substance abuse, and community violence have been attributed to increase of abuse; however, abuse occurs in all social strata
  - Document all pertinent findings, managements, and interventions (for legal purposes)

Special Considerations for Specific Injuries

Head and Neck Injury

- Larger relative mass of the head and lack of neck muscle strength provide increased momentum in acceleration-deceleration injuries.
- Fulcrum of cervical mobility in the younger child is at the C2–C3 level (60–70% of fractures in children occur in C1 or C2).
- Head injury is the most common cause of death in pediatric trauma victims.
- Diffuse head injuries are common in children; focal injuries are rare.
- Soft tissues, skull, and brain are more compliant in children than in adults.
- Due to open fontanelles and sutures, infants up to 12 months of age may be more tolerant to increased ICP and can have delayed signs.
- Subdural bleeds in an infant can produce hypotension (extremely rare).
- Significant blood loss can occur through scalp lacerations and should be controlled immediately.
- Modified GCS should be used for assessing infants and young children.

Traumatic Brain Injury

- Early recognition and aggressive management can reduce mortality and morbidity.
- May be classified as mild (GCS 13–15), moderate (GCS 9–12), or severe (GCS less than or equal to 8).

Signs and symptoms

- Signs of increased ICP include elevated blood pressure, bradycardia, irregular respirations progressing to Cheyne-Stokes respirations, and bulging fontanelle in infants.
- Signs of herniation include asymmetrical pupils and abnormal posturing.

Management

- Administer high-concentration oxygen for mild to moderate head injury (GCS 9–15).
- Intubate and ventilate at a normal breathing rate with 100% oxygen for severe head injury (GCS 3–8).
- Administer lidocaine per medical direction to blunt rise in ICP (controversial) before intubation.
- Hyperventilate in the presence of asymmetric pupils, active seizures, neurologic posturing.

Chest Injury

- Chest injuries in children less than 14 years of age are usually the result of blunt trauma.
- Because of thoracic compliance of the chest wall, severe intrathoracic injury can be present without signs of external injury.
- Tension pneumothorax is poorly tolerated and is an immediate threat to life.
- Flail segment is an uncommon injury in children; when noted without a significant mechanism of injury, child abuse should be suspected.
- Many children with cardiac tamponade will have no physical signs of tamponade other than hypotension.

Abdominal Injury

- Musculature is minimal and poorly protects the viscera.
- Organs most commonly injured are liver, kidney, and spleen.
- Onset of symptoms may be rapid or gradual.
- Because of the small size of the abdomen, palpation should be performed in one quadrant at a time.
- Any child who is hemodynamically unstable without evidence of obvious source of blood loss should be considered to have an abdominal injury until proven otherwise.

Extremity Injury

- These injuries are relatively more common in children than adults.
- Growth plate injuries are common.
- Compartment syndrome is an emergency in children.
- Any sites of active bleeding must be controlled.
- Splinting should be performed to prevent further injury and blood loss.
- Pneumatic antishock garments (PASG) may be useful in unstable pelvic fracture with hypotension (per protocol).

Burns

- Burns may occur from thermal, chemical, or electrical.
- Management priorities include prompt management of the airway; required because swelling can develop rapidly.
- If intubation is indicated, an ET tube one-half size smaller than expected may be required.
- Suspect musculoskeletal injuries in electrical burn patients and perform spine immobilization.

Trauma Management Considerations for Pediatric Patients

Besides general patient care guidelines, which are appropriate for all injured patients, special consideration for airway control, immobilization techniques, and fluid management must be given to injured children.

Airway Control

- Maintain the airway in an in-line or neutral position (vs. a sniffing position appropriate for older children and adults).
- Padding may need to be placed under the shoulders to maintain a neutral airway position.
- Provide high-concentration oxygen to all patients, while keeping the airway patent through jaw-thrust positioning and suctioning (if needed).
- Perform ET intubation (followed by gastric tube insertion) if airway and ventilation remain inadequate.
- Needle cricothyroidotomy is rarely indicated for traumatic upper airway obstruction.

Immobilization

- Appropriately size spinal immobilization devices for infants and children.
- Equipment that may be used:
  - Rigid cervical collar
  - Towel/blanket roll
  - Child safety seat
  - Pediatric immobilization device
  - Vest-type/short backboard
  - Long backboard
  - Straps, cravats
  - Tape
  - Padding
- Place patient supine and immobilize in a neutral in-line position.
- Infants, toddlers, and preschoolers should be padded from shoulders to hips.

Fluid Management

- Airway and breathing management take priority over management of circulation because circulatory compromise is less common in children than adults.
- Special considerations apply when vascular access is indicated.
- Large-bore IV catheters should be inserted into large peripheral veins.
- Transport should not be delayed to obtain vascular access.
- IO access in children less than 6 years of age (and occasionally older children) can be used if IV access fails.

- An initial fluid bolus of 20 mL/kg of LR or NS should be given to manage volume depletion.
- Reassess vital signs and repeat the bolus if needed.
- Vital signs that do not improve after a second bolus indicate the need for rapid surgical intervention.

SUDDEN INFANT DEATH SYNDROME

- Leading cause of death in American infants under 1 year of age.
- Defined as the sudden death of an apparently healthy infant that remains unexplained by history and a thorough autopsy.
- Occurs an average of 1.1 times for every 1000 live births and is responsible for more than 7000 deaths in the United States each year.
- Cannot be predicted or prevented, although positioning during sleep may be a factor.
- Occurs during periods of sleep, usually between midnight and 6 a.m.
- Typical age is the first year of life, but the majority (85%) of SIDS deaths occur within the first 6 months.
- Seasonal distribution is October through March (during cool weather world wide).
- Frequently, the infant has a history of minor illness, such as a cold, within two weeks before death.
- Classic signs are usually present:
  - Lividity
  - Frothy, blood-tinged drainage from the nose and mouth
  - Rigor mortis
- With most cases, there are no external signs of injury.
- There will often be evidence that the baby was active just before death (e.g., rumpled bed clothes, unusual position or location in the bed).

Pathophysiology

- Cause is unknown—Studies have failed to confirm many physiological, environmental, genetic, and social factors as causes.
- Studies have confirmed that SIDS is not caused by external suffocation, regurgitation or aspiration of vomitus, hereditary factors, or allergies.
- A small percentage of SIDS deaths are thought to be abuse related.
- Factors suggested to explain SIDS:
  - Immaturity of the CNS secondary to a prenatal event
  - Idiopathic apnea
  - Brain stem abnormalities
  - Upper airway obstruction
  - Hyperactive upper airway reflexes
  - Cardiac conduction disorders
  - Abnormal responses to hypoxia and hypercarbia
  - Abnormal responses to hyperthermia
  - Alterations in fat metabolism
- Risk factors associated with the syndrome:
  - Maternal smoking
  - Young maternal age (under age 20)
  - Infants of mothers who received poor or no prenatal care
  - Social deprivation

  - Premature births and low–birth-weight infants
  - Infants of mothers who used cocaine, methadone, or heroin during pregnancy
- Confirmation of SIDS:
  - Confirmed by excluding other causes of death
  - Autopsy findings that occur in most SIDS deaths
    - — Smooth muscle thickening in small pulmonary arteries and right ventricular hypertrophy

      Both findings are thought to be secondary to hypoxia and pulmonary vasculature constriction
    - — Brain stem tumors that may be associated with respiratory center dysfunction
    - — Neuroepithelial bodies in the tracheobronchial tree along with distal atelectasis
    - — In about 80% of victims—Intrathoracic petechiae, especially on the thymus, pleura, and pericardium

Management

- EMS providers can do little to help the SIDS infant.
- The primary role of the paramedic is to provide emotional support for parents or other caregivers and loved ones.
- If the infant is potentially or questionably viable, resuscitation should proceed as for any other infant in cardiac arrest.
- Though resuscitation probably will be unsuccessful, it is important for the parents or other caregivers to see that everything possible is being done for their child.
- Follow pediatric resuscitation protocols and consult with medical direction regarding decisions to initiate or continue resuscitation efforts.
- Expect a variety of grief reactions from those who witness the event (parents, family members, neighbors, babysitters).
  - These reactions may vary from shock and disbelief to anger, rage, and self-blame.
  - Arrangements should be made for a relative or neighbor to stay with the family or accompany them to the hospital so that they are not left alone.
  - Many areas have SIDS resource services that provide immediate counseling and support for the family of a SIDS infant.
- Because of the mysterious nature of SIDS deaths and classic signs such as postmortem lividity and frothy fluid in the infant's nose and mouth, SIDS victims may appear to have been abused or neglected.
  - Regardless of the circumstances, avoid comments or questions that may imply a suspicion of inappropriate child care.
  - Determining the cause of death is not the responsibility of the EMS crew (although careful scene observation is crucial).
  - Document all findings objectively, accurately, and completely.
  - Medical direction and other authorities (per protocol) should be advised if inappropriate child care is suspected.

CHILD ABUSE AND NEGLECT

- More than 2.4 million cases of suspected child abuse and neglect are reported each year in the United States, resulting in about 4000 deaths.
- Follow local protocol in reporting suspected abuse and discuss any suspicions of child abuse or neglect with medical direction.
- Agencies that may be involved in cases of child abuse or neglect include state, regional, and local child protection services; and hospital social service departments.

Elements of Child Abuse

- Child abuse and neglect are the maltreatment of children by their parents, guardians, or other caregivers.
- Forms of maltreatment:
  - Infliction of physical injury
    - — Battered child syndrome
    - — Shaken baby syndrome
  - Sexual exploitation
  - Infliction of emotional pain and neglect
    - — Medical neglect
    - — Safety neglect
    - — Nutritional deprivation
- Factors implicated in the potential for child abuse
  - Caregiver with the potential to abuse
  - Child with particular characteristics that place him or her at risk for abuse
  - Element of crisis

Characteristics of Abusers

- Child abuse usually reflects a pattern of maladjusted behavior rather than an isolated act of violence. Often, the abuser is the child's parent, although other caregivers may also be responsible.
- In physical abuse, most abusers tend to be unhappy, angry adults under tremendous stress.
- Abusers are usually isolated and incapable of using support agencies or an extended family in times of crisis.
- Often, abusers experienced physical or emotional abuse themselves as children.
- Abusers come from all ethnic, geographical, religious, educational, occupational, and socioeconomic groups.
- Other factors include impoverishment (low socioeconomic conditions) and alcohol or other drug dependence.

Characteristics of an Abused Child

- Abused children often have certain traits or characteristics that increase their risk for abuse:
  - Demanding and difficult behavior
  - Decreased level of functioning
  - Hyperactivity
  - Precociousness with intellectual ability equal to or superior to the parent
- Often, the abused child is viewed by the parent as "special" or "different" from other siblings.
- Other factors that tend to increase the potential for child abuse are age (child is usually under 5 years old), gender, and illegitimacy.
- Crises that may precipitate abuse:
  - Physical abuse or neglect can occur constantly during a child's life.
    - — More often, it is intermittent and unpredictable
  - Abuse is frequently precipitated by stressors in the adult caregiver's life, particularly in situations when the caregiver expects the child to fill emotional needs created by the stress.

- Failure of the child to respond in an ideal way to the caregiver's needs may lead to an abusive episode
- Some specific crises are associated with episodes of child abuse:
  - Financial stress
  - Loss of employment
  - Eviction from housing
  - Marital or relationship stress
  - Physical illness in a child that leads to intractable crying
  - Death of a family member
  - Diagnosis of an unwanted pregnancy
  - Birth of a sibling

History of Injuries Suspicious for Abuse

- Physical abuse or neglect is often difficult to determine.
- Ultimate diagnosis usually begins with suspicions based on unexplained injuries, discrepant history, delays in seeking medical care, and repeated episodes of suspicious injuries.
- If at any time an injured child indicates that a particular adult caused him or her physical harm, take the report seriously and consult with medical direction.
- Often these accusations are true.
- Remember the following 15 indicators:
  - Any obvious or suspected fractures in a child under 2 years of age
  - Injuries in various stages of healing, especially burns and bruises
  - More injuries than usually seen in other children of the same age
  - Injuries scattered on many areas of the body
  - Bruises or burns in patterns that suggest intentional infliction
  - Suspected increased intracranial pressure in an infant
  - Suspected intra-abdominal trauma in a young child
  - Any injury that does not fit the description of the cause
  - Accusation that the child injured himself or herself intentionally
  - Long-standing skin infections
  - Extreme malnutrition
  - Extreme lack of cleanliness
  - Inappropriate clothing for the situation
  - Child who withdraws from parent
  - Child who responds inappropriately to the situation (e.g., quiet, distant, withdrawn)

Physical Findings Suggestive of Abuse

- Multiple, widely dispersed bruises, welts, and burns suggest nonaccidental trauma. Such physical findings, with a vague history or delays in seeking medical care for the child, should alert the paramedic to the possibility of abuse or neglect.
- Bruises that predominate on the buttocks or lower back are usually related to punishment.
- Genital area or inner thigh bruises are usually inflicted for toileting mishaps.
- Facial bruises or numerous petechiae on the ear lobe are usually caused by slapping.
- Bruises of the upper lip and labial frenulum are usually caused by forced feedings or from jamming a pacifier into the mouth of a screaming infant.

- Pressure bruises in shapes resembling fingertips, fingers, or the entire hand of the abuser are usually caused by squeezing.
- Human bite marks result in paired, crescent-shaped bruises that often contain individual teeth marks. The size of the arc distinguishes adult bites from a child bite.
- Welts:
  - Strap marks 1–2 in. wide are usually caused by a belt.
  - Bizarre-shaped welts or bruises are usually inflicted by a blunt object that resembles its shape.
- Choke marks may be seen on the neck.
- Circumferential bruising or abrasions on the ankles or wrist may be caused by a rope, a cord, or a dog leash.
- Burns:
  - Cigarette burns are often found on the palms, soles, or abdomen.
  - A lighted cigarette, a hot match, or burning incense is sometimes applied to the hand to stop the child from sucking the thumb or to the genital area to discourage masturbation.
  - Burns may be inflicted with lighters or other sources of open flame (a gas stove) to teach a child not to play with fire.
  - Dry contact burns may result from forcibly holding a child against a heating device.
  - The most common hot-water burns or scalds occur from forcible immersion of the hands, feet, or buttocks in scalding water.
    - These injuries often involve both arms or both legs, or they may be circular burns restricted to the buttocks.
    - Such burns are incompatible with falling or stepping into a tub of hot water.

Subdural Hematoma

Brain injury is the leading cause of death in battered children.

Signs and symptoms

- Various pathological lesions
  - Cerebral contusions
  - Intraparenchymal hemorrhage
  - Subdural or even epidural hematomas
- Should be suspected in any young child who is in a coma or having convulsions, particularly if there is no history of seizure disorder
- In many cases, associated with skull fractures or scalp bruises caused by a direct blow from a caregiver's hand or by the child being hit against a wall or door
- Can also result from vigorous shaking of the child (shaken baby syndrome)
- Acceleration and deceleration forces on the brain associated with shaking cause tearing of the bridging cerebral veins with bleeding into the subdural space

Signs and symptoms of shaken baby syndrome

- Retinal hemorrhages
- Irritability
- Altered level of consciousness
- Vomiting
- A full fontanelle

Abdominal Visceral Injury

- Intra-abdominal injuries are the second most common cause of death in battered children.
- These injuries are usually produced by a blunt force such as a punch or blow to the abdomen.

Signs and symptoms

- Recurrent vomiting
- Abdominal distention
- Absent bowel sounds
- Localized tenderness with or without abdominal bruising
- History of trauma to the child's abdomen—Routinely denied by caregivers in these cases

Bone Injury

- More than 20% of physically abused children have a positive radiological bone survey from previous abusive episodes.
- Injuries that may be obvious only through radiography include fractures of the ribs, lateral portion of the clavicle, scapula, sternum, and extremities.
- Multiple fractures in various stages of healing are highly suspicious for physical abuse.

Injuries from Sexual Abuse

- Sexual abuse of a child is a symptom of a seriously disturbed family relationship, usually associated with physical or emotional neglect or abuse.
- Often, the sexually abusive adult experienced similar abuse as a child and justifies this maladaptive behavior subconsciously.
- Family relationships are complex, and silent complicity by at least one parent is often involved.
- Injuries from sexual abuse may be physical and psychological.
  - Sexual abuse may include vaginal intercourse, sodomy (anal intercourse), oral-genital contact, or molestation (fondling, masturbation, or exposure)
- In many cases, the victimized child is female.
- Over half the victims are under 12 years of age at the time of the first offense.
- Since many of these incidents are chronic and occur without force, an EMS response is seldom initiated. If a physical injury results from the abuse, emergency care may be summoned.
- Physical findings suggestive of sexual abuse:
  - Pregnancy or venereal disease in a child 12 years of age or younger
  - Painful urination or defecation
  - Tenderness or lacerations to the perineal area
  - Bleeding from the rectum or vagina
  - Presence of dried blood, semen, or pubic hair in the genital area of a child
- Emergency management for child victims of sexual abuse:
  - Care should be limited to managing life-threatening injury and providing emotional support during transport to the receiving hospital.
  - These children undergo extensive interviews and examination by the emergency department physician and others.

- Carefully document any statements made by the patient, family member, or caregiver; findings should be reported to medical direction.
- These children require compassionate support:
  - A sexually abused child should never receive the impression that she or he is responsible for any of the abuse or that discussion of the event is inappropriate
  - If possible, the child should be interviewed and cared for by a paramedic of the same gender

INFANTS AND CHILDREN WITH SPECIAL NEEDS

- Some infants are born with, and some children develop conditions that require special needs and medical equipment to sustain life:
  - Infants born prematurely.
  - Those who have altered functions from birth.
  - Those who have chronic or acute disease of the lung, heart, or CNS.
- These children are often cared for at home by family and home health services.
- Many are technologically dependent and are on special medical equipment:
  - Tracheostomy tubes
  - Home artificial ventilators
  - Central venous lines
  - Gastrostomy tubes
  - Shunts

Tracheostomy Tubes

- The patient with a complete tracheostomy has had the airway surgically interrupted so that the larynx is no longer connected to the trachea.
- Modern tracheostomy tubes are flexible and relatively comfortable for the patient and have few associated risks.
- Complications that can occur with the tracheostomy tube (all of which may lead to inadequate ventilation) include:
  - Obstruction
  - Air leak
  - Bleeding
  - Dislodgement
  - Infection

Management

- Aseptic technique and respiratory support are always high priorities in caring for these patients.
- Should the tracheostomy tube fail to provide a patent airway because of obstruction or dislodgement, it will need to be cleaned with sterile water or saline, or removed and reinserted.
  - Medical direction may recommend that a tracheostomy tube be replaced with an ET tube as a temporary measure.
- Tracheal suction (using sterile technique) may be necessary to remove secretions and mucus.
  - If tracheal intubation becomes necessary in these patients, it will need to be performed via the stoma.

Home Artificial Ventilators

- When a patient needs help breathing, the child may be put on a mechanical ventilator that can simulate the normal bellows action usually provided by the diaphragm and thoracic cage.
- The type of home ventilator used will depend on the patient's specific needs.
- Ventilators are classified by function based on the variables they deliver during certain phases of the respiratory cycle.
- Complications can occur from a machine malfunction and alarms, airway obstruction, and respiratory distress.

Management

- Because the many types of artificial ventilators operate differently, never try to "troubleshoot" a ventilator problem or adjust the machine's settings.
- The EMS crew should always manage the patient—not try to correct the machine's malfunction.

Central Venous Lines

- Some patients with chronic illnesses require prolonged and frequent access to venous circulation for drug or fluid therapy.
- Types of vascular access devices (VADs) that may frequently be encountered in the prehospital setting for both child and adult patients who are cared for in the home include:
  - Surgically implanted medication delivery devices such as Mediports
  - Peripheral vascular access devices such as peripherally inserted central catheters (PICC)
  - Central venous access devices (e.g., Hickman, Groshong)
- Complications that may occur with VADs:
  - Cracked line
  - Air embolism
  - Bleeding
  - Obstruction
  - Local infection

Management

- A torn or leaking catheter (cracked line) may allow fluids or medications to infiltrate into the surrounding tissues; this can lead to an air embolism.
- If a torn catheter is suspected (evidenced by leaking fluid, complaint of a burning sensation, or swollen and tender skin near the insertion site), stop the infusion immediately and clamp the catheter between the tear and the patient.
- Position the patient who develops an altered level of consciousness (indicating a possible air embolism) on the left side with the head slightly lowered to help prevent the embolism from traveling to the brain.
- High-concentration oxygen, IV access, and rapid transport for physician evaluation are indicated.
- Any bleeding at the site should be controlled with direct pressure.
- Occasionally, the lumen port will become obstructed by a blood clot that disrupts the flow of fluids or medications.
- Signs and symptoms of obstruction include a sluggish flow and swelling and tenderness at the site.

- When this occurs, transport the patient to the hospital so that the catheter can be cleared with thrombolytics or replaced.
- Attempts to clear a VAD require special training and authorization from medical direction.

Gastric Tubes and Gastrostomy Tubes

- A gastric tube is used as a temporary measure to provide liquid feeding to a patient who cannot swallow or absorb nutrients (often used for feeding premature infants).
  - Inserted through the nose or mouth into the stomach; can cause irritation to the nasal and mucous membranes.
  - Designed for short-term use.
- A gastrostomy tube provides a permanent route for gastric feeding in patients who cannot usually be fed by mouth (e.g., a patient with facial burns or paralysis).
  - The tube is surgically placed into the stomach and can be visualized in the upper left quadrant of the abdomen.
  - The opening (stoma) has a flexible silicone "button" (covered with a protective cap) that allows for regular feedings.

Management

- Serious complications with gastric or gastrostomy tubes are rare and seldom require emergency care.
- Be aware of potential complications (all of which can result in inadequate nutrition and fluid needs):
  - Obstruction
  - Pulmonary aspiration
  - GI disturbances (vomiting and diarrhea)
  - Irritation to the mucous membranes
  - Electrolyte imbalances
- Emergency care primarily is supportive and may include transportation for physician evaluation.
- If not contraindicated, the patient will be most comfortable lying on the right side with the head elevated.

Shunts

- A shunt is a surgical procedure performed to relieve abnormal fluid pressures from excess CSF around the brain in children with hydrocephalus (ventricular shunt) or in the portal veins in patients with portal hypertension.
- The shunt for hydrocephalus consists of two catheters, a reservoir, and a valve to prevent backflow. The first catheter is inserted through the skull to drain fluid from the ventricles of the brain. The second catheter is passed into another body cavity (usually the abdomen or right atrium of the heart through the jugular vein), where the excess fluid is absorbed. The reservoir can usually be palpated over the mastoid area, just behind the ear.

Management

- Be aware of complications from this procedure:
  - The need for catheter replacement as the child grows (requiring several surgeries in the first 10 years of life)
  - Obstruction from clotted blood or fluid
  - Catheter displacement

- Infection is a complication that occurs within several weeks of surgical placement.
- Signs and symptoms of obstruction or displacement are those of increased ICP including:
  - Headache
  - Nausea and vomiting
  - Visual disturbances
  - Cushing's triad (elevated systolic pressure, irregular respirations, bradycardia)
- Children who have a complication from a ventricular shunt are surgical emergencies, and require immediate care to prevent brain stem herniation.
- The paramedic should first ensure adequate airway, ventilatory, and circulatory support for these patients. Medical direction may recommend additional therapies, including IV access, ET intubation, and hyperventilation to lower ICP.
- These patients are prone to respiratory arrest and require immediate transportation to an appropriate facility for physician evaluation.
  - If possible, the patient's head should be elevated during transport.

CHAPTER QUESTIONS

1. When caring for a toddler, it is important to remember that a toddler:
   a. does not mind being separated from his caregiver
   b. has little fear of anything
   c. may apologize for being hurt
   d. does not mind being touched
2 You are caring for a 16-year-old male who was the driver of a car involved in a collision. While assessing your patient, remember that adolescents:
   a. are very cautious and rarely take risks
   b. are overly concerned with modesty or about their appearance
   c. may be reluctant to disclose information about their personal habits
   d. usually do not want their peers around when they are hurt
3. Because an infant has a smaller circulating blood volume than an adult:
   a. a comparatively small blood loss in an infant would constitute a major hemorrhage for an adult
   b. external bleeding must be stopped as quickly as possible
   c. the respiratory rate is slower than an adult's
   d. the heart rate is slower than an adult's
4. Your responsive 4-year-old male patient has swallowed a marble that is causing a complete airway obstruction. Your immediate care should include:
   a. CPR
   b. oxygen by pediatric non-rebreather
   c. backblows and chest thrusts
   d. abdominal thrusts (Heimlich maneuver)
5. You are caring for a 10-month-old female patient. She has swallowed a piece of a hot dog that is causing a complete airway obstruction. Your treatment should include:
   a. backblows and chest thrusts
   b. blind finger sweeps to attempt removal of the object
   c. high-concentration oxygen by blow-by or non-rebreather
   d. CPR

6. When caring for a pediatric patient in respiratory failure, general guidelines include:
   a. performing blind finger sweeps to relieve airway obstructions
   b. suctioning the airway for 20–30 seconds
   c. using a 750 mL BVM device for infants
   d. padding beneath the shoulder blades to maintain an open airway
7. One of the most reliable signs of early hypoperfusion in a 2-year-old is:
   a. a decreased blood pressure
   b. strong peripheral pulses
   c. delayed capillary refill
   d. excessive tear production
8. In infants and children, the primary cause of cardiac arrest is:
   a. shock
   b. respiratory failure
   c. hypothermia
   d. seizures
9. The number-one killer of American children from ages 1 to 14 is:
   a. motor vehicle crashes
   b. firearms
   c. airway obstruction
   d. burns
10. If you suspect your pediatric patient has been physically abused, you should:
    a. transport the child and report your suspicions to the emergency department staff
    b. have local law enforcement respond to the scene to question the parents
    c. ask the child if he has been abused
    d. make your suspicions known to both the parents and the child at the scene

Suggested Reading

US Department of Transportation, National Highway Traffic Safety Administration. *EMT-Paramedic: National Standard Curriculum*. Washington, DC: US Department of Transportation, National Highway Traffic Safety Administration; 1998.

Chapter 36
Geriatrics

An 82-year-old male with a history of congestive heart failure presents with dyspnea that has gradually increased over the past week. He has a productive cough with brown sputum. Vital signs are BP 110/66, HR 96, RR 20, and temperature is 100.6°F. He is unable to walk and has not eaten in 2 days.

What would be the most likely assessment?

IMPACT OF AGING ON SOCIETY

- According to the National Institute of Aging, the number of Americans age 55 and older will almost double between now and 2030—from 60 million today (21% of the total U.S. population) to 107.6 million (31% of the population)—as the Baby Boomers reach retirement age.
- During that same period of time, the number of Americans over 65 will be more than double, from 34.8 million in 2000 (12% of the population) to 70.3 million in 2030 (20% of the total population).
- The next generation of retirees will be the healthiest and longest lived.
- Americans reaching age 65 today have an average life expectancy of an additional 17.9 years (19.2 years for females and 16.3 years for males).
- The likelihood that an American who reaches the age of 65 will survive to the age of 90 has nearly doubled over the past 40 years—from just 14% of 65-year-olds in 1960 to 25% at present. By 2050, 40% of 65-year-olds are likely to reach age 90.
- This creates great challenges as society attempts to provide quality, cost-effective health care and support the increasing health and living expenses for older adults. For the requirements of this population to be met adequately, certain goals must be accomplished.
- The public must become better educated about the needs of the older adult population, as care-giving responsibilities often fall to families and friends.
- Current and new health-care professionals must be educated regarding the special needs of this population.
- Older persons have unique characteristics that differentiate them from younger populations, such as higher level of adverse drug reactions and urinary incontinence.
- Thus, special training is needed to treat the frail, older adult population.
- The aging of the U.S. population demands continued and expanded research efforts into chronic diseases that affect frail older adults and their families.
- Health-care financing, delivery, and administrative structures need to be reformed to accommodate the predominance of chronic illness among the aging population.
- Solutions must be developed for long-term care needs of the growing aging population, addressing the emotional and financial needs of older adults and their families and the financial impact of long-term care on the country.

PHYSIOLOGICAL CHANGES OF AGING

- Gerontology is the study of aging.
- The aging process proceeds at different rates in different people, and organ systems age at differing rates within the individual. In certain areas, however, predictable functional declines occur in all people with increasing age.
- As a rough guideline, these changes begin to occur at a rate of 5–10% for each decade of life after the age of 30.
- Although all body systems are affected by the aging process, the effects on specific organ systems particularly relevant to the older adult are those that occur in the respiratory, cardiovascular, renal, nervous, and musculoskeletal systems.

Respiratory System Changes

- Respiratory function in the older adult generally is compromised because of changes in pulmonary physiology that accompany the aging process. Reduced pulmonary capacity is related to alterations in lung and chest wall compliance. With aging, the chest wall becomes increasingly stiff as the bony thorax becomes more rigid and lung elasticity decreases.
- Variable increases in alveolar diameter and the tendency for distal airways to collapse on expiration lead to an increase in residual volume and a decrease in vital capacity.
- Several changes occur by age 75; vital capacity may decrease by as much as 50%. Maximum breathing capacity may decrease by as much as 60%. Maximum work rate and maximum oxygen uptake may decrease by as much as 70%.
- Arterial oxygen pressure (PaO_2) also slowly decreases with age, but arterial carbon dioxide pressure ($PaCO_2$) remains unchanged.
- At age 30, the PaO_2 of a healthy person breathing ambient air at sea level is about 90 torr; at age 70, the expected PaO_2 is 70 torr. These findings, combined with the normal decline in central and peripheral chemoreceptor function, produce a diminished ventilatory response to hypoxic and hypercapnic challenge.
- Other factors may impair the body's defense against inhaled bacteria and particulate matter.
    - Loss of cilia in the airways
    - Diminished cough reflex
    - Impaired gag reflex
- The decline in pulmonary defense mechanisms makes infectious pulmonary diseases of the older adult more common and more difficult to eliminate.

Cardiovascular System Changes

- Cardiac function declines with age from nonischemic physiological changes and the high incidence of atherosclerotic coronary artery disease.
- Structural and physiological changes occur in the cardiovascular system that limits cardiac function. A diminished ability to raise the heart rate even in response to exercise or stress, a decrease in compliance of the ventricle, a prolonged duration of contraction, and decreased responsiveness to catecholamine stimulation.
- Between the ages of 30 and 80, resting cardiac output decreases about 30%.
- This, combined with the progressive increase in peripheral vascular resistance that occurs after age 40, yields a significant drop in organ perfusion. When the cardiovascular system is placed under unexpected stress, myocardial hypertrophy, coronary artery disease, and hemodynamic changes predispose the geriatric patient to dysrhythmias, heart failure, and sudden cardiac arrest.

- Changes also occur in the heart's electrical conduction pathways. These physiological changes often lead to dysrhythmias, including chronic atrial fibrillation, sick-sinus syndrome, and various types of bradycardias and heart blocks, all of which can contribute to the decline in cardiac output.

Renal System Changes

- Structural and functional changes occur in the kidneys during the aging process. Renal blood flow is reduced an average of 50% between the ages of 30 and 80. This reduction is associated with a proportional decrease in the glomerular filtration rate of about 8 mL/min per decade.
- Renal mass decreases by about 20% between the ages of 40 and 80.
- Steady decline in kidney function places the older patient at greater risk of renal failure from trauma, obstruction, infection, and vascular occlusion.
- As decades pass, significant impairment develops in renal concentrating ability, sodium conservation, free water clearance (diuresis), glomerular filtration, and renal plasma flow.
- Hepatic blood flow also decreases, limiting the effectiveness of liver metabolism. These decreases in renal and hepatic function, combined with changes in lean body mass and body water, make the older person more susceptible than younger adults to electrolyte abnormalities or toxic manifestations in response to medications or drugs.

Nervous System Changes

- It is now well known that intellectual functioning deteriorates selectively in the older adult and may result from many organic causes. Beginning at about age 30, the total number of neurons in certain cortical areas decreases gradually. By age 70, a 10% reduction in brain weight has occurred.
- These factors, along with decreased cerebral blood flow and alterations in the location and amounts of specific neurotransmitters, probably contribute to alterations in the central nervous system (CNS).
- With aging, the velocity of nerve conduction in the peripheral nervous system also decreases.
- Toxic or metabolic factors can affect mental functioning. They include use of medications; electrolyte imbalances; hypoglycemia; acidosis; alkalosis; hypoxia; liver, kidney, or lung failure; pneumonia; congestive heart failure; cardiac dysrhythmias; infection anywhere in the body; or neoplastic syndromes.

Musculoskeletal System Changes

- As the body ages, there is muscle shrinkage, calcification of muscles and ligaments, and thinning of the intervertebral disks. Osteoporosis is common in older adults (especially women), and an estimated 68% of older patients show some degree of *kyphosis*.
- Other significant changes occur as a result:
  - A decrease in total muscle mass
  - A decrease in height of 2–3 in.
  - Widening and weakening of certain bones
  - A posture that impairs mobility and alters the body's balance
- Because of these changes, falls are common.

Other Physiological Changes

- Other physiological changes that occur with aging include alterations in body mass and total body water, a decreased ability to maintain internal homeostasis, a decrease in the function of immunological mechanisms, possible nutritional disorders, and decreases in hearing and visual acuity.

- As an individual approaches age 65, lean body mass may decrease as much as 25%, and fat tissue may increase as much as 35%.
- Changes in body composition can influence the dosage and frequency of administration of fat-soluble drugs, because there is more drug per weight of metabolically active tissue and a larger reservoir for accumulation of the drug.
- The decrease in total body water is likely to increase the concentration of water-soluble drugs.
- The body's ability to maintain internal homeostasis through normal thermoregulatory mechanisms declines over time in a linear fashion beginning at about age 30.
- This and other factors predispose the older adult to cold- and heat-related conditions such as hypothermia, heat exhaustion, and hyperthermia.
- Several factors contribute to the increased risk of thermoregulatory disorders.
  - Impaired sympathetic nervous system function, resulting in decreased capacity for peripheral vasoconstriction
  - Lowered metabolic rate
  - Poor peripheral circulation
  - Chronic illness
- Aging causes a decrease in primary antibody response and cellular immunity.
- Older adults consume less than the minimum daily requirement of most vitamins.
- Other factors that are associated with poor nutrition include:
  - Poor dentition and reduced mastication
  - Decreased esophageal motility
  - Frequent hypochlorhydria
  - Decreased intestinal secretions that tend to reduce absorption
- Elderly patients easily can become victims of malnutrition, leading to dehydration and hypoglycemia.

ASSESSMENT OF THE GERIATRIC PATIENT

- Normal physiological changes and underlying acute or chronic illness may make evaluation of an ill or injured older person a challenge.
- Besides the components of a normal physical assessment, consider special characteristics of older patients that can complicate the clinical evaluation.
- Geriatric patients are likely to suffer from concurrent illness.
- Aging may affect an individual's response to illness or injury.
- Social and emotional factors may have greater impact on health than in any other age group.

History Taking

- Gathering a history from an older patient usually requires more time than with younger patients.
- Use the following techniques to effectively communicate with older patients:
  - Always identify yourself
  - Talk at eye level to ensure that the patient can see you as you speak
  - Locate hearing aid, eyeglasses, and dentures (if needed)
  - Turn on lights
  - Speak slowly, distinctly, and respectfully

- Use the patient's surname, unless he or she requests otherwise
- Listen closely
- Be patient
- Preserve dignity
- Use gentleness

Physical Examination

- When conducting the physical examination of an older patient, consider the following points:
  - The patient may fatigue easily
  - Patients commonly wear many layers of clothing for warmth, which may hamper the examination
  - Respect the patient's modesty and need for privacy unless it interferes with patient care procedures
  - Explain actions clearly before examining all patients, especially those with diminished sight
  - Be aware that the patient may minimize or deny symptoms through fear of being bedridden or institutionalized or losing self-sufficiency
  - Try to distinguish symptoms of chronic disease from acute immediate problems
- If time permits, evaluate the patient's immediate surroundings for the following:
  - Evidence of alcohol or medication use
  - Presence of food items
  - General condition of housing
  - Signs of adequate personal hygiene
- Ask friends or family members about the patient's appearance and responsiveness now versus his or her normal appearance, responsiveness, and other characteristics.
- Ensure gentle handling and adequate padding for patient comfort if ambulance transport is necessary.

SYSTEM PATHOPHYSIOLOGY, ASSESSMENT, AND MANAGEMENT

Pulmonary System

Pneumonia

- Pneumonia is a leading cause of death in the geriatric age group, and is often fatal in frail adults. Older patients are more likely to develop bacteremia and are more susceptible to many respiratory pathogens. This, associated with the presence of chronic disease, impairs respiratory tract clearance and allows pharyngeal colonization by pathogens that may be aspirated into the lungs. Because of the decreased pulmonary reserve in older patients, pneumonia may commonly be associated with respiratory failure.
- Risk factors for bacterial pneumonia include the following:
  - Institutionalized environments
  - Chronic diseases
  - Immune system compromise
- Unlike in younger patients with bacterial pneumonia, the usual clinical picture of pyrexia, productive cough, pleurisy, and signs of pulmonary consolidation is often absent in the older patient. This atypical presentation is responsible for the common delay in diagnosis.

- The following signs and symptoms may be present:
  - Fever (variable)
  - Cough
  - Shortness of breath
  - Alterations in mental status
  - Tachycardia
  - Tachypnea
- Emergency care is directed toward managing life threats, maintaining oxygenation, and providing transportation for physician evaluation.

Chronic Obstructive Pulmonary Disease

- Chronic obstructive pulmonary disease (COPD) in the geriatric patient is a major health problem in the United States. COPD is a common finding in the older patient who has a long history of cigarette smoking; usually associated with a variety of disease processes that result in reduced expiratory airflow.
- An exacerbation of COPD often follows an acute respiratory infection that causes airway edema, bronchial smooth muscle irritability, and increased mucous secretion. These airway abnormalities may lead to factors associated with acute decompensation, limited airflow, increased work of breathing, dyspnea, ventilation-perfusion mismatching, hypoxemia, respiratory acidosis, and hemodynamic compromise.
- Signs and symptoms of COPD in the geriatric patient include the following:
  - Cyanosis
  - Wheezing
  - Abnormal or diminished breath sounds
  - Dysrhythmias
  - Paradoxical breathing
  - Jugular vein distention
  - Decreased oxygen saturation levels
  - Extreme anxiety
- Obtain a thorough history of the event (including a history of prior intubation or steroid therapy), and be prepared for aggressive airway management.
- Emergency management of COPD is aimed at correcting life-threatening hypoxemia and improving airflow that may be accomplished through airway and ventilatory support with supplemental oxygenation and bronchodilators administered by inhalation or injection (per medical direction).

Pulmonary Embolism

- Pulmonary embolism is a life-threatening cause of dyspnea associated with venous stasis, heart failure, COPD, malignancy, and immobilization, all of which are common in older adults.
- Most pulmonary emboli in the geriatric age group arise indirectly from the leg veins with propagation to the iliofemoral veins.
- Signs and symptoms may range from a presentation of left ventricular failure with sudden tachypnea, unexplained tachycardia (a hallmark sign), and atrial fibrillation to signs and symptoms solely of the underlying venous thrombosis.
- Pulmonary embolism may precipitate congestive heart failure (CHF) and may also masquerade as bacterial pneumonia in this age group.
- Emergency care is directed at ensuring adequate airway, ventilatory, and circulatory support; immobilization and elevation of an affected extremity; and rapid transport for physician evaluation.

Cardiovascular System

Myocardial Infarction (MI)

- Chest pain as a symptom of MI becomes less frequent by age 70, and only 45% of patients over age 85 with MI have this complaint. Lack of typical chest pain can cause MI to go unrecognized in the older patient.
- Six major risk factors should be evaluated when assessing an older adult patient for MI:
  - Previous MI
  - Angina
  - Diabetes
  - Hypertension
  - High cholesterol
  - Smoking
- Although some older patients will have chest pain or discomfort, many complain only of vague symptoms such as dyspnea, abdominal or epigastric distress, and fatigue.
- For many patients, the event is completely "silent," which may be a result of decreased visceral sensory function or higher incidences of mental deterioration in this age group.
- Silent MIs are usually marked by an atypical complaint:
  - Fatigue
  - Breathlessness
  - Nausea
  - Abdominal pain

Emergency management

- Airway, ventilatory, and circulatory support
- Oxygen administration and pain management therapy
- Management of serious dysrhythmias according to advanced life support (ALS) protocol
- Rapid and gentle transport for physician evaluation

Heart Failure

- Heart failure is more frequent in older adults and has a larger incidence of noncardiac causes. Occurs when ventricular output is insufficient to meet the metabolic demands of the body.
- Common causes:
  - Ischemic heart disease
  - Valvular heart disease
  - Cardiomyopathy
  - Dysrhythmias
  - Hyperthyroidism
  - Anemia

Signs and symptoms

- Dyspnea
- Fatigue (often the first symptom of left-sided heart failure)
- Orthopnea
- Dry, hacking cough progressing to productive cough with frothy sputum

- Dependent edema due to right-sided heart failure
- Nocturia
- Anorexia, hepatomegaly, ascites
- Conditions associated with heart failure must be reversed as soon as possible to prevent cardiac damage
- In addition to oxygen administration and electrocardiogram (ECG) monitoring, management may include intubation, intravenous (IV) therapy, and drug therapy (furosemide, nitroglycerin, morphine)

Dysrhythmias

- The most common cause of dysrhythmias in the older patient is heart disease.
- Several factors should be considered when assessing dysrhythmias in the geriatric patient:
  - PVCs are frequently present in most adults over age 80
  - Atrial fibrillation is the most common dysrhythmia
  - Dysrhythmias may result from electrolyte imbalances
- In addition to the serious implications of some dysrhythmias, there are other associated complications:
  - Traumatic injury from falls due to cerebral hypoperfusion
  - Transient ischemic attacks (TIAs)
  - Heart failure
- Emergency management is directed at ensuring adequate airway, ventilatory, and circulatory support; oxygen administration; and transport for physician evaluation.
- Serious dysrhythmias should be managed according to advanced cardiac life support (ACLS) protocol.

Abdominal and Thoracic Aneurysm

- Atherosclerotic disease is a common cause of abdominal and thoracic aneurysm. Abdominal aortic aneurysm affects about 2–4% of the U.S. population over 50 years of age.
- Acute dissecting aortic aneurysm is more common than abdominal aneurysm and is associated with a high mortality rate.
- Signs and symptoms will vary according to the site of rupture or extent of dissection:
  - Abdominal aneurysm
    - — Unexplained hypotension
    - — Sudden onset of abdominal or back pain
    - — Syncope
    - — Low back pain or flank pain
    - — Pulsatile, tender mass
    - — Diminished distal pulses
  - Thoracic aneurysm
    - — Chest pain
    - — Syncope
    - — Stroke
    - — Hypotension
    - — Absent or reduced pulses
    - — Heart failure
    - — Pericardial tamponade
    - — Acute MI

- The goals of prehospital care are relief of pain and immediate transport to a medical facility.
- Airway, ventilatory, and circulatory support may be required if the patient decompensates.
- Other prehospital management includes the following measures:
  - Gentle handling of the patient
  - Decreasing anxiety
  - High-concentration oxygen administration
  - Large-bore IV access (restrict fluids unless severe hypotension is present)
  - Pain medication (per medical direction)

Hypertension

- The incidence of hypertension in older adults increases with atherosclerosis.
- Associated risk factors:
  - Advanced age
  - Diabetes
  - Obesity
- Hypertension is often defined by a resting blood pressure consistently greater than 140/90 mmHg. Blood pressures greater than 160/95 doubles mortality in men. Chronic hypertension is associated with many medical conditions, including:
  - Myocardial ischemia and infarction
  - Cardiac hypertrophy and left ventricular failure
  - Kidney failure
  - Blindness
  - Stroke
  - Peripheral vascular disease
  - Aneurysm formation
- Other signs and symptoms that may suggest chronic hypertension include epistaxis, tremors, and nausea and vomiting.
- Prehospital management primarily is supportive. In severe cases, medical direction may recommend the administration of antihypertensives.

Neurology

Cerebrovascular Disease

- Stroke is the third leading cause of death in the United States and the leading cause of brain injury in adults. Neurological impairment is caused either by an ischemic or hemorrhagic interruption in the blood supply to the brain.
- Associated risk factors for cerebral vascular disease in the older adult:
  - Smoking
  - Hypertension
  - Diabetes
  - Atherosclerosis
  - Hyperlipidemia
  - Polycythemia
  - Heart disease

Signs and symptoms of stroke and TIA

- Unilateral paralysis.
- Numbness.

- Language disturbance.
- Visual disturbance.
- Monocular blindness.
- Vertigo.
- Diplopia.
- Ataxia.
- Once the diagnosis of a stroke is suspected, time in the field must be minimized because there is limited time to initiate therapy (less than 3 hours from onset is required for thrombolytics).
- Prehospital management is directed at managing the patient's airway, breathing, and circulation and monitoring vital signs.
- In addition to supporting vital functions, the most important element of prehospital care for a stroke victim is to identify the patient with stroke and to rapidly transport the patient for definitive care to the appropriate emergency receiving facility. In some states, emergency medical service (EMS) services are obligated to transport stroke patients to specialty stroke referral centers, bypassing a closer emergency receiving facility.

Delirium

- Delirium is an abrupt disorientation for time and place, usually with illusions and hallucinations. The patient's mind may "wander," speech may be incoherent, and the patient may be in a state of mental confusion or excitement.
- Delirium is commonly brought on by physical illness.
- Signs and symptoms vary according to personality, environment, and severity of illness.
- Causes of delirium are associated with organic brain dysfunction.
  - Tumor
  - Metabolic disorders
  - Fever
  - Drug reactions
  - Alcohol intoxication or withdrawal
- Delirium is potentially life threatening and requires emergency care.
- The condition may be reversible (if diagnosed early) but can progress to chronic mental dysfunction.
- Prehospital management includes the following measures:
  - Ensure adequate airway, breathing, and circulatory support
  - Treat hypoxia with oxygen
  - Treat hypotension with IV fluids (if appropriate)
  - Reduce agitation and anxiety
  - Avoid patient injury and ensure personal safety
    - — Restrain if necessary (per protocol)
    - — Sedate as a last resort
  - Consider hypoglycemia or a narcotic state
    - — Measure blood glucose
    - — Administer dextrose 50% or naloxone per protocol
  - Assess for CNS injury (trauma or stroke)
    - — Perform a careful neurological exam
  - Look for signs of CNS infection (e.g., encephalitis)
  - Transport the patient for physician evaluation

Dementia

A slow, progressive loss of awareness of time and place, usually with an inability to learn new things or remember recent events. Often a result of brain disease. Possible causes include stroke, genetic or viral factors, and Alzheimer's disease. Generally considered irreversible and eventually results in a person becoming totally dependent on others because of the progressive loss of cognitive functioning.

Behaviors associated with dementia

- During the course of the disease, patients often attempt to "cover up" their memory loss by confabulation (making up stories to fill gaps in memory).
- Sudden outbursts or embarrassing behaviors may be the first obvious signs of the illness.
- Some patients may eventually regress to a "second childhood" and require total care for feedings, toilet, and physical activity.
- Dementia may be difficult to differentiate from delirium in the prehospital setting.
- The key difference between the two conditions is that delirium is "new" with a rapid onset; dementia is progressive (see Table 36-1).
- A history of the event from a rational witness such as a friend or family member is the best source of information. If a rational witness is not available, the patient should be treated for delirium, which may be a life-threatening emergency.

Alzheimer's Disease

- A progressive brain disorder that gradually destroys a person's memory and ability to learn, reason, make judgements, communicate, and carry out daily activities. As Alzheimer's progresses, individuals may also experience changes in personality and behavior, such as anxiety, suspiciousness or agitation, as well as delusions or hallucinations.
- Although there is currently no cure for Alzheimer's, new treatments are on the horizon as a result of accelerating insight into the biology of the disease. Research has also shown that effective care and support can improve quality of life for individuals and their caregivers over the course of the disease from diagnosis to the end of life.
- Alzheimer's disease is a condition in which nerve cells in the cerebral cortex die and the brain substance shrinks. It is the single most common cause of dementia, and is responsible for the majority of cases in persons over age 75.
- Alzheimer's disease does not directly cause death; patients ultimately stop eating and become malnourished and immobilized so that they are prone to infections.
- Several theories have been suggested as possible causes:
  - Abnormalities in glutamate metabolism
  - Chronic infection
  - Toxic poisoning by metals
  - A reduction in brain chemicals such as acetylcholine
  - Genetics

TABLE 36-1: Differential Diagnosis for Delirium and Dementia

Delirium	Dementia
Abrupt	Gradual
Reduced attention span	Impaired recent memory
Disorganized thinking	Regression
Hallucinations	Poor judgement

- Early symptoms of the disease primarily are related to memory loss, particularly the ability to make and recall new memories.
  - As the disease progresses, agitation, violence, and impairment of abstract thinking begin.
  - Judgement and cognitive abilities begin to interfere with work and social interactions.
  - In advanced stages, patients often become bedridden and totally unaware of their surroundings.
  - Once the patient is bedridden, the complications of bedsores, feeding problems, and pneumonia make life expectancy very short.
- There is no specific treatment for Alzheimer's disease apart from the provision of nursing and social care for the patient and relatives.
- In the prehospital setting, patients with Alzheimer's disease are managed similarly to those with dementia.

Parkinson's Disease

- Parkinson's disease is a brain disorder (caused by degeneration of or damage to nerve cells in the basal ganglia) that causes muscle tremor, stiffness, and weakness.
- There are several characteristic signs of the disease:
  - Trembling (usually beginning in one hand, arm, or leg)
  - A rigid posture
  - Slow movements
  - A shuffling, unbalanced walk
- Untreated, the disease progresses more than 10–15 years to severe weakness and incapacity.
- Emergency care for these patients primarily is supportive and includes airway, ventilatory, and circulatory support and transport for physician evaluation.
- Although there is no cure for Parkinson's disease, counseling, exercise, special aids in the home, and drug therapy can improve the patient's morale, mobility, and quality of life.

Endocrinology

Diabetes

- About 20% of older adults have diabetes, and almost 40% have some impaired glucose tolerance.
- Type 2 diabetes (non–insulin-dependent) is most common in older adult patients, especially when the person is overweight.
- Associated risk factors for complications related to diabetes:
  - Decreased ability to care for self
  - Living alone
  - Decline in renal function
  - Polydrug use

Hyperglycemic Hyperosmolar Nonketotic Coma (HHNK)

- HHNK is a serious complication of older adult, non–insulin-dependent diabetics with a mortality rate of 20–50%.
- Patient is often found comatose or complaining of profound polydipsia and polyuria from osmotic diuresis, leading to dehydration and electrolyte loss.
- Several predisposing factors make the older adult patient susceptible to HHNK:
  - Infection
  - Noncompliance with medications

- Polydrug use
- Pancreatitis
- Stroke
- Hypothermia
- Heat stroke
- MI

- If HHNK is suspected, vigorously search for an underlying cause; ensure adequate airway, ventilatory, and circulatory support; initiate IV therapy; and rapidly transport the patient for physician evaluation.
- Control of diabetes:
  - A combination of dietary measures, weight reduction, and oral hypoglycemic agents can usually keep type 2 diabetes under control.
  - Insulin injections are not usually required for type 2 diabetes.
  - If uncontrolled, diabetes can lead to complications:
    - Retinopathy
    - Peripheral neuropathy (ulcers on the feet are common)
    - Kidney damage
  - Diabetics also have a higher-than-average risk of atherosclerosis, hypertension and other cardiovascular disorders, and cataracts.

Management

Emergency care includes airway, ventilatory, and circulatory support; blood glucose screening; IV dextrose (if indicated, and in the absence of cerebral damage); and transport for physician evaluation.

Thyroid Disease

Thyroid disease appears to be more common in the older adult patient and is thought to be related to the aging process. Thyroid dysfunction should be suspected in any older adult patient who is ill.

Signs and symptoms

"Characteristic" signs and symptoms of thyroid disorders are often not present in the geriatric patient.

Hyperthyroidism

- Weight loss
- Mental status changes
- CHF
- Tachydysrhythmias
- Lethargy
- Constipation

Hypothyroidism

- Weight loss
- Nonspecific musculoskeletal complaints
- CHF
- Anemia
- Altered mental status (dementia, depression, coma, seizures)
- Hyponatremia

Management

- Emergency care primarily is supportive to ensure vital functions.
- Following physician evaluation, patients with thyroid disease are treated with various thyroid drugs, radioactive iodine treatments, and sometimes surgery.
- Severe complications from thyroid disease include thyroid storm and myxedema coma that may be complicated by coexisting coronary artery disease.

Gastroenterology

Gastrointestinal (GI) Hemorrhage

- GI bleeding most commonly affects patients 60–90 years of age and has a mortality rate of about 10%. The older the patient, the higher the risk of death. This is due to several characteristics of older adult patients:
  - Less able to compensate for acute blood loss
  - Less likely to feel symptoms, so they seek treatment at later stages of disease
  - More likely to be taking aspirin or nonsteroidal anti-inflammatory drugs (NSAIDs), placing them at higher risk for ulcer disease and bleeding
  - At higher risk for colon cancer, intestinal vascular abnormalities, and diverticulitis
  - More likely to be on blood-thinning medications
  - Abdominal pain in an older adult patient should always be considered a serious complaint
- Life-threatening causes of abdominal pain in this age group include:
  - Abdominal aortic aneurysm
  - GI hemorrhage
  - Ruptured viscus
  - Dead or ischemic bowel
  - Acute bowel obstruction

Signs and symptoms of GI bleeding

- Vomiting of blood or coffee-ground emesis.
- Blood-tinged stools or black, tarry stools.
- Weakness.
- Syncope.
- Pain.
- If bleeding is suspected or confirmed in a patient with signs and symptoms of shock, measures to ensure adequate airway, ventilatory, and circulatory support should be initiated and the patient rapidly transported for definitive care.

Bowel Obstruction

Bowel obstruction generally occurs in patients with prior abdominal surgeries or hernias and in those with colonic cancer.

Signs and symptoms

- Complaints of constipation
- Abdominal cramping
- Inability to pass gas
- Protracted vomiting of foodstuffs or bile
- Vomiting of fecal material

- Heart rate and blood pressure—often in normal ranges
- Sometimes, abdomen mildly distended and tender in all four quadrants (abdominal pain is variable)

Management

- Prehospital care primarily is supportive to ensure vital functions.
- After physician evaluation, most patients are treated conservatively with bowel rest, nasogastric suction, and hydration.
- Surgery will sometimes be required to lyse the offending adhesions (which may result in a cycle of new scarring and obstruction) or for hernia repair (most commonly in men).

Problems with Continence

- Continence is the ability to control bladder or bowel function.
- Several factors are required for continence:
  - An anatomically correct GI/GU tract
  - Competent sphincter mechanisms
  - Cognitive and physical function
  - Motivation
- Some factors associated with continence are affected by age:
  - A decrease in bladder capacity
  - Involuntary bladder contractions
  - Decreased ability to postpone voiding
  - Medications that can affect bladder and bowel control
- All forms of incontinence are usually embarrassing for the patient and if chronic, can lead to skin irritation, tissue breakdown, and urinary tract infection.
- Some cases of incontinence are managed surgically to restore sphincter function.
- Persons with mild cases often wear absorptive undergarments to relieve discomfort and embarrassment.

Bladder Incontinence

- Injury or disease of the urinary tract.
- Prolapse of the uterus.
- Decline in sphincter muscle control surrounding the urethra (common in older adults).
- Damage to the brain or spinal cord/seizures.
- Pelvic fracture.
- Prostate cancer.
- Dementia.
- Urinary incontinence can vary in severity from mild incontinence (the escape of small amounts of urine) to total incontinence (the complete loss of bladder control).

Bowel Incontinence

- Fecal impaction.
- Severe diarrhea.
- Injury to anal muscles (e.g., from childbirth or surgery).
- Damage to the brain or spinal cord/seizures.
- Dementia.
- Bowel incontinence in older adults is usually the result of fecal impaction.

- Feces lodged in the rectum irritate and inflame the lining and may allow fecal fluid and small feces to pass involuntarily.

Problems with elimination

- Older adults may have problems with urination and/or bowel elimination.
  - Common causes of difficulty in urination:
    - — Enlargement of the prostate (male patients)
    - — Urinary tract infection (more prevalent in female patients)
    - — Urethral strictures
    - — Acute or chronic renal failure
  - Conditions associated with difficulty in bowel elimination:
    - — Diverticular disease
    - — Constipation
    - — Colorectal cancer
- Problems with elimination can cause extreme pain and anxiety for older adult patients, and their complaints should be taken seriously.
- These conditions require physician evaluation to identify the cause and to select an appropriate therapy.

Integumentary Changes

- As people age, the skin gradually becomes dry, transparent, and wrinkled.
- Aging results in a gradual decrease in epidermal cellular turnover and reduced rate of nail and hair growth.
- The associated loss of deep, dermal vessels and capillary circulation leads to common complaints such as dry, itchy skin, alterations in thermal regulation, and skin-related complications. Common skin complications include:
  - Slow healing
  - Increased risk of secondary infection
  - Increased risk of fungal or viral infections
  - Increased susceptibility to abrasions and tears
- Be gentle with the skin of an older adult patient when performing medical procedures. Use aseptic technique during wound management. Gently place and remove ECG electrodes, and use careful taping procedures when securing IV catheters or tubing.

Pressure Ulcers

- Pressure ulcers are a common finding in older adult patients.
- Often develop on the skin of patients who are bedridden or immobile.
- Most pressure ulcers occur in the lower legs, back, and buttocks, and over bony areas such as the greater trochanter or the sacrum.
- Pressure ulcers commonly affect victims of stroke or other illnesses that result in a loss or alteration in the sensation of pain.
- Skin exposure to moisture, poor nutrition, and friction or shear also may be factors for developing pressure ulcers.
- Other causes of pressure ulcers in older adult patients include vascular and metabolic disorders, trauma, and cancer.
- Pressure ulcers result from tissue hypoxia. They generally start as red, painful areas that become purple before the skin breaks down, developing into open sores. Once integrity of the skin has been breached, the sores often become infected, after which they are slow to heal.

- Pressure ulcers should be covered with sterile dressing, using aseptic technique.
- Transport the patient for physician evaluation and wound care.

Musculoskeletal Changes

Osteoarthritis

- Osteoarthritis (degenerative arthritis) is a common form of arthritis in older adult patients that results from cartilage loss and wear and tear on the joints. Osteoarthritis leads to pain, stiffness, and occasionally loss of function of the affected joint.
- The affected joint often becomes large and distorted from the outgrowth of new bone that tends to develop at the margins of the joint surface.
- Osteoarthritis evolves in middle years and occurs to some extent in most people over age 60, although some have no symptoms.
- Following physician evaluation, treatment may include medications (analgesics, NSAIDs, corticosteroids), physical therapy, and sometimes joint-replacement surgery.

Osteoporosis

- Osteoporosis is considered a natural part of aging.
- This condition is especially common in older women after menopause because of a decrease in the estrogen hormone that helps to maintain bone mass.
- The loss in bone density causes bones to become brittle and easily fractured (which is often the first sign of the disease).
- Typical sites for fractures are just above the wrist, at the head of the femur, and at one of several vertebras (often a spontaneous fracture).
- Once diagnosed, osteoporosis is treated with preventive measures such as a diet high in calcium, calcium supplements, exercise, and hormone replacement therapy after menopause.

Special Problems with Sensation

As people age, they most likely will experience problems with vision, hearing, and speech.

Problems with Vision

- Vision changes begin to occur at age 40 and gradually increase over time.
- The effects of aging on vision include reading difficulties and the following:
  - Poor depth perception
  - Poor adjustment of the eyes to variations in distance
  - Altered color perception
  - Sensitivity to light
  - Decreased visual acuity
- Two common eye conditions that develop with age are cataracts and glaucoma.
- A cataract is a loss of transparency of the lens of the eye that results from changes in the delicate protein fibers within the lens.
  - A cataract never completely causes blindness, but clarity and detail of an image progressively are lost
  - Cataracts usually occur in both eyes, but in most cases, one eye is more severely affected than the other
  - Surgery to remove the cataract is a common procedure in the United States
- Glaucoma is a condition in which intraocular pressure increases and causes damage to the optic nerve.
  - Results in nerve fiber destruction and partial or complete loss of peripheral and central vision

- May result from aging (rarely seen before age 40), a congenital abnormality, or trauma to the eye
- Symptoms of acute glaucoma include dull, severe, aching pain in and above the eye; fogginess of vision; and the perception of "rainbow rings" (halos) around lights at night
- Testing for glaucoma is part of most eye examinations in adults
- If detected early, the condition can be treated with oral medications and eye drops to relieve intraocular pressure

Problems with Hearing

- Although not all older adult patients have hearing loss, overall hearing tends to decrease with age from degeneration of the hearing mechanism (sensorineural deafness).
- Hearing problems also can be caused by the following:
  - Meniere's disease (increased fluid pressure in the labyrinth)
  - Certain drugs
  - Tumors
  - Some viral infections
- Hearing loss can interfere with the ability to perceive speech, thereby limiting the person's ability to communicate.
  - Hearing can sometimes be restored or improved through hearing-aid devices and surgical implants
- Tinnitus can occur as a symptom of many ear disorders.
  - The noise in the ear (e.g., ringing, buzzing, whistling) may sometimes change in nature and intensity
  - In most cases it is present at all times with intermittent awareness by the person
  - Tinnitus is usually associated with hearing loss, especially hearing loss that develops from aging

Problems with Speech

- Speech is the most commonly used method of human communication.
- Common problems with speech in older adults are often associated with:
  - Difficulty in word retrieval
  - Decreased fluency of speech
  - Slowed rate of speech
  - Changes in voice quality
- There are several possible causes of these disorders:
  - Damage to the language centers of the brain (usually because of stroke, head injury, or brain tumor)
  - Degenerative changes in the nervous system
  - Hearing loss
  - Disorders of the larynx
  - Poor-fitting dentures

Toxicology

- Older adult patients are at increased risk for adverse drug reactions because of age-related alterations in body composition, drug distribution, metabolism, and excretion—and because they are often prescribed multiple medications.
- Several drugs that commonly cause toxicity in the geriatric patient:
  - Lidocaine
  - Beta-blockers

- Antihypertensives
- Diuretics
- Digitalis
- Psychotropics
- Antidepressants

- The adverse reactions associated with these and other drugs often result from "accidents" or "mishaps" in the prescribed drug regimen.
- Common causes of drug-induced illness in the geriatric patient:
  - Medication noncompliance
  - Confusion, forgetfulness
  - Vision impairment
  - Self-selection of drugs
  - Multiple prescriptions from more than one physician
  - Improper resumption of old medications in addition to newly prescribed ones
  - Excessive dosing of over-the-counter drugs with synergistic or cumulative effects
  - Changes in habits regarding alcohol, diet, and exercise that may affect drug metabolism
  - Dispensing error
- Symptoms of drug toxicity and adverse drug reactions in older adults:
  - Acute delirium
  - Akathisia
  - Altered vision
  - Bradycardia
  - Cardiac dysrhythmias
  - Chorea
  - Coma
  - Confusion
  - Constipation
  - Fatigue
  - Glaucoma
  - Hypokalemia
  - Orthostatic hypotension
  - Paresthesias
  - Psychological disturbances
  - Pulmonary edema
  - Severe bleeding
  - Tardive dyskinesia
  - Urinary hesitancy
- Emergency care for patients with adverse drug reactions may vary from "transport only" to full advanced cardiac life support interventions.

Alcohol Abuse

- Alcohol abuse is a common problem in older adults and is often attributed to severe stress as the primary risk factor.
- Signs and symptoms of alcohol abuse may be very subtle:
  - Mood swings
  - Denial
  - Hostility

    - Confusion
    - Frequent falling
    - Anorexia
    - Insomnia
- If alcohol abuse is suspected, discretely interview friends and family members about the patient's alcohol or other drug use.
    - Identification of these patients and appropriate referral by a physician for treatment are the cornerstones of therapy
- Management of the acutely intoxicated patient may include resuscitative measures to manage the patient's airway, ventilation, and circulation.
- In addition, the patient who has signs and symptoms of acute alcohol intoxication should be carefully assessed for occult trauma and coexisting medical conditions.
    - Hypoglycemia
    - Cardiomyopathy and dysrhythmias
    - GI bleeding
    - Polydrug abuse (especially barbiturates and tranquilizers)
    - Ethylene glycol or methanol ingestion

Environmental Considerations

Hypothermia

- Unlike younger patients who experience hypothermia often from environmental extremes, older adults may develop hypothermia while indoors because of cold surroundings and/or accompanying illness that alter heat production or conservation.
- Factors contributing to hypothermia in older adults may be physiological, socioeconomic, and/or medical.
- Physiological characteristics of older adults that make them susceptible to hypothermia:
    - Less able to compensate for environmental heat loss
    - Decreased ability to sense changes in ambient temperature
    - Less total body water to store heat
    - Less likely to develop tachycardia to increase cardiac output in response to cold stress
    - Decreased ability to shiver to increase body heat
- In addition to physiological factors, older adult patients are more prone to develop hypothermia because of socioeconomic factors such as fixed incomes to pay for the cost of heat in the home.
- This often results in lower ambient temperatures in the home, inefficient insulation (cool and drafty homes), and poorly functioning furnaces.
- Malnutrition (and an associated decrease in fat stores) also may be a factor in hypothermia in older adult patients who live alone.
- Medical causes of hypothermia in older adults:
    - Arthritis
    - Drug overdose
    - Hepatic failure
    - Hypoglycemia
    - Infection

    - Parkinson's disease
    - Stroke
    - Thyroid disease
    - Uremia
- The signs and symptoms of hypothermia may be subtle:
    - Altered mental state
    - Slurred speech
    - Ataxia
    - Dysrhythmias
- In severe cases, coma without signs of life may be present.
- Rapid and gentle transport for in-hospital rewarming and life support measures is crucial for the patient's survival.

Hyperthermia

- Hyperthermia in older adults is less common than hypothermia but carries a significant mortality rate. The condition is most likely to result from exposure to high environmental temperatures that continue for several days.
- As in hypothermia, the thermoregulatory mechanisms of older persons render them unable to control body temperature even in moderate environmental heat.
- Hyperthermia also may result from medical conditions:
    - Hypothalamic dysfunction
    - Spinal cord injury
- Certain medications can lead to hyperthermia by inhibiting heat dissipation, increasing motor activity, and impairing cardiovascular function.
- Hyperthermic illness may present as heat cramps, heat exhaustion, or heat stroke.
- Emergency management is directed at removing the patient from the warm environment, cooling the patient, and ensuring the patient's vital functions through airway, ventilatory, and circulatory support.
- Rapid transport for physician evaluation is indicated to manage the systemic manifestations that may result from serious heat-related illness.

Behavioral/Psychiatric Disorders

Depression

Depression is common in older persons, and can result from both physiological and psychological causes.

Physiological causes

- Dehydration
- Electrolyte imbalance
- Fever
- Hyponatremia
- Hypoxia
- Medications
- Metabolic disturbances
- Organic brain disease
- Reduced cardiac output
- Thyroid disease

Psychological

- Fear of dying
- Financial insecurity
- Loss of a spouse
- Loss of independence
- Significant illness
- Signs and symptoms of depression vary by individual.
  - Feelings of hopelessness
  - Extreme isolation
  - Loss of energy, fatigue
  - Irritability
  - Sleeplessness
  - Loss of appetite.
  - Significant weight loss
  - Decreased libido
  - Deep feelings of worthlessness and guilt
  - Recurrent thoughts of death
  - Suicide attempts
- A major goal of prehospital care is to identify the patient who may be depressed so that appropriate resources can be provided.
- After determining there are no physical threats to life, try to establish a rapport with these patients so that their mood can be evaluated.
- If possible, family members should be interviewed to gather information about the patient's mental state and any history of depression.

Suicide

- The rate of completed suicides for older people is higher than that of the general population, and the majority of these people visit their primary care physician in the month before the suicide.
- Usually, they are suffering from their first episode of major depression, which is only moderately severe, yet the depressive symptoms go unrecognized and untreated. Be aware of the increased risk for suicide when evaluating older adult patients who are depressed.
- There is no evidence that questions about suicidal thoughts and feelings increase the risk of suicide.
- Many depressed people are willing to discuss their suicidal thoughts.
- It is important to question the patient about suicidal thoughts if he or she is suspected of being at high risk.
- These three questions are appropriate to ask the patient:
  - Do you have thoughts about killing yourself?
  - Have you ever tried to kill yourself?
  - Have you thought about how you might kill yourself?
- After assessing the risk for suicidal tendencies, the patient should be transported for physician evaluation.
- While en route to the hospital, the patient should be encouraged to discuss feelings and should be reassured that he or she can be helped through the crisis.

Trauma

- Trauma is the fifth leading cause of death for persons over age 65.
- One-third of traumatic deaths in people aged 65–74 are secondary to vehicular trauma, and 25% result from falls.
- In those older than 80, falls account for 50% of injury-related deaths.
- Burns also are a major cause of disability and death in older adult patients.

Vehicular Trauma

The following facts are based on analysis of data from the U.S. Department of Transportation's Fatality Analysis Reporting System:

- 7078 people 65 years and older died in motor vehicle crashes in 1996, 1% more than in 1995 and 32% more than in 1975.
- Eighty percent of elderly deaths in 1996 motor vehicle crashes were passenger vehicle occupants, and 17% were pedestrians.
- People 65 years and older represented 13% of the population in 1996 and 17% of motor vehicle deaths.

Head Trauma

- Head injury with loss of consciousness in older patients is often associated with poor outcome.
- Among other physiological changes, the aging process may be associated with cerebral atrophy that produces a notable distance between the surface of the brain and the inner tables of the skull.
- As bridging veins stretch across this subdural space, they more easily are torn, resulting in subdural hematomas.
- The extra space within the cranial vault often allows an older person to sustain a significant amount of internal hemorrhage before the volume-pressure relationship of the cranium is exceeded and symptoms are manifested.
- Older patients are also particularly susceptible to injuries of the cervical spine because of progressive arthritic and degenerative changes associated with aging.
- These structural alterations lead to increased stiffening and decreased flexibility of the spine with narrowing of the spinal canal. This renders the spinal cord more susceptible to damage from relatively minor trauma.

Chest Injuries

- Mechanism of injury that suggests thoracic trauma in an older patient must be considered potentially lethal. The aged thorax is less elastic and more susceptible to injury.
- The pulmonary system has marginal reserve because of several physiological changes related to aging.
  - A reduced alveolar surface area
  - Decreased patency of small airways
  - Diminished chemoreceptor response
- Injuries to the heart, aorta, and major vessels are a greater risk to older patients than younger adults because of decreased functional reserve and anatomical alterations that make injury in these areas more likely of greater significance.
- Myocardial contusion may be a complication of blunt injury to the chest and, if severe, may result in pump failure or life-threatening dysrhythmias.
- Cardiac rupture, valvular injury, and aortic dissection may also occur with significant blunt chest injury. The first two entities are rare but rapidly fatal.

- Dissecting aortic aneurysm should always be considered when the mechanism of injury produces rapid deceleration. Aortic dissections are often not immediately fatal, and proper evaluation and management can be life-saving.
- Because of impaired coronary response to increased oxygen demands and commonly occurring underlying conduction disturbance, older patients may develop ischemia and dysrhythmias from significant trauma, even if the heart has not been directly affected.

Abdominal Injuries

- Abdominal injuries in older adults have more serious consequences than those in any other age groups.
- The older patient also is less likely to tolerate surgery and is more susceptible to postoperative pulmonary and septic complications.

Musculoskeletal Injuries

- The osteoporotic bones of older patients are vulnerable to fracture with even mild trauma.
- Pelvic fractures are highly lethal in this age group, causing severe hemorrhage and associated soft tissue injury.
- When evaluating for skeletal trauma, remember that the older patient may have decreased pain perception and often surprisingly little tenderness with major fractures.
- Even with appropriate care, the mortality rate for older patients with musculoskeletal injury is increased by delayed complications:
  - ARDS
  - Sepsis
  - Renal failure
  - Pulmonary embolism

Falls

- Falls are a major cause of morbidity and mortality in older adults, accounting for about 10,000 deaths each year. It has been estimated that one-third of older adults living at home fall each year and 1 in 40 of these persons is hospitalized.
- A major cause of falls in older adults results from the use of prescribed sedative-hypnotics that affect balance and postural control, such as alprazolam, diazepam, chlordiazepoxide, and flurazepam.

Fractures

- Fractures are the most common fall-related injury.
- A hip fracture is the most common fracture resulting in hospitalization.
- In those who survive hip fracture, a majority will have significant mobility problems and may become more functionally dependent.
- Falls that do not result in physical injury may lead to self-imposed immobility resulting from the fear of falling again.
- Strict and prolonged immobility may result in other conditions:
  - Joint contractures
  - Pressure sores
  - Urinary tract infection
  - Muscle atrophy
  - Depression
  - Functional dependency

Assessment

- Assume that any fall indicates an underlying problem.
- Attempts should be made to uncover the multitude of medical, psychological, and environmental factors that may have been responsible for the fall. So that as much information as possible is obtained about the falling episode, the patient history should include the following details:
  - A comprehensive review of all medical problems and medications
  - A precise recounting of the fall
    - — Previous history of falling
    - — Time of fall and location
    - — Symptoms experienced
    - — Activity in which the victim was engaged
    - — Use of devices
    - — Presence of witnesses
- Evaluating the patient's cardiovascular, neurological, and musculoskeletal systems should be emphasized.

Burns

- More than 1000 older adults die as a result of fires and burns in the United States each year.
- Reasons for the increased risk of morbidity and mortality from burn trauma in older adults:
  - Preexisting disease
  - Skin changes that result in increased burn depth
  - Altered nutrition
  - Decreased ability to fight infection

Management

- After initial care and resuscitation, older adult patients with thermal injury require special considerations in fluid therapy to prevent renal tubular damage.
- Hydration is assessed in initial hours after burn injury by monitoring pulse and blood pressure and by striving to maintain a urine output of at least 50–60 mL/hr.

Trauma Management Considerations

Priorities of trauma care for older patients are similar to those for all trauma patients. Special consideration should be given to transport strategies and to evaluating the older adult patient's cardiovascular, respiratory, and renal systems.

Cardiovascular system

- Recent or past MI contributes to the risk of dysrhythmias and congestive heart failure. Adjustment of heart rate and stroke volume may be decreased in response to hypovolemia.
- Older patients may require higher arterial pressures than younger patients for perfusion of vital organs because of atherosclerotic peripheral vascular disease.
- Rapid IV fluid administration to older patients may precipitate volume overload. Care must be taken not to overhydrate these patients, since older adults as a group are more susceptible to congestive heart failure; however, hypovolemia and hypotension are also poorly tolerated.

- Monitor lung sounds and vital signs carefully and frequently during fluid administration.

Respiratory system

- Physical changes decrease chest wall compliance and movement and thus diminish vital capacity. PaO_2 decreases with age! Lower PO_2 at the same fractional inspired oxygen concentration occurs with each passing decade. Remember, all organ systems have less tolerance to hypoxia.
- COPD (common in older patients) requires that airway management and ventilation support be carefully adjusted for appropriate oxygenation and carbon dioxide removal. High-concentration oxygen may suppress hypoxic drive in some patients, but this therapy should never be withheld from a patient with clinical signs of cyanosis.
- Dentures may need to be removed for adequate airway and ventilation management.

Renal system

- The kidneys have decreased ability to maintain normal acid-base balance and to compensate for fluid changes. Any preexisting renal disease may further decrease renal ability to compensate. Decreased renal function (along with decreased cardiac reserve) places the injured older patient at risk for fluid overload and pulmonary edema secondary to IV fluid therapy.

Transport strategies

- Positioning, immobilization, and transport of an older trauma patient may require modifications to accommodate physical deformities. Packaging should include bulk and extra padding to support and provide comfort for the patient.
- Prevent hypothermia by keeping the patient warm.

Elder Abuse

- Refers to the infliction of physical pain, injury, debilitating mental anguish, unreasonable confinement, or willful deprivation by a caretaker of services that are necessary to maintain mental and physical health of an older adult patient. Elder abuse has become increasingly recognized as a growing problem in the United States, affecting more than 1 million older people.
- There are several classifications of elder abuse; they include physical abuse, psychological abuse, and/or financial or material abuse.

Neglect

- All 50 states have elder abuse statutes, and in most states, reporting of suspected elder abuse is mandatory under law. If abuse or neglect of an older person is suspected, advise medical direction and follow the procedures established by local protocol.
- In addition to suspicious physical injuries, several other warning signs indicate that an older adult person might be the victim of abuse or neglect:
  - An upset or agitated state
  - Dehydration, malnutrition, poor personal hygiene
  - Hazardous or unsafe living conditions
  - Unsanitary and unclean living conditions

CHAPTER QUESTIONS

1. Which of the following medications poses the greatest risk of adverse effects in the geriatric patient if given at normal adult doses?
   a. Lidocaine
   b. Adenosine
   c. Midazolam
   d. Narcan
2. The most common psychiatric disorder among geriatric patients is:
   a. schizophrenia
   b. paranoia
   c. depression
   d. posttraumatic stress disorder
3. A 90-year-old female has been experiencing episodes of nocturnal confusion for several weeks. Her lower extremities are swollen, with large, translucent, fluid-filled areas resembling blisters on the skin. These areas probably are caused by:
   a. an allergic reaction to medication
   b. toxicity from an antidepressant medication the patient is taking
   c. increased hydrostatic pressure caused by right-sided CHF and sleeping sitting up
   d. degenerative effects of old age on the skin of the lower extremities
4. A 77-year-old male has been experiencing dizziness and weakness when he attempts to stand quickly. Causes that should be considered include:
   a. beta blocker use
   b. use of vasodilators for treatment of hypertension
   c. hypovolemia secondary to diuretic use or depressed thirst mechanisms
   d. all of the above
5. A 99-year-old female presents with multiple bruises on her face and upper extremities. She lives with her 65-year-old son, who tells you that the patient is always falling down and is just generally clumsy. The patient appears malnourished and frightened. She cowers when you approach and is reluctant to allow you to examine her. Her son seems to be hostile toward you and your partner and nervously attempts to explain each bruise. In this case you should do all of following except:
   a. obtain a complete patient and family history
   b. report suspicions of elder abuse to the emergency department staff
   c. be honest and open with the patient's son about your concerns
   d. listen carefully for inconsistencies in stories

Suggested Reading

US Department of Transportation, National Highway Traffic Safety Administration. *EMT-Paramedic: National Standard Curriculum*. Washington, DC: US Department of Transportation, National Highway Traffic Safety Administration; 1998.

Chapter 37

Patients with Special Challenges

You are treating a 59-year-old morbidly obese female with a history of congestive heart failure who presents with dyspnea that has gradually increased over the past week. She has a productive cough with brown sputum.

Vital signs are BP 110/66, HR 96, RR 20, and temperature is 100.6°F.

What would be the most likely assessment?

Paramedics frequently provide care to patients with special challenges. Patients who are physically challenged may require special considerations in patient assessment and management.

PHYSICAL CHALLENGES

Hearing Impairments

- Deafness is a complete or partial inability to hear. Total deafness is rare and usually congenital. Partial deafness may range from mild to severe, and most commonly is the result of disease, injury, or degeneration of the hearing mechanism that occurs with age.
- Conductive deafness refers to the faulty transportation of sound from the outer to the inner ear. This type of deafness is often curable and usually results from accumulation of earwax that blocks the outer ear canal, infection such as otitis media, or injury to the eardrum or middle ear.
- Sensor neural deafness is when sounds that reach the inner ear fail to be transmitted to the brain because of damage to the structures within the ear or to the acoustic nerve, which connects the inner ear to the brain. It is often incurable. Causes include:
  - Sensorineural deafness that is present in early life; may be congenital
  - Birth injury or damage to the developing fetus
  - Severe jaundice soon after birth
- Sensorineural deafness that occurs in later life may be caused from:
  - Prolonged exposure to loud noise
  - Disease, such as Meniere's disease
  - Tumors
  - Medications
  - Viral infections
  - Natural degeneration of the cochlea and/or labyrinth in old age

- Recognizing a patient with a hearing impairment may be possible by noting the following:
  - Presence of hearing aids
  - Poor diction
  - Inability to respond to verbal communication in the absence of direct eye contact

Visual Impairments

- Normal vision depends on the uninterrupted passage of light from the front of the eye to the light-sensitive retina at the back.
- Any condition that obstructs the passage of light from the retina can cause vision loss. Visual impairments may be present at birth from a congenital disorder or result from:
  - Cataracts
  - Degeneration of the eyeball, optic nerve, or nerve pathways
  - Eye or brain injury
  - Infection (cytomegalovirus [CMV], herpes simplex virus [HSV], bacterial ulcers)
  - Vitamin A deficiency in children living in poor countries
- Patients with visual impairment may be totally blind or have a partial loss of vision that affects central vision, peripheral vision, or both.
- Patient who has central loss of vision is usually aware of the condition.
- Those who have a loss of peripheral vision may be more difficult to identify since the loss often goes unnoticed by the person until it is well advanced.

Speech Impairments

- Speech impairments include disorders of language, articulation, voice production, or fluency (blockage of speech), all of which can lead to an inability to communicate effectively.
- Language disorders result from damage to the language centers of the brain (usually from stroke, head injury, or brain tumor). These patients often demonstrate aphasia with a slowness to understand speech, and problems with vocabulary and sentence structure.
- Aphasia can affect both children and adults and may affect their ability to speak and/or comprehend written or spoken words.
- Delayed development of language in a child may result from hearing loss, lack of stimulation, or emotional disturbance.

Articulation Disorders (Dysarthria)—Inability to Produce Speech Sounds

- Result from damage to nerve pathways passing from the brain to the muscles of the larynx, mouth, or lips. Patient's speech will often be slurred, indistinct, slow, or nasal.
- Disorders of articulation may result from brain injury and from diseases such as multiple sclerosis and Parkinson's disease.
- In children, they commonly are the result of delayed development from hearing problems.

Voice Production Disorders

- Characterized by hoarseness, harshness, inappropriate pitch, and abnormal nasal resonance, and are often a result from disorders that affect closure of the vocal cords.

- Some disorders are caused by hormonal or psychiatric disturbances, and by severe hearing loss.

Fluency Disorders

- Marked by repetitions of single sounds or whole words, and by the blocking of speech. Stuttering is an example of a fluency disorder.

Obesity

- Abnormal increase in the proportion of fat and cells, mainly in the viscera and the subcutaneous tissues of the body. Although reasons for obesity in some people are unclear, known causes for the condition include the following:
  - Caloric intake that exceeds calories burned
  - Low basal metabolic rate
  - Genetic predisposition for obesity
- Associated with an increased risk for the following:
  - Hypertension
  - Stroke
  - Heart disease
  - Diabetes
  - Some cancers
  - Osteoarthritis is also aggravated by increased body weight
- Managed with weight-loss programs, exercise, counseling, medications, and sometimes surgery. The goal of long-term treatment is permanent weight loss.

Paraplegia/Quadriplegia

- Paraplegia is weakness or paralysis of both legs and sometimes part of the trunk.
- Quadriplegia is weakness or paralysis of all four extremities and the trunk.
- Conditions result from nerve damage in the brain and spinal cord, usually caused by the following:
  - Motor vehicle crash
  - Sports injury
  - Fall
  - Gunshot wound
  - Medical illness
- Both paraplegia and quadriplegia are accompanied by a loss of sensation and urinary control.
- Patients with extremity and trunk paralysis may require accommodations in patient care.
- Patient may have a halo traction device to stabilize the spine, which may complicate airway management and make patient transport difficult.
- Ostomies:
  - Trachea
  - Bladder
  - Colon
- Priapism may be present in some male patients.
- Transport:
  - Additional manpower may be needed to move special equipment and prepare patient for transport.

MENTAL CHALLENGES

Mental illness refers to any form of psychiatric disorder.

- Psychoses—Comprises a group of mental disorders in which the individual loses contact with reality. Thought to be related to complex biochemical disease that disorders brain function. Examples include:
  - Schizophrenia
  - Bipolar disorder (manic-depressive illness)
  - Organic brain disease
- Neuroses—Refers to diseases related to upbringing and personality in which the person remains "in touch" with reality. Neurotic symptoms generally do not limit work or social activity and tend to fluctuate in intensity with stress. Examples include:
  - Depression
  - Phobias
  - Obsessive-compulsive behavior
- Recognizing a patient who is mentally challenged may be difficult, especially when caring for mildly neurotic patients whose behavior may be unaffected.
- Patients with more serious disorders may present with signs and symptoms consistent with mental illness.
- When obtaining the patient history, do not be hesitant to ask about:
  - History of mental illness
  - Prescribed medications
  - Compliance with prescribed medications
  - Concomitant use of alcohol or other drugs
- If the patient appears to be paranoid or shows anxious behavior, ask the patient's permission before beginning any assessment or performing any procedure. Once rapport and trust have been established, care should proceed in the same manner as for a patient who does not have mental illness. These patients experience illness and injury like all other patients.

Developmentally Disabled

- Person who is developmentally disabled has impaired or insufficient development of the brain that causes an inability to learn at the usual rate.
- Causes include the following:
  - Unsatisfactory parental interaction (lack of stimulation)
  - Severe vision or hearing impairment
  - Mental retardation
  - Brain damage before, during, or after birth, or in infancy
  - Severe diseases of body organs and systems

Signs of Developmental Delay

- Delays may be of varying severity and may affect any or all of the major areas of human achievement, including development of the following abilities:
  - Walking upright
  - Fine hand-eye coordination
  - Listening, language, and speech
  - Social interaction

Down Syndrome

- Down syndrome results from a chromosomal abnormality that causes mild to severe mental retardation and a characteristic physical appearance.
- Features of the patient with Down syndrome typically include:
  - Eyes that slope upward at the outer corners
  - Folds of skin on either side of the nose that cover the inner corners of the eyes
  - Small face and small facial features
  - Large and protruding tongue
  - Flattening on back of the head
  - Hands that are short and broad
- Commonly, Down syndrome occurs from the failure of the two chromosomes numbered 21 in a parent cell to go into separate daughter cells during the first stage of sperm or egg cell formation.
- Results in a triplet of chromosome 21 (trisomy 21) rather than the usual pair.
- Extra number 21 chromosome is passed on to the child, leading to Down syndrome.
- Incidence of affected fetuses increases with increased maternal age (mothers over age 35), and those with a family history of Down syndrome.
- Persons with Down syndrome usually do not survive past their middle years.
- About 25% of children born with Down syndrome have a heart defect at birth.
- Many have congenital intestinal disorders, hearing defects, and other illnesses.
- Persons with Down syndrome are capable of limited learning, and are often affectionate and friendly.
- Extra time must be allowed for obtaining a history and for performing assessment and patient care procedures.

Emotionally Impaired

- Persons with emotional impairments include those with the following:
  - Neurasthenia (nervous exhaustion)
  - Anxiety neurosis
  - Compulsion neurosis
  - Hysteria
- These disorders can result in a wide range of physical or mental symptoms attributed to mental stress in someone who is not psychotic.
- Signs and symptoms that may result from emotional impairment include somatic complaints such as chest discomfort, tachycardia, dyspnea, choking, and syncope.
- It is important to gather a complete history from the patient and perform a thorough examination to rule out serious illness.
- Prehospital care (in the absence of serious illness) is primarily supportive and includes calming measures and transport for physician evaluation.

Emotionally/Mentally Impaired (EMI)

- Refers to persons who have impaired intellectual functioning (mental retardation) that results in an inability to cope with normal responsibilities of life.
- Mental retardation can be further classified with IQ assessment as:
  - Mild (IQ 50–70)
  - Moderate (IQ 35–59)
  - Profound (IQ less than 20)

Causes of Mental Retardation

- Genetic conditions
  - Phenylketonuria (PKU); a single-gene disorder caused by a defective enzyme
  - Chromosomal disorder (Down syndrome)
  - Fragile X syndrome (a single-gene disorder on the Y chromosome; the leading inherited cause of mental retardation)
- Problems during pregnancy
  - Use of alcohol, tobacco, or other drugs by the mother
  - Illness and infection (toxoplasmosis, cytomegalovirus, rubella, syphilis, HIV)
- Problems at birth
  - Brain injury
  - Prematurity, low birth weight
- Problems after birth
  - Childhood diseases (whooping cough, chicken pox, measles, HIV disease)
  - Injury (head injury, near drowning)
  - Exposure to lead, mercury, and other environmental toxins
  - Poverty and cultural deprivation
  - Malnutrition
- Disease-producing conditions
  - Inadequate medical care
  - Environmental health hazards
  - Lack of stimulation
- Special considerations
  - Accommodations that may be necessary during patient care will vary by the patient's level of retardation
  - Many with mild retardation will show no psychological symptoms apart from slowness in carrying out mental tasks
- Those with moderate-to-severe retardation may have the following:
  - Limited to absent speech
  - Neurological impairments are common
  - These patients may require extra time and care in patient assessment, management, and transportation

PATHOLOGICAL CHALLENGES

Physical injury and disease may result in pathological conditions that require special assessment and management skills.

Arthritis

- Arthritis refers to inflammation of a joint, characterized by pain, stiffness, swelling, and redness. Arthritis has many forms and varies widely in its effects.
- Osteoarthritis results from cartilage loss and wear and tear of the joints (common in elderly patients).
- Rheumatoid arthritis is an autoimmune disorder that damages joints and surrounding tissues.

Cancer

- A group of diseases that allow for an unrestrained growth of cells in one or more of the body organs or tissues.

- Malignant tumors most commonly develop in major organs, like the lungs, breasts, intestine, skin, stomach, and pancreas, but may also occur in cell-forming tissues of the bone marrow, and in the lymphatic system, muscle, or bone.
- Patients with cancer are often very ill. Signs and symptoms depend on the cancer's primary site of origin.
- Try to obtain a thorough history from the patient, including a list of all medications. Many cancer patients take anticancer drugs and pain medicine through surgically implanted ports, such as a Mediport. Transdermal skin patches that contain analgesic agents are also very common.

Cerebral Palsy (CP)

- General term for nonprogressive disorders of movement and posture resulting from damage to the fetal brain during later months of pregnancy, during birth, during the newborn period, or in early childhood.
- Most common cause is cerebral dysgenesis (abnormal cerebral development) or cerebral malformations.
- Less common causes include the following:
  - Fetal hypoxia
  - Birth trauma
  - Maternal infection
  - Kernicterus (excessive fetal bilirubin, associated with hemolytic disease)
  - Postpartum encephalitis, meningitis, or head injury

Spastic Paralysis

- Produces abnormal stiffness and contraction of groups of muscles.
- Child may be categorized as having one of the following conditions:
  - Diplegia—Affecting all four limbs, the legs more severely than the arms
  - Hemiplegia—Affecting limbs only on one side of the body; the arm usually more severely than the leg
  - Quadriplegia—Affecting all four limbs severely; not necessarily symmetrically
  - Athetosis—Producing involuntary writhing movements
  - Ataxia—Producing a loss of coordination and balance
  - Hearing defects, epilepsy, and other central nervous system (CNS) disorders are commonly present with the disease
- Weakness, paralysis, and developmental delay vary by the type and severity of disease.
- Some children with mild CP attend regular schools.
- Those with more severe forms of the disease never learn to walk or effectively communicate, and require lifelong skilled nursing care.
- Accommodations that may be required during an emergency call include allowing additional scene time for the physical examination and extra resources and manpower to facilitate transport.

Cystic Fibrosis (CF) (Mucoviscidosis)

- Inherited metabolic disease of the lungs and digestive system that manifests itself in childhood. Caused by a defective recessive gene inherited from each parent. The defective gene causes the glands in the lining of the bronchi to produce excessive amounts of thick mucus and predisposes the individual to chronic lung infections.

Additionally, the pancreas of a patient with CF fails to produce the enzymes required for the breakdown of fats and their absorption from the intestine.

- These alterations in metabolism cause classic symptoms of CF that include the following:
  - Pale, greasy-looking, and foul-smelling stools (often noticeable soon after birth)
  - Persistent cough and breathlessness
  - Lung infections that often develop into pneumonia, bronchiectasis, and bronchitis
- Other features of the disease include stunted growth and sweat glands that produce abnormally salty sweat.
- In some cases, the child with CF may fail to thrive. Many patients survive into adulthood, although poor health is common.
- Older patients with CF are generally aware of their disease.
- Some may be oxygen-dependent and will require respiratory support and suctioning to clear the airway of mucus and secretions.
- Expect a lengthy history and physical exam due to the nature of the disease and associated medical problems.
- Some patients will have received heart and lung transplants, and may require transfer to specialized medical facilities for treatment.
- If parents are unaware of the possibility of CF in the presence of signs and symptoms described above, the paramedic should advise the physician at the receiving hospital of his or her suspicions.

Multiple Sclerosis (MS)

- Progressive and incurable autoimmune disease of the CNS, in which scattered patches of myelin in the brain and spinal cord are destroyed.
- Scarring and destruction of the tissues causes symptoms that range from numbness and tingling to paralysis and incontinence.
- Cause of MS is unknown; however, it may have a heritable or viral component.
- Disease usually begins early in adult life, becomes active for a brief time, and then resumes years later.
- Symptoms vary with the affected areas of the CNS and may include:
  - Brain involvement
    - — Fatigue
    - — Vertigo
    - — Clumsiness
    - — Muscle weakness
    - — Slurred speech
    - — Ataxia
    - — Blurred or double vision
    - — Numbness, weakness, or pain in the face
  - Spinal cord involvement
    - — Tingling, numbness, or feeling of constriction in any part of the body
    - — Extremities that feel heavy and become weak
    - — Spasticity
- Symptoms of MS may occur singly or in combination, and may last from several weeks to several months.
- Attacks vary in intensity and may be precipitated by injury, infection, or physical or emotional stress.
- Some patients become disabled, bedridden, and incontinent early in middle life.

- Disabled patients also often suffer from painful muscle spasms, constipation, urinary tract infection, skin ulcerations, and mood swings.
- Disease is managed with medications, physical therapy, and counseling.
- Some patients with MS may be difficult to examine and may be unable to provide a complete medical history due to the nature of their illness.
- Allow extra time for patient assessment and to prepare the patient for transport. Patient should not be expected to ambulate.
- Respiratory support may be indicated in severe cases.

Muscular Dystrophy

- Inherited muscle disorder that results in a slow but progressive degeneration of muscle fibers.
- Classified according to the following:
  - Age that symptoms first appear
  - Rate at which the disease progresses
  - Way in which it is inherited
- Muscular dystrophy is incurable.
- Most common form of the disease is Duchenne muscular dystrophy.
  - Caused by a sex-linked, recessive gene that affects only males
  - Rarely diagnosed before 3 years of age
- Signs and symptoms include:
  - Child slow in learning to sit up and walk
  - Unusual gait
  - Curvature of the spine
  - Muscles that become bulky as they are replaced by fat
  - Eventually, most children will be unable to walk
    - Many do not live past their teenage years because of chronic lung infections and congestive heart failure
- Accommodations that may be required during emergency care will depend on the person's age, weight, and severity of disease.
- Young children will be relatively easy to examine and prepare for transport.
- Older patients may require additional manpower and resources to assist with moving the patient to the ambulance.
- Respiratory support may be indicated in severe cases.

Poliomyelitis (Polio)

- Infectious disease caused by poliovirus hominis. Virus is spread through direct and indirect contact with infected feces and by airborne transmission.
- It attacks with variable severity, ranging from asymptomatic infection to a febrile illness without neurological sequelae to aseptic meningitis and finally to paralytic disease (including respiratory paralysis) and possible death.
- Incidence has declined since the Salk and Sabin vaccines were made available in the 1950s.
- May affect nonimmune adults and indigent children.
- Signs and symptoms of polio in both the nonparalytic and paralytic forms include the following:
  - Fever
  - Malaise

  - Headache
  - Intestinal upset
- Often, persons with the nonparalytic form of polio recover completely.
- In the paralytic form, extensive paralysis of muscles of the legs and lower trunk can occur.
- Caring for a patient with paralytic polio who has respiratory paralysis may require advanced airway support to ensure adequate ventilation.
- If the lower body is paralyzed, urinary catheterization may be indicated.
- Additional resources and manpower may be needed to prepare the patient for transport.

Previously Head-Injured Patients

- Traumatic brain injury can result from many mechanisms of trauma.
- These injuries can affect many cognitive, physical, and psychological skills.
- Cognitive deficits of language and communication, information processing, memory, and perceptual skills are common.
- Physical deficit can include ambulation, balance and coordination, fine motor skills, strength, and endurance.
- Psychological status also is often altered.
- Depending on the patient's area of brain injury, obtaining a history and performing assessment and patient care procedures may be very difficult.
- Some patients may require restraint.
- Family members and other caregivers should:
  - Be involved in managing the patient (when appropriate)
  - Be interviewed to determine if the patient's actions and responses are "normal" for the patient
  - Expect to spend additional time at the scene to provide care to these patients

Spina Bifida

- Congenital defect in which part of one or more vertebrae fails to develop, leaving part of the spinal cord exposed. Condition ranges in severity from minimal evidence of a defect to severe disability. In severe cases, the legs of some children may be deformed with partial or complete paralysis and loss of sensation in all areas below the level of the defect.
- Associated abnormalities may include:
  - Hydrocephalus with brain damage
  - Cerebral palsy
  - Epilepsy
  - Mental retardation
- Because of the varying degrees of spina bifida, prehospital care will need to be tailored to the patient's specific needs.
- Some patients will require no special accommodations.
- Others will need extended on-scene time for assessment and management, and perhaps additional resources and manpower to prepare the patient for transport.

Myasthenia Gravis

- Autoimmune disorder in which muscles become weak and tire easily.
- Damage occurs to muscle receptors that are responsible for transmitting nerve impulses, commonly affecting muscles of the eyes, face, throat, and extremities.

- Rare disease that can begin suddenly or gradually.
- Can occur at any age, but usually appears in women between age 20 and 30, and in men between 70 and 80 years of age.
- Classic signs and symptoms include:
  - Drooping eyelids, double vision
  - Difficulty in speaking
  - Difficulty in chewing and swallowing
  - Difficult extremity movement
  - Weakened respiratory muscles
- Affected muscles become worse with use, but may recover completely with rest.
- May be exacerbated by infection, stress, medications, and menstruation.
- Can often be controlled with drug therapy to enhance the transmission of nerve impulses in the muscles.
- In a small number of patients, the disease will progress to paralysis of the throat and respiratory muscles, and may lead to death.
- Accommodations required for care vary based on the patient's presentation.
- In most cases, supportive care and transport will be all that is required.
- In the presence of respiratory distress, measures should be taken to ensure adequate airway and ventilatory support.

CULTURALLY DIVERSE PATIENTS

- Individuals vary in many ways, and there is enormous diversity in populations of all cultures. Diversity (a term once used primarily to describe "racial awareness") now refers to differences of any kind: race, class, religion, gender, sexual preference, personal habitat, and physical ability.
- Experiences of health and illness vary widely because of different beliefs, behaviors, and past experiences, and may conflict with the paramedic's learned medical practice.
- By revealing awareness of cultural issues, the paramedic will convey interest, concern, and respect.
- When dealing with patients from different cultures, remember the following key points:
  - The individual is the "foreground"—the culture is the "background".
  - Different generations and individuals within the same family may have different sets of beliefs.
  - Not all people identify with their ethnic cultural background.
  - All people share common problems or situations.
  - Respect the integrity of cultural beliefs.
  - Realize that people may not share your explanations of the causes of their ill health, but may accept conventional treatments.
  - You do not have to agree with every aspect of another's culture, nor does the person have to accept everything about yours for effective and culturally sensitive health care to occur.
  - Recognize your personal cultural assumptions, prejudices, and belief systems and do not let them interfere with patient care.
- Regardless of the patient's cultural background, educational status, occupation, or ability to speak English, most patients will be anxious during an emergency event.

- Attempt to communicate in English first to determine whether the patient understands or speaks some English words or phrases.
- Bystanders, coworkers, or family members may be available to provide assistance.
- If the patient does not speak or understand English, attempt to communicate with signs or gestures.
- Notify the receiving hospital as soon as possible to arrange for an interpreter.
- If time permits, all assessment procedures should be performed slowly and with the patient's permission.
- Be aware that "private space" is culturally defined.
- Pointing to the area of the body to be examined before touching the patient is best.
- Respect the patient's need for modesty and privacy at the scene and during transport.

TERMINALLY ILL PATIENTS

Paramedics will care for terminally ill patients (patients with advanced stages of disease with an unfavorable prognosis and no known cure). These will often be emotionally charged encounters that will require a great deal of empathy and compassion for the patient and his or her loved ones. If emotions at the scene are out of control, it will be important for the paramedic to take control and to calm the people involved. If emergency medical service (EMS) has been summoned to assess late stages of a patient's terminal illness or a change in the patient's condition, gather a complete history and ask the patient or family about advance directives and the appropriateness of resuscitation procedures. Carefully review any documentation made available to the EMS crew (a DNR order) and consult with medical direction so that appropriate patient care decisions can be made.

Special Considerations

- Care of a terminally ill patient will often be primarily supportive and limited to calming and comfort measures, and perhaps transport for physician evaluation.
- Pain assessment and management are important in caring for these patients.
- Attempt to gather a complete pain medication history.
- Examine the patient for the presence of transdermal drug patches or other pain-relief devices.
- Following an assessment of the patient's vital signs, level of consciousness, and medication history, medical direction may recommend the administration of analgesics or sedatives to ensure the patient's comfort.

PATIENTS WITH COMMUNICABLE DISEASES

- Exposure to some infectious diseases can pose a significant health risk to EMS providers. It is important to ensure personal protection on every emergency response. Required precautions will depend on the mode of transmission and the pathogen's ability to create pathological processes.
- In some cases gloves will provide for necessary protection.
- In other cases, respiratory barriers will also be indicated.

Special Considerations

- Some infectious diseases (acquired immunodeficiency syndrome [AIDS]) will take a toll on the emotional well-being of affected patients, their families, and loved ones.

- Psychological aspects of providing care to these patients include an emphasis on the following:
  - Recognizing each patient as an individual with unique health-care needs
  - Respecting each person's personal dignity
  - Providing considerate, respectful care focused upon the person's individual needs

FINANCIAL CHALLENGES

- It is estimated that 41 million Americans and one-third of persons living in poverty have no health insurance, and insurance coverage held by many others would not carry them through a catastrophic illness.
- Financial challenges for health care can quickly result from loss of a job and depletion of savings.
- Financial challenges combined with medical conditions that require uninterrupted treatment (tuberculosis [TB], HIV/AIDS, diabetes, hypertension, mental disorders) or that occur in the presence of unexpected illness or injury can deprive the patient of basic health-care services.
- In addition, poor health is closely associated with homelessness, where rates of chronic or acute health problems are extremely high.
- Persons with financial challenges are often apprehensive about seeking medical care.
- Fortunately, the patient's ability to pay for emergency health care generally is not a concern for EMS providers.
- When caring for a patient with financial challenges who is concerned about the cost of receiving needed health care, explain the following:
  - Patient's ability to pay should never be a factor in obtaining emergency health care.
- Federal law mandates that quality, emergency health care be provided, regardless of the patient's ability to pay.
- Payment programs for health-care services are available in most hospitals.
- Government services are available to assist patients in paying for health care.
- Free (or near-free) health-care services are available through local, state, and federally-funded organizations.
- In cases where no life-threatening condition exists, counsel the patient with financial challenges about alternative facilities for health care that do not require ambulance transport for emergency department evaluation.
- Consider providing an approved list of alternative heath-care sites that can provide medical care at less cost than those charged by emergency departments.

? CHAPTER QUESTIONS

1. Cystic fibrosis is an inherited metabolic disease of the lungs and digestive system that manifests itself in childhood; it is caused by a defective recessive gene inherited from each parent.
   a. True
   b. False

2. Congenital defect in which part of one or more vertebrae fails to develop, leaving part of the spinal cord exposed.
   a. Spina bifida
   b. Myasthenia gravis
   c. Polio
   d. None of the above

Suggested Reading

US Department of Transportation, National Highway Traffic Safety Administration. *EMT-Paramedic: National Standard Curriculum*. Washington, DC: US Department of Transportation, National Highway Traffic Safety Administration; 1998.

Chapter 38

Acute Interventions for the Home Health-Care Patient

Your 93-year-old patient fell from her bed in a nursing home, is confused, complains of lower back pain, and has a lateral rotation of her right lower extremity. Her pelvis is intact and she states the pain is severe. Her chart reveals she has a history of renal disease and suffers from a decrease in cardiac reserve.

What do you conclude from this history?

HOME HEALTH-CARE SERVICES IN THE UNITED STATES

- Services are required by an estimated 8 million people.
- Reasons for home health-care service:
  - Acute illness
  - Long-term health conditions
  - Permanent disability
  - Terminal illness
- The role of a paramedic is providing acute interventions.

OVERVIEW OF HOME HEALTH CARE

- Home health care started in the United States in the late 1800s.
  - Direct result of rapid growth of city and an increase in the number of immigrants moving into large cities
  - Emphasis of home health care then was on personal hygiene and preventive care
- Heath services were provided by visiting nurse groups.
  - Worked in tenements to help the poor
  - Few physicians were associated with most of these home health-care groups
- Home health care continued to focus on the poor until mid-1960s.
  - Rest of the population received care in hospitals and doctors' offices
- Social Security Act of 1965.
  - Home health care became a benefit to elderly patients receiving Medicare
  - Greatly accelerated industry's growth
- 1973—Services were extended to certain disabled younger Americans.
- 1983—Hospice benefits were added.
- 1997—An estimated 38.5 million elderly and disabled Americans were enrolled in Medicare programs. 3.4 million Medicare recipients received home health services.

Advanced Life Support (ALS) Response to Home Care Patients

- About 25% of home health patients have conditions related to diseases of the circulatory system as their primary diagnosis.
- People with heart disease, including congestive heart failure, make up about half this group.
- Other common diagnoses of home care patients include:
  - Cancer
  - Diabetes
  - Chronic lung disease
  - Renal failure/dialysis
  - Hypertension

Role of the Home Health-Care Provider

- Home health care incorporates a variety of health and social services.
- Services are provided at home to recovering, disabled, or chronically ill persons in need of medical, nursing, social, or therapeutic treatment and/or assistance with the essential activities of daily living, including:
  - Skilled nursing services
  - Physical, speech, and occupational therapy
  - Medical social services
  - Home health aides
  - Nutritional counseling

Examples of Home Health-Care Problems

- Home care problems requiring intervention by a home health practitioner or physician
  - Chemotherapy
  - Pain management
  - Hospice care
  - Cardiopulmonary care
  - Dermatological and wound care
  - Gastroenterological and ostomy care
  - Catheter management/IV therapy
  - Orthopedic care
  - Rehabilitative care
  - Urological and renal care
  - Specimen collection
  - Acquired immunodeficiency syndrome (AIDS)
  - Organ transplantation
- Home care problems requiring acute intervention
  - Inadequate respiratory support
  - Acute respiratory events
  - Vascular access complications
  - Acute cardiac events
  - Gastrointestinal/genitourinary (GI/GU) crisis
  - Acute infections

- Maternal/child conditions
- Hospice/comfort care

Injury Control and Prevention in the Home Care Setting

- Injury (and illness) control is an epidemiological-based, scientific approach that attempts to minimize morbidity and mortality.
- Three components to injury control:
  - Primary prevention
  - Acute care (secondary prevention designed to reduce the sequelae of acute illness or injury)
  - Rehabilitation (tertiary prevention)
- Infection control in the home care setting:
  - Infection control measures include applying principles of standard precautions and body substance isolation when indicated
    - — All patients should be treated as though they have an infectious disease
- Recommended equipment for infection control in the home setting includes the following:
  - Mask
  - Gown
  - Goggles, glasses, or face shield
  - Resuscitation mask
  - Specimen bags
  - EPA-approved disinfectant effective against HBV, HIV, TB
  - Soap and water
  - Disposable paper towels
  - Impervious trash bags and labels

Types of Home Care Patients

- Major classifications of home care patients and associated complaints include the following:
  - Airway pathologies
  - Inadequate pulmonary toilet
  - Inadequate alveolar ventilation
  - Inadequate alveolar oxygenation
  - Circulatory pathologies
  - Alterations in peripheral circulation
  - GI/GU pathologies
  - Ostomies
  - Catheters
  - Home dialysis
  - Infections
  - Cellulitis
  - Sepsis
  - Wound care
  - Surgical wound closure
  - Decubitus wounds

- Drains
- Hospice care
- Maternal/child care
- Apnea monitors
- The new parent
- Progressive dementia in the patient at home
- Psychosocial support of the home care family
- Chronic pain management
- Home chemotherapy
- Transplant candidate

GENERAL PRINCIPLES OF ASSESSMENT AND MANAGEMENT

- Scene size-up
- Body substance isolation, use standard precautions
- Emergency medical service (EMS) crew should ensure that infectious waste found in the home environment is properly contained and disposed of per protocol
- Scene safety
  - Pets
  - Firearms and other home protection devices
  - Home hazards
  - Surroundings
  - Ability to maintain a healthy environment
  - Adequate nutritional support available
  - Adequate basic needs (heat, water, shelter, electricity, etc.) available
- Initial assessment
  - Focus on life-threatening illness or injury
  - Take appropriate measures as indicated
- Focused history and physical examination
- Noncritical findings
- Medication interactions
- Available home health history
- Compliance issues
- Assessing for possibility of dementia
- Other intervention and transport considerations
- Notification of family or caretakers
- Securing the home
- On-going assessments—Evaluate any changes in the patient's status while at the scene or en route to the hospital
- Differential diagnosis and continued management

Prehospital Management

- Depending on the patient's condition, home health treatment may need to be replaced with advanced life support treatment.
  - Airway and ventilatory support
  - Circulatory support

- Pharmacological intervention.
- Nonpharmacologic interventions.
- Transport considerations:
  - Hospital for physician evaluation
  - Home care follow-up
  - Referral to other public service agencies
  - Notification of family medical doctor or home health agencies

SPECIFIC ACUTE HOME HEALTH SITUATIONS

Respiratory Support

- More than 600,000 patients are discharged to home care with diseases of the respiratory system each year.
- Respiratory support patients have an increased risk for airway infections.
- Progression of some respiratory diseases may lead to an increased respiratory demand, making current support inadequate.
- Examples of chronic pathologies that require home respiratory support include the following:
  - Chronic lung disease
  - Asthma
  - Bronchopulmonary dysplasia
  - Patients awaiting a lung transplant
  - Cystic fibrosis
  - Sleep apnea
  - Infection causing exacerbation of condition
- Problems that may lead to a request for EMS assistance include the following:
  - Increased respiratory demand
  - Increased bronchospasm
  - Increased secretions
  - Obstructed or malfunctioning respiratory devices
  - Improper application of medical devices to support respirations
- Three common ways to provide oxygen therapy in the home:
  - Compressed gas—Refers to oxygen stored under pressure in oxygen cylinders equipped with a regulator that controls flow rate.
  - Liquid oxygen.
  - Very cold and stored in a container similar to a thermos.
  - When released, the liquid converts to gas and is used like compressed gas.
  - Oxygen concentrators—An electrically powered device that separates oxygen from air, concentrates it, and stores it. This system does not have to be resupplied.
  - A cylinder of oxygen must be available as a backup in case of power failure.

Oxygen Delivery Devices

- Oxygen is delivered to patients in the following ways:
  - Nasal cannulas
  - Oxygen masks
  - Tracheostomy collars (a device that delivers high humidity and oxygen to a patient with a surgical airway)

 - Some patients may require continuous positive airway pressure (CPAP)
 - Delivered by ventilatory support systems through mask CPAP, nasal CPAP, or bilevel positive airway pressure (BiPAP)
- Support ventilator management may be indicated in the following situations:
  - To prevent nocturnal hypoxemia caused by sleep hypoventilation in patients with neuromuscular disorders
  - To prevent respiratory fatigue in patients with chronic obstructive pulmonary disease (COPD)
  - To improve ventilation and oxygen saturation in patients with obstructive apnea

Home Ventilators

- Home ventilators can be classified in the following ways:
  - Volume ventilators
  - Pressure ventilators
  - Negative pressure ventilators

Volume Ventilators (Volume-Preset)

- Deliver a predetermined volume of gas with each cycle, after which inspiration is terminated
- Deliver a constant tidal volume regardless of changes in airway resistance or in the compliance of the lungs and thorax
- Volume remains the same unless excessively high peak airway pressures are reached, in which case, safety release valves stop the flow

Pressure Ventilators (Pressure-Preset)

- Pressure-cycled devices that terminate inspiration when a preset pressure is achieved
- When the preset pressure is reached, the gas flow stops and the patient passively exhales
- Most commonly are used for patients whose ventilatory resistance is not likely to change

Negative Pressure Ventilators

- Have settings for respiratory rate and the pressure of the negative force exerted.
- Use negative pressure to raise the rib cage and lower the diaphragm to create negative pressure within the lungs so that air flows into the lungs.
- Used for patients with healthy lungs, but who have a muscular inability to inhale.
- Examples of this type of ventilator are the "iron lung" and the plastic wrap or poncho ventilators.

Causes of ventilator alarms

- Ventilators are equipped with alarms to alert of problems with ventilator function including the following:
  - Loss of power alarms
  - Frequency alarms (indicating changes in respiratory rate)
  - Volume alarms (indicating low-exhaled volume, low/high-minute ventilation)
  - High-pressure alarms
- If alarms are sounding, check for the following possible causes:
  - Kinks in endotracheal (ET) tube
  - Disconnected ventilator tubing or poor connections

  - Water in ventilator tubing
  - Excessive secretions
  - Pneumothorax
  - Patient anxiety
- After consulting with medical direction, acute interventions may include:
  - Providing temporary ventilation assistance with a bag-valve mask device
  - Repositioning the ET tube
  - Correcting poor ventilator tube connections
  - Emptying water from tube or water traps
  - Suctioning the airway
  - Thoracic decompression
  - Possible sedation

Assessment

- When caring for a patient who requires oxygen therapy, evaluate the patient for the following:
  - Work of breathing
  - Tidal volume
  - Peak flow
  - Oxygen saturation
  - Quality of breath sounds
- This assessment can be performed with:
  - Visual inspection (chest rise and fall)
  - Peak flow meters
  - Pulse oximetry
  - Auscultation
- Be constantly aware of signs and symptoms of hypoxia that include:
  - Restlessness
  - Headache
  - Confusion and mental status changes
  - Hyperventilation
  - Tachycardia
  - Hypertension
  - Dyspnea
  - Cyanosis
- Management goals for a patient receiving oxygen therapy who requires acute intervention are improvement of the following:
  - Airway patency
  - Ventilation
  - Oxygenation
- Improving airway patency
  - Reposition airway devices to ensure they are properly applied and well-fitted
  - Clear secretions that obstruct airflow from the airway with suction and from any airway device with sterile water
  - If necessary, the home airway device should be replaced with a new device
  - A tracheostomy tube that has become blocked and that cannot be cleared may need to be replaced with another tracheostomy tube (or temporarily replaced with an ET tube) to ensure adequate ventilation

- Improving ventilation and oxygenation
  - If ventilation does not improve after providing a patent airway remove the home care device
  - Assist the patient's ventilations with positive pressure ventilation via a bag-valve device and supplemental oxygen
  - Monitor oxygen saturation with pulse oximetry
  - Administer supplemental oxygen as necessary to maintain oxygen saturation at 90% or higher
  - Medical direction may recommend adjusting the settings of a home care device or changing the flow rate of an oxygen delivery device to improve ventilation and oxygenation
  - Additional manpower may be needed to assist with moving the patient who has airway devices to the ambulance for transport for physician evaluation

Psychological Support and Communication Strategies

- Respiratory insufficiency can be a horrifying experience for the patient, particularly for a patient who is ventilator-dependent.
- Attempt to calm the patient.
- Assure him or her that respirations will be adequately supported by other means.
- Loss of verbal communication is a major source of anxiety in the patient who has a tracheostomy.
- The ability to communicate with these patients will be based on the following characteristics of the patient:
  - Level of cognition
  - Level of consciousness
  - Language
  - Fine and gross motor skills
- Methods of communication may include signing and writing on notepads.

Vascular Access Devices (VADs)

- Many patients in the home care setting will have indwelling vascular devices. VADs are used to do the following:
  - Provide nutritional support
  - Administer medications
  - Provide long-term vascular access
    - — Dialysis patients
    - — Patients receiving chemotherapy
- Those with indwelling vascular devices may experience problems such as the following:
  - Anticoagulation associated with percutaneous or implanted devices
  - Embolus formation associated with indwelling devices, stasis, and inactivity
  - Air embolus associated with central venous access devices
  - Obstructed or malfunctioning vascular access devices
  - Infection at the access site
  - Obstructed dialysis shunts
- Types of VADs:
  - Surgically implanted medication delivery devices (e.g., Mediports)

- Peripheral vascular access devices (peripherally inserted central catheters [PICC], midline catheters)
- Central venous tunneled catheters, such as Hickman, Groshong, or Broviac
- Dialysis shunts

Assessment Findings for Vascular Access Devices

Infection

- Common problem of VADs is infection near the entry site, tunnel, or port.
- Signs and symptoms of site infection include pain, redness, and swelling.
- Signs and symptoms of systemic infection (which may result from a site infection):
  - Fever
  - Tachycardia
  - General weakness
  - Malaise
  - Mental status changes
  - Body aches
  - Possible septicemia
  - Drainage from the site
  - Tenderness and warmth at the site
- General principles in managing the site infection are to:
  - Ensure sterile technique when assessing and manipulating the line
  - Clean site with alcohol and then povidone-iodine solution (per protocol)
  - Apply antimicrobial ointment if required per local protocol
  - Cover site with a transparent, sterile dressing (per protocol)
- Document procedure and label dressing with date, time, and your initials.
  - Consult with medical direction

Hemorrhage

- Control bleeding at the site of a VAD by applying gentle, direct pressure with aseptic technique. These patients will often need to be transported for physician evaluation or referred to a home health practitioner for definitive care.
- Hemodynamic compromise:
  - May result from circulatory overload
  - Can develop from too much IV fluid or from IV fluid that is delivered too fast
- Signs and symptoms:
  - Rise in blood pressure
  - Distended neck veins
  - Pulmonary congestion (crackles and/or wheezes)
  - Dyspnea
- Management:
  - Slow the infusion to a keep-open rate
  - Provide high-concentration oxygen
  - Elevate the patient's head
  - Maintain body warmth to promote peripheral circulation and ease the stress on the central veins
  - Monitor vital signs

- ◦ Consult with medical direction for patient management and disposition
- ◦ May result from embolus
- ◦ Displacement of a surgically implanted catheter or port is rare

Causes of embolus formation

- Air embolism:
  - ◦ IV fluid containers that run dry
  - ◦ Air in IV tubing
  - ◦ Loose connections in catheter tubing
  - ◦ Catheter tears and breakage
- Thrombus:
  - ◦ Clot formation from inactivity or stasis
- Plastic or catheter tip migration:
  - ◦ Plastic or catheter fragment from tugging or shearing forces
  - ◦ Wire from central line placement
- Signs and symptoms:
  - ◦ Hypotension
  - ◦ Cyanosis
  - ◦ Weak, rapid pulse
  - ◦ Loss of consciousness
- Management:
  - ◦ Stop the IV infusion
  - ◦ Position the patient on the left side with the head down (in an attempt to keep the embolus in the right side of the heart)
  - ◦ Administer high-concentration oxygen
  - ◦ Notify medical direction
  - ◦ Obstruction of the vascular device
- An indwelling vascular device may become obstructed, disrupting the flow of fluids and medications. Immediate intervention is required to clear the device by irrigation or by administering thrombolytic agents.
- Flushing and irrigation.
- Vascular access devices and medication ports require regular irrigation with normal saline and/or heparin depending on the type of VAD.
- Frequency of irrigation depends on the specific device.
- If a VAD is obstructed, consult with medical direction and follow these steps:
  - ◦ Explain the procedure to the patient
  - ◦ Prepare prescribed irrigation solutions (normal saline and heparin)
  - ◦ Clean the injection cap(s) with an antiseptic and alcohol wipe and allow to air dry
  - ◦ Release the clamp from the catheter (if present)
  - ◦ Irrigate the lumen with normal saline and then flush with heparin solution (no faster than 0.5 mL/sec)
  - ◦ Maintain positive pressure on the syringe plunger when withdrawing the needle to prevent a backflow of blood into the catheter tip and to ensure a heparin lock
  - ◦ Clamp the catheter
  - ◦ Loop the catheter with the cap pointing upward on the dressing
    - — Secure with tape

  - Properly dispose of all equipment
    - Anticoagulant therapy
      - There may be occasions when a medication port or other vascular device will require declotting with thrombolytic agents (e.g., Urokinase [Abbokinase])
      - Always consult with medical direction before administering anticoagulant therapy
- Steps to follow in declotting a Port-A-Cath device:
  - Explain the procedure to the patient
  - Prepare necessary solutions—1 mL of Urokinase and 1 mL of normal saline solution in a 3-mL syringe with a noncoring (Huber) needle
    - Consult with medical direction for dosage
  - Using sterile technique, clean the injection cap or area of skin over the Port-A-Cath septum with alcohol followed by povidone wipe (per protocol), and allow to air dry
  - Connect the syringe to the integrated extension tubing
    - Unclamp the tubing
  - Slowly inject the medication solution into the occluded lumen and port of the Port-A-Cath
    - Wait 30 minutes
  - Attempt to aspirate the residual clot
  - Repeat the procedure with a 15-minute dwell time if patency is not achieved
  - Notify medical direction if the catheter cannot be aspirated
    - If patency is achieved, follow the above procedure for flushing and irrigation
  - Properly dispose of all equipment
- Catheter damage
  - A damaged (cracked or torn) catheter can do the following:
    - Allow fluids or medications to infiltrate into the surrounding tissues
    - Lead to an air embolism
- Signs and symptoms of a damaged catheter:
  - Leaking fluid
  - A complaint of a burning sensation
  - Swollen and tender skin near the insertion site
    - If catheter damage is suspected:
      - Stop the infusion immediately
      - Clamp the catheter between the crack or tear in the catheter and the patient
      - Administer high-concentration oxygen
      - Establish IV access through a peripheral vein
      - Transport for physician evaluation

GI/GU Crisis

- About 500,000 patients with diseases of the digestive or genitourinary systems are discharged to home care each year.
- Medical therapy found in the home setting for patients with GI/GU disease.
  - Devices for gastric/intestinal emptying or feeding
    - Nasogastric (NG) tube
    - Feeding tube
    - Peg tubes, J-tubes, G-tubes
    - Colostomy

- Devices for the urinary tract
  - External urinary catheters (Condom catheter, Texas catheter)
  - Indwelling urinary catheter (Foley catheter, Coudé catheter)
  - Surgical urinary catheters (suprapubic catheters)
  - Urostomy
- Acute interventions that may be required for these patients can result from the following:
  - Urinary tract infection
  - Urosepsis
  - Urinary retention
  - Problems with gastric emptying or feeding

Urinary Tract Infection (Urosepsis)

- Urinary tract infection (UTI) is common and occurs in all age groups and both genders.
- Organisms most frequently associated with UTI are gram-negative organisms normally found in the GI tract:
  - *Escherichia coli*
  - *Klebsiella*
  - *Proteus*
  - *Enterobacter*
  - *Pseudomonas*
- Such organisms are frequently introduced from the hands of health personnel at the time of bladder catheterization.
- Other factors that increase a person's risk for UTI include:
  - Obstructions (urethral strictures, calculi, tumors, blood clots)
  - Trauma (abdominal injury, ruptured bladder, local trauma related to sexual activity)
  - Congenital anomalies (polycystic kidneys, horseshoe kidney, spina bifida)
  - Abdominal or gynecological surgery
  - Acute or chronic renal failure
  - Immunocompromised state (HIV, the elderly)
  - Postpartum state
  - Aging changes, particularly in the female
  - If allowed to progress, UTI may lead to septic complications (urosepsis)
  - Managed with antibiotic therapy

Urinary Retention (The Inability to Urinate)

- May result from the following:
  - Urethral stricture
  - Inflammation
  - Enlarged prostate
  - Central nervous system (CNS) dysfunction
  - Foreign body obstruction
  - Use of certain medications such as parasympatholytic or anticholinergic agents
- These patients need physician evaluation to determine the cause of urine retention.
- If the cause is not easily correctable, the patient may require hospitalization.
- Some patients may require bladder catheterization with an indwelling Foley catheter device.

- This procedure may be indicated to do the following:
  - Empty the bladder of a patient with urinary retention
  - Replace a nonfunctioning indwelling urinary catheter device

Indwelling foley catheter insertion

- Personal protective equipment
- Urinary catheterization set containing:
  - Sterile gloves
  - Antiseptic solution
  - Sterile cleansing sponges
  - Sterile drapes or towels
  - Syringe containing 5-mL sterile water
  - Connecting tubing and collection bag
  - Water-soluble sterile lubricant
  - Urinary catheter with 5-mL Foley balloon
  - Usually a No. 16 F for males or a 14 F for females
  - Standard length is 18 in.

Male catheterization

- Explain procedure to patient.
- Place patient in supine position and remove patient's pants and undergarments.
- Open catheterization set using sterile technique.
- Don sterile gloves.
- Place one sterile drape over the thighs, just below the patient's penis, and another above the penis to cover the abdomen.
- Open package of antiseptic solution and saturate sterile sponges (or cotton balls).
- Open package of water-soluble lubricant and lubricate the first several inches of the catheter.
- Grasp the patient's penis with one hand and retract the foreskin (if present).
- With the other hand, cleanse the glans with a sterile sponge (maintaining hand sterility) and then discard the sponge.
  - Repeat the procedure
- Raise the shaft of the penis upright to straighten the penile urethra and pass the tip of the catheter through the meatus.
- Continue passing the catheter with gentle, steady pressure into the urethra until it is fully inserted (near the point of catheter bifurcation to ensure that the balloon is in the bladder).
  - If mild resistance is felt at the external sphincter, slightly increase traction on the penis and continue with steady, gentle pressure on the catheter
  - If significant resistance is met, withdraw the catheter and consult with medical direction
- Attach the syringe to the catheter and inflate the balloon.
- Gently pull on the catheter to feel resistance.
  - Reposition the retracted foreskin of an uncircumcised patient
- Run the catheter tubing along the patient's leg and tape the connecting tubing to the patient's thigh.
  - Do not place any tension on the catheter
- Attach the collection bag to the bed or stretcher at a level below that of the patient to facilitate drainage by gravity.

Female catheterization

- Prepare patient and equipment as previously described.
- Female patients should be positioned with knees bent, hips flexed, and feet resting about 24 in. apart.
- With one hand, separate patient's labia to expose urethral meatus.
- Cleanse surrounding area with a sterile sponge or cotton ball (maintaining hand sterility) in downward strokes from anterior to posterior, and discard sponge.
  - Repeat procedure
- Introduce the tip of well-lubricated catheter into urethra using sterile technique.
  - Continue to advance catheter with gentle, steady pressure until it is fully inserted (near the point of catheter bifurcation to ensure the balloon is in the bladder)
- Attach syringe to catheter and inflate the balloon.
- Run the catheter tubing along the patient's leg and tape the connecting tubing to the patient's thigh. Do not place any tension on the catheter.
- Attach the collection bag to the bed or stretcher at a level below that of the patient to facilitate drainage by gravity.

Problems with Gastric Emptying or Feeding

- Gastric tubes found in the home care setting are devices inserted into the stomach or intestines for the following reasons:
  - Removing fluids and gas by suction or gravity
  - Instilling irrigation solutions or medications
  - Administering enteral feedings
- Aspiration of gastric contents.
- Causes of aspiration of gastric contents:
  - A nonpatent gastric tube
  - Improper nutritional support via a feeding tube
  - Patient positioning
- Patients at greatest risk for aspiration of tube feedings:
  - Unconscious patients
  - Confused patients
  - Seriously debilitated patients
  - Elderly patients
  - Patients with a tracheostomy or large-bore feeding tube
  - Patients with an impaired gag reflex
  - Patients not able to sit upright
- Patients with feeding tubes should be closely monitored for:
  - Respirations that represent minimal respiratory effort
  - Lung sounds that are clear on auscultation
- Other problems that can occur in patients with feeding tubes:
  - Diarrhea
  - Choking
  - Irritable bowel syndrome
  - Bowel obstruction

Obstructed or malfunctioning gastric devices

- Causes of a gastric device obstruction and malfunction:
  - A kinked or clogged tube
  - Displacement of a surgically implanted feeding tube

TABLE 38-1: Types and Placement of Feeding Tubes

Type of Tube	Placement
Nasogastric tube (NG tube)	Passed via nose into stomach
Nasointestinal tube	Passed via nose into intestine
Esophagostomy tube	Passed into the esophagus though a surgically created opening in the anterior neck
Gastrostomy tube (G-tube)	Passed directly into the stomach through an opening created in the abdominal wall
Jejunostomy tube (J-tube, PEG tube)	Passed into the jejunum through an opening created in the abdominal wall

- Acute interventions:
  - Unkinking a tube
  - Irrigating a clogged tube
  - Reinserting a displaced tube (per medical direction)

(See Table 38-1 for types and placement of feeding tubes.)

Ostomies

- An ileostomy or colostomy is a surgical procedure in which part of the intestine is brought through an incision in the abdominal wall and formed into an artificial opening to allow the discharge of intestinal contents into a bag attached to the skin.
  - An ileostomy is an opening into the small intestine
  - A colostomy is an opening into the large intestine
- The bowel usually discharges liquid or solid feces into a bag (pouch) once or twice a day; the bag is then changed.
- Potential complications associated with ostomies:
  - Infection
  - Hemorrhage
  - Obstruction
  - Stomal problems
- Colostomy irrigation, ostomy care, and pouch changes are usually performed for home care patients by family members and home health practitioners.
- These procedures require special training and are usually not considered an acute intervention for paramedic practice.

Assessment and Management of Patients with GI/GU Crisis

- Evaluate patient to determine need for immediate transport for physician evaluation by doing the following:
  - Obtaining a focused history
  - Performing a physical examination
- Physical examination may include assessment for:
  - Abdominal pain
  - Abdominal distention
  - Aspiration
  - Intestinal obstruction
  - Urinary infection
  - Urinary retention

- Fever
- Peritonitis

Acute Infections

- More than 160,000 patients with infectious and parasitic diseases are discharged to home care in the United States each year.
- Home care patients with acute infections have an increased mortality rate from sepsis and severe peripheral infections. Many have a decreased ability to perceive pain or perform self-care.
- Conditions that may result in the need for acute interventions in the homebound population:
  - Airway infections in the immunocompromised patient
  - Delayed healing and increased peripheral infection from poor peripheral perfusion
  - Skin breakdown and peripheral infections from immobility or sedentary lifestyle
  - Infection and sepsis from implanted medical devices
  - Wounds and incisions
  - Abscesses
  - Cellulitis

Open Wounds

- Patients with open wounds who are discharged to home care may have a variety of dressings, wound packings, drains that permit drainage of fluid or air, and wound closure devices.

Wound Care Devices Found in Home Care Patients

- Dressings and wound-packing material:
  - Cotton dressings (gauze)
  - Impregnated cotton dressings
  - Combination dressings
  - Paste bandages
  - Exudate absorptive dressings
  - Foam dressings
  - Hydrocolloid dressings
  - Hydrogel dressings
  - Hydrophilic powder dressings
  - Transparent film (adhesive or nonadhesive)

Drains

- Penrose drains
- Jackson-Pratt drains

General Principles in Wound Care Management

- Wound care management requires an assessment of the wound and surrounding tissues and an evaluation for infection or sepsis.
- General principles in wound care management include an assessment for:
  - Location and size
  - Color of the wound bed
    - — Red or pink granular wound bed indicates healing
    - — Green, yellow, or black wound bed suggests infection or necrosis (tissue death)

- Drainage
  - — Clear or serosanguineous drainage is common in a healing wound
  - — Green or yellow drainage suggests infection
- Wound odor
  - — A sweet smell may indicate decay
  - — A foul smell may indicate infection
    - Occlusive and transparent adhesive dressings will cause a wound odor
- Surrounding skin
  - — Assess for redness, inflammation, or signs of breakdown

Changing (redressing) wounds

- Dressing should be changed after wound evaluation if it has become wet or contaminated.
- Medical direction may recommend cleaning the wound with normal saline and/or antiseptic solution before redressing.
- Some patients may require transportation for physician evaluation if severe infection or sepsis is suspected.

Maternal/Child Conditions

- Insurance company control of hospital stays for childbirth.
- In the early 1990s, many insurance companies began paying only for 24-hour hospital stays for uncomplicated vaginal childbirth ("drive-by deliveries").
- In the wake of complaints about inadequate care, states began passing laws in 1995 and 1996 requiring insurance to pay for 48-hour stays.
- Similar federal law passed in 1996 (effective in January 1998) mandated hospital stays of the following:
  - At least 48 hours for women who give birth naturally
  - Up to 4 days for those who deliver by caesarean section
- Possible problems encountered by mother/child patient groups when they return to the home care setting.
- Postpartum pathophysiologies:
  - Postpartum hemorrhage
    - — Occurs in about 5% of all deliveries
    - — Frequently takes place within the first few hours after delivery, but can be delayed up to 6 weeks
    - — Causes
      - Incomplete contraction of uterine muscle fibers
      - Retained pieces of placenta or membranes in the uterus
      - Vaginal or cervical tears during delivery (rare)
  - Postpartum infection (endometritis)
    - — Affects 2–8% of all pregnancies
    - — Occurs when bacteria proliferate and invade the uterus or other tissues along the birth canal
    - — Symptoms
      - Usually develop on the second or third day after delivery
      - Fever and abdominal pain are the most common signs of infection

- Pulmonary embolism
  - Pulmonary embolism during pregnancy, labor, or the postpartum period is one of the most common causes of maternal death
  - Embolus is frequently the result of a blood clot in the pelvic circulation
  - Embolism is more commonly associated with cesarean section than with vaginal delivery
- Postpartum depression
  - Affects 10–15% of mothers
  - Probably caused by a combination of sudden hormonal changes and a variety of psychological and environmental factors
  - Ranges from an extremely common and short-lived attack of mild depression ("baby blues") to a depressive psychosis that requires in-hospital supervision
  - Risk factors for postpartum depression
    - Low self-esteem
    - Anxiety
    - Poor marital adjustment
    - Adverse socioeconomic conditions
    - Previous episodes of depression
    - Complicated pregnancy or delivery
    - Fetal complications
    - Recent life stressors
  - Thoughts of many women with postpartum depression
    - Fear they will harm their babies
    - Often feel ashamed and guilty for these feelings
  - Signs and symptoms of postpartum depression
    - Severe sleep disturbance
    - Fear of harming self or baby
    - Lack of interest in previously enjoyed activities
    - Anxiety
    - Forgetfulness or memory loss
    - Hostility
    - Unexplainable crying—Joy or sadness
    - Desire to leave—Feelings of being trapped
    - Hopelessness
    - Panic attacks
    - Change of appetite—Loss of appetite or overindulgence
    - Lack of sexual interest
    - Over or under concern for baby
    - Fantasies of disaster or bizarre fears
    - Rapid mood swings
    - Irritability
    - Fatigue or exhaustion
    - Increased alcohol consumption or other drug use
    - Difficulty making decisions
    - Hatred of spouse, self, or baby
    - Inability to care for baby
    - Loss of hope
  - Sensitivity to the possibility of depression is crucial to successful diagnosis and treatment

- Septicemia in the newborn
  - Healthy newborns are vulnerable to several conditions that can require hospital treatment
  - Jaundice that results from physiological immaturity of bilirubin metabolism
  - Dehydration that can lead to serious electrolyte abnormalities
- Sepsis
  - Septicemia in the newborn is usually caused by group B streptococci, *Listeria monocytogenes*, or gram-negative enteric organisms (especially *Escherichia coli*)
  - Signs and symptoms of sepsis
    - May be minimal and nonspecific
    - "In the newborn, anything can be a sign of anything"
  - Examples of signs and symptoms of sepsis in the newborn
    - Temperature instability
    - Respiratory distress
    - Apnea
    - Cyanosis
    - GI changes (vomiting, distention, diarrhea, anorexia)
    - CNS features (irritability, lethargy, weak suck)
  - Risk factors for sepsis
    - Prematurity
    - Prolonged rupture of membranes
    - Chorioamnionitis
      - An inflammatory reaction in the amniotic membranes caused by bacterial viruses in the amniotic fluid
      - Diagnosis is generally confirmed by a positive blood, urine, or cerebrospinal fluid (CSF) culture
- Infantile apnea
  - Apnea is defined as periods of cessation of respirations for more than 10–15 seconds with or without cyanosis, pallor, hypotonia, and/or bradycardia, or for less than 10 seconds accompanied by bradycardia
  - Often reflects the immature respiratory control centers in some infants
  - Other causes of infantile apnea
    - Metabolic derangements (hypoglycemia, hypocalcemia, hypothermia)
    - Infection (sepsis, pneumonia, meningitis)
    - CNS damage (hemorrhage, hypoxic injury, seizures)
    - Pulmonary disorders (respiratory distress, hyaline membrane disease, pneumonia, obstruction, upper respiratory abnormalities)
    - Intentional poisoning
  - The presence of apnea must be assessed carefully and documented
  - Observation with electronic apnea monitoring devices
    - Most infants with the presumptive diagnosis of apnea will be hospitalized and observed closely using electronic apnea monitoring devices
    - Apnea monitoring devices detect changes in thoracic or abdominal movement and heart rate
  - Managing apnea in these patients may include the home-care use of:
    - Apnea monitors
    - Oscillating waterbeds
    - CPAP with supplemental oxygen
  - Some patients may be prescribed respiratory stimulants (e.g., Doxapram, methylxanthines)

- Failure to thrive (FTT)
  - The abnormal retardation of the growth and development of an infant resulting from conditions that interfere with normal metabolism, appetite, and activity
  - Causative factors
    - Chromosomal abnormalities
    - Major organ system defects that lead to deficiency or malfunction
    - Systemic disease or acute illness
    - Physical deprivation (primarily malnutrition related to insufficient breast milk, poverty, poor knowledge of nutrition)
    - Various psychosocial factors (e.g., maternal deprivation)
  - Can result in permanent and irreversible retardation of physical, mental, or social development
  - Any suspicions of FTT should be carefully documented and reported to medical direction

Well Baby Care

- Some infants and children will have periodic health assessments through well baby care programs that specialize in medical supervision and services for healthy infants.
- Well baby care promotes optimal physical, emotional, and intellectual growth and development.
- Such health-care measures include the following:
  - Routine immunizations to prevent disease
  - Screening procedures for early detection and treatment of illness
  - Parental guidance and instruction in proper nutrition, accident prevention, and specific care and reading of the child at various stages of development
  - Recommended preventive health-care schedule for children who are developing normally
    - Monthly for the first 6 months of life
    - Every 2 months until 1 year of age
    - Every 3 months during the second year
    - Every 6 months during the third year, followed by annual visits
- Types of well baby care facilities
  - Clinic ("well baby clinics")
  - Doctor's office
  - Office of a community health nursing service, or a school
- Nurses or nurse practitioners frequently provide the care in these programs

Hospice/Comfort Care

- In 1996, hospices served nearly 450,000 patients throughout the United States.
- Hospice services include supportive social, emotional, and spiritual services to the terminally ill, and support for the patient's family.
- Hospice care:
  - Relies on the combined knowledge and skill of an interdisciplinary team of professionals that includes physicians, nurses, medical social workers, therapists, counselors, chaplains, and volunteers who coordinate an individualized plan of care for each patient and family.
  - The need for hospices will likely continue to rise as a result of:
    - Aging population
    - Increasing number of people with AIDS
    - Rising health-care costs

  - Medical professionals and the general public are increasingly choosing hospice care over other forms of health care for terminally ill patients because of its holistic, patient-family, in-home-centered philosophy.
- Palliative care (comfort care):
  - Unique form of health care primarily directed at providing relief to a terminally ill person through symptom and pain management.
  - Focuses on the needs of the patient and the family when a person with a life-threatening illness has reached the terminal stage of the illness.
  - A primary goal of palliative care is to improve the quality of a person's life as death approaches and to help patients and their families move toward this reality with comfort, reassurance, and strength.
  - Palliative care is not focused on death; it is about specialized care for the living—Some programs also address mental health and spiritual needs.
  - May be delivered in hospices, home care settings, and hospitals.
  - Because medical needs vary depending on the disease that is leading toward death, specialized palliative care programs exist for common conditions such as cancer and AIDS.
- Rights of the terminally ill:
  - Bill of Rights and Responsibilities for Terminally Ill Patients
- Medical therapy found in the home setting:
  - Medical therapy that may be found in the home of a patient receiving hospice care:
    - Medication delivery devices for the relief of pain (e.g., narcotic infusion devices)
    - Medical and legal documents

      Do Not Resuscitate (DNR) orders

      Advance directives
  - Concerns of the paramedic about effective pain management, overmedication, or interpreting medical or legal documents should be discussed with medical direction.
    - EMS and medical direction should work closely with the families and private physicians of terminally ill patients in private homes and hospice programs so that they will use the EMS system appropriately (i.e., when to call 911).
    - Though resuscitation may not be indicated, EMS may be needed to:

      Manage pain

      Treat acute medical illness or traumatic injury

      Provide transportation to a hospital
    - If the patient is not to receive medical intervention to prolong life, measures of comfort should be provided to the patient and emotional support should be provided to family members and loved ones.

? CHAPTER QUESTIONS

1. You are treating a geriatric nursing home patient who has been diagnosed with a urinary tract infection. Which of the following measurements might be considered unreliable just because of the patient's age?

   a. Body temperature

   b. Blood pressure

   c. Poor skin turgor

   d. Level of consciousness

2. Upon examination of a 76-year-old assisted living patient, her vital signs reveal pale skin, BP 100/60, and a pulse of 110. Electrocardiogram (ECG) shows atrial fibrillation. When you repeat vital signs with the patient in a seated position, BP drops to 80/60 and pulse increases to 130. The patient has been having diarrhea with black stools. You suspect she is experiencing:
   a. uncontrolled atrial fibrillation
   b. dehydration
   c. a bowel obstruction
   d. a GI hemorrhage

Suggested Reading

US Department of Transportation, National Highway Traffic Safety Administration. *EMT-Paramedic: National Standard Curriculum*. Washington, DC: US Department of Transportation, National Highway Traffic Safety Administration; 1998.

Section 7

Operations

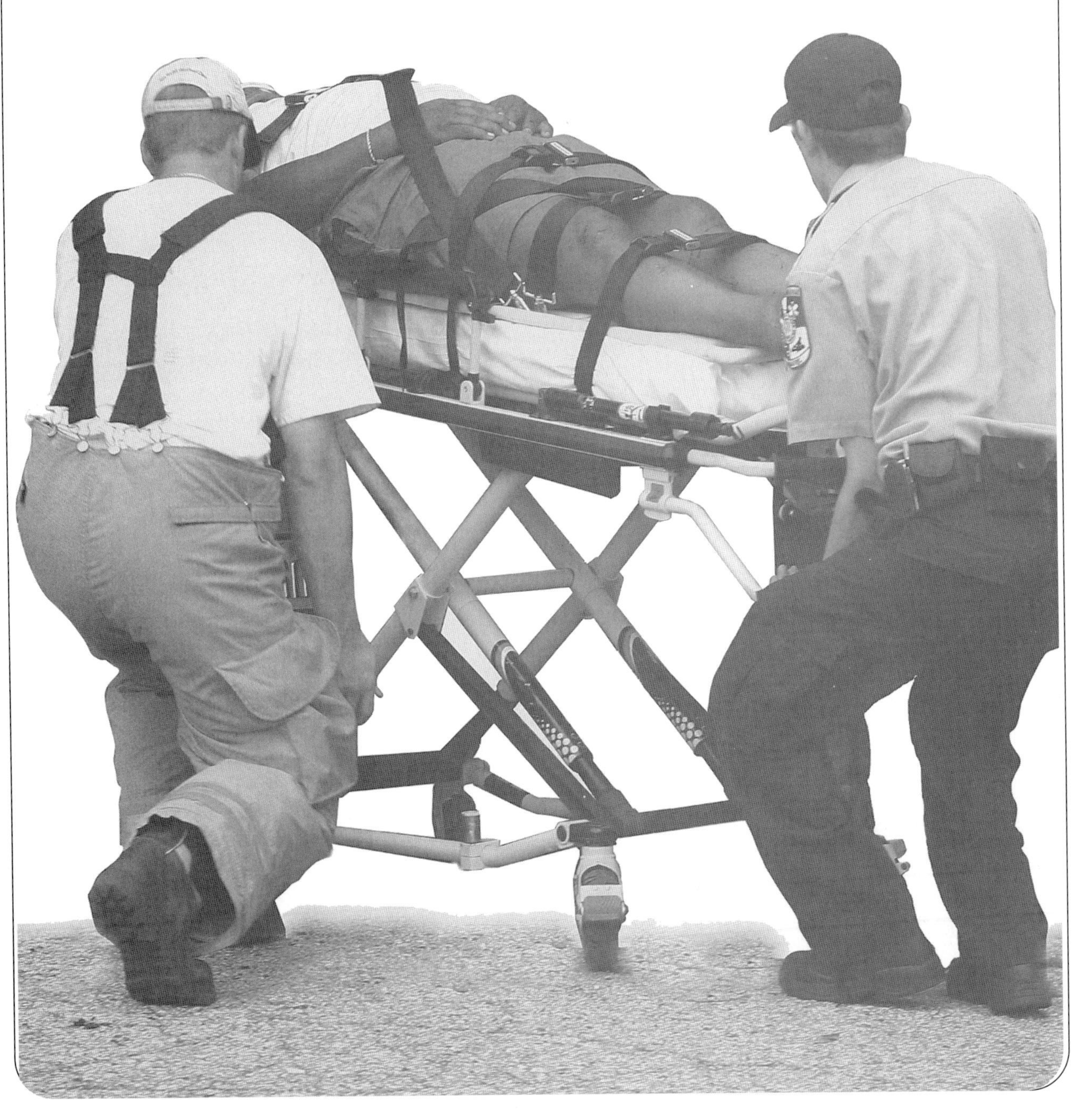

Chapter 39
Ambulance Operations

It is the beginning of your ambulance shift. Your dispatch center summons you to respond to a remote area of your response area for an advanced life support (ALS) intercept at a landing zone (LZ). The patient is a 42-year-old male who was involved in a rollover motor vehicle collision and was airlifted from the accident scene to a landing zone, where you will transport the patient to the regional trauma center. What concerns should you have regarding setting up the LZ?

The modern ambulance is much more than just a vehicle for transporting a patient to the hospital. Today's ambulances are well equipped and efficiently organized vehicles or aircraft with advanced communications systems and technology that can bring needed medical supplies, personnel, and advanced life support care to the emergency scene.

AMBULANCE STANDARDS

- In 1968, the National Academy of Sciences-National Research Council (NAS-NRC) recommended ambulance design standards including size, shape, color, electrical systems, and emergency equipment; this led to the development of the current federal specifications used by many states for their current ambulance requirements.
- The national standards developed by NAS-NRC and National Highway Traffic Safety Administration (NHTSA) are known as the KKK Standards. These standards (and associated revisions) provide the foundation of uniformity among ambulance vehicles.
- The standards pertain to the three basic ambulance designs:
  - Type I—Conventional, truck-cab–chassis with modular ambulance body
  - Type II—Standard van, forward control integral cab-body ambulance
  - Type III—Specialty van, forward control integral cab-body ambulance
- Other federal standards, state statutes, administrative rules, and city/county/district ordinances that influence ambulance design, equipment, and staffing include the following:
  - Air ambulance standards
  - Operational staffing standards
  - Operational driver standards
  - Operational driving standards
  - Operational equipment standards

CHECKING AMBULANCES

- Checklists and record keeping:
  - Completing an ambulance equipment and supply checklist at the beginning of every work shift is important.
  - This should be done to address safety, patient care, and risk-management issues.

  - This will also ensure the appropriate handling and safekeeping of scheduled medications.
  - Record keeping can be performed with pen and paper checklists or with specialized computer software.
- Some equipment may require routine maintenance, testing, and cleaning to ensure safe and effective operation.
- The procedure for vehicle maintenance and routine care will vary by emergency medical service (EMS) agency.

AMBULANCE STATIONING

Characteristics of Appropriate Ambulance Stationing

- In the 1970s, methods for estimating ambulance service needs and stationing in a community were developed on the basis of ambulance availability and the average response time to the emergency scene.
- Methods for estimating needs have now shifted toward determining the percentage of compliance in providing EMS services within time frames that meet national standards.
- The American Heart Association recommends that advanced life support be available at the scene within 8 minutes of a cardiac arrest.
- Factors that affect these estimates include the following:
  - Geographical area
  - Population and patient demand
  - Traffic conditions
  - Time of day
  - Appropriate placement of emergency vehicles
- The strategies are based on call volumes and locations.
- Computers and other sophisticated technologies may be used to formalize strategic unit deployment and decrease response times.
- Deployment strategies vary by EMS agency, from simple deployment of one vehicle stationed in the middle of a response area to comprehensive automated deployment plans for each hour of the day and each day of the week, complete with "mini-deployment" plans within each hour, depending on the number of ambulances left in the system.
- The optimal deployment system generally is a compromise between these two extremes.

SAFE AMBULANCE OPERATIONS

- Safe ambulance operation is crucial for the safety of patients, the EMS crew, and others near an emergency response. Many EMS agencies require personnel to do the following:
  - Complete an emergency driving course
  - Participate in periodic evaluations of their emergency driving skills
- Factors that influence safe ambulance operations:
  - Size and weight of the emergency vehicle
  - Driver's experience level
  - Appropriate use of escorts
  - Environmental conditions
  - Appropriate use of lights, sirens, and air horns

- Proceeding safely through intersections
- Parking at an emergency scene
- Driving with "due regard for the safety of all others"

- Guidelines for safe ambulance driving:
  - Be tolerant and observant of other motorists and pedestrians
  - Always use occupant safety restraints (both driver and passenger)
  - Be familiar with the characteristics of the emergency vehicle
  - Be alert to changes in weather and road conditions
  - Exercise caution in the use of audible and visible warning devices
  - Drive within the speed limit, except in circumstances allowed by law
  - Select the fastest and most appropriate route to and from the incident scene
  - Maintain a safe following distance
  - Drive with due regard for the safety of all others
  - Always drive in a manner consistent with managing acceptable levels of risk

Appropriate Use of Escorts

- Police escorts during an emergency response can be dangerous and should be used sparingly. Collisions can occur from confusion when motorists in the area wrongly assume that only one emergency vehicle is on the roadway.
- As a rule, police escorts should only be used when the EMS crew is responding to a scene in an unfamiliar area. A safe distance between the ambulance and the police escort should be observed.
- Use of lights, sirens, and air horns when police escorts are used should be guided by protocol. If audible and visual warning devices are used, the ambulance and police escort should use different siren tones (per protocol) to alert motorists that a second emergency vehicle is in the area.

Environmental Conditions

- Adverse environmental conditions pose significant dangers for those responding to an emergency call.
- Factors that can affect safe ambulance operation include road and weather conditions:
  - Fog and heavy rain decrease visibility
  - Ice, snow, mud, oil, or water on the roadway may cause slippery surfaces, or they may cause the ambulance to hydroplane
- When adverse environmental conditions are present, proceed at safe speeds that are appropriate for the road and weather conditions.
- Low-beam headlights should be used during all emergency responses.
  - Headlights increase visibility for the EMS crew
  - They allow for easier identification of the ambulance by other motorists

Appropriate Use of Warning Devices

- Characteristics of use of audible and visual warning devices during an emergency response and during patient transport:
  - Use should be guided by protocol
  - It should also be based on state motor vehicle laws
- Most EMS agencies authorize the use of audible and visual warning devices during all emergency responses in which the cause or severity of the emergency is unknown.

- Use of warning devices during patient transport is generally reserved for patients with limb- or life-threatening illness or injury.
- When audible and visual warning devices are indicated, remember that motorists may not be able to hear the audible devices for the following reasons:
  - Car windows rolled up
  - Using audio system
  - Using air conditioning or heating system
- Always proceed with caution and never assume that the vehicle's lights, sirens, and air horns provide an absolute right-of-way or privileged immunity to proceed.
- Proceeding through intersections.
  - It has been estimated that 53% of all ambulance crashes in the United States occur in intersections when an ambulance goes against a red light.
  - The driver of an emergency vehicle should do the following:
    - — Stop at all controlled intersections
    - — Attempt to make eye contact with all drivers before proceeding through an intersection
  - Other safety precautions for proceeding through intersections include the following:
    - — Making a secondary stop before crossing the intersection
    - — Using the siren's "yelp" mode or air horn to alert nearby traffic
- Parking at an emergency scene.
- When parking the ambulance at an accident scene, ensure that the vehicle's location allows for adequate traffic flow around the area.
- If law enforcement and fire service personnel have secured the scene, the ambulance should be parked in the following way:
  - About 100 ft past the accident scene (on the same side of the road)
  - Uphill (about 200 ft) and upwind if the presence of hazardous materials is suspected
- If the scene has not been secured by law enforcement and fire service personnel, the ambulance should be positioned about 50 ft in front of the scene ("fend-off" position) so that it deflects and averts from the scene other vehicles that might strike the ambulance or providers.
- Other safety precautions for parking at an emergency scene include the following:
  - Leaving emergency warning devices on (particularly at night)
  - Setting the parking brake
- When choosing an appropriate parking area for the ambulance, consider the possibility of the following:
  - Collapsing structures
  - Fires
  - Explosive hazards
  - Downed electrical wires

Operating with Due Regard for All Others

- Most states allow the following privileges for drivers of emergency vehicles:
  - Driving slightly above the speed limit
  - Proceeding through controlled intersections (after a stop) during an emergency response
- These privileges must take into consideration the safety of all other people using the roadway. This "due regard for all others" carries legal responsibility.
- It can result in liability for the paramedic and EMS agency if damage, injury, or death results from its failure.

The "Two-Second" Rule

- Most rear-end collisions are caused by drivers who follow too closely behind the vehicle in front of them.
- Ensure that there is sufficient space (following distance) between the emergency vehicle and the vehicle in front of it.
- The "two-second" rule can be used to "gauge" the recommended distance required for sufficient space between vehicles.
- Look at an object by the side of the road (e.g., a tree or sign) that will soon be passed by the vehicle ahead.
- Count "one thousand and one, one thousand and two"
- If you reach the object before you have said it, you are traveling too close to the vehicle in front of you.
- This rule applies with good road and weather conditions.
- If road and weather conditions are not good, following distance should be increased to a four- or five-second count.

Braking Distance

- Braking distance is based on the following:
  - Average reaction time
  - Average vehicle weight
  - Average road conditions
  - Average brake quality
- Braking distance is adversely affected by the following:
  - Wet roadways
  - Poor brakes
  - Poor tires
  - Heavy vehicle weight
  - Poor reaction time
- Be aware of local and state laws and regulations concerning the operation of an emergency vehicle.

AEROMEDICAL TRANSPORT

- Air evacuation is rooted in military history. During the Prussian siege of Paris in 1870, soldiers and civilians were evacuated by hot air balloon.
- In 1928, a Marine pilot used an engine-powered aircraft to evacuate the wounded in Nicaragua.
- The first full-scale use of motorized aircraft for medical evacuation did not occur until 1950 during the Korean conflict.
- Experience gained in Korea was the basis for developing helicopter rescue in Vietnam. Nearly a million casualties were transported by air in Vietnam.
- Recent military confrontations involving the United States in Panama, Grenada, and the Middle East had massive advanced aeromedical support capabilities and plans onsite before the confrontations started.
- Response times of 25 minutes were achieved for aeromedical evacuation of wounded solders in Operation Desert Storm.
- Field surgical units were set up to handle the estimated 1500–3000 casualties that occurred within the first 24 hours of the war.
- Most of those who were injured in the conflict arrived by air transport.

- Characteristics of aeromedical transport today:
  - There are about 300 civilian EMS flight programs that use fixed-wing and/or rotary-wing (helicopter) aircraft throughout the United States.
  - Fixed-wing aircraft services:
    - — Fixed-wing aircraft services are not usually as high-profile as helicopters
    - — They are frequently used for the following:

      Interhospital transfer of patients

      Vital organ delivery when the distance is greater than 100 miles

Aeromedical Crew Members and Training

- Air ambulance staffing:
  - Pilot
  - Various health-care professionals with specialized training in flight physiology and advanced medical equipment and procedures
    - — Emergency medical technicians (EMTs)
    - — Paramedics
    - — Respiratory therapists
    - — Nurses
    - — Physicians
- Guidelines for personnel qualifications have been established by the American College of Surgeons Committee on Trauma and the Association of Air Medical Services.
- Department of Transportation National Highway Traffic Safety Administration (DOT-NHTSA):
  - DOT-NHTSA funded the development of the Air Medical Crew National Standard Curriculum in 1988
  - It is used by many flight programs to teach the following:
    - — Flight physiology
    - — Aircraft components and construction
    - — Safety regulations
    - — Aviation and navigation terminology
    - — Operational safety
- Sampling of organizations associated with the air medical industry:
  - Air Medical Physicians Association (AMPA)
  - Association of Air Medical Services (AAMS)
  - Commission on Accreditation of Air Medical Services (CAAMS)
  - Commission on the Accreditation of Medical Transport Services (CAMTS)
  - International Society of Air Medical Services (Australasia) (ISAMS)
  - National Association of Air Medical Communications Specialists (NAAMCS)
  - National EMS Pilots Association (NEMSPA)
  - National Flight Nurses Association (NFNA)
  - National Flight Paramedics Association (NFPA)

Utilization of Aeromedical Services

- Criteria for requesting aeromedical services to the scene of an emergency are developed by the appropriate authority of the local EMS system.
- Air transportation generally should be considered when emergency personnel have found the following:

  - That the time needed to transport a patient by ground to an appropriate facility poses a threat to the patient's survival and recovery
  - That weather, road, or traffic conditions would seriously delay the patient's access to ALS
  - That critical care personnel and specialized equipment are needed to adequately care for the patient during transport
- Notification of aeromedical services.
  - Requests for medical services are accepted by most aeromedical transport providers from the following sources:
    - — Physicians
    - — EMS and fire service personnel
    - — Other on-scene public service agency personnel
- If air service is requested for medical, trauma, or search and rescue events, advise the flight crew of the following:
  - Type of emergency response
  - Number of patients
  - Location of LZ
  - Any prominent landmarks or hazards, such as vertical structures, power lines
- Direct ground-to-air communications must be available between a designated LZ officer and the aeromedical staff on board the responding aircraft.
- Landing site preparation.
  - Space requirements for a helicopter LZ generally must be 100 by 100 ft.
  - Characteristics of the ideal LZ:
    - — It has no vertical structures that could impair takeoff or landing
    - — It is relatively flat and free of high grass, crops, or other factors that may conceal uneven terrain or hinder access
    - — It is free of debris that may injure people or damage structures or the helicopter
  - If patients are close to the LZ, provide protection by covering their wounds and eyes.
  - Rescue personnel close to the landing site should wear the following protective equipment:
    - — Helmets with lowered face shields
    - — Safety glasses
  - If a nighttime LZ is used, emergency vehicles with lighted bar lights should be situated at the perimeters of the LZ.
    - — If white lights are used, direct them down to the center of the LZ as spotlights
  - Traffic cones with reflectors can help identify the LZ.
  - Dusty LZs should be wetted down by a fire crew, especially if vehicle traffic is moving in the area.
  - Helpful radio communications with the pilot include notification about the following conditions:
    - — Wind direction
    - — Any possible obstructions or hazards
  - If hazardous materials are present, advise the flight crew of the following:
    - — The substance
    - — The location of the hazardous materials site
    - — The possibility of any patient contamination
  - One emergency responder should stand facing the LZ so that the pilot can see the landing area.

- Safety precautions:
  - Clear everyone from the landing area during takeoffs and landings
  - Keeping all people a distance of 100–200 ft from the area is best
- Patient preparation:
  - Preparing a patient for aeromedical transport requires the following special considerations:
    - Airways must be established and secured before loading
    - Pneumatic antishock garments must be applied before loading (per local protocol)
    - External cardiopulmonary resuscitation devices should be positioned according to aircraft configuration
    - Restraints or pharmacological control may be required for combative patients

CHAPTER QUESTION

1. Planning scene safety is essential, because using proper safety techniques will:
   a. ensure that there will be no risk of injuries to the paramedic
   b. provide immunity from allegations of negligence
   c. maximize the chance for a successful outcome for all involved
   d. none of the above

Suggested Reading

US Department of Transportation, National Highway Traffic Safety Administration. *EMT-Paramedic: National Standard Curriculum*. Washington, DC: US Department of Transportation, National Highway Traffic Safety Administration; 1998.

Chapter 40
Medical Incident Command

It is early February at 1 p.m. and the superintendent is currently meeting with all school principals in the district about more proposed budget cuts. The meeting is taking place at the local school district building.

A call was received at the Picking Prep School from a group that identified itself as TUFF-ONE. The caller stated that a bomb (with an unknown amount of nuclear material) was placed somewhere in the building in a backpack.

The secretary quickly called 911, then the superintendent's office, and is now consulting the school's emergency procedures.

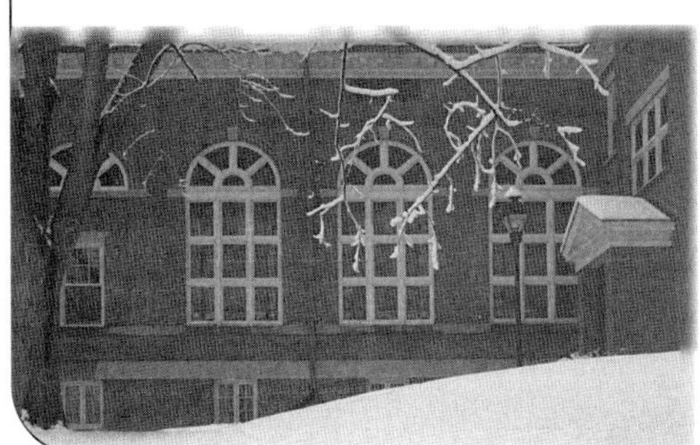

Four inches of snow fell overnight and the temperature is predicted to reach only 9° with 25 mph winds, as a cold snap continues throughout the entire northeast.

As a responder, you are dispatched to standby at the local church to set up a staging area. As preliminary reports are radioed into the communication center, why is common terminology so important when responding to a multiagency mass casualty incident?

- A major incident is classified as an event for which available resources are insufficient to manage the number of casualties or the nature of the emergency.
- Major incidents, such as the following, may stress and overwhelm local, regional, state, and even national and international resources:
  - Highway accidents
  - Air crashes
  - Major fires
  - Train derailments
  - Building collapses
  - Acts of violence or terrorism
  - Search and rescue operations
  - Hazardous materials releases
  - Natural disasters

HOMELAND SECURITY PRESIDENTIAL DIRECTIVE 5

To prevent, prepare for, respond to, and recover from terrorist attacks, major disasters, and other emergencies, the United States government shall establish a single, comprehensive approach to domestic incident management. The objective of the United States government is to ensure that all levels of government across the nation have the capability to work efficiently and effectively together, using a national approach to domestic incident management.

WHAT IS THE NATIONAL INCIDENT MANAGEMENT SYSTEM (NIMS)?

- A core set of:
  - Doctrine
  - Concepts
  - Principles
  - Terminology
  - Organizational processes that are applicable to all hazards
- NIMS has six components.
  - Command and management
  - Preparedness
  - Resource management
  - Communications and information management
  - Support technologies
  - Ongoing management and maintenance

Command and Management

NIMS standardizes incident management for all hazards across all levels of government. It is based on three key constructs:

- Incident command system
- Multiagency coordination systems
- Public information systems

Preparedness

NIMS establishes measures and capabilities that all agencies should develop.

Resource Management

NIMS standardizes describing and tracking inventory before, during, and after an incident.

Communications and Information Management

Effective communications, information management, and intelligence sharing are paramount in operating at a domestic incident.

Supporting Technologies

Ability to provide architecture for science and technology support to the incident management system during a crisis.

Ongoing Management

The Department of Homeland Security will establish a multijurisdictional, multidisciplinary NIMS integration center.

MASS CASUALTY INCIDENTS

- **Disasters**—Some people call these types of incidents disasters. It is important to remember that the term disaster has a specific legal meaning. States and localities declare a "state of emergency." The president declares a "major disaster."

- **Types of disasters**—Several events have the potential to cause mass casualty incidents:
  - Natural disasters (floods, winter storms, hurricanes, tornados)
  - Technical hazards (Haz-mat incidents, building collapse)
  - Transportation accidents (road, rail, aircraft, ship, etc.)
  - Civil and political disorder (demonstrations, strikes, riots)
  - Criminal or terrorist incidents
- **Mass casualty incidents**—A mass casualty incident (or MCI) is any incident that injures or causes illness in enough people to overwhelm the resources usually available in a particular system or region.

Goals of MCI Management

1. Do the greatest good for the greatest number
2. Manage scarce resources
3. Do not relocate the disaster

- MCIs place great demands on resources, including equipment, rescuers, and facilities. Our goal as responders is not to relocate the disaster!
- Patient prioritization at the scene is important for effective patient distribution.
- Don't send all of the red patients to one hospital.

Stages of an Incident

- Initial notification
- Implementation
- Operations
- Escalation
- Stabilization
- De-escalation
- Termination

EMS Initial Response Roles and Responsibilities

- **Initial response roles**—EMS is a specific component of the overall incident management system. The first arriving unit should start the following actions:
- **First arriving unit**—The first emergency response unit to arrive at a mass casualty incident is by default "in charge" (the incident commander) until relieved. As a result, the individuals on the first emergency response unit must take immediate actions to begin to manage the entire incident. These actions may be the most important steps taken in the entire incident. The initial unit must resist the "temptation" to begin one-on-one patient care.
- **Assess scene for safety**—The object is to ensure no one else gets hurt. Assess the scene for safety much as you would for a normal response to any EMS incident—except that the scene is much bigger and requires a wider look. The following may pose a hazard:
  - Fire
  - Electrical hazards
  - Spilled or contained flammable liquids
  - Hazardous materials
  - Nuclear, chemical or biological agents
  - Other life threats
  - Debris that poses a threat to rescuers or their vehicles
  - Secondary explosions

- **Scene size-up:**
  - How big is the incident and how bad is it?
  - What type of incident?
  - Approximate number of patients.
  - Severity of injuries.
  - Area involved, including problems with scene access.
- **Confirmation of incident:**
  - Report situation—Contact dispatch with your size-up information.
  - Request assistance—Resources and mutual aid if needed.
  - Notify the Medical Command Center to insure rapid hospital notification.
- **Setup**—Setup the scene for the best management of mass casualties by on-scene and responding resources, including:
  - Staging
  - Secure access and egress
  - Secure adequate space for work areas
    - — Triage, treatment, transportation

Simple Triage and Rapid Treatment (START)

Triage—Triage is a French word meaning "to sort."

Purpose of triage

1. Assigns treatment priorities
2. Separates MCI victims into easily identifiable groups
3. Determines required resources for treatment, transportation, and definitive care
4. Prioritization of patient distribution and transportation

Benefits of triage

1. Identifies patients who require rapid medical care to save life and limb.
2. Provides rational distribution of casualties.
3. Separating the minor injuries reduces the urgent burden on each hospital—An average of 10–15% of MCI patients are serious enough to require extended hospitalization.

What is START?

- START was developed by Hoag Hospital and the Newport Beach Fire Department to be used in the event of an MCI.
- START enables EMS providers to triage patients at an MCI in less than 60 seconds and is based on three observations:
  - Respirations
  - Circulation
  - Mental Status
- This triage method assures rapid initial assessment of all patients as the basis for assignment to treatment and as the first medical assessment of the incident.
- So how does it work?
  - Begin where you are.
  - Relocate green (minor) tag patients.
  - Move in an orderly pattern, taging patients as you go.
  - Maintain count (how many red, yellow, black, and green tags).
  - Provide minimal treatment.

- START permits rescuers to quickly and accurately categorize patients into four treatment groups:
  - **Red**—Immediate (highest priority). Typical problems are:
    - — R = Respirations/airway
    - — P = Perfusion/pulse
    - — M = Mental status
  - **Yellow**—Delayed (second priority). Typical problems are:
    - — Burn patients without airway problems
    - — Major or multiple bone or joint injuries
    - — Back and spine injuries
  - **Green**—Minor (third priority). Typical problems are:
    - — "Walking wounded." (The ability to "walk" does not necessarily mean that this is a "minor" patient. Minor cuts and bruises are acceptable criteria for this type of patient.)
    - — Minor painful swollen deformities
    - — Minor soft tissue injuries
  - **Black**—Dead/nonsalvageable (lowest priority). These are nonbreathing patients to whom resuscitation would normally be attempted but who are not salvageable given the resources available early in an MCI response.

The START Process

- Begin where you stand.
- Identify those injured who can walk. Make a clear announcement that those who can walk should get up and do so to an easily recognized point.

Relocate green patients

- Relocate to a designated area (away from immediate danger and outside the initial triage area).
- Tag each of these as a green patient.

Triage patients in an orderly pattern

- Move through the patients in an orderly pattern.
- Assess each casualty and mark the category using triage ribbons or triage tags.

Maintain a patient count

- Maintain a count of the casualties.
- Mark on 2–3 in. tape on thigh.
- Save a small piece of triage ribbon and place in your pocket.

Steps in START Assessment (Figure 40-1)

Step 1—Move green tag patients.

Step 2—Respiration. Check for respiratory compromise.

- If airway is closed, open the airway.
- None—**black** tag (dead).
- More than 30 per minute—**red** tag (immediate).
- Less than 30 per minute—**further evaluation required**—go to step 3 (perfusion).

Step 3—Perfusion. Radial pulse check.

- Not palpable—**red** tag (immediate).

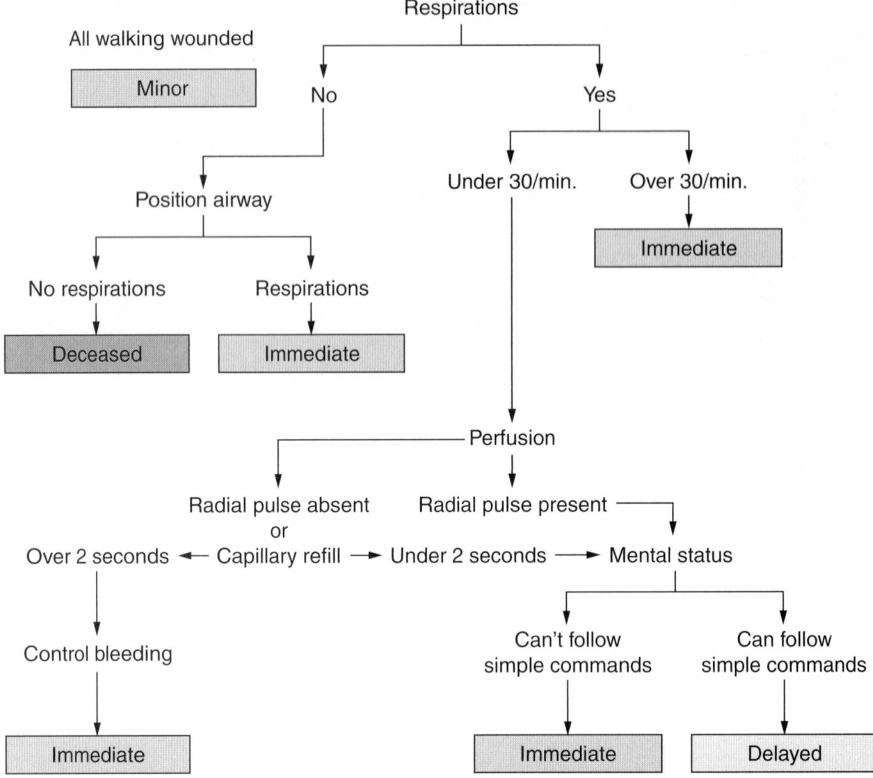

Figure 40-1 START flowchart. (*From* http://www.citmt.org/start/flowchart.htm#Detailed.)

- Control severe bleeding—bystanders use direct pressure, raise legs.
- Palpable—**further evaluation required**—go to step 4 (mental status).

Step 4—Mental status. Check for compromise of mental status.

- Altered mental status—**red** tag (immediate).
- Mental status appropriate—**yellow** tag (delayed) or **green** (minor) according to other findings (obvious injuries or illnesses).

Late in the evening, an F-3 tornado touched down in your county. Radar tracking reported that the tornado moved approximately 15 miles along the ground, including traveling across the edge of one town of approximately 50,000 people. First reports from the scene indicate that multiple homes in the town were destroyed or damaged extensively and there could be injuries or fatalities.

It is still raining in places and a tornado watch still exists in your county. Reports from the first arriving units are still coming in but there are numerous casualties reported on Main Street. Your unit arrives on scene; the incident commander summons you to a group home were civilians went to seek refuge. There are reports of multiple patients with injuries. You and your partner are sent to begin utilizing the START system. Utilizing the START system, triage and give each patient a priority.

? CHAPTER QUESTIONS

Based on the preceding scenario, utilizing the START system, triage and give each patient a priority tag.

1. **Patient Description:**
   Female patient, 42 years old
   Visible presenting problem:
   Partial amputation of 1st, 2nd, and 3rd digits on right hand, burns to both hands
   Respirations:
   Regular, 22/minute
   Radial pulse:
   Weak, 112 bpm
   Mental status:
   Alert
   a. Red tag
   b. Green tag
   c. Yellow tag
   d. Black tag
2. **Patient Description:**
   Female patient, 2 years old
   Visible presenting problem:
   Right radius/ulna fracture
   Respirations:
   Shallow, 34 bpm
   Radial pulse:
   Thready weak, 142 bpm
   Mental status:
   Confused
   a. Red tag
   b. Green tag
   c. Yellow tag
   d. Black tag
3. **Patient Description:**
   Male patient, 65 years old
   Visible presenting problem:
   Difficulty breathing
   Respirations:
   Shallow, 28 bpm
   Radial pulse:
   Weak, 100 bpm
   Mental status:
   Confused
   a. Red tag
   b. Green tag
   c. Yellow tag
   d. Black tag

4. **Patient Description:**
   Male patient, 42 years old
   Visible presenting problem:
   Partial thickness burns to both hands and arms, respiratory track irritation
   Respirations:
   Regular, 20 bpm
   Radial pulse:
   Thready weak, 114 bpm
   Mental status:
   Alert
   a. Red tag
   b. Green tag
   c. Yellow tag
   d. Black tag
5. **Patient Description:**
   Male patient, 22 years old
   Visible presenting problem:
   Difficulty breathing, coughing up blood-tinged sputum
   Respirations:
   Shallow, 28 bpm
   Radial pulse:
   Thready weak, 114 bpm
   Mental status:
   Confused
   a. Red tag
   b. Green tag
   c. Yellow tag
   d. Black tag
6. **Patient Description:**
   Female patient, 25 years old
   Visible presenting problem:
   Contusion to left side of forehead
   Respirations:
   Absent (even after repositioning)
   Radial pulse:
   Thready weak, 114 bpm
   Mental status:
   Unresponsive
   a. Red tag
   b. Green tag
   c. Yellow tag
   d. Black tag
7. **Patient Description:**
   Male patient, 14 years old
   Visible presenting problem:
   Scalp laceration

Respirations:
Steady, 24 bpm
Radial pulse:
Strong, 112 bpm
Mental status:
Alert, but anxious
a. Red tag
b. Green tag
c. Yellow tag
d. Black tag

8. **Patient Description:**
Female patient, 72 years old
Visible presenting problem:
Right ankle fracture
Respirations:
Steady, 12 bpm
Radial pulse:
Weak, thready, irregular, 62 bpm
Mental status:
Alert
a. Red tag
b. Green tag
c. Yellow tag
d. Black tag

9. **Patient Description:**
Male patient, 35 years old
Visible presenting problem:
Abrasion on posterior thorax
Respirations:
Steady, 16 bpm
Radial pulse:
Strong, 90 bpm
Mental status:
Alert
a. Red tag
b. Green tag
c. Yellow tag
d. Black tag

10. **Patient Description:**
Male patient, 21 years old
Visible presenting problem:
Partially decapitated
Respirations:
Absent
Radial pulse:
Absent

Mental status:

Unresponsive

a. Red tag

b. Green tag

c. Yellow tag

d. Black tag

Suggested Readings

US Department of Transportation, National Highway Traffic Safety Administration. *EMT-Paramedic: National Standard Curriculum*. Washington, DC: US Department of Transportation, National Highway Traffic Safety Administration; 1998.

www.fema.gov/emergency/nims/index.shtm.

www.usfa.dhs.gov/training/. Accessed on May 23, 2007.

Chapter 41

Rescue Awareness and Operations

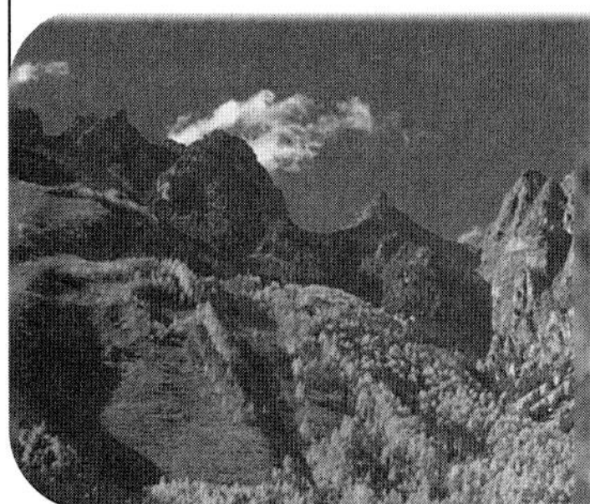

During an extended rescue operation in a remote wilderness area, you are treating a patient who has fallen 150 ft into a valley. The patient has been stabilized and you have treated any immediate life-threatening problems. You are notified by the incident commander that it may be an hour before the helicopter is able to extract the patient from the accident scene.

During this time, what is your highest priority?

- Rescue is defined as "the act of delivery from danger or imprisonment."
- Many day-to-day activities of emergency medical service (EMS) providers and other public service agencies are embraced by this definition when they are called to care for persons who are traumatized or stranded.
- Rescue is a patient-driven event (no patient, no rescue), and requires specialized medical and mechanical skills, with the right amount of each being applied at the appropriate time.

APPROPRIATE TRAINING FOR RESCUE OPERATIONS

- Requires training and expertise so that medical and mechanical skills are carefully balanced. Success of a rescue is dependent on a coordinated effort between medical care and specialized rescue effort that allows for the following:
  - Patient access and assessment for treatment needs
  - Treatment to begin at the site
  - Release from entrapment or imprisonment
  - Medical care to continue throughout the incident

Role of the Paramedic in Rescue Operations

- Systems operations approach.
  - Most rescue operations in the United States are provided by this approach. Extrication activities are usually performed by fire service personnel, specialized units, or both.
  - Patient care activities are the responsibility of the EMS provider.
- Second type of system provides rescue services by fire, EMS, or law-enforcement agencies that have "cross-trained" personnel. Roles and responsibilities for rescue and patient care are shared in this system.

- Primary role of the paramedic in rescue operations.
  - Have proper training and appropriate personal protective equipment (PPE) to allow access and the provision of treatment at the site and continuing throughout the incident.
- As first responders, the paramedic should:
  - Understand hazards associated with various environments
  - Know when gaining access or attempting rescue is safe or unsafe
  - Have skills to effect a rescue when safe and necessary
  - Understand the rescue process and when certain techniques are indicated or contraindicated
  - Be skilled in patient packaging techniques to allow for safe extrication and medical care
- Safety is important because of the potential for associated risks that may involve:
  - Hazardous materials
  - Inclement weather
  - Temperature extremes
  - Fire
  - Electrical hazards
  - Toxic gases
  - Unstable structures
  - Heavy equipment
  - Road hazards
  - Sharp edges and fragments
- Initial scene assessment for hazards, personal protective measures, and constant monitoring throughout the operation are essential.
- Safety priorities include:
  - Personal safety
  - Safety of the crew
  - Safety of bystanders
  - Rescue of the trapped and injured
- When the well-trained and properly equipped rescuer acts safely, remaining vigilant for hazards, he or she minimizes the risk of personal injury and of complicating the scene by becoming another patient who requires care and possibly extrication.
- Crew is the support team for the rescuer.
  - Crew safety is essential to ensure an effective operation and provide mutual support for each member of the team.
  - Operating with disregard for the safety of fellow team members increases risk of injuries and complications of the operation.
- Uninvolved people must be evacuated and kept clear of hazards.
  - Bystanders or untrained *helpers* only increase the risk of additional injuries and complications of the rescue operation.
- Rescue of the trapped or injured is the last priority.
  - These people are already trapped or injured.
  - Carrying out the first three priorities safely maximizes the chance for a successful rescue.

PHASES OF A RESCUE OPERATION

- The seven phases of a rescue operation include:
  - Arrival and scene size-up
  - Hazard control

- Gaining access to the patient
- Medical treatment
- Disentanglement
- Patient packaging
- Transportation

Arrival and Scene Size-Up

- Requires the paramedic to determine what is needed at a particular emergency event. This is performed quickly by gathering facts about the situation, analyzing the problems, and determining the appropriate response.
- Scene size-up involves continuous evaluation of the emergency scene.
- The paramedic must constantly be alert to situations that may change the needs of a particular incident.
- Paramedics should establish command and conduct a scene assessment.
- Determine the number of patients and triage as necessary.
- Determine if the situation is a search, rescue, or body recovery.
- Perform a risk versus benefit analysis.
- Request additional resources as required by the situation.
- ICS should be used as a command/control mechanism.
- Make a realistic *time* estimate in accessing and evacuating.
- En route, gather as much information about the situation as possible.
- Essential information includes the following:
  - Exact location
  - Type of occupancy (manufacturing, mercantile, residence)
  - Number of victims
  - Type of situation
  - Hazards
- Weather conditions can affect rescue attempts, patient status, and the need to expedite the operation.

Description of the Scene

- Highly populated areas (high-rise school, shopping mall) may require specialized vehicles and equipment.
- Rural or wilderness settings may require helicopter rescue or special resources.
- Hazardous materials may require specialized response.
- Decontamination may be needed for bystanders, patients, and rescue personnel.
- Time of day may dictate scene requirements.
  - Rush-hour traffic
  - Crowd control
  - Additional lighting
- Resources that may be needed to handle an emergency event include:
  - Additional emergency vehicles for large numbers of patients
  - Area hospital availability and personnel
  - Aeromedical services
  - Law enforcement
  - Fire service for auto extrication, fire suppression, or lighting
  - Water rescue, teams with self-contained underwater breathing apparatus (SCUBA), and other specialized rescue units

  - Hazardous materials teams
  - Urban search and rescue teams

Hazard Control

- Identify and control as many hazards as possible.
- Manage, reduce, and minimize the risks from the uncontrollable hazards.
- Make the scene as safe as possible.
- Ensure all personnel are in PPE appropriate for the situation.

Gaining Access to the Patient

- Critical component in patient's eventual outcome.
- The trauma patient may require the following:
  - Rapid assessment
  - Stabilization
  - Extrication
  - Rapid transportation
- Extrication tools and equipment:
  - Use minimum force needed to reduce risk of injury
  - Clear the area of unnecessary people
  - Keep extraneous noise to a minimum
- Safety officer should stay alert for stresses of the operation.
  - Rotate personnel to avoid heat exposure and injuries related to fatigue
- Use personal protective clothing.
- Use protective covering for the patient.
- Paramedics have primary responsibility for patient care, and serve an important role as observers for potentially hazardous procedures.

Medical Management

- Provide medical management appropriate for the situation; this may include the following:
  - Spinal immobilization
  - Airway management and ventilation
  - Oxygen administration
  - Intravenous (IV) fluid therapy
- If a rapidly fatal or potentially fatal condition is recognized, "load and go."
- Physical examination should be performed after the initial assessment is complete and life-threatening conditions have been stabilized.
- Another crew member may perform the examination simultaneously if it does not interrupt the initial assessment and emergency interventions.

Disentanglement

- Involves making a pathway through the wreckage of an accident and removing wreckage from patients (release from physical entrapment)
- Methods must be driven by patient's needs
- Perform a "risk versus benefit" analysis that considers personal safety
- Assess the need for specialized equipment and techniques
- Be aware of available resources and how to mobilize them

Patient Packaging

- Packaging refers to physical stabilization and preparation for transport
- May require special rescue capabilities (moving patients over hazardous terrain, lifting patients by hoist to a helicopter)
- Coordination of activities and patient care responsibilities offer greatest chance of successful outcome
- Coordination of the removal phase
  - Paramedic responsibilities
    - Ensure that the patient is ready to be removed
    - Protect the patient from additional injury during disentanglement and egress
    - Provide the patient with protective cover
      - Blankets
      - Tarpaulins
      - Ear and eye protection
    - Apply supplemental oxygen via a face mask to patient
      - Protects patient from toxic fumes when present
    - Stabilize the cervical spine
    - Immobilize patient on long spine board
    - Secure IV lines, oxygen tubing
    - Immobilize extremity fractures and cover open wounds if time permits
- Consider use of other patient care equipment as the patient is removed from the area of entrapment
- Communication and coordination with other rescuers should continue during this process
- Exit pathway must be clear and secure
- There should be no additional danger for the patient or the rescuers during the removal phase

Transportation

- Have a wheeled stretcher, basket stretcher, or long spine board available
- Consider equipment needs and personnel for moving the patient
- Transport vehicle should be appropriately warmed or cooled for patient comfort
- During transport, continue patient care and advise medical direction of patient status

RESCUER PERSONAL PROTECTIVE EQUIPMENT

Rescuer Protection

- EMS PPE historically has been adapted from other fields.
- EMS does not have a national uniform trauma reporting system to identify potential work-related exposures.
- Risk management and PPE design need to be driven by data.
- It generally is agreed that EMS providers involved in rescue and other rescue personnel should have access to the following PPE:
  - Impact-resistant protective helmet with ear protection and chin strap
  - Safety goggles with an elastic strap and vents to prevent fogging
  - Lightweight "turnout" coat that is puncture resistant
  - Slip-resistant, waterproof gloves

  - Boots with steel insoles and steel toe protection
  - Self-contained breathing apparatus (SCBA)
- The same PPE is not appropriate in all situations.
  - PPE must be appropriate for the situation encountered
  - PPE may not prevent exposure to infectious disease but it does minimize risk
- PPE that may be appropriate in some rescue situations:
  - Head protection that meets safety standards for the appropriate application
    - Compact firefighters' helmet meeting NFPA standards adequate for most vehicle/structural applications
    - Climbing helmet for confined space and technical rescue applications
    - Padded rafting/kayaking helmet for water rescue
  - Eye protection
    - Adequate face shield (face shields on most fire helmets are inadequate)
    - ANSI-approved safety glasses/goggles with solid shields are preferred
  - Hearing protection
    - Required for high-noise areas
    - Ear plugs or ear muffs should be available
  - Hand protection
    - Gloves that allow for adequate dexterity and protection from cuts/punctures
  - Foot protection
    - Gear that provides ankle support to limit range of motion
    - Tread to provide traction and prevent slips
    - Insulation from environmental extremes
    - Steel toe/shank that meets safety requirements
  - Flame/flash protection when danger from fire exists
    - Nomex/PBI/flame-retardant cotton to provide limited flash protection, turnout clothing, jumpsuits/flyers/coveralls
  - Personal flotation device (PFD) when operating on or around water
    - Must meet coast guard standards for flotation
    - Type III preferred for most water rescue work
    - Should have whistle and strobe light attached
    - Knife for cutting should be attached
  - Visibility
    - Reflective trim should be on all outerwear
    - Orange clothing or safety vests should be used during highway operations
  - Extended, remote, or wilderness protection
    - Additional/different PPE must be considered for bad weather conditions not normally encountered (e.g., cold, rain, snow, wind)
    - Personal drinking water and snacks
    - Possible shelter needs

Personal Protection from Bloodborne Pathogens

- Occupational Safety and Health Administration (OSHA) has established criteria for workplace protection from bloodborne and airborne diseases.
- Measures for personal protection should be observed whenever there is a potential for exposure to communicable diseases.

SURFACE WATER RESCUE

- People are drawn to moving water for recreation. Many people (including rescuers) underestimate the power and hazards of water.
- Hydraulics of moving water is affected by:
  - Depth and velocity of water
  - Obstructions to flow

Obstructions to Flow

- Water that moves over a uniform obstruction can create recirculating currents ("drowning machines") that can trap victims and make escape difficult.
- Recirculating currents are commonly found in rivers and on "low head" dams.
  - Height of the dam is no indication of the degree of hazard
- Force of the moving water is very deceptive and makes for a hazardous rescue.
- Trapped victims often succumb to fatigue, hypothermia, and drowning.
- Strainers are obstructions (e.g., trees, grating, wire/mesh) that allow current to flow through, yet can trap objects such as boats or people.
  - Force of the water against the victim makes escape difficult
  - Rescuers must cautiously approach strainers to avoid their own entrapment
- Foot/extremity pin:
  - It is considered unsafe to walk in fast moving water over knee depth
    - — Extremity may become trapped in a strainer
    - — Victim is dragged under the surface of the water
  - If a foot or extremity pin occurs, body part must be extricated from entrapment in the same way it went in

Flat Water

- About 3900 deaths occur each year in flat (static) water (lakes, ponds, and marsh) from drowning. Factors that contribute to these deaths include:
  - Alcohol or other drug use
  - Cool water temperature that leads to hypothermia
- PFDs routinely worn and fastened properly when on or around the water can save lives by decreasing the likelihood of drowning.

Water Temperature

- Immersion in water that has a temperature less than 98°F (36.67°C) can cause hypothermia.
  - A human cannot maintain body heat in water below 92°F (33.33°C).
  - Water causes heat loss 25 times faster than exposure to air at the same temperature. The colder the water, the faster the rate of heat loss.
- A person who experiences a 15- to 20-minute immersion in 35°F (1.67°C) water will likely die from hypothermia and drowning.
- Sudden immersion in cold water may trigger laryngospasm that can lead to:
  - Aspiration
  - Severe hypoxia
  - Unconsciousness
- Hypothermic patients rapidly lose the ability for self-rescue.
  - Sudden immersion in cold water may trigger laryngospasm
  - Hypothermic victims are unable to follow directions (e.g., grab a safety device)

- ◦ Hypothermia increases the likelihood of drowning
  - ◦ Victims become incapacitated and unable to help themselves to safety
- Water temperature varies widely with seasons and runoff.
  - ◦ Even on warm days water temperature can be very low.
- PFDs lessen heat loss and energy required for flotation.
  - ◦ If sudden immersion occurs, a single victim should assume HELP position.
  - ◦ If multiple people are in the water, they should huddle to decrease heat loss.
- Cold protective response or mammalian diving reflex increases the chance of a victim's survival in cold water.
  - ◦ Protective physiological response
    - — Face immersion in cold water causes parasympathetic stimulation. Heart rate decreases (bradycardia)
    - — Peripheral vasoconstriction shunts blood to the core.
    - — Hypotension.
  - ◦ Effectiveness of this response is affected by
    - — Victim's age
    - — Posture in the water
    - — Lung volume
    - — Temperature of the water
  - ◦ Rapid development of hypothermia can sometimes improve brain viability in patients with prolonged submersion
    - — Hypothermic patients should be presumed salvageable
    - — "A victim is never cold and dead—only warm and dead"
    - — Patient must be rewarmed in a hospital before an accurate assessment can be made

Rescue vs. Body Recovery

- Besides water temperature, other factors that affect a patient's clinical outcome after a submersion incident include:
  - ◦ Length of time of submersion
  - ◦ Known or suspected trauma
  - ◦ Environmental conditions
  - ◦ Age and physical condition
  - ◦ Time until rescue or removal has been achieved
- Because successful resuscitation with full neurological recovery has occurred in near-drowning victims with prolonged submersion in extremely cold water, resuscitation should be initiated by rescuers at the scene unless there is obvious physical evidence of death.
  - ◦ Putrefaction
  - ◦ Dependent lividity
  - ◦ Rigor mortis

In-Water Spinal Immobilization

- Requires special training. Only rescuers trained in water rescue should enter the water.
- Steps for in-water spinal immobilization:
  - ◦ Primary rescuer maintains spinal immobilization and the patient's airway
  - ◦ Second rescuer determines cervical collar size and holds open collar under the victim's neck

- ◦ Second rescuer brings collar up to back of victim's neck
  - — Primary rescuer allows second rescuer to bring collar around victim's neck and throat while maintaining the airway
- ◦ Second rescuer secures fastener on collar while primary rescuer maintains the airway
- ◦ Second rescuer secures victim's hands at victim's waist
- ◦ Patient is back-boarded and extricated
  - — Submerge the board under the victim at the waist.
  - — Never lift the victim to the board. Allow the board to float up to the victim.
  - — Secure the victim with straps, cravats, or other devices.
  - — Move the victim to an extrication point at shore or boat.
  - — Extricate the victim headfirst so that body weight will not compress possible spinal trauma.
  - — Avoid extrication of victim through surf because the board could collapse.
  - — Maintain the patient's airway during extrication.

Summary of Rescue Techniques

- Never underestimate the power of moving water.
  - ◦ Moving water is very deceptive
  - ◦ Do not enter without highly specialized training
- Water rescue model is reach-throw-row-go.
  - ◦ If the victim is close to shore, reach with an oar, large branch, pole, or other long rescue device.
  - ◦ Throw a flotation device to the victim such as, a water throw bag attached to polypropylene rope. Become proficient with a water throw bag.
  - ◦ Row out to the victim in a boat (if one is available).
  - ◦ Go—If a boat is unavailable and reach and throw methods are not options, trained rescuers should go to the patient by wading or swimming.
- For a first responder, a shore-based rescue attempt (by talking the victim into self-rescue, reaching, or throwing) is the method of choice.
- Even with shore-based rescue techniques a PFD must be worn.
- Ensure secure footing to avoid being pulled into the water by the victim.
- Self-rescue techniques if fallen into flat or moving water:
  - ◦ Cover mouth/nose during entry
  - ◦ Protect your head and keep face out of the water
  - ◦ If in flat water, assume the HELP position
  - ◦ If in moving water, do not attempt to stand up
  - ◦ Float on back with feet downstream and head pointed toward the nearest shore at a 45° angle

HAZARDOUS ATMOSPHERES

- Oxygen-deficient environments can occur in confined spaces. A confined space is one with limited access or egress, not designed for human occupancy or habitation. Examples of confined spaces include the following:
  - ◦ Grain bins and silos
  - ◦ Wells and cisterns
  - ◦ Storage tanks

- Manholes and pumping stations
- Drainage culverts
- Underground vaults
- Trenches and cave-ins

Hazards Associated with Confined Spaces

- Six major hazards are associated with confined spaces:
  - Oxygen-deficient atmospheres
  - Chemical/toxic exposure/explosion
  - Engulfment
  - Machinery entrapment
  - Electricity
  - Structural concerns

Oxygen-Deficient Atmospheres

- Oxygen-deficient atmospheres are not a visible problem.
- Rescuers often presume an atmosphere is safe.
- Available oxygen in confined spaces must be tested by trained personnel using an atmospheric monitoring meter at the top, middle, and bottom of a confined space before entry.
  - Any confined space that has an oxygen concentration less than 19.5% must be considered an atmospheric hazard.
  - Oxygen level that is too high (above 22%) in a confined space also may produce rapid combustion and is a serious safety hazard.
  - Be aware that increased oxygen content can give atmospheric monitoring meters a false reading.

Chemical/Toxic Exposure/Explosion

- Oxygen can be removed from the atmosphere by certain chemical reactions.
  - Chemical reactions that occur during the formation of rust on steel structures and while pouring concrete
  - Natural decaying processes that displace oxygen by producing dangerous gases (e.g., methane)
- The presence of some chemicals and gases can lead to toxic exposure, and many carry a high risk of explosion.
- Toxic gases that may be found in confined spaces:
  - Hydrogen sulfide (H_2S)
  - Carbon dioxide (CO_2)
  - Carbon monoxide (CO)
  - Chlorine (Cl)
  - Low/high oxygen (O_2) concentrations
  - Methane (CH_4)
  - Ammonia (NH_3)
  - Nitrogen dioxide (NO_2)
- Some dusts and particulate materials found in grain bins, silos, and storage tanks can be highly explosive when mixed with air.
- Presence of toxic or explosive gases in confined spaces should be monitored by trained personnel with an appropriate testing device.

Engulfment

- Mechanical entrapment can occur when earth, grain, coal, or any other dry material that can flow engulfs a person in a confined space.
- Can produce an oxygen-deficient atmosphere and subsequent suffocation.
- Persons trapped by engulfment may be victims of physical (crushing) injury.
  - Are at increased risk for explosive hazards

Machinery Entrapment

- Machinery found in some structures (e.g., grain bins and silos) often have augers, screws, conveyors, and other machinery to move material stored in them.
- These and other mechanical devices can entrap a person, requiring extrication.
- Before attempting rescue, trained and experienced personnel should identify and secure all mechanical devices.

Electricity

- Electrical hazards from the power supply of motors and materials management equipment may be present.
- All electrical devices (e.g., electrical boxes and switches) must be identified and secured by experienced personnel.
- This "lockout process" must prevent any unauthorized person from entering the area or gaining access to the controls that have been shut off.
- Motors and other electrical devices can "store" power that can lead to entrapment or injury.

Structural Concerns

- Supporting structures of a confined space must be identified before entry.
- Most cylindrical structures are supported by central I-beams that make for relatively easy maneuvering.
- Noncylindrical structures may have L-, T-, and X-shaped spaces.
  - Can affect entry and rescue procedures and compound the extrication pathway

Crush Compartment Syndromes Secondary to Entrapment

- Compartment syndromes can be caused by crushing mechanisms leading to:
  - Ischemic muscle damage
  - Tissue necrosis
  - Crush syndrome
- Injuries can be severe and are associated with the following:
  - Internal organ rupture
  - Major fractures
  - Hemorrhagic shock
- Degree of injury produced by the crushing force depends on the following:
  - Amount of pressure applied to the body
  - Amount of time the pressure remains in contact with the body
  - Specific body region in which the injury occurs
- Massive crush injury to vital organs may cause immediate death.
- Patients with crush syndrome are victims of compressive forces that crush tissue, causing prolonged hypoxia.

- Patients may appear stable for hours or days, as long as the compressive forces remain in place.
- When the patient is released from the entrapment, reperfusion to the trapped body part may lead to the following:
  - Volume loss into the tissue
  - Release of myoglobin, lactic acid, and other toxins into the circulation
- These events occur simultaneously, and may ultimately lead to death.
- If the patient's condition or mechanism of injury is suspicious for compartment syndrome or crush injury, consult with medical direction.

- Management of crush syndrome is controversial.
- Prehospital care must be supervised through a medical direction physician familiar with this pathological process.

Emergencies in Confined Spaces

- OSHA requires a permit process before workers may enter a confined space.
  - Area must be made safe or workers must don PPE
  - Fall-arresting and retrieval devices must be in place
  - Environmental monitoring must be available at the site before entry
- Nonpermitted sites are likely locations for emergencies.
  - No atmospheric monitoring is done
  - Entrants are likely to encounter oxygen-deficient atmosphere
- Other types of emergencies that can occur in confined spaces (in both permitted and nonpermitted locations) include the following:
  - Falls
  - Medical emergencies
  - Explosion
  - Entrapment
  - Exposure to toxic gases and chemicals
- Safe entry for rescuers.
  - Safe entry for rescuers in a confined space operation requires specialized training
  - No rescuer should make entry until a rescue team has made the area safe
  - Safe entry cannot be made without the following:
    - Proper and thorough training in confined space rescue
    - Atmospheric monitoring to determine oxygen concentration, hydrogen sulfide level, carbon monoxide, explosive limits, flammable atmosphere, and toxic air contaminants
    - Proper ventilation
    - Secured electrical systems (lockout/tagout of all power)
    - Dissipation of stored energy
    - Disconnection of all pipes (blinding/blanking) to prevent flow into the site
    - Appropriate respiratory protection
- Supplied air breathing apparatus (SABA).
  - Because close quarters make gaining access and extrication difficult in confined space rescue, use of the typical "bottle-on-back" SCBA is usually dangerous
    - Provides limited air supply
    - Can cause entrapment
    - May have to be removed to make some entries

- ◦ Supplied air or air-line breathing apparatus is preferred in confined space operations
  - — Lightweight device
  - — Provides a nearly unlimited supply of air from an air-supply device located outside the confined space
  - — Potential complications of the SABA
    - Damaged or entangled air lines
    - Limitations imposed by the length of the air hose
  - — Trained rescuers carry a small, personal reserve air supply ("escape bottle") that can be used for a short time if needed
- Arriving at the scene.
  - ◦ Perform a scene size-up
    - — Determine the nature of the emergency by obtaining a copy of the OSHA permit for the site from the permit/entry supervisor
    - — Determine the number of workers (victims) in the confined space
  - ◦ Request specialized rescue teams
  - ◦ Establish a safe perimeter away from the incident and allow only rescue team members to enter the space
  - ◦ Assist workers at the site with any remote retrieval devices they may be using

Rescue from Trenches/Cave-Ins

- Most trench collapses occur in trenches less than 12 ft deep and 6 ft wide.
- Federal law requires either shoring or a "trench box" for evacuations that are 5 ft or deeper.
  - ◦ These collapses often occur when contractors forsake safety measures because of the increased costs in providing them
- Factors that contribute to collapse include the following:
  - ◦ Lips on one or both sides of the trench that cave in
  - ◦ Walls that shear away and cave in
  - ◦ Excavated dirt piled too close to the edge, causing collapse
  - ◦ Presence of intersecting trenches
  - ◦ Ground vibrations
  - ◦ Water seepage
- Arriving at the scene.
  - ◦ When arriving at the scene where a collapse has occurred, causing burial, be aware that a second collapse is likely to occur and one should not approach the lip.
  - ◦ Rescue attempts by EMS personnel should not be made unless the trench is less than waist deep.
  - ◦ Steps in scene management include:
    - — Securing the scene, establishing command, and securing a safe perimeter
    - — Shutting down nonessential equipment that can cause vibrations
    - — Requesting specialized rescue teams
    - — Preventing entry into the trench or cave-in area
  - ◦ Access to the patient should be attempted by trained personnel only after proper shoring is in place.
  - ◦ Shoring and excavating can be labor and time intensive.
  - ◦ Scene safety is necessary for a successful recovery.

HIGHWAY OPERATIONS

- Traffic flow is the largest hazard in EMS highway operations.
  - Associated highway hazards:
    - — Emergency responses to limited and unlimited access highways
    - — Emergency vehicle crashes
    - — Backed-up traffic that impedes access and egress from the incident scene.
  - Because of the potential problems in traffic flow, EMS personnel must work closely with law enforcement to help ensure a safe response.
  - Techniques to reduce traffic hazards:
    - — Position an apparatus (pumper, rescue, or other emergency vehicle) across the traffic way ("fend-off" position) to protect the scene from traffic hazards
    - — Stage unnecessary apparatus off of highway (essential on limited access highways); establish staging area away from scene
    - — Position an apparatus to reduce traffic flow and provide for a safe ambulance loading area
    - — Use only essential warning lights so that drivers are not distracted or confused

      Consider the use of amber scene lighting

      Turn off headlights that might blind nearby motorists
    - — Use traffic cones and flares to redirect traffic away from workers and to create a safe zone

      Use flares safely in proximity to the scene

      Do not extinguish once ignited
    - — Ensure all rescuers wear high-visibility clothing (e.g., orange highway vests, reflective trim)
  - Other scene hazards associated with highway operations include:
    - — Fuel/fire hazards
    - — Electrical power
    - — Unstable vehicles
    - — Air bags/supplemental restraint systems (SRS)
    - — Hazardous cargoes

Fuel/Fire Hazards

- Gasoline spills are a common fire hazard for EMS providers.
- Decrease risk that flammable liquids will ignite by one of the following methods:
  - Turning off the vehicle ignition switch
  - Forbidding smoking
  - Avoiding use of flares near the spill
- Approach the scene with fire extinguishers and have the extinguishers ready throughout extrication.
- Ideally, a fire apparatus with a charged hose line should be on the scene.
- Car battery of a crashed car generally should be left connected to operate power electric door locks, windows, seat mechanisms, and trunks.
  - If the battery is to be disabled, disconnect the "ground" cable first to reduce the chance of "sparking," which may ignite spilled fuel or leaking battery gases
  - Battery cable can be cut with wire cutters or disconnected with battery pliers
  - Disconnected cable should be folded back onto itself and securely taped to insulate it from any bare metal contact that might reestablish the electrical ground to the system
  - Both cables should be disconnected and secured

- Vehicle fires.
  - Most result from ruptured fuel tanks or fuel lines.
  - Do not attempt to fight fully involved vehicle fires unless trained to do so.
  - Trapped victims should be removed if possible.
  - All actions must be directed toward rescuer safety and protection.
    - Crouch low and approach vehicle from side
    - Stay clear of bumpers that may "fly off" during fire conditions
    - Wear personal protective equipment

Electrical Power

- Downed electrical wires are dangerous
  - Modern transformers are programmed to retest broken circuits at certain intervals
    - "Dead" lines may suddenly surge with lethal current
  - Only utility workers and trained rescuers should secure downed electrical wires
- If a vehicle is in contact with downed wires
  - Advise persons inside to remain inside unless there is risk of explosion or fire
  - Leaving vehicle poses significant risk of electrical injury
- Never approach the patient until scene is safe
- Do not proceed into area if a tingling sensation in the feet, legs, or thorax is experienced
- If patient contact is necessary, use nonconductive equipment
  - Leather gauntlets
  - Wooden poles
  - Polypropylene rope
  - Other special equipment
- No equipment will provide absolute safety from electrical injury

Unstable Vehicles

- Must be stabilized before gaining access
- Standard methods include the following:
  - Supporting vehicle with wooden cribbing, wheel chocks, air bags
  - Securing vehicle with ropes and cables
  - Chaining vehicle to poles, trees, other vehicles and structures
- Management requires specialized training

Air bags/Supplemental Restraint Systems (SRS)

- Air bags as a supplemental restraint system have become a required safety feature in the United States.
- Three types of air bags:
  - Frontal-impact
  - Side-impact
  - Head-protection bags
- Air bags are generally considered an effective safety device in vehicle crashes.
  - Children and small adults in the passenger seat have, however, been fatally injured after air bag deployment
- Deployed air bags are not dangerous.

- Residue may cause minor skin or eye irritation
  - Wear gloves and eye protection
  - Keep residue away from patient/rescuer eyes and wounds
  - Wash thoroughly after exposure
- Incident with fire
  - Use the normal fire-extinguishing procedures
  - Although heat may trigger an undeployed air bag, it will not cause the activating canister to explode
- Incident with a deployed air bag
  - Use normal rescue procedures and equipment
  - Do not delay medical attention
  - Deployed air bags are not dangerous
  - Wear gloves and eye protection
  - Keep residue away from patients' eyes and wounds
  - Remove gloves and wash hands after exposure to residue
- Incident with an undeployed air bag
  - Undeployed air bag is unlikely to deploy after a crash
  - When a patient is pinned directly behind an undeployed air bag, special procedures should be followed:
    - — Disconnect or cut both battery cables
    - — Avoid placing your body or objects in front of the air bag module (the deployment path of the air bag)
    - — Do not mechanically displace or cut through the steering column until after the system has been fully deactivated
    - — Do not cut or drill into the air bag module
    - — Do not apply heat around the steering wheel hub

Hazardous Cargoes

- Most hazardous substances transported in the United States travel by road.
- Be suspicious of crashes involving commercial vehicles.
- Methods that can be used to identify carriers of hazardous cargoes include:
  - UN numbers
  - Placards

Auto Anatomy

- Basic understanding of auto anatomy is required during vehicle rescue operations. Important considerations:
  - Roof and roof support posts (A, B, C, and D posts)
    - — Cutting the supports interrupts the unibody construction
  - Fire wall
    - — Separates single engine and occupant compartment
    - — Frequently collapses onto occupants' legs during high-speed, head-on collisions
  - Engine compartment and power train
    - — Battery is usually in the engine compartment
  - Undercarriage and unibody versus frame construction
    - — Roof posts, floor, fire wall, trunk support are integral to unibody
    - — Most cars are of unibody construction
    - — Light trucks are usually of frame construction

- Safety glass versus tempered glass
  - — Safety glass (glass-plastic laminate glass), usually in windshield, is designed to stay intact when shattered or broken; fractures into long strands
  - — Tempered glass (high tensile strength) does not stay intact when shattered or broken; fractures into small pieces
- Doors
  - — Reinforcing bar in most car doors
  - — Designed to provide structural integrity during front and side collisions
  - — Case hardened steel "Nader" pin/latch is designed to prevent car door from opening during collisions
  - — If pin is engaged, it may be difficult to pry door open; it must be disengaged first

Rescue Strategies

- Should begin during initial size-up.
- Can sometimes be based on information provided by the dispatching center before arrival.
- After arriving on the scene:
  - Employ hazard control
  - Establish command
  - Call for appropriate backup
- Important elements of scene size-up include:
  - Scene safety (including protecting the scene from traffic hazards)
  - Location of the crash
  - Vehicle stability
  - Electrical hazards
  - Fire hazards
  - Hazardous materials
  - Special rescue needs
  - Number and location of patients
- After initial scene size-up and ensuring scene safety, assess the degree of entrapment and the fastest means of extrication.
- Attempt to gain access to trapped victims by first trying to open all car doors.
  - When a door cannot be readily opened by the patient or rescuer, try the side windows.
- Initial patient care can be provided until trained rescue personnel with extrication tools can safely remove the patient from the vehicle through:
  - Door removal
  - Roof removal
  - Front or rear windshield openings
  - Dash roll-up maneuver

HAZARDOUS TERRAIN

- Hazardous terrain can pose significant difficulties during rescue operations.
- Three common classifications of hazardous terrain are low-angle, high-angle, and flat terrain with obstructions.
  - Low-angle (steep slope)
    - — Refers to terrain that is capable of being walked on without the use of hands
    - — Secure footing may be difficult

— Difficult to carry a litter even with multiple rescuers
— Low-angle rescue
Rope used to counteract gravity during litter carry
Consequence of error likely to be a fall and tumble
◦ High-angle (vertical)
— Refers to cliff, building side, or terrain so steep hands must be used for balance when scaling it (slopes greater than 40°)
— Total dependence on rope or aerial apparatus for litter movement
— Consequence of error likely to be fatal
— Rappelling by trained personnel to retrieve victims is required in high-angle rescue
◦ Flat terrain
— May have various obstructions that can make rescue difficult
— Examples include level land with large rocks, loose soil (scree), and waterbeds or creeks
— Additional manpower and resources may be needed to safely extricate a victim and ensure safe litter movement

Patient Packaging Using Litters

- Basket stretcher standard for rough terrain evacuation
- Rigid frame provides protection for the victim
- Relatively easy to carry with adequate personnel
- Patients immobilized on a long backboard and secured in the basket
- Alternative spinal immobilization devices (vest-type devices) can be used with the basket stretcher
- Two basic designs: wire mesh (Stokes) and plastic
  - Wire mesh
    - Strongest of the baskets
    - Relatively inexpensive
    - Design allows for air and water to flow through the device, making it ideal in water rescue operations when used with supplemental flotation
  - Plastic basket stretchers
    - Weaker than steel mesh, but provide better protection for the patient
    - Plastic bottoms with steel frames are considered superior designs
- Most basket stretchers are equipped with adequate restraints
  - All require additional strapping or lacing (e.g., harness, leg stirrups) to prevent movement and padding for rough-terrain evacuation or extraction
  - A plastic helmet or litter shield should be available for patient protection
- Patient movement
  - Nontechnical/nonrope evacuation is usually faster
  - Flat rough terrain
    - Litter-carrying procedures
    - Leapfrogging
    - Adequate numbers of bearers
    - Load-lifting straps to assist with carry
  - Low-angle/high-angle evacuation
    - Secure anchors
    - Rope-lowering systems

- Rope-hauling systems
- Specialized knowledge and skill required for use
- Use of aerial apparatus
  - Tower-ladder or bucket trucks
    - Litter belay during movement to bucket
    - Attachment of litter to bucket
  - Aerial ladders
    - Upper sections not wide enough to slot litter
    - Litter must be belayed if being slid down ladder
  - Ladder or aerial apparatus should not be used as a crane to move a litter
- Moving a patient during low-angle and high-angle evacuations requires specialized knowledge and skills

- Litter-carrying procedures
  - Carrying a litter across rough, flat terrain requires a minimum of six rescuers
    - Four to carry the litter
    - Two to observe or "scout" for potential hazards (e.g., loose rocks, holes, tree branches)
  - Team members should be matched in height to ensure that equal weight is shared and that the litter remains level
  - Load-lifting straps are sometimes used to spread the weight of the load over other parts of the rescuer's body (e.g., around the rescuer's shoulders and back)

Helicopter Use in Hazardous Terrain Rescue

- Helicopters can be used for patient transport and for rescue operations.
- When used for rescue, the mission, crew, and capabilities of the helicopter team (civilian and military) are specific for rescue techniques versus providing medical care and transport.
- Rescue helicopter team has specialized knowledge and skills required to hover or land in tight places and to transport people and equipment.
- Special rescue techniques that these helicopters employ may include:
  - Cable hoisting to extract people from the ground
  - Short-haul ("sling loads") operations that allow personnel and equipment to be carried beneath the helicopter as an external load

ASSESSMENT PROCEDURES DURING RESCUE

Environmental Issues Affecting Assessment

- Weather and temperature extremes
  - Difficulty in completely exposing patients for full assessment and treatment
  - Physical examination compromised
  - Patients susceptible to hypothermia or hyperthermia
  - Rescuer mobility restricted due to clothing or PPE
- Access to patient may be limited
  - Parts may not be accessible for examination
  - Cramped space
  - Limited lighting
- Equipment limitations
- Patient may be trapped for an extended period
- Rescuer PPE essential but cumbersome

Specific Assessment/Management Considerations

During rescue operations, it may be necessary to downsize initial assessment and management equipment from normal boxes and "street packaging" so that it can be transported to the patient. Besides ensuring adequate lighting to perform assessment and treatment, the paramedic should have access to the necessary equipment to treat a patient during rescue operations.

Advanced Life Support (ALS) Skills

- Should only be provided if necessary. Good basic life support (BLS) skills, however, are mandatory.
- ALS equipment such as IV lines, endotracheal (ET) tubes, and electrocardiogram (ECG) leads will complicate the extrication process.
- Definitive airway control and volume replacement may, however, be essential.
- Airway control with supplemental oxygen administration must be a priority throughout the rescue event.
- Patient monitoring:
  - Monitor patient's vital signs and level of consciousness
  - In high-noise and limited-space areas take blood pressure (BP) by palpation
  - Compact devices such as pulse oximeter helpful
  - ECG cumbersome during extrication
  - Continue talking to patient
  - Explain what is being done and answer questions
  - Provide emotional support
- Improvisation:
  - Upper extremity fractures tied to torso
  - Lower extremity fractures tied to uninjured leg (buddy splinting)
  - Formable splints are very useful to secure extremity fractures or dislocations

Pain Control

- Nonpharmacological management
  - Splinting
  - Distraction—Talking to the patient and asking questions
  - Scratching or creating sensory stimuli when doing painful procedure
- Pharmacological agents
  - May be indicated to control pain that results from trauma
  - Pain medication can mask serious injury and alter a patient's level of consciousness
  - Consult with medical direction or follow established protocol regarding the appropriateness of drug therapy in these situations

? CHAPTER QUESTIONS

1. You are operating at the scene of a motor vehicle crash; patient access should not be made until:

   a. batteries of the involved vehicles have been disconnected

   b. patients have been located and counted

c. power sources for rescue equipment have been started
d. the scene is adequately protected from possible hazards

2. You are operating at an extended rescue operation in a wilderness area; you have entered the patient into the trauma system, and cared for immediate problems. You know there may be an hour before the helicopter and the ambulance will intersect. During this time, what is your highest priority?
   a. Removing the patient from the trauma system because the "golden hour" has been lost
   b. Completing your prehospital care report to accompany the patient
   c. Anticipating and preparing for changes in patient condition
   d. Expediting your estimated time of arrival (ETA) by using local law enforcement escort services
3. Upon arrival at the scene of a motor vehicle crash, the paramedic's first priority is to:
   a. gain entry into the automobile to triage victims
   b. size up the situation for hazards, injuries, and additional resources needed
   c. stabilize the vehicles
   d. immediately remove bystanders from the scene

Suggested Reading

US Department of Transportation, National Highway Traffic Safety Administration. *EMT-Paramedic: National Standard Curriculum.* Washington, DC: US Department of Transportation, National Highway Traffic Safety Administration; 1998.

Chapter 42

Paramedic Response to Hazardous Materials Incidents

It is a midsummer day; the temperature has peaked at 98°F, and the humidity is 58%. Dispatch summons your ambulance to an overturn on Interstate 1 involving a tanker tractor trailer. As information is gathered by the dispatcher, she relays the information to your unit. Reports are coming in to central dispatch of rollover motor vehicle collision with people trapped. Upon arrival you find an overturned 18-wheel tanker truck. Your partner notices, during your scene survey, that a green haze is emanating from the tanker portion of the truck. You notify dispatch that you are relocating to a safe location, and set up a staging area about a half-mile away. You let incoming units know of the staging area and request the response of the county hazardous materials (haz-mat) unit. Bystanders are reporting the driver is trapped, and seriously injured. You use the binoculars to survey the scene from a distance and confirm the driver is pinned in the vehicle. You also notice a UN placard number on the side of the vehicle. The UN number is 3355.

Is this the appropriate response for this incident so far?

PARAMEDIC RESPONSIBILITIES AT A HAZARDOUS MATERIALS INCIDENT

- Incident size-up (first priority is *scene safety*).
- Recognition and/or confirmation that incident involves haz-mat.
- Maintain a high index of suspicion when responding to incidents involving:
  - Transportation incidents (rail, waterway, air)
  - Highway crashes
  - Storage facilities
  - Manufacturing plants
  - Acts of terrorism
- Use the following resources to identify the substance:
  - Department of Transportation (DOT) North American Emergency Response Guide (NAERG)
  - United Nations (UN) numbers
  - National Fire Protection Agency (NFPA) 704 placard system
  - DOT placards

  - Shipping papers (found in the driver's compartment of tractor trailers, also known as the shipping manifest)
  - Material safety data sheets (MSDS)
- The above resources will assist the first responder in determining:
  - Immediate need for evacuation
  - Immediate action with ambulatory patients
  - Zones such as:
    - Hot zone—Dangerous area
    - Warm zone—Entry/decontamination point
    - Cold zone—Safe area
  - Assessment of toxicological risk
  - Type of chemical
  - Specific actions of a chemical and its reactivity to water
  - Potential for secondary contamination
  - Specific out-of-hospital medical treatment
  - Specific appropriate techniques in decontamination of patients
- Priority is to treat decontaminated patients and to transport patients that pose no risk of contaminating you, your equipment, and the receiving emergency room.
- NFPA outlines levels of response, including what level of training is required by all personnel who may arrive first. All first responders must be trained to an awareness level.
- Paramedics who may transport "semidecontaminated patients" must be trained to the NFPA 473 "Level-1"
- Paramedics who may have to rapidly "decon" and assist in the decontamination corridor must be trained to the 473 "Level-2"
- Haz-mat scene size-up includes a high degree of awareness. Responding to any one of the following incidents could be a potential haz-mat incident and should be approached with caution:
  - Vehicle crashes involving commercial vehicles, pest control vehicles, tankers, cars with alternative fuels, and tractor-trailers
  - Mass transportation such as railroads
  - Pipelines
  - Mass storage facilities
  - Tanks/storage vessels
  - Warehouses
  - Hardware/agricultural stores
  - Agriculture
  - Manufacturing operations
  - Chemical plants
  - All manufacturing operations
  - Known or unknown acts of terrorism
  - Shopping centers
  - Public environments
  - Health-care facilities
  - Laboratories

- The paramedic should recognize hazards by utilizing:
  - Placarding of vehicles (required by law, but be aware that some vehicles are not placarded)
  - The NAERG, which could assist the paramedic in determining the specific chemical
- Common UN/DOT placard classifications are listed below:
  - Explosives
  - Gasses
  - Flammable liquids
  - Flammable solids
  - Oxidizers and organic peroxides
  - Poisonous and etiologic agents
  - Radioactive materials
  - Corrosives
  - Miscellaneous haz-mat
- NFPA 704 System for fixed facilities (Figure 42-1)
  - Blue—Health hazard
  - Red—Fire hazard
  - Yellow—Reactivity hazard

Identification of Substances

Dealing with a haz-mat is often difficult, especially with unknown substances. Using resources such as the MSDS may reveal detailed substance information. Shipping papers may also assist in revealing substance identification. Other resources used in responding to haz-mat include:

- Poison control centers
- CAMEO computer database information
- Computer modeling for plumes
- CHEMTREC (1-800-424-9300 24-hour toll-free hotline)
- Other reference sources such as textbooks, handbooks, or technical specialists

Haz-mat response teams utilize specialized recognition equipment to monitor and recognize unknown chemicals. Common equipment used includes:

- Air-monitoring equipment
- Gas-monitoring equipment
- Ph testing
- Chemical testing
- Colormetric tube testing

THE IMPORTANCE OF HAZARDOUS MATERIAL ZONES (FIGURE 42-2)

Hot Zone

- Contamination actually present
- Site of incident/release
- Entry with high level PPE
- Entry limited to trained haz-mat team members

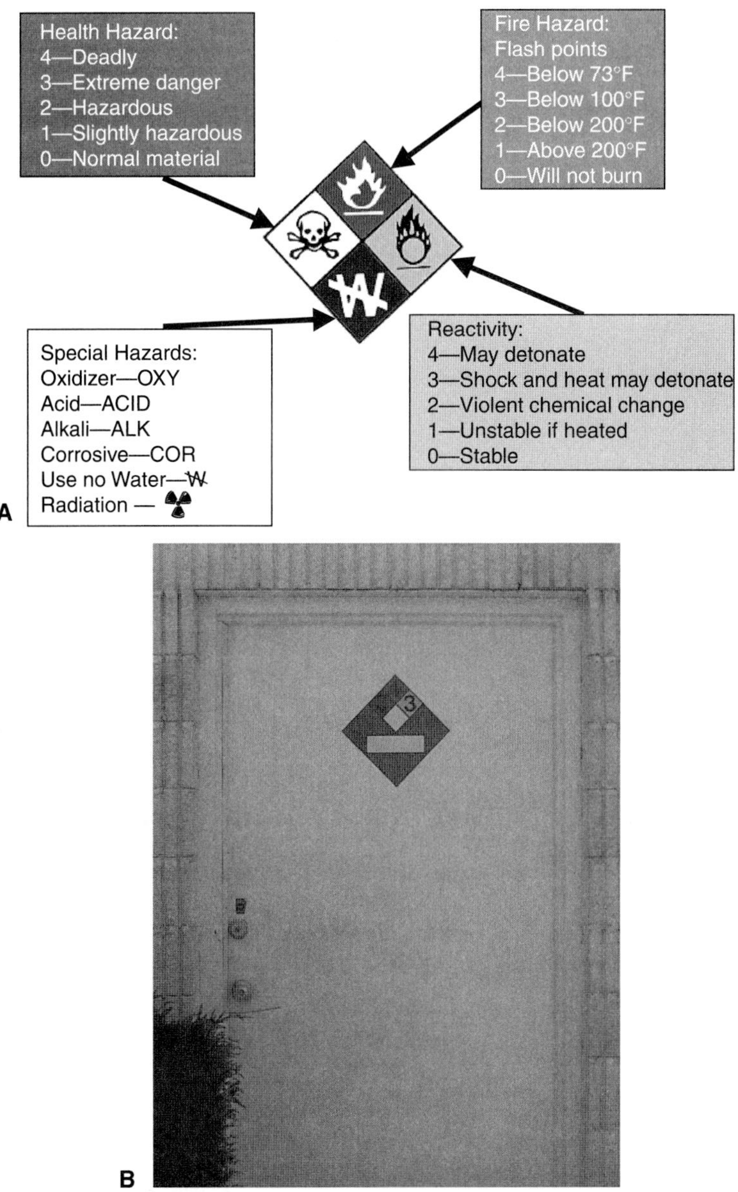

Figure 42-1 NFPA 704. A. From http://hazmat.dot.gov/pubs/erg/gydebook.htm. B. Courtesy of Peter DiPrima.

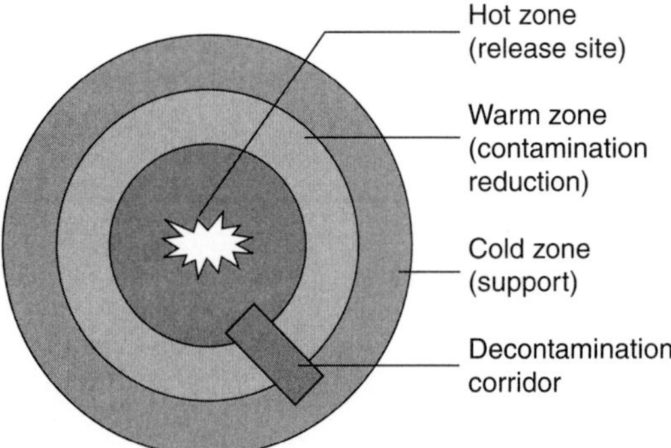

Figure 42-2 Hazardous materials zones.

Warm Zone

- Buffer zone outside of hot zone
- Where decontamination corridor is located
- Corridor has "hot" and "cold" ends
- Authorized trained haz-mat team members

Cold Zone

- Safe area
- Staging for personnel and equipment
- Where medical monitoring occurs
- Safe operation area for EMS personnel

Specific Terminology for Medical Haz-mat Operations

- Boiling point (BP)—The temperature at which the vapor pressure of the maerial being heated equals atmospheric pressure
- Flammable/explosive limits—The highest and lowest concentrations of a substance that can explode or burn
- Flash point (FP)—The lowest temperature at which the vapor given off by a substance forms an ignitable mixture with air
- Ignition temperature
- Specific gravity—The ratio of the density of a solid or liquid to the density of water
- Vapor density (VD)—The relative density of a vapor compared to air
- Vapor pressure—A measure of how readily a solid or liquid mixes with air at its surface (Vapor pressure approaching 760 mmHg indicates a volatile substance and suggests that there will be high concentration in the air)
- Water solubility—The degree to which a material or its vapors dissolve in water
- Alpha radiation—Massive and travel only 3–4 inches from their radioactive source
- Beta radiation—More energetic and less massive than alpha particles. Beta particles can travel up to 100 ft from their source
- Gamma radiation—Not particles but forms of pure energy that can travel great distances from their source

Specific Toxicological Terms

- Threshold limit value (TLV)
- Lethal concentration and doses (LD)
- Parts per million/billion (ppm/ppb)
- Immediately dangerous to life and health (IDLH)
- Permissible exposure limit (PEL)
- Short-term exposure limit (TLV-STEL)
- Ceiling level (TLV-C)

TYPES OF CONTAMINATION

Primary Contamination

- Exposure to substance
- Only harmful to individual
- Little chance of exposure to others

Secondary Contamination

- Exposure to substance
- Substance easily transferred
- Touching patient results in contamination
- Key concept in haz-mat medical operations
- Gas exposure rarely results in secondary contamination
- Liquid and particulate matter more likely to result in secondary contamination

HOW POISONS ARE ABSORBED

- Topical absorption
  - Skin and mucous membranes
  - Not all skin absorbs at same rate
  - Not all poisons easily absorbed
- Respiratory inhalation
  - Absorption through bronchial tree
  - Oxygen-deficient atmospheres
- Gastrointestinal ingestion
  - Ingestion of substances
  - Factors affecting absorption
- Parenteral injection
  - Injection
  - Wound entry
  - Invasive medical procedures

Cycle of Poison Actions

Absorption

- Time to delivery into blood stream

Distribution

- Distribution to target organs
- Poison or drug binds to tissues/molecules
- Actions
- Deposits

Biotransformation

- Liver

Elimination Through

- GI
- Kidneys
- Respiratory system

Actions of Poisons are Determined by Several Factors

- Acute toxicity
  - Immediate effect from substance
- Delayed toxicity
  - No immediate effect

  - Symptoms appear later
  - Delayed pathology or disease
- Local effects
  - Effect immediate at the contaminated site
  - Burn model
  - Progression of effects like burn
  - Topical or respiratory
  - Skin irritation—acute bronchospasm
- Systemic effects
  - Cardiovascular
  - Neurological
  - Hepatic
  - Renal
- Dose response
  - Physiologic response to dosage
  - How much to get an effect
  - Essential concept for decontamination
- Synergistic effects
  - Combinations may react synergistically
  - Standard pharmacologic approach
  - Standard treatment can result in synergy
  - Medical control/poison control reference

COMMONLY ENCOUNTERED HAZARDOUS MATERIALS

- Corrosives (acids/alkalis)
- Pulmonary irritants (ammonia/chlorine)
- Pesticides (carbamates/organophosphates)
- Chemical asphyxiants (cyanide/CO)
- Hydrocarbon solvents (xylene/methlyene chloride)

CONSIDERATIONS FOR PERFORMING INVASIVE PROCEDURES

- Risk versus benefit (will treating the patient contaminate you or further contaminate the patient?)
- Purpose of decontamination is to reduce the patient's dosage of material, decrease the threat of secondary contamination, and reduce the risk of rescuer injury and contamination.
- Environmental considerations are a consideration if there are no life threats.
- Trained haz-mat response team members will prevent runoff of material. If there are life threats, patient's comes first. Remember, only trained and fully protected haz-mat response team members should rescue victims of a haz-mat incident.

Modes of Decontamination

- Dilution
  - Lavage with copious amounts of water
  - Water is universal decontamination solution

- Dilution decreases dose and action
- Reduction of topical absorption
- Absorption
  - Use of pads to "blot" up the material
  - Towels to dry the patient after lavage
  - Usually a secondary method to lavage
  - Common for environmental cleanup
- Neutralization
  - Almost never used in patient decontamination
  - Hazard of exothermic reactions
  - Time to determine neutralizing substance
  - Lavage usually dilutes and removes faster
- Disposal/isolation
  - Removal of clothing
  - Removal of substances

Decontamination Decision Making

- Field considerations include flight of walking contaminated victims to rescuer
  - "Fast break" event—action required now
- Conscious, contaminated people will "self-rescue" by walking out of hot zone
- Immediate decontamination often not avoidable
- Speed of haz-mat team response may hinder walking contaminated

EMS Gross Decontamination and Treatment

- All EMS needs gross decontamination capability
- EMS preparedness for quick decontamination
- Need for rapid EMS PPE
- Need quick transport isolation methods

"Fast break" Incident Decision Making

- Critical patient—Unknown/life-threatening material (remember patients who are contaminated are a risk to the EMS crew as well as equipment, and the emergency department)
- Decontamination and treatment simultaneous
- Remove clothing (80% of contamination is removed by having the patient remove their clothing)
- Treat life-threatening problems
- Lavage—Water is universal decontamination solution
- Contain/isolate patient
- Transport

Noncritical—Unknown/Life-threatening Material

- More contemplative approach
- Decontamination and treatment simultaneous
- Remove clothing
- Treat life-threatening problems
- Lavage—Water is universal decontamination solution

- Contain/isolate patient
- Transport

Noncritical—Substance Known

- Slower approach
- Environmental/privacy considerations
- More thorough decontamination
- Clothing removal
- Thorough lavage/wash
- Drying/reclothing PRN
- Medical monitoring
- Patient isolation PRN
- Transport

Longer Duration Event Decision Making

- Patients in hot zone—Nonambulatory
- No rescue attempted
- Wait for haz-mat team
- Team will set up decontamination corridor

Haz-mat Team Will Not Make Entry Until

- Medical monitoring of entry team
- Decontamination corridor established
- Longer duration event
- Often 60 minutes for team deployment
- Setup time slow and organized
- Better opportunity for thorough decontamination
- Better PPE
- Less chance of secondary contamination
- Better environmental protection

LEVELS OF HAZARDOUS MATERIALS PERSONAL PROTECTION (FIGURE 42-3)

- Level "A" protection
  - Highest level of personal protection
  - Highest degree of protection from chemical breakthrough
  - Fully encapsulated suit
  - Covers everything including SCBA
  - Impermeable/sealed
  - Typically used by haz-mat team for entry into hot zone
- Level "B" protection
  - Level of protection typically worn by decontamination team
  - Decontamination wears one level below entry
  - Usually nonencapsulating protection
  - SCBA worn outside suit
  - Easier entry and SCBA bottle changes
  - Easier to work in
  - High degree of repellence

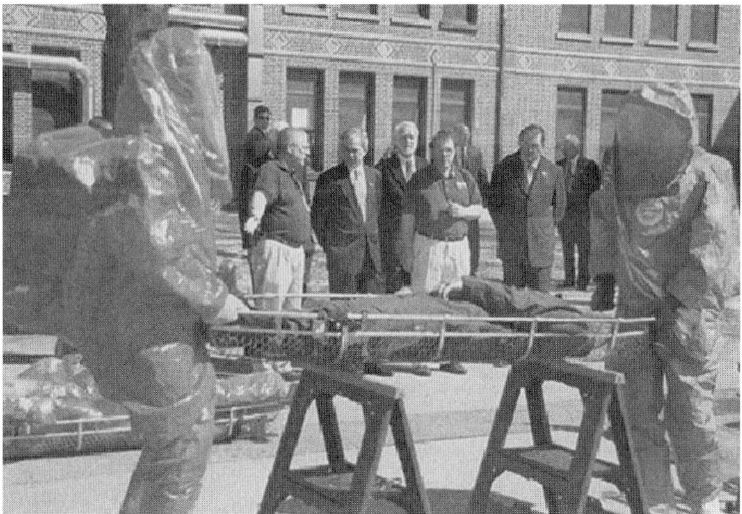

A

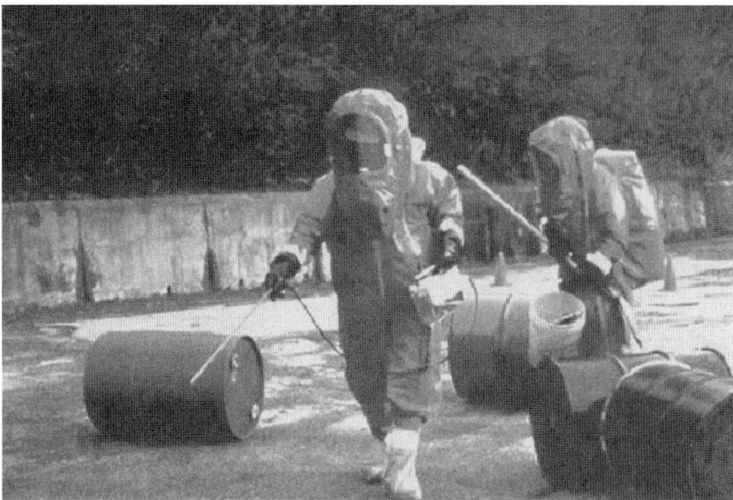

B

Figure 42-3 Levels of protection. A. Level A protective HAZMAT suit. B. Level B protective haz-mat suit. C. Level C protective HAZMAT suit. D. Level C with personnel using Powered Air Purifying Respirators (PAPR) and CBRNE gas masks. (Parts A and C from Grey MR, Spaeth KR. *The Bioterrorism Sourcebook.* Part B from http://www.epa.gov/superfund/programs/er/resource/d1_04.htm. Part D, Courtesy of Peter DiPrima.)

- Level "C" protection
  - Nonpermeable clothing
  - Eye and hand protection
  - Foot covering
  - Used during transport of patients with potential of secondary contamination
- Level "D" protection
  - Firefighter turnout clothing

Determining Appropriate PPE

- Depends on if the chemical is known.
- A permeability chart is consulted to determine "breakthrough" time.

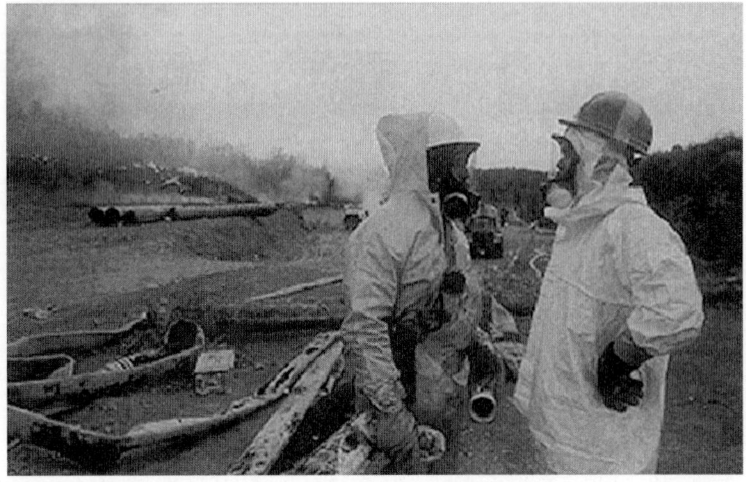

C

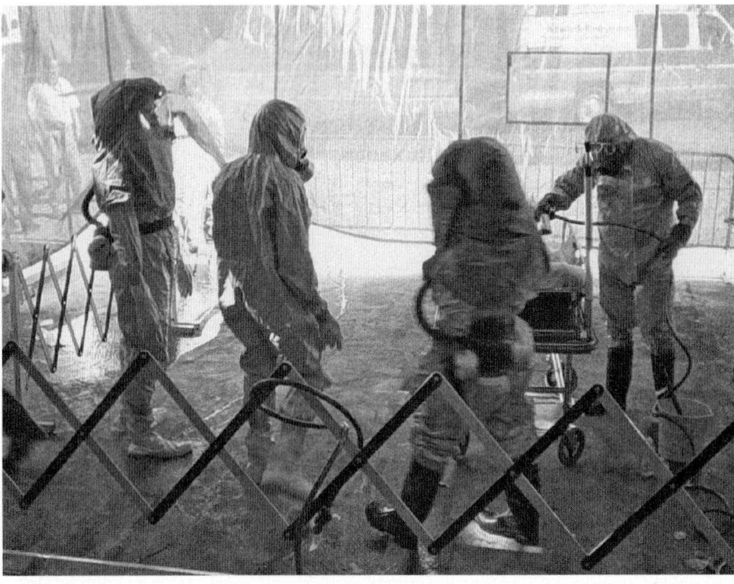

D

Figure 42-3 *(Continued)*

- Double or triple gloves or chemical resistant gloves are used.
- Nitrile gloves have a high resistance to chemicals.
- If situation is emergent, take maximal barrier precautions, using full turnouts or Tyvek suits/gowns.
- Use HEPA filters and eye protection.
- Remove leather shoes, use rubber boots.
- Ideally at least level "B" protection should be used.
- Ideally use disposable protection.

PROCEDURES IN TRANSPORTING A SEMIDECONTAMINATED PATIENT (AS A LAST RESORT)

- Use as much disposable equipment as possible
  - Reduces decontamination later

- Practicality of lining an ambulance interior with plastic
  - Impractical
  - Time consuming

If airborne contaminants can permeate cabinets, it is unsafe for the driver to operate the ambulance. Patients who are "off-gassing" should not be placed in the patient compartment of an ambulance because of the risk of injuring the crew.

Medical Monitoring and Rehabilitation

Entry team/decontamination team readiness prior to entry:

- Assessment of vital signs and documentation (blood pressure, pulse, respiratory rate, temperature, body weight, ECG, and mental/neurological status).
- Team members should have normal values on file.
- Rescuer PPE can cause considerable heat stress. Prehydration prior to entry should include 8–16 oz of water or sport drink.

After Exit, Personnel Should Return to the Medical Sector for "Rehab"

- Assessment of vital signs and documentation (blood pressure, pulse, respiratory rate, temperature, body weight, ECG, and mental/neurological status).
- Rescuer PPE can cause considerable heat stress. Prehydration prior to entry should include 8–16 oz of water or sport drink.
- Use weight to estimate fluid losses.
- No reentry until vital signs are back to normal.

Heat stress factors include prehydration of the member, degree of physical fitness, ambient air temperature, degree of activity, and duration in the PPE.

CHAPTER QUESTIONS

1. During a haz-mat incident, the paramedic will establish a patient decontamination area, which is also called the:
   a. hot zone
   b. cold zone
   c. warm zone
   d. triage zone
2. To find out if a truck that is leaking some type of fluid is carrying haz-mat, look for information from the following source first:
   a. MSDS
   b. placards
   c. waybill
   d. shipping papers

Suggested Reading

US Department of Transportation, National Highway Traffic Safety Administration. *EMT-Paramedic National Standard Curriculum*. Washington, DC: US Department of Transportation, National Highway Traffic Safety Administration; 1998.

Chapter 43
Crime Scene Awareness

On a relatively quiet morning, a frantic call enters the 911 system for a student who entered a local high school and began to open fire with a shotgun. Upon beginning your response and awaiting clearance to enter the crime scene, the local police department is reporting that a 16-year-old student opened fire with a shotgun in a common area of the high school. So far the reports are saying the principal and a student were DOA. Two other students are wounded, and there are multiple kids missing or unaccounted for.

When entering this crime scene, what are some scene safety and crime scene awareness issues that you may encounter?

- Many violent crimes require an EMS response.
- EMS crews often arrive at the scene before law enforcement personnel.
- Hazard awareness control and avoidance are issues of concern for emergency responders.
- National studies have reported a decline in violent crimes in recent years; but violence against EMS personnel that arises from street gangs, threat groups, domestic disputes, and drug users is on the rise.
- Personal safety and crime scene awareness must be the priority on every emergency call of this nature.

APPROACHING THE SCENE

- Approach is part of scene size-up.
- Determining personal safety is an integral part of scene size-up.
- Size-up begins before arrival at the scene with information provided by the dispatch center. Information that may be available from a dispatching center and that should alert the EMS crew to possible dangers includes:
  - Known locations of unsafe scenes, and/or the presence of:
    - — Large crowds
    - — People under the influence of alcohol or other drugs
    - — On-scene violence
    - — Weapons
  - Previous experience with calls at this location or area
- Be aware of additional hazards that may exist at the scene, such as:
  - Downed power lines
  - Busy roadways
  - Toxic substances
  - Potential for fire
  - Dangerous pets
  - Vehicle hazards and dangers

- Begin observation several blocks from the scene.
- Use audible and visual warning (AVW) devices appropriate for the call.
  - Urban scene—Excess use could draw a crowd.
  - Highway scene—Lights required for safety.
  - Joint fire—EMS-law enforcement response postures should be defined with preplanning.
    - — Fire—EMS response with full use of AVW devices
    - — Law enforcement responding without AVW devices and at normal speed
    - — Need for interagency cooperation and understanding
- Scene safety considerations must continue throughout the call.
- Violence can resume.
- Crowds gather or turn violent.
- Additional persons can enter the scene.
- Violence may occur even with police present.
- EMS personnel may be mistaken for police.
  - Uniform colors.
  - Badges.
  - Exiting a vehicle with lights and sirens.
  - This could cause aggression toward the EMS crew authority figures.
  - Others may expect the EMS crew to intervene in violent situations.
  - Remember to include an "escape and strategic escape plan" in your protocols.

Known Violent Scenes

- If the scene is known to be violent, remain at a safe and out-of-sight distance from the area until it has been secured.
- Remaining at a safe staging area away from a violent scene is important for several reasons:
  - If you can be seen, people will come to you.
  - Entering an unsafe scene adds another potential victim(s).
  - You may be injured or killed.
  - You may become a hostage.
  - You may become another patient in a scene that is already a multiple casualty incident.

Approach to Residences

- Everyday response—All calls require a certain level of caution. Even calls that appear "routine" require size-up.
- Begin assessment of scene even before exiting the emergency vehicle.
- Warning signs of danger in residential calls include:
  - Past history of problems or violence
  - Known drug or gang area
  - Loud noises (screams, items breaking, possible gunshots)
  - Seeing or hearing acts of violence
  - The presence of alcohol or other drug use
  - Evidence of dangerous pets (exotic snakes and reptiles, vicious breeds of dogs)
  - Unusual silence or darkened residence
- Approach—Choose tactics that match threat or situation.
- If actual danger is present, retreat and call for police.

- Avoid use of lights/sirens.
- Avoid using unconventional pathways.
- Avoid a position between the emergency vehicle's lights and residence.
- Listen for signs of danger before announcing presence or entering the residence.
- Stand to the side of the entry door opposite the hinges (doorknob side).
- When actual danger becomes evident, immediately retreat from the scene.

Approach to Vehicles

- One-person approach—Driver remains in ambulance, which is elevated and provides greater visibility.
- If nighttime, use ambulance lights to illuminate interior of the vehicle and surrounding area.
- Notify dispatch of situation, location, license plate number, and state.
- Approach passenger side of vehicle.
  - Protection from vehicular traffic
  - Opposite approach that a driver would expect from law enforcement personnel
- Do not walk between ambulance and other vehicle.
  - Ambulance lights cause backlighting
  - Could be injured if vehicle backs up
  - When approaching passenger side of vehicle, walk around rear of ambulance, then to passenger side of vehicle
- Car posts A, B, and C may provide best ballistic protection.
  - Observe rear seat
    - — Do not move forward of "C" post unless there are no threats in the back seat
  - Observe front seat from behind "B" post
    - — Move forward only after ensuring safety
- Retreat to a safe staging area at the first sign of violence or problem and request law-enforcement assistance.
  - Weapons
  - Suspicious behavior or movements in the vehicle
  - Arguing or fighting among passengers

VIOLENT STREET INCIDENTS

- Murder, assault, robbery
  - Involve dangerous weapons
  - Violence may be directed toward EMS personnel from
    - — Perpetrators at the scene or who return to scene
    - — Injured and distraught patients
- Dangerous crowds and bystanders
  - May quickly become large in number and volatile
  - Violence directed toward everyone and everything in surrounding area
- Warning signs of danger—Street scenes
  - Voices become louder
  - Pushing, shoving
  - Hostilities toward people at scene (perpetrator, police, victim, etc.)
  - Rapid increase in crowd size
  - Inability of law enforcement to control crowds

- Safety actions—Crowds
  - Constantly monitor crowd
  - Retreat from scene if necessary
  - When possible and safe to do so, remove patient from scene as the crew retreats
    - Negates the need to return to the scene later

VIOLENT GROUPS AND SITUATIONS

Street Gang Awareness

- Most gangs and other threat groups operate on the premise of intimidation and extortion.
- Gang characteristics:
  - A gang can be defined as any group of people who engage in socially disruptive or criminal behavior
  - Usually territorial
  - Often, but not always, of the same gender
  - Operate by creating an atmosphere of fear in a community
  - May choose a name, logo, specific color, or method of dress used for purposes of identification for their own members and their counterparts
- Graffiti (probably the most visible sign of gang criminal activity)
- Clothing
  - Unique clothing—Specific to group
  - Identifies affiliation and rank within group

Clandestine Drug Laboratories

The illegal manufacture of drugs can pose significant hazards for emergency providers.

Types of Drug Laboratories

- Synthesis—Creating drugs from chemical precursors (LSD, methamphetamine)
- Conversion—Changing a drug's form (cocaine HCl to base form)

Safety Hazards

- Can produce highly explosive and toxic gases.
- Can readily be absorbed through the skin in quantities that can be fatal.
- Can produce oxygen-depleted atmospheres.
- Toxic solvents used in drug-making process can lead to laboratory explosions and exposure to dangerous chemicals.
- "Booby traps" can maim or kill an intruder.
- Laboratories with armed or otherwise violent occupants.
- Usually located in an area that ensures privacy, and is well ventilated.
- Has access to water, electric, and gas utilities required for drug manufacturing.
- Suspicious persons, activities, deliveries.
- Be alert for chemical odors, and chemical equipment.
- If a drug laboratory is identified, the EMS crew should:
  - Leave the area immediately.
  - Notify law enforcement and request appropriate agencies and personnel.

  - Initiate an incident management system and haz-mat procedures (per protocol).
  - Assist law enforcement personnel to coordinate an orderly evacuation of the surrounding area for public safety.

DOMESTIC VIOLENCE

- Domestic violence is violence that occurs between persons in a relationship.
- Perpetrator may be male or female in an opposite-sex or same-sex relationship.
- Results in physical, emotional, sexual, verbal, or economic abuse and may occur in multiple combinations.
- Indicators of domestic violence and abuse include:
  - Apparent fear of a household member.
  - Different or conflicting accounts by parties at the scene.
  - One party preventing another from speaking.
  - A patient who is reluctant to speak.
  - Injuries that do not match the reported mechanism of injury.
  - Unusual or unsanitary living conditions or personal hygiene.
- Be aware that acts of violence may be directed toward EMS personnel by the perpetrator—Take safety precautions.
- If the scene is considered safe for the EMS crew:
  - Treat the patient.
  - Notify authorities.
  - Medical direction.
  - Other authorities per standard operating procedures and protocol.
  - Mandatory reporting may be required.
  - Do not be judgmental about the relationship.
  - Do not direct accusations toward the abuse.
  - Provide phone number for domestic violence hot line, community support programs, and available shelters.

TACTICS FOR SAFETY

Avoidance

- Avoidance is always preferable to confrontation.
- Be observant. Be knowledgeable of warning signs that may indicate a dangerous situation. Be knowledgeable of proper tactical response.
- Staging—Dispatcher learns of danger and advises not to approach scene until danger is handled and scene is secured by appropriate authorities.

Tactical Retreat

- Leaving the scene when danger is observed.
- Violence or indicators of violence displayed.
- Requires immediate, decisive actions.
- May be accomplished on foot or by vehicle (in a calm and safe manner) by choosing the mode and route of retreat that provides the least exposure for danger.
- Be aware that the risks faced by the EMS crew are now located behind them.
  - Stay alert for associated dangers
- Required distance from danger for a safe tactical retreat is guided by the nature of the incident.

- In general, a safe distance must:
  - Protect the crew from any potential danger.
  - Be out of immediate line of sight.
  - Be protected from gunfire (cover).
  - Be far enough away to react if danger reapproaches.
- Once tactical retreat has been achieved:
  - Notify other responding units and agencies of danger per interagency EMS/law enforcement standard operating procedures and agreements.
- Documentation is key to reducing liability should injuries or deaths occur.
  - Observations of danger at the scene.
  - Who was notified of the danger?
  - Your actions at the scene.
  - Time left/time returned to scene.

Cover and Concealment

- Cover and concealment are means to provide protection from injury.
- Cover—Hides your body behind large and heavy structures.
  - Provides ballistic protection.
- Concealment—Hides your body.
  - Offers little or no ballistic protection
  - Examples—Hiding behind
    - Bushes
    - Wallboard
    - Vehicle door
- When the need for cover or concealment arises, the paramedic should:
  - Constantly be aware of surroundings.
  - Place as much of the body as possible behind adequate cover.
  - Constantly look for ways to improve protection and location.
  - Be aware of reflective clothing (e.g., trim, badges) that may draw attention or serve as a target.

Distraction and Evasive Maneuvers

- Distraction and evasive tactics can be used as self-defense measures during retreat, or when retreat and cover and concealment are not available options.
- Distraction—A self-defense measure that creates diversion in a person's attention.
  - Wedge stretcher in doorway to block aggressor.
  - Throw equipment to trip or slow aggressor.
- Evasive tactics—A self-defense measure where the moves and actions of an aggressor are anticipated, and whereby unconventional pathways are used during retreat for personal safety.
  - Use unconventional path while retreating.
  - Anticipate moves of aggressor.
- Warning signs that can indicate impending violence from an aggressor may include a person who does the following:
  - Conspicuously ignores emergency responders.
  - Becomes verbally abusive.

- Invades personal space.
- Has a violent history or background.
- Shifts weight from side to side or foot to foot ("boxer stance").
- Clenches fists.
- Has tightened musculature.
- Maintains eye contact by staring.

- Crews trained in tactical EMS often employ preassigned roles for specific distraction and evasive maneuvers.
  - Threats of physical violence
  - Firearms encounters
  - Edged weapons encounters
- Contact provider:
  - Crew member that initiates and provides direct patient care
  - Performs patient assessment
  - Handles most interpersonal scene contact
- Cover provider:
  - Crew member whose main function is to "cover" or observe scene for danger while "contact" provider takes care of patient
  - Generally avoids patient care duties that would prevent observation of the scene
  - In small crews "cover" provider likely to have other functions (e.g., ensuring safe-keeping of equipment, drugs, and supplies while at the scene)
- Communication between providers.
  - Warning signals
    - — Crews should develop methods of alerting other providers to danger without alerting aggressors.
    - — Verbal and nonverbal signals needed.
      Coded terms
      Scratching the neck
      Rubbing the nose
  - Involve dispatch in danger signal process

TACTICAL PATIENT CARE

- *Refers to providing patient-care activities inside the scene perimeter or "hot" zone*
  - Special training and authorization
  - Body armor and a tactical uniform
  - Compact and functional equipment
  - In some operations, personal defensive weapons
  - May require risks not taken in standard EMS situations

Body Armor

- Soft body armor (also known as "bulletproof vests").
- Offers protection from most handgun bullets, most knives, and some blunt trauma.
- Does not offer protection from high velocity (rifle) bullets, thin or dual-edged weapons (ice pick).
- Wearer may feel false sense of security.
  - Body armor does not cover the entire body.
  - Severe injury may still result from the forces of cavitation (in the absence of penetration) even when the vest is properly worn.

EMS Care in the Hot Zone

- Most tactical medics (emergency medical technician-tactical [EMT-T] and Special Weapons and Tactics [SWAT]) are trained in:
  - Care under fire
  - Hostage survival
  - Medicine across the barricade
  - Medical aspects of extended operations
  - Wound ballistics, weapons, and their effects
  - Medical threat assessment and medical intelligence
  - Clinical forensic medicine and evidence preservation
  - Toxic hazards—Identification, risks, and management
- Several hands-on laboratories are included in most training programs such as:
  - Physical assessment under sensory deprivation/overload conditions
  - Medical threat assessment
  - Advanced medical-tactical techniques
  - Field expedient decontamination
  - New technologies for safe searches
  - Management of dental injuries
  - "Officer down" rescue and extraction
  - Aeromedical evacuation
  - Medical management of clandestine drug laboratory raids
  - Safe search techniques
  - Remote physical assessment

Patient Care Differences

- Extraction of patient from the area safely is a major concern.
- Frequent care of trauma patients.
- Care may be modified to meet tactical considerations.
- Medical and transport interventions must be coordinated with incident commander.
- Tactical EMS providers often function under protocols and standing orders that differ from those of more "standard" EMS practice.
  - Medical direction issues regarding patient care are dictated by
    - The nature of the event
    - The uncontrolled and hazardous scene in which EMS is delivered

EMS AT CRIME SCENES

Crime Scene

- A location where any part of a criminal act occurred
- A location where evidence relating to a crime may be found
- Evidence
  - Fingerprints
    - Unique—No two people have identical fingerprints.
    - Ridge characteristics left behind on a surface with oils and moisture from skin.
  - Footprints
  - Blood and body fluids
    - Can be tested for DNA and ABO blood typing

    - Also have unique characteristics that may be individual specific
    - Blood spatter evidence
  - Particulate evidence (hairs, carpet, and clothing fibers)
  - EMS provider's observations of the scene
    - Patient (victim) position
    - Patient's injuries
    - Conditions at the scene
      - Lights
      - Curtains
      - Signs of forced entry
    - Statements of persons at the scene
    - Statements of the patient/victim
    - Dying declarations

Preserving Evidence

- Patient care is the ultimate priority.
- Evidence protection is performed while caring for the patient.
- Evidence preservation techniques:
  - Be observant.
  - Touch only what is required for patient care.
  - If necessary to touch something, remember it and tell police.
  - Wear latex gloves.
    - Infection control
    - Prevents you from leaving your fingerprints
    - Will not prevent you from smudging other fingerprints
  - Report pertinent observations.
- Approach no crime scene until it has been secured for your safety.
- Park your vehicle as far away as conveniently possible to preserve skid marks, tire prints, or other evidence.
- Survey and assess the scene before proceeding to the victim.
- Try to approach the victim from a route different from the assailant's probable route.
- Follow the same path to and from the victim.
- Avoid stepping on blood stains or splatter if possible.
- Disturb the victim and the victim's clothing as little as possible while performing your assessment and during treatment.
- When cutting the clothing from a victim, try to do it in a way to preserve the points of wounding.
- Report your actions and any disturbances you make to the crime scene investigator.
- Keep all unnecessary people away from the victim.
- Do not smoke or eat at the crime scene.
- Do not touch any evidence if at all possible.
- Make no comments to bystanders about the situation.
- Save the victim's clothes and personal items in a paper bag.
  - The bag should be labeled, sealed, and turned over to law enforcement personnel.
- Be aware of any dying declarations made by your patient.
- Keep accurate, detailed records.
- Law enforcement personnel are in charge of the crime scene—You are in charge of the patient.

CHAPTER QUESTION

1. When responding to a crime scene, the first responsibility of the paramedic is:
   a. gathering evidence
   b. scene safety
   c. patient care
   d. capturing the criminal

Suggested Reading

US Department of Transportation, National Highway Traffic Safety Administration. *EMT-Paramedic National Standard Curriculum*. Washington, DC: US Department of Transportation, National Highway Traffic Safety Administration; 1998.

ANSWERS TO CHAPTER QUESTIONS

Chapter 1 EMS Systems/Roles and Responsibilities

1. **The correct answer is a.**
2. **The correct answer is d.**
3. **The correct answer is d.** All skills listed in this question are advanced-level care that only can be performed by an EMT-Paramedic.

Chapter 2 The Well-Being of the Paramedic

1. **The correct answer is b.** Latex or nonlatex gloves such as Nitrile gloves should be worn with every patient to protect from infectious disease.
2. **The correct answer is d.**
3. **The correct answer is a.**
4. **The correct answer is b.**
5. **The correct answer is d.**

Chapter 3 Illness and Injury Prevention

1. **The correct answer is b.**
2. **The correct answer is d.**
3. **The correct answer is c.**
4. **The correct answer is a.**

Chapter 4 Medical/Legal Issues

1. **The correct answer is c.** Regardless of being paid or volunteering, the same components are required to establish negligence.
2. **The correct answer is a.**
3. **The correct answer is a.**
4. **The correct answer is d.**

Chapter 5 Ethics

1. **The correct answer is a.**
2. **The correct answer is b.**
3. **The correct answer is b.**

Chapter 6 General Principles of Pathophysiology

1. **The correct answer is c.**
2. **The correct answer is a.**
3. **The correct answer is d.** The visceral pleura cover the outer layer of the lungs.
4. **The correct answer is d.**
5. **The correct answer is b.**

Chapter 7 Pharmacology

1. **The correct answer is d.**
2. **The correct answer is c.**
3. **The correct answer is a.** Enteral drugs are administered along any portion of the gastrointestinal tract.
4. **The correct answer is c.**
5. **The correct answer is d.**
6. **The correct answer is c.**
7. **The correct answer is c.**

8. **The correct answer is c.**
9. **The correct answer is b.**
10. **The correct answer is c.**
11. **The correct answer is e.**
12. **The correct answer is d.**
13. **The correct answer is b.**
14. **The correct answer is a.**

Chapter 8 Venous Access and Medication Administration

1. **The correct answer is 7.5 mL.**
2. **The correct answer is 1 tablet.**
3. **The correct answer is 3 tablets.**
4. **The correct answer is 200 mg.**
5. **The correct answer is 2 mL.**
6. **The correct answer is 0.8 mL.**
7. **The correct answer is 1.2 mL.**
8. **The correct answer is 42 drops minute.**
9. **The correct answer is 75 drops per minute.**
10. **The correct answer is 44 drops per minute.**
11. **The correct answer is 0.8 L.**
12. **The correct answer is 480 mL.**
13. **The correct answer is 50 drops per minute.**
14. **The correct answer is 25 mL/hour.**
15. **The correct answer is 8 hours.**
16. **The correct answer is 10 hours.**
17. **The correct answer is 56 drops per minute.**
18. **The correct answer is 44 drops per minute.**
19. **The correct answer is 21 drops per minute.**
20. **The correct answer is 2 ampoules.**
21. **The correct answer is d.**
22. **The correct answer is c.**
23. **The correct answer is a.**
24. **The correct answer is c.**
25. **The correct answer is d.**
26. **The correct answer is b.**
27. **The correct answer is d.**
28. **The correct answer is d.**
29. **The correct answer is c.**
30. **The correct answer is b.**
31. **The correct answer is d.** Remember to divide the weight in pounds by 2.2.
32. **The correct answer is a.**

Chapter 9 Therapeutic Communications

1. **The correct answer is e.**
2. **The correct answer is a.**

Chapter 10 Life Span Development

1. **The correct answer is a.**
2. **The correct answer is b.** Gonadotropins in men promote production of the male hormone testosterone.

Chapter 11 Airway Management and Ventilation

1. **The correct answer is d.**
2. **The correct answer is b.**
3. **The correct answer is a.**
4. **The correct answer is c.**
5. **The correct answer is d.**
6. **The correct answer is b.**
7. **The correct answer is a.**

Chapter 12 Patient Assessment

1. **The correct answer is b.**
2. **The correct answer is c.**
3. **The correct answer is d.**
4. **The correct answer is b.**
5. **The correct answer is b.**
6. **The correct answer is c.**
7. **The correct answer is b.**
8. **The correct answer is a.**
9. **The correct answer is a.**
10. **The correct answer is c.** All life-threatening injuries should be treated as they are found.

Chapter 13 Trauma Systems and Mechanism of Injury

1. **The correct answer is d.**

Chapter 14 Hemorrhage and Shock

1. **The correct answer is b.**
2. **The correct answer is c.**
3. **The correct answer is b.** Orthostatic vital signs are classified as a rise from a recumbent position to a sitting or standing position associated with a fall in systolic pressure (after 1 minute) of 10–15 mm Hg and/or a concurrent rise in pulse rate (after 1 minute) of 10–15 beats/min, which indicate a significant volume depletion and a decrease in perfusion status.
4. **The correct answer is a.**
5. **The correct answer is d.**
6. **The correct answer is b.**
7. **The correct answer is b.**
8. **The correct answer is c.**
9. **The correct answer is d.** A very important question to ask a trauma patient would be if he or she takes anticoagulation medicines. This would increase the patient's risk of uncontrollable bleeding.

Chapter 15 Soft Tissue Trauma

1. **The correct answer is c.**

Chapter 16 Burns

1. **The correct answer is d.**
2. **The correct answer is a.**

Chapter 17 Head and Facial Trauma

1. **The correct answer is b.**

Chapter 18 Spinal Trauma

1. The correct answer is a.

2. The correct answer is d.

Chapter 19 Thoracic Trauma

1. The correct answer is d.

2. The correct answer is a.

Chapter 20 Abdominal Trauma

1. Appendix: Hollow
Gallbladder: Hollow
Liver: Solid
Pancreas: Solid
Stomach: Hollow
Sigmoid Colon: Hollow
Spleen: Solid
Right Kidney: Solid

2. Appendix: RLQ
Gallbladder: RUQ
Liver: RUQ
Pancreas: LUQ
Stomach: LUQ

Chapter 21 Musculoskeletal Trauma

1. The correct answer is b.

2. The correct answer is e.

3. The correct answer is d.

4. The correct answer is a.

Chapter 22 Pulmonary Emergencies

1. The correct answer is a.

2. The correct answer is a.

3. The correct answer is d.

4. The correct answer is a.

5. The correct answer is d.

6. The correct answer is c.

7. The correct answer is c.

Chapter 23 Cardiology

1. The correct answer is b.

2. The correct answer is c.

3. The correct answer is e.

4. The correct answer is e.

Chapter 24 Neurology

1. The correct answer is b.

2. The correct answer is d.

3. The correct answer is c.

4. The correct answer is a.

Chapter 25 Endocrinology

1. The correct answer is b.
2. The correct answer is a.

Chapter 26 Allergies and Anaphylaxis

1. The correct answer is c.
2. The correct answer is b.

Chapter 27 Gastroenterology

1. The correct answer is a.
2. The correct answer is b.

Chapter 28 Toxicology

1. The correct answer is a.
2. The correct answer is c.
3. The correct answer is c.
4. The correct answer is d.

Chapter 29 Hematology

1. The correct answer is b.
2. The correct answer is a.

Chapter 30 Infectious and Communicable Diseases

1. The correct answer is b.
2. The correct answer is a.

Chapter 31 Behavioral and Psychiatric Disorders

1. The correct answer is b.
2. The correct answer is a.
3. The correct answer is c.

Chapter 32 Gynecology

1. The correct answer is b.
2. The correct answer is a.

Chapter 33 Obstetrics

1. The correct answer is c.
2. The correct answer is d.
3. The correct answer is a.

Chapter 34 Neonatology

1. The correct answer is c.
2. The correct answer is d.
3. The correct answer is a.
4. The correct answer is c.
5. The correct answer is b.

Chapter 35 Pediatrics

1. The correct answer is c.
2. The correct answer is b.
3. The correct answer is a.
4. The correct answer is d.
5. The correct answer is d.

6. **The correct answer is d.**
7. **The correct answer is c.**
8. **The correct answer is b.**
9. **The correct answer is a.**
10. **The correct answer is a.**

Chapter 36 **Geriatrics**

1. **The correct answer is a.** Lidocaine toxicity should be monitored when administering this medicine to any patient over 75 years old.
2. **The correct answer is c.**
3. **The correct answer is c.**
4. **The correct answer is d.**
5. **The correct answer is c.**

Chapter 37 **Patients with Special Challenges**

1. **The correct answer is a.**
2. **The correct answer is a.**

Chapter 38 **Acute Interventions for the Home Health-Care Patient**

1. **The correct answer is a.**
2. **The correct answer is d.**

Chapter 39 **Ambulance Operations**

1. **The correct answer is a.**

Chapter 40 **Medical Incident Command**

1. **The correct answer is b.**
2. **The correct answer is a.** This patient is triaged as a RED tag because his respiratory rate is 34 breaths/min. When triaging using START, respirations greater than 30 are automatically triaged as RED tag patients.
3. **The correct answer is a.** The patient's mental status is confused, which makes the patient a RED tag under the START triage system.
4. **The correct answer is b.**
5. **The correct answer is a.** The patient's mental status is confused, which makes the patient a RED tag under the START triage system.
6. **The correct answer is d.** This patient is triaged as a BLACK tag because after repositioning the patient's airway the patient still does not breathe.
7. **The correct answer is b.**
8. **The correct answer is b.**
9. **The correct answer is b.**
10. **The correct answer is d.**

Chapter 41 **Rescue Awareness and Operations**

1. **The correct answer is d.**
2. **The correct answer is c.**
3. **The correct answer is b.**

Chapter 42 **Paramedic Response to Hazardous Materials Incidents**

1. **The correct answer is c.**
2. **The correct answer is b.**

Chapter 43: **Crime Scene Awareness**

1. **The correct answer is b.**

PRACTICE EXAM

Questions 1 through 6: Match the term with the definition.

a. P-wave
b. PR interval
c. QRS complex
d. ST segment
e. T-wave
f. QT interval

1. The interval representing total duration of ventricular electrical systole.

2. A small deflection representing depolarization of the atria.

3. A deflection that represents ventricular repolarization or recovery.

4. A large waveform representing ventricular depolarization.

5. The interval representing conduction time through the atria, AV node, bundle of His, and bundle branches, up to the point of activation of the ventricular muscle tissue.

6. The segment between the end of the QRS complex and the beginning of the T-wave.

7. Interpret the electrocardiogram (ECG) below:

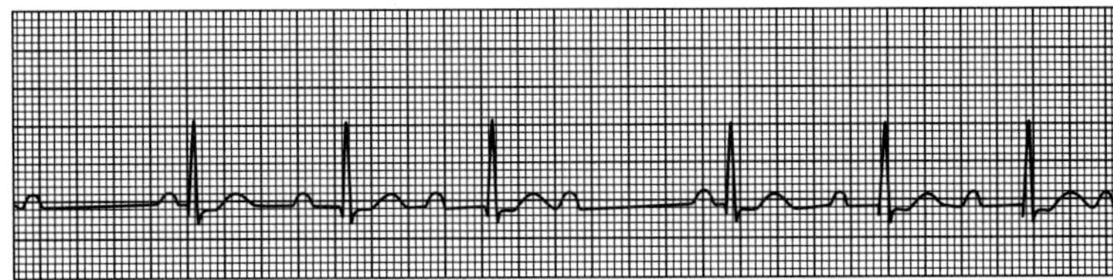

a. first degree heart block
b. second degree heart block (Wenckebach)
c. third degree heart block
d. second degree heart block (Mobitz type-II)

8. Interpret the ECG below:

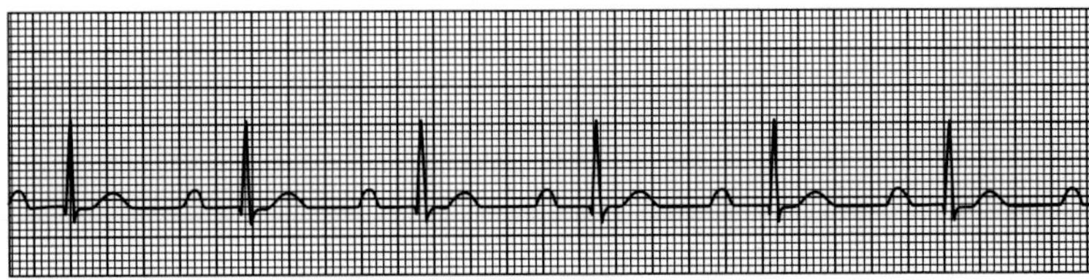

a. first degree heart block
b. second degree heart block (Wenckebach)
c. third degree heart block
d. second degree heart block (Mobitz type-II)

9. Interpret the ECG below:

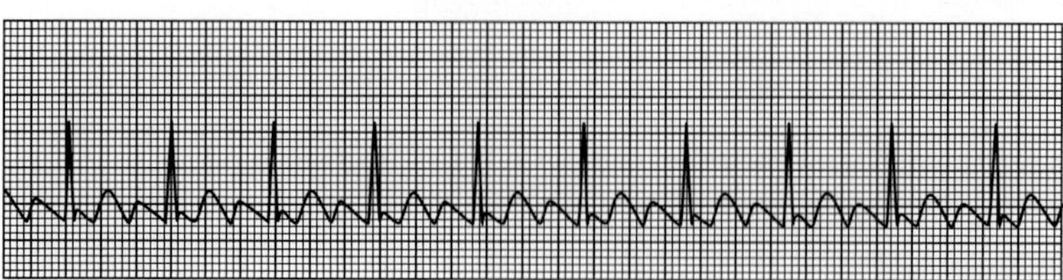

a. atrial fibrillation
b. atrial tachycardia
c. atrial flutter
d. none of the above

10. Interpret the ECG below:

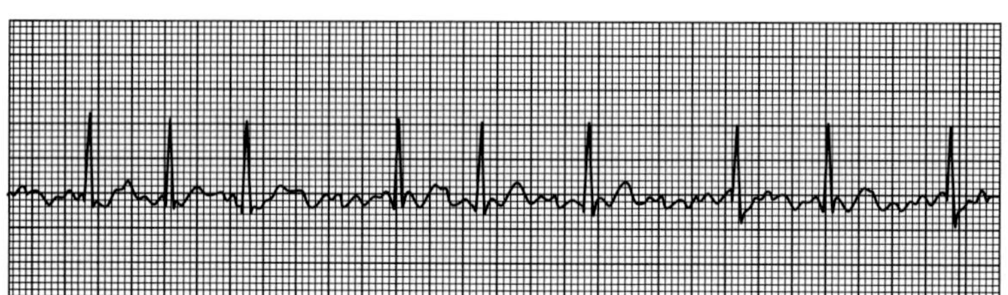

a. atrial fibrillation
b. atrial tachycardia
c. atrial flutter
d. none of the above

11. Interpret the ECG below:

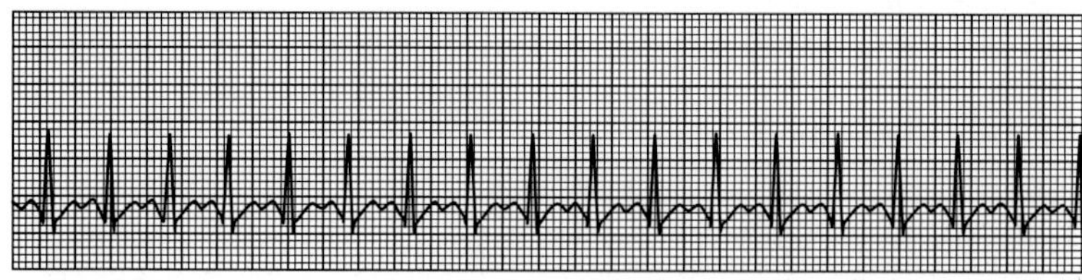

a. sinus tachycardia
b. ventricular tachycardia
c. supraventricular tachycardia (SVT)
d. junctional tachycardia

12. Interpret the ECG below:

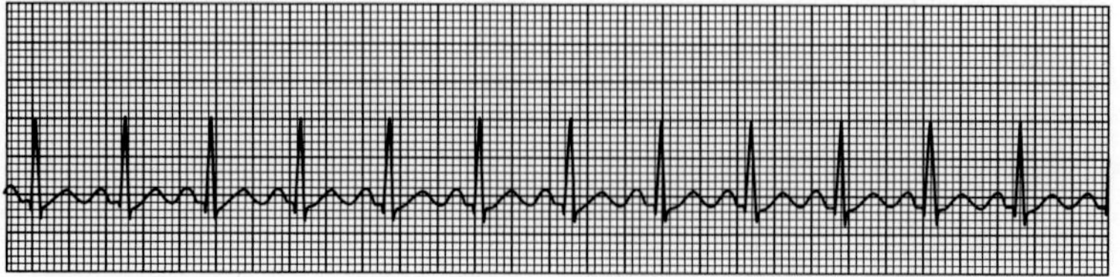

a. sinus rhythm
b. sinus bradycardia
c. sinus arrest
d. sinus tachycardia

13. Interpret the ECG below:

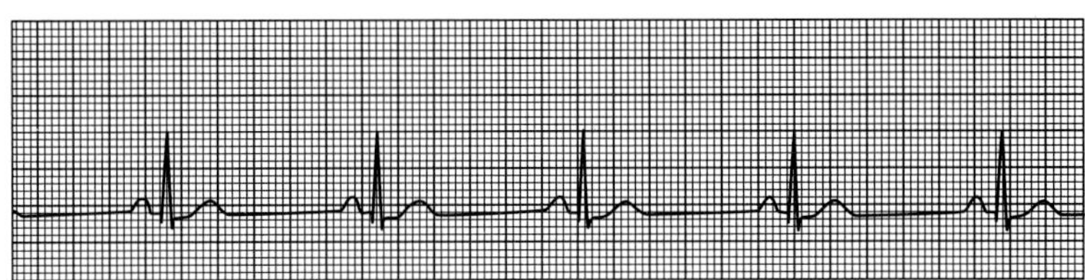

a. sinus rhythm
b. sinus bradycardia
c. sinus arrest
d. sinus tachycardia

14. Interpret the ECG below:

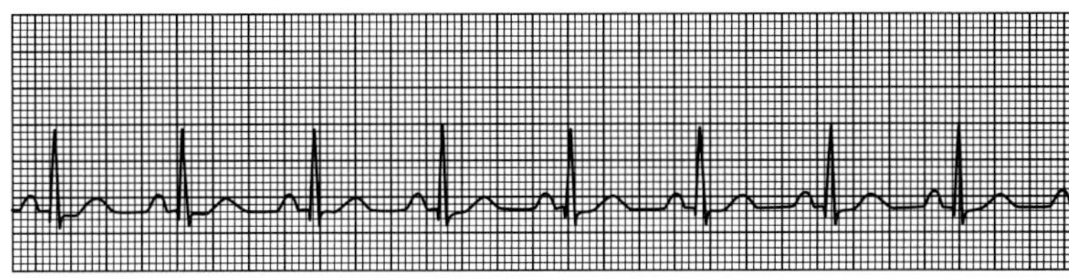

a. sinus rhythm
b. sinus bradycardia
c. sinus arrest
d. sinus tachycardia

15. Interpret the ECG below:

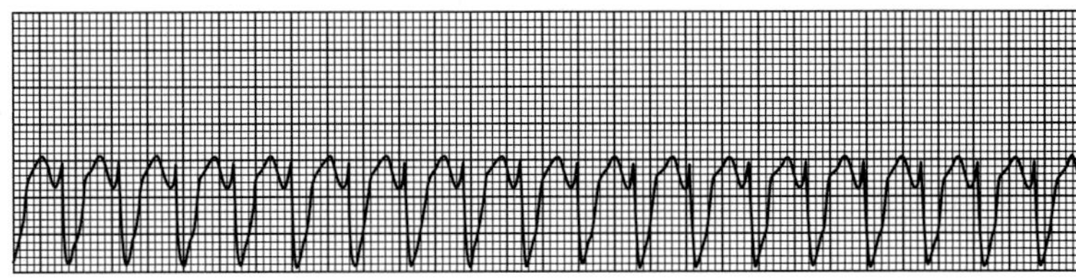

a. supraventricular tachycardia
b. ventricular tachycardia
c. torsades de pointe
d. normal sinus rhythm

16. Interpret the ECG below:

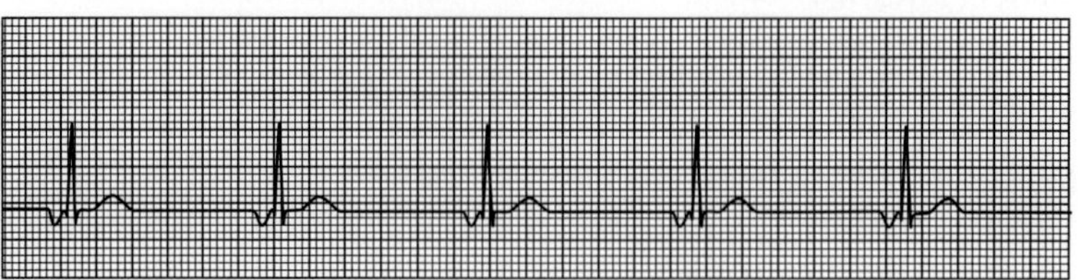

a. junctional rhythm
b. sinus bradycardia
c. atrial arrest
d. none of the above

17. Interpret the ECG below:

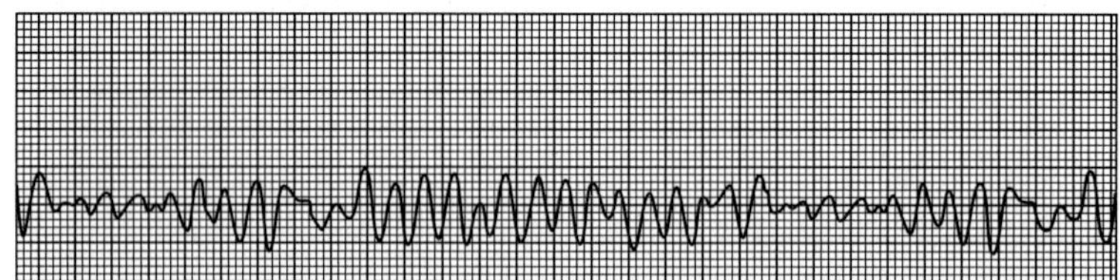

a. supraventricular tachycardia
b. ventricular tachycardia
c. ventricular fibrillation
d. normal sinus rhythm

18. Interpret the ECG below:

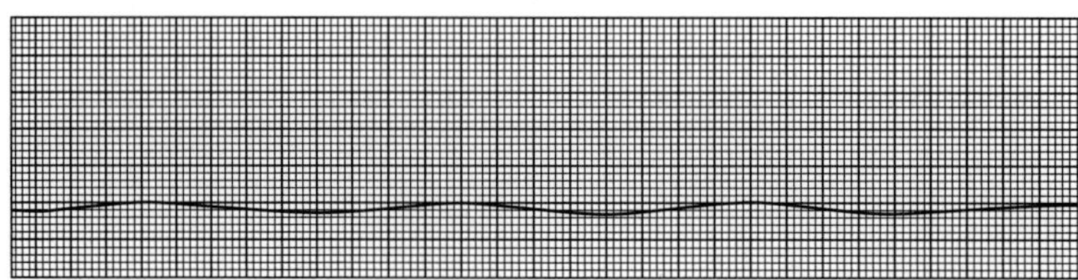

a. supraventricular tachycardia
b. ventricular tachycardia
c. ventricular fibrillation
d. asystole

19. Interpret the ECG below:

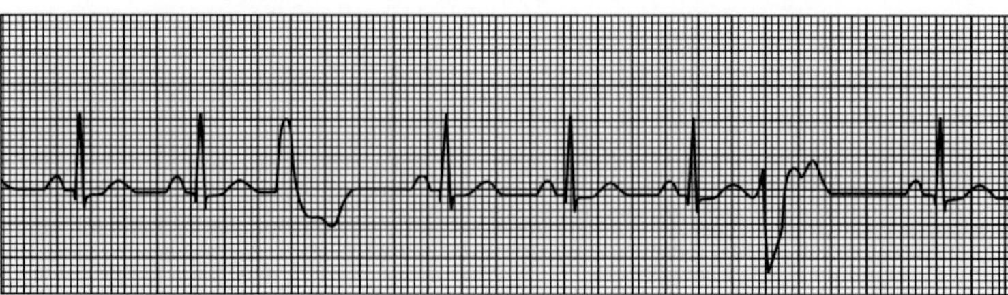

a. junctional rhythm
b. sinus bradycardia
c. atrial arrest
d. sinus rhythm with multifocal premature ventricular contractions (PVCs)

20. Interpret the ECG below:

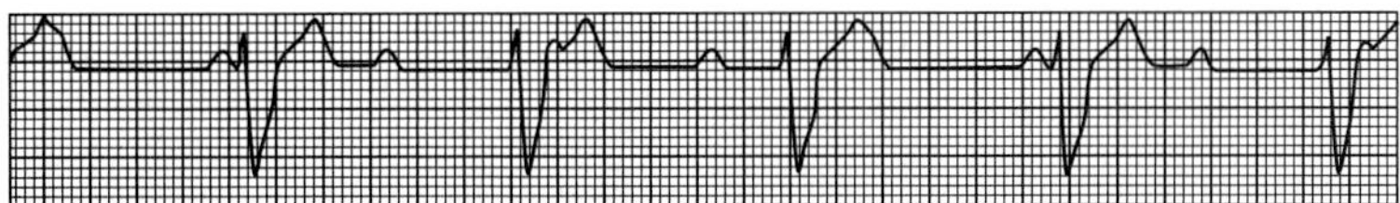

a. first degree heart block
b. second degree heart block (Wenckebach)
c. third degree heart block
d. second degree heart block (Mobitz type-II)

21. Interpret the ECG below:

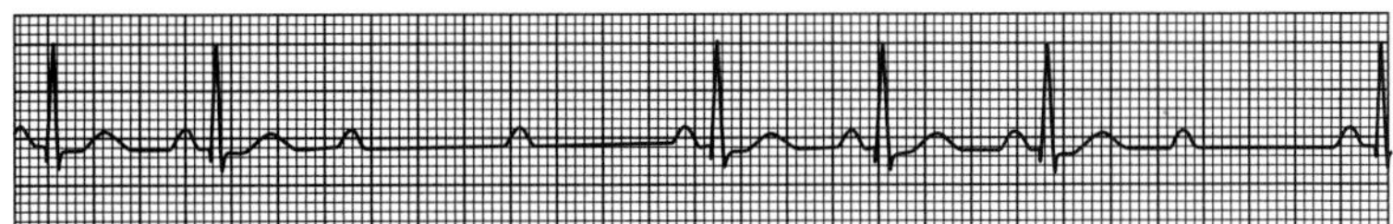

a. first degree heart block
b. second degree heart block (Wenckebach)
c. third degree heart block
d. second degree heart block (Mobitz type-II)

22. You have successfully intubated your patient and your partner has been performing bag-valve-mask ventilation for the past few minutes when she tells you the bag is becoming harder to squeeze. You notice distended jugular veins and cyanosis. Upon auscultation, the right chest is silent, and the left has diminished sounds. What do you do immediately?
a. Insert an oropharyngeal airway as a bite block
b. Extubate the patient
c. Decompress the right chest with a large bore catheter
d. Perform a cricothyrotomy

23. Your patient is a 69-year-old male who presents sitting at the kitchen table in moderate respiratory distress. His elbows are on the table allowing him to be seated in a tripod position, and he appears to be really working at breathing. Although this problem came on gradually today, his family states that he has had lung disease for a long time. He is a lifetime smoker and is on home oxygen at 2-L/min via nasal cannula. He takes the following medications:
• Atrovent MDI
• Theolair (theophylline)
• Proventil MDI
He appears very thin and barrel chested with a pink complexion. You immediately notice pronounced accessory muscles in his neck and chest along with retractions. He labors to breathe, pursing his lips during exhalation. His vital signs are pulse 90 regular, blood pressure (BP) 140/80, respiratory rate (RR) of 40 labored, skin is warm and pink, diffuse wheezes, and his SpO2 is 90%.
Your prehospital presumptive diagnosis is:
a. asthma
b. congestive heart failure
c. chronic bronchitis
d. emphysema

24. The landmark for needle decompression is:

a. third intercostal space, midaxillary line

b. sixth intercostal space, midclavicular line

c. second intercostal space, midclavicular line

d. second intercostal space, midaxillary line

25. After locating the second intercostal space, midclavicular line, you insert the catheter:

a. above the second rib

b. below the second rib

c. above the third rib

d. none of the above

26. Signs and symptoms of cyanide poisoning may include odor or taste of bitter or burnt almonds (40% of population cannot detect odor), extreme difficulty in breathing, cyanosis (extremely late sigh), cardiac arrhythmias, seizures, altered mental status, and cardiac arrest.

a. True

b. False

27. When administering drugs via the endotracheal (ET) tube:

a. the patient should be hyperventilated

b. CPR must be halted

c. the patient should be hyperventilated after drug administration, and cardiopulmonary resuscitation (CPR) should be resumed

d. all of the above

28. All of the following drugs may be administered via the ET tube except:

a. lidocaine

b. epinephrine

c. albuterol

d. atropine

e. naloxone

29. You are treating a patient who is a 54-year-old male, complaining of crushing substernal chest pain, radiating to his left neck and down his left arm, for the past 20 minutes. The patient presents with a BP of 124/80, a heart rate (HR) of 84, respirations of 12, with cool, clammy skin, nausea, and vomiting. Your presumptive diagnosis is that the patient is experiencing a/an:

a. acute myocardial infarction

b. flulike symptoms

c. exacerbation of chronic obstructive pulmonary disease [COPD]

d. cardiogenic shock

30. Your patient is a 70-year-old female, found sitting in a chair, complaining of sudden onset of shortness of breath. The patient presents with a BP of 240/130, HR of 110, with respirations of 40 and labored; denies chest pain, nausea, or vomiting. The patient's lung sounds reveal bilateral rales 1/3 from the bases and expiratory wheezes over remaining lung fields. The patient is cool, pale, and extremely diaphoretic. This patient is most likely suffering from:

a. exacerbation of COPD

b. acute myocardial infarction

c. acute pulmonary edema

d. chronic asthma

31. Your patient is a 72-year-old male, found lying on a bed, complaining of severe difficulty breathing. The patient presents with a BP of 200/120, with a HR of 120, respiratory rate of 36, rales 2/3 full, and is cool, pale, and diaphoretic. The patient has a history of CHF. The patient is placed on oxygen, and an IV is established. The medication of choice is:

a. NTG 1/150 g SL

b. magnesium sulfate 2 g IVB

c. lidocaine 1.5 mg/kg IVB

d. atropine 1.0 mg IVB

32. The solution concentration of albuterol sulfate is:

a. 0.83%

b. 0.083%

c. 1.0%

d. 0.1%

33. Diphenhydramine (Benadryl) should be used in caution for patients suffering:

a. severe allergic reaction

b. dystonic reaction

c. extra pyramidal reaction

d. closed angle glaucoma

34. When an ambulance crew is assigned or happens upon a scene where the release of hazardous materials (haz-mat) or the use of weapons of mass destruction (WMD) is suspected, and the crew has not been contaminated, the ambulance crew should:

a. remain on-scene and contain any contaminated victims

b. immediately withdraw to a safe distance upwind

c. isolate crew and unit, and await decontamination instructions

d. establish a staging, triage, and mobilization center

35. For pediatric patients, the correct position to maintain the optimal airway is age dependent.

a. True

b. False

36. Oxygen should always be provided at high concentration with pediatric patients and should be humidified when possible.

a. True

b. False

37. The criterion for the definition of an MCI is not primarily dependent upon the number of patients.

a. True

b. False

38. All of the following are accepted routes of administration for pharmacological agents except:

a. intravenous

b. intraoccular

c. intramuscular

d. oral

39. The fastest route of administration, where the drug goes directly to the target organ, is:

a. intravenous

b. intramandibular

c. subcutaneous

d. oral

40. The preferred site for intramuscular (IM) administration in the field is:

a. quadriceps muscles

b. gluteus muscle

c. trapezoid muscle

d. deltoid muscle

41. Subcutaneous administration occurs:

a. in a muscle of the target site

b. in a vein

c. under the skin in connective tissue

d. in the alveoli

42. Which of the following is an example of drug administration via inhalation?

a. 10–15 L/min oxygen in a nonrebreather mask

b. 1/150 grain nitroglycerin sublingual

c. 50 cc of 25% dextrose, bolus

d. 10 cc epinephrine, 1/10,000 bolus

43. All of the following drugs can be administered via the endotracheal route except:

a. narcan

b. valium

c. adenosine

d. epinephrine

44. One kilogram is equal to _____ pounds.

a. 1.2

b. 0.12

c. 0.22

d. 2.2

45. The volume to administer equals the desired dose (grams, milligrams, or micrograms) divided by the concentration of medication.

a. True

b. False

46. In a microdrip infusion set, _____ is equal to _____ drops/minute.

a. 0.1 cc, 6

b. 1.0 cc, 60

c. 0.5 cc, 30

d. all of the above

47. Medications affect the _______________ nervous system, which affects the patient.

a. parasympathetic

b. sympathetic

c. both a and b

d. none of the above

48. Acetylcholine is the main neurotransmitter of the __________ nervous system in the pre- and postganglion spaces.

a. parasympathetic
b. sympathetic
c. both a and b
d. none of the above

49. Norepinephrine and epinephrine are the main neurotransmitters of the ________ nervous system.

a. parasympathetic
b. sympathetic
c. both a and b
d. none of the above

50. The "fight or flight" mechanism of the sympathetic nervous system results in:

a. decreased BP
b. dilated pupils
c. decreased pulse rate
d. all of the above

51. The initial assessment is a chronological search for and the immediate correction of life-threatening problems.

a. True
b. False

52. The correct order of assessment priorities in the initial assessment are:

a. circulation, breathing, airway/c-spine, disability, expose, and examine
b. airway, breathing, circulation, c-spine, expose, and examine
c. airway/c-spine, breathing, circulation, disability, expose, and examine
d. none of the above

53. Air exchange is best assessed by:

a. looking, listening, and feeling for air exchange at the mouth and nose
b. watching very closely for any movement of the chest wall
c. holding a mirror over the mouth and checking for condensation
d. asking family members if there is a history of respiratory illness

54. The most common cause of airway obstruction in the unconscious patient is:

a. pulmonary edema
b. congestive heart failure
c. foreign bodies
d. the tongue

55. Other causes of airway obstruction (besides the most common cause) may be due to:

a. facial trauma
b. inhaled or ingested substances
c. oropharyngeal trauma
d. all of the above

56. The swelling of tissues or injury to the airway structures may be a result of:
a. trauma
b. a severe allergic reaction
c. illness
d. all of the above

57. You respond to a call that involves a motor vehicle accident with injuries. Your patient is unconscious and unresponsive. You would open this patient's airway by utilizing:
a. the head-tilt-chin lift maneuver
b. the prone (face down) method
c. the hyperextension of the head and neck method
d. the modified jaw thrust method

58. Which of the following is *not* an airway adjunct?
a. BVM with oxygen reservoir
b. Endotracheal tube
c. Nasopharyngeal airway
d. Seizure "bite stick"

59. Which of the following "pulse sites" is *not* to be used for the assessment of the presence of a pulse during CPR? (Consider *all* patient categories.)
a. Carotid artery
b. Pedal artery
c. Brachial artery
d. Femoral artery

60. The "V" in the "AVPU" scale of the neurological examination stands for:
a. vice addictive
b. voice commands are followed
c. the fact that the patient responds to verbal stimulus
d. the fact that the patient is alert and oriented

61. The objective secondary survey includes which of the following?
a. Inspection, palpation, auscultation and percussion
b. Looking for anything abnormal
c. Pertinent negatives
d. All of the above

62. A blood pressure may be taken only after examination of the extremity rules out any contraindication of such an action.
a. True
b. False

63. An ECG detects:
a. the mechanical action of the heart
b. imminent respiratory arrest or compromise
c. when a myocardial infarction is about to occur
d. none of the above

64. Obtaining the "chief complaint" is completed in what part of the patient assessment?
a. During the initial assessment
b. During the taking of vital signs

c. During the secondary, subjective assessment
d. None of the above

65. The nasal cannula is best utilized with an oxygen flow rate set at:
a. 10–12 L/min to deliver 90% inspired oxygen concentration
b. 2–6 L/min to deliver 25–40% inspired oxygen concentration
c. 1–2 L/min to deliver 50% inspired oxygen concentration
d. 15 L/min to deliver 100% inspired oxygen concentration

66. Proper use of the nonrebreather oxygen mask includes:
a. inflating the resevoir bag *prior* to patient application
b. using a 3–6 L/min flow rate
c. inflating the resevoir bag *after* patient application
d. using a demand-valve positive pressure device to inflate the resevoir bag

67. Which of the following airway adjuncts is the best, ideal airway for the acutely intoxicated, unconscious patient?
a. Oropharyngeal airway (OPA)
b. Nasopharyngeal airway (NPA)
c. Endotracheal tube (ETT)
d. Esophageal gastric tube airway (EGTA)

68. Shock is defined as
a. an electrical disruption of tissues
b. an inadequate perfusion of oxygen to the tissues
c. a temporary loss of consciousness
d. blood loss of one pint or less

69. Shock involves a sympathetic reflex in which continuous blood flow to the coronary and cerebral circulatory systems is increased or maintained. Based on this fact, which of the following statements is correct?
a. Arterioles dilate in most parts of the body
b. The veins and venous reservoirs constrict
c. Heart activity decreases dramatically
d. The veins and venous reservoirs dilate

70. In nonprogressive shock, the compensatory mechanisms involved that attempt to return blood volume back to normal include:
a. baroreceptor reflexes
b. water and salt conservation by the kidneys
c. increased thirst mechanism
d. all of the above

71. In progressive shock, a vicious cycle occurs resulting in:
a. a progressive increase in cardiac output
b. vasomotor improvement
c. a progressive decrease in cardiac output
d. an increase in coronary blood flow

72. After shock has progressed to a certain stage, transfusion or any other type of therapy becomes ineffective. This stage is referred to as

a. anaphylactic shock

b. septic shock

c. irreversible shock

d. compensated shock

73. Which of the following signs/symptoms are *not* found in the early phases of shock?

a. Restlessness, apprehension

b. Decreased systolic blood pressure

c. Strong, rapid pulse

d. Pallor

74. Which of the following signs/symptoms are *not* found in the late stages of shock?

a. Strong, rapid pulse

b. Metabolic acidosis

c. Hyperventilation

d. Weak, thready pulse

75. Cardiogenic shock occurs when a percentage of functioning myocardial tissue is lost. This critical mass of myocardial tissue that is lost must be at least __________ or more of the total myocardial mass of the heart in order for cardiogenic shock to occur.

a. 5%

b. 10%

c. 20%

d. 35%

76. Even with the best treatment possible, the mortality rate for patients in cardiogenic shock is approximately:

a. 25%

b. 35%

c. 50%

d. 85%

77. Treatment of cardiogenic shock includes all of the following except:

a. fluid challenges

b. the use of vasopressors (dopamine, dobutamine)

c. control of pain and apprehension

d. maintenance of an adequate airway and oxygenation

78. The average adult male has approximately ________ L of circulating blood volume.

a. 30

b. 20

c. 10

d. 5

79. Mild hemorrhage (class I) is usually defined by a blood loss of ____________.

a. 1000 cc

b. 750 cc

c. 250 cc

d. 100 cc

80. Moderate hemorrhage (class II) is usually defined by a blood loss of __________.

a. 1000–1250 cc

b. 750 cc

c. 250 cc

d. 100 cc

81. Clinical manifestations of severe hypovolemia (blood loss of 1500–1800 cc) include all of the following except:

a. tachypnea

b. hypotension

c. widened pulse pressure

d. decreased urinary output

82. The fluid treatment for severe hypovolemia includes:

a. colloidal infusions

b. crystalloid infusions

c. neither a nor b

d. both a and b

83. Hypotension, tachycardia, itching hives, and difficulty breathing are reliable signs that the patient is in ____________ shock.

a. septic

b. neurogenic

c. cardiogenic

d. anaphylactic

84. A critical incident stress debriefing should occur ________ after the incident.

a. <12 hours

b. 12–24 hours

c. immediately

d. 24–72 hours

85. The triple-layered sac which surrounds and protects the heart is the:

a. epicardium

b. pericardium

c. endocardium

d. myocardium

86. Blood which has collected carbon dioxide and wastes from the coronary circulation drains into the:

a. coronary sinus

b. coronary vein

c. coronary artery

d. coronary sulcus

87. Parasympathetic control of the heart occurs through the:

a. cardiac plexus

b. thoracic nerve

c. vagus nerve

d. trigeminal nerve

You arrive on the scene at the local bar and find a 22-year-old female patient who is agitated and confused. Her airway is open and she is breathing. Her blood pressure is 240/180 mmHg. Her radial pulse is present and bounding and the respiratory rate is 32 bpm. Her blood glucose is 82 mg/dL. Her skin is slightly pale, cool, and clammy. Her pupils are equal and reactive but sluggish to respond to light. The pulse oximeter reading is 86%. The monitor shows a sinus tachycardia at 128 bpm, with an occasional unifocal premature ventricular contraction.

Questions 88 through 91: Answer based on the scenario above.

88. The agitation and confusion experienced by the patient is most likely due to:
a. hypoglycemia
b. hypotension
c. hypoxia and hypercarbia
d. sympathetic nervous system discharge

89. Your priority treatment for this patient should be:
a. administration of oxygen via nonrebreather mask
b. administration of 25g of 50% Dextrose
c. administration of 0.4 mg of Narcan
d. intubate the patient with a tracheal tube

90. Upon further assessment, you note bilateral rales in all lung fields. The patient is becoming more agitated and confused. It is likely the patient is suffering from:
a. aspiration pneumonia
b. an asthma attack with exacerbation
c. chronic hypertension with cor pulmonale
d. acute pulmonary edema secondary to hypertensive crisis

91. As you continue your assessment and treatment, one of the bar patrons admits that he and the patient were doing drugs. Which of the following drugs may cause this type of presentation in a patient?
a. Talwin
b. Cocaine
c. Heroin
d. Ruffanol

92. The primary goal in the management of the traumatic-brain-injured patient in the prehospital environment is to:
a. reduce the intracranial blood pressure as quickly as possible
b. maintain the systolic blood pressure and prevent hypotension
c. decrease hypertensive states
d. reduce the extra-cellular fluid volume

93. The best method to correct metabolic acidosis in the prehospital setting is to:
a. ensure a patent airway and provide positive ventilation with 100% oxygen
b. administer sodium bicarbonate every 5 minutes at 1 mEq/kg
c. administer oxygen via a nasal cannula at 4 L/min
d. administer lactated Ringer's with a buffer agent

94. You encounter a patient suffering from a significant pneumothorax. You would expect a(n) __________ PaO_2 and a(n) __________ $PaCO_2$.
a. decreased, increased
b. increased, decreased

c. increased, increased
d. decreased, decreased

95. The outer layer of the pleural space is referred to as:
a. visceral
b. parietal
c. humoral
d. effusional

96. Failure of the vasomotor center will result in which type of shock?
a. Hypovolemic
b. Obstructive
c. Distributive
d. Cardiogenic

97. In a patient with severe chronic lung disease (such as COPD), the main stimulus for breathing is:
a. hypoxia
b. acidosis
c. hypercapnia
d. alkalosis

Questions 98 through 103: Match the following phases of the infectious process with their respective definitions.
a. Exposure to appearance of symptoms
b. Onset of symptoms to resolution
c. Cannot transmit infectious agent
d. Exposure to seroconversion
e. Creation of antibodies
f. Transmission of infectious agent is possible

98. Latent period

99. Communicable period

100. Incubation period

101. Seroconversion

102. Window phase

103. Disease period

104. You arrive at the scene of a fall. You find a 42-year-old woman lying on the ground under a ladder. She says she fell a couple of feet. She is complaining of pain in her ankle. Which of the following components of the initial assessment are you unable to determine from the information given?
a. General impression
b. Airway
c. Breathing
d. Transport priority

105. You have just delivered an infant. The baby is limp with central cyanosis. There is no apparent respiratory effort. You should:

a. begin basic life support resuscitation immediately

b. withhold resuscitation for one minute so the Apgar score can be used to guide your efforts

c. give oxygen by blow-by, but withhold other resuscitative measures until a 1-minute Apgar score can be determined

d. position, dry, warm, suction, and stimulate the infant, but withhold other resuscitation until a 1-minute Apgar score can be determined

106. Which of the following memory aids would be used to solicit a medical history from an asthmatic patient?

a. AVPU

b. SOAP

c. SAMPLE

d. ICE

107. The National Highway Act charged the______with developing an emergency medical services (EMS) system and upgrading prehospital emergency care.

a. Department of Transportation

b. American Red Cross

c. Department of Health and Human Services

d. State EMS Agencies

108. In hypoperfusion caused by dehydration, oxygen deprivation at the cellular level results in:

a. respiratory acidosis

b. respiratory alkalosis

c. metabolic acidosis

d. metabolic alkalosis

109. During an overnight shift on advanced life support (ALS) Ambulance 7, you're dispatched to a suicide attempt. On arrival, you find a 33-year-old female who took an unknown amount, but possibly up to 60 tablets (0.5 mg/each), of clonazepam 30 minutes before calling 911. She has also consumed alcohol tonight. A physical exam reveals her to be somnolent (drowsy) but arousable, and she has an intact gag reflex.

Vital signs: BP 120/palpation; pulse 90; RR 12; O_2 sat 95% on room air.

What is your primary treatment goal?

a. Maintaining a patent airway

b. Establishing an IV, and administer fluid boluses

c. Administering nalaxone 2.0 mg IV or IM

d. None of the above

110. The diameter of the endotracheal tube for an average adult is:

a. 9.0–11.0 mm

b. 5.0–7.0 mm

c. 7.0–9.0 mm

d. 2.5–5.0 mm

111. Homeostatic mechanisms are regulated through which of the following?

a. Hypothalamus

b. Adrenal glands

c. Kidneys and lung
d. All of the above

112. Which of the following is one of the "six" rights of medication administration?
a. The right container
b. The right doctor
c. The right route
d. The right pharmacy

113. An example of the enteral route of drug administration is:
a. sublingual
b. intravenous
c. subcutaneous
d. topical

114. Buccal administration of a drug is accomplished:
a. by nasal spray
b. through a newborn's umbilical vein or artery
c. between the cheek and gum
d. through an intraosseous needle

115. A liquid form of a drug prepared using an alcohol extraction process is called a/an:
a. solution
b. tincture
c. emulsion
d. spirit

116. How many grams of dextrose are contained in a 500 mL bag of D_5W?
a. 5
b. 10
c. 100
d. 25

Questions 117 through 121: Match the term with the definition.
a. Proventil
b. Drug used to treat high cholesterol
c. Antidote for organophosphate poisoning
d. Secreted from the beta cells in the pancreas
e. Beta-2 medication used for asthma treatment

117. Atropine
118. Terbutaline
119. Insulin
120. Antihyperlipidemics
121. Beta2 Medication

122. The predominant extracellular cation is:
a. calcium (Ca^{+2})
b. magnesium (Mg^{+2})
c. sodium (Na^{+})
d. potassium (K^{+})

123. The primary cause for ketoacid production in a hyperglycemic patient is:
a. glycogen metabolism
b. carbohydrate metabolism
c. fat metabolism
d. none of the above

124. You respond to a 28-year-old male, unconscious, and gasping for breath on the ground next to a lawnmower. Neighbors report that he has suffered multiple bee stings. He has obvious airway swelling, and his tongue is protruding from his mouth. He is deeply cyanotic. Vital signs: heart rate of 40 and blood pressure of 50 by palpation. What is your primary drug of choice for treating this patient?
a. Oxygen
b. Epinephrine
c. Atropine
d. Proventil

125. An obese 58-year-old female presents with upper right quadrant abdominal pain that worsens after meals, nausea, and vomiting. The most likely cause of these signs and symptoms is:
a. appendicitis
b. cholecystitis
c. tubal pregnancy
d. pancreatitis

126. A 46-year-old male is having difficulty breathing, is diaphoretic, and complains of tightness in his chest. Upon your arrival, his level of consciousness is decreased. Which one of the following is *least* likely to be the cause of his signs and symptoms?
a. Myocardial infarction
b. Severe asthma attack
c. Hypoglycemia
d. Spontaneous pneumothorax

127. A common sign/symptom of cardiovascular compromise in anaphylaxis is:
a. hypotension
b. diaphoresis
c. hypertension
d. bradycardia

128. The primary reason for performing the Sellick's maneuver during endotracheal intubation is to:
a. prevent regurgitation
b. decrease dead air space
c. avoid having to hyperextend the neck
d. make intubation easier

129. One small box on ECG paper equals:
a. 0.20 seconds
b. 0.02 seconds
c. 0.04 seconds
d. 0.40 seconds

130. When the core temperature of the body drops below ______, an individual is considered to be hypothermic.

a. 99°F

b. 98.6°F

c. 97°F

d. 95°F

131. An 89-year-old female presents with multiple bruises on her face and upper extremities. She lives with her son, who tells you that the patient is always falling down and is just generally clumsy. The patient appears malnourished and frightened. She cowers when you approach and is reluctant to allow you to examine her. Her son seems to be hostile toward you and your partner and nervously attempts to explain each bruise. In this case you should do all of the following except:

a. obtain a complete patient and family history

b. report suspicions of elder abuse to the emergency department staff

c. be honest and open with the patient's son about your concerns

d. listen carefully for inconsistencies in stories

132. The constructive or "building up" phase of metabolism is called:

a. catabolism

b. aerobolism

c. anabolism

d. ionolism

133. The term "status epilepticus" refers to:

a. a chronic seizure patient taking anticonvulsant medication regularly

b. a generalized seizure lasting more than 1 minute

c. two or more seizures with no intervening periods of consciousness

d. a patient experiencing a seizure for the first time

134. A stroke caused by the gradual development of a blood clot in a cerebral artery is called a/an:

a. thrombotic stroke

b. embolic stroke

c. hemorrhagic stroke

d. aneurism

135. The most common psychiatric disorder among geriatric patients is:

a. schizophrenia

b. paranoia

c. depression

d. posttraumatic stress disorder

136. A dopamine drip is ordered at 5 mcg/kg/minute. You are to set up your IV drip by injecting 400 mg of dopamine into a 500 mL IV bag of normal saline. You are using a standard microdrop administration set. The patient weighs 176 lb. What is the patient's weight in kilograms?

a. 100 kg

b. 70 kg

c. 50 kg

d. 80 kg

137. The acronym SLUDGE is helpful in remembering the effects of cholinergic medication. The effects include:

a. sedation

b. lactation

c. urination

d. dilation

138. A 99-year-old nursing home patient is found to have severe pedal edema. His neck veins are flat. No adventitious sounds are present in the lung fields. There is no abdominal distension. The patient reportedly spends 12–14 hours a day sitting in front of the TV with his feet in a dependent position. The edema of his ankles and feet probably results from:

a. right-sided heart failure

b. immobility and the dependent position of his feet

c. liver disease

d. left-sided heart failure

139. How many milligrams are in a gram?

a. 10

b. 100

c. 1,000

d. 10,000

140. A patient is to receive 1 L of normal saline over 6 hours. The IV set delivers 20 drops/mL. What is the infusion rate?

a. 37 drops per minute

b. 100 drops per minute

c. 56 drops per minute

d. 33 drops per minute

141. Capnography depicts respiration.

a. True

b. False

142. Normal range for ETCO2 is:

a. 30–40 mmHg

b. 35–45 mmHg

c. 45–50 mmHg

d. 55–60 mmHg

143. Monitoring $ETCO_2$ during resuscitation can alert EMS professionals to a return of spontaneous circulation.

a. True

b. False

144. Oxygenation is the process of getting oxygen into the body and to the tissues for metabolism.

a. True

b. False

145. Pulse oximetry cannot be used to measure ventilation.

a. True

b. False

146. Capnography is used to measure oxygenation.

a. True

b. False

147. The most common cause of burn injury is:

a. chemical

b. scald

c. contact

d. thermal

148. A 5 ft 6 in., 210 lb, 64-year-old male business executive had a physical exam prior to his retirement from corporate work. His blood pressure was >180/115 on three separate days. Further examination showed normal to low plasma renin activity, elevated total peripheral resistance (TPR), cardiac output (CO) of 7.2 L/min, x-ray evidence of left ventricular hypertrophy, retinal hemorrhages, and mild polyuria. Recommended therapy was weight reduction to his ideal level, a low-salt diet (<2 g/day sodium), prudent exercise, and a reduction in alcohol consumption (<3 oz whiskey/day). This change in lifestyle did little to change the condition. Medication was initiated in the form of an oral diuretic and progressed to a beta-blocker; eventually a vasodilator was included to reduce the blood pressure to <140/90.

What is the prehospital diagnosis for this individual?

a. Uncontrolled hypertension

b. Controlled hypertension

c. Diabetes mellitus

d. Myocardial infarction

149. An HbCO level of 40–60% results in:

a. death

b. confusion, ataxia, hallucinations, coma

c. headache, decreased function

d. nausea, irritability

150. A patient who has been diagnosed with hypokalemia with serum levels below 3 mEq/L usually shows an ECG with ____________ of the ST segment.

a. depression

b. elevation

c. narrowing

d. widening

151. You have just delivered an infant. The baby is limp with central cyanosis. There is no apparent respiratory effort. You should:

a. begin basic life support resuscitation immediately

b. withhold resuscitation for one minute so the APGAR score can be used to guide your efforts

c. give oxygen by blow-by, but withhold other resuscitative measures until a 1-minute APGAR score can be determined

d. position, dry, warm, suction, and stimulate the infant, but withhold other resuscitation until a 1-minute APGAR score can be determined

152. In the presence of a myocardial infarction (MI), a positive creatinine phosphokinase (CPK)-MB is present.
 a. True
 b. False

153. Subgroups of the population at increased risk for burn injuries are:
 a. infants and patients older than 60
 b. infants and toddlers
 c. toddlers and teenagers
 d. teenagers and young adults

154. Transient headache, postural syncope, and hypotension are side effects of what medication?
 a. Lidocaine
 b. Atropine
 c. Nitroglycerine
 d. Amiodorone

155. Patients who have suffered high-voltage injuries are at risk for:
 a. myoglobin release, damaging the kidneys
 b. brain injury due to increasing intracranial pressure
 c. hidden inhalation injuries
 d. fluid overload if too much fluid is given quickly

156. A 57-year-old man summons EMS because he has had "crushing" chest pain for the past half hour with no relief at rest. He describes the pain as 7/10, radiating to his left arm, and states he is nauseous. His wife states he came into the house looking very "gray." When asked what he was doing before the chest pain occurred she states, "He was shoveling snow." Interpret the 12-lead ECG below:

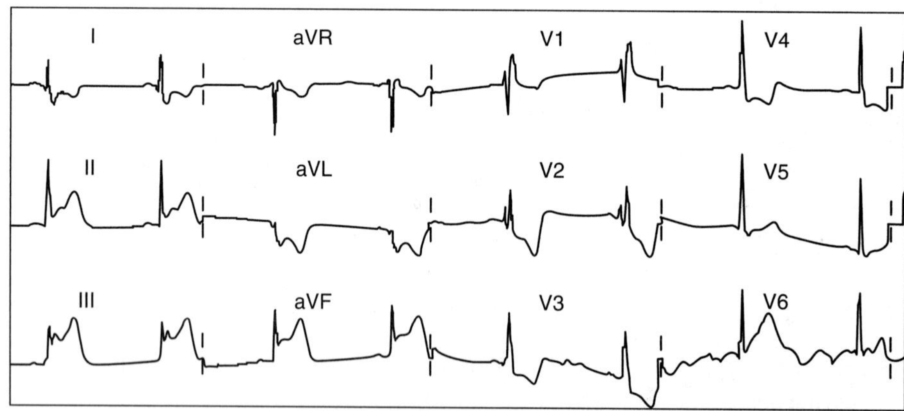

 a. pericarditis
 b. acute inferior wall MI
 c. anterior wall MI
 d. hypokalemia

157. One kilogram is equal to:
 a. 1.2 lb
 b. 12 lb
 c. 22 lb
 d. 2.2 lb

158. The volume to administer equals the desired dose divided by the concentration of medication.

a. True

b. False

159. In a microdrip infusion set, _____ is equal to _____ drops per minute.

a. 0.1 cc, 6

b. 1.0 cc, 60

c. 0.5 cc, 30

d. all of the above

160. Medications affect the _______________ nervous system, which thus affects the patient.

a. parasympathetic

b. sympathetic

c. both a and b

d. none of the above

161. Acetylcholine is the main neurotransmitter of the _______________ nervous system.

a. parasympathetic

b. sympathetic

c. both a and b

d. none of the above

162. Norepinephrine and epinephrine are the main neurotransmitters of the ____________ nervous system.

a. parasympathetic

b. sympathetic

c. both a and b

d. none of the above

163. The best indication of brain perfusion is:

a. pupillary response

b. pulse rate

c. mental status

d. skin color

164. The ____________________ nervous system originates in the cranial nerves and sacral spinal chord.

a. parasympathetic

b. sympathetic

c. both a and b

d. none of the above

165. Vasoconstriction of arteries and mild bronchoconstriction in the lungs are the effects of ___________ adrenergic receptors.

a. beta

b. delta

c. gamma

d. alpha

166. Vasodilatation of arteries, bronchodilation in the lungs, and increased myocardial rate and force of contraction are the effects of _____________ adrenergic receptors.
a. beta
b. delta
c. gamma
d. alpha

167. All of the following are effects of the parasympathetic nervous system except:
a. decreased force of atrial contraction
b. bronchial constriction
c. increased heart rate
d. increased defecation

168. Atropine sulfate is considered:
a. a parasympathomimetic drug
b. a parasympathetic blocker
c. a parasympatholytic drug
d. both b and c

169. Atropine sulfate is indicated for which of the following conditions?
a. Symptomatic bradycardia
b. Asystole
c. Organophosphate poisoning
d. All of the above

170. The correct dosage of atropine for organophosphate poisoning patients is:
a. 0.1- to 0.2-mg bolus initially, repeat as necessary
b. 2.0- to 5.0-mg bolus initially, every 10–15 minutes, repeat as necessary
c. 2.0-g bolus not to be repeated
d. 1.0- to 2.0-mg bolus, repeat as necessary

171. The indications for calcium chloride are:
a. acute myocardial infarction
b. digitalis intoxication
c. acute hypocalcemia
d. none of the above

172. 50% dextrose contains:
a. 25 mg of dextrose in 50 cc of water
b. 25 g of dextrose in 50 cc of water
c. 50 mg of dextrose in 50 cc of water
d. 50 g of dextrose in 50 cc of water

173. Diazepam (Valium) is:
a. a minor tranquilizer
b. a CNS depressant
c. an anticonvulsant
d. all of the above

174. Indications for diazepam include all of the following except:

a. to calm a suicidal patient that is threatening to take his/her life

b. to "break" status epilepticus

c. to induce amnesia during synchronized cardioversion

d. acute alcohol withdrawal

175. Dopamine, at low dosages:

a. stimulates beta and dopaminergic receptors, increasing inotropic action and renal mesenteric dilation

b. causes increased heart rate

c. causes vasoconstriction and decreased renal flow

d. is contraindicated in cardiogenic shock

176. Which solution would tend to stay in the vascular space *longest* in treating a hypovolemic patient?

a. Lactated Ringer's solution

b. D_5W

c. $D_{10}W$

d. Half normal saline

177. The cool and pale skin assessed in a patient with hypoperfusion (shock) results from:

a. loss of thermoregulatory mechanisms

b. vasovagal response

c. generalized vasoconstriction

d. blood being shunted from the arms

178. Blood returning to the left side of the heart from the lungs usually has concentrations which, compared to blood in the right side of the heart, are:

a. higher pO_2 and pCO_2 concentrations

b. lower in both concentrations of pO_2 and pCO_2

c. lower pO_2 and higher pCO_2

d. higher pO_2 and lower pCO_2

e. none of the above

179. Interpret the ECG below:

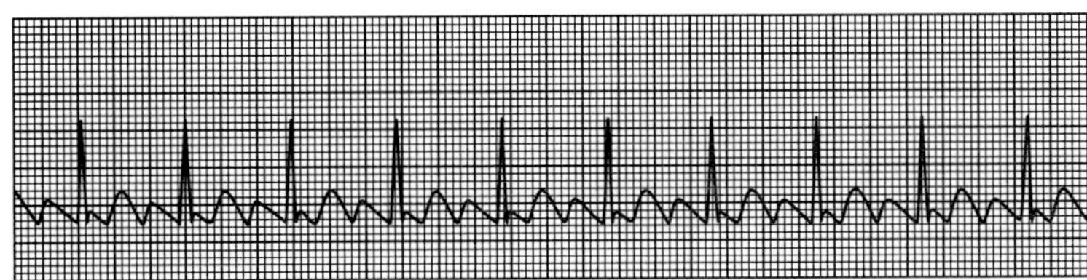

a. atrial flutter

b. atrial fibrillation

c. second degree heart block type II

d. none of the above

180. Interpret the ECG below:

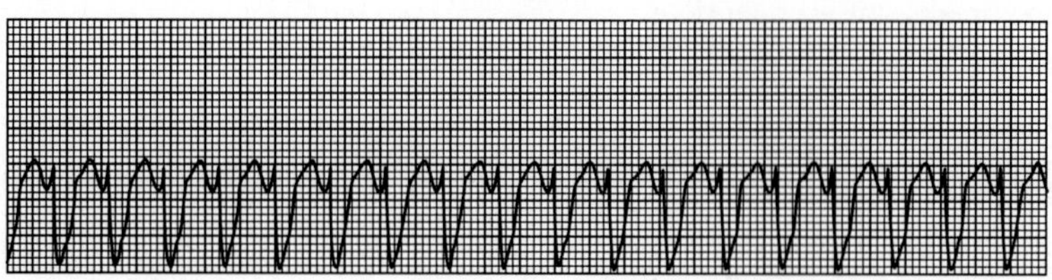

a. atrial flutter
b. atrial fibrillation
c. second degree heart block type II
d. ventricular tachycardia

PRACTICE EXAM ANSWERS

1. **The correct answer is f.** The QT interval is measured from the beginning of the QRS complex to the end of the T-wave. A normal QT does not usually exceed 0.42 seconds.

2. **The correct answer is a.** The P-wave is normally seen before the QRS complex at a consistent interval.

3. **The correct answer is e.** The T-wave appears after the QRS complex.

4. **The correct answer is c.** Each component of the waveform has a specific connotation. The initial negative deflection is a Q-wave, the initial positive deflection is an R-wave, and the negative deflection after the R-wave is an S-wave. Not all QRS complexes have all three components, even though the complex is commonly referred to as the QRS complex.

5. **The correct answer is b.** The interval is measured from the beginning of the P-wave to the beginning of the QRS complex. A normal PR interval is 0.12–0.20 seconds.

6. **The correct answer is d.** Normally it is isoelectric at baseline, but may be elevated or depressed in a variety of conditions.

7. **The correct answer is b.**
   - Rhythm—Regularly irregular
   - Rate—Normal or slow
   - QRS duration—Normal
   - P-wave—Ratio 1:1 for 2, 3, or 4 cycles then 1:0
   - P-wave rate—Normal but faster than QRS rate
   - P-R interval—Progressive lengthening of P-R interval until a QRS complex is dropped

8. **The correct answer is a.**
   - Rhythm—Regular
   - Rate—Normal
   - QRS duration—Normal
   - P-wave—Ratio 1:1
   - P-wave rate—Normal
   - P-R interval—Prolonged (>5 small squares)

9. **The correct answer is c.**
   - Rhythm—Regular
   - Rate—Around 110 beats per minute
   - QRS duration—Usually normal
   - P-wave—Replaced with multiple F (flutter) waves, usually at a ratio of 2:1 (2F—1QRS) but sometimes 3:1
   - P-wave rate—300 beats per minute
   - P-R interval—Not measurable

10. The correct answer is a.

- Rhythm—Irregularly irregular
- Rate—Usually 100–160 beats per minute but slower if on medication
- QRS duration—Usually normal
- P-wave—Not distinguishable as the atria are firing off all over
- P-R interval—Not measurable
- The atria fire electrical impulses in an irregular fashion causing irregular heart rhythm.

11. The correct answer is c.

- Rhythm—Regular
- Rate—140–220 beats per minute
- QRS duration—Usually normal
- P-wave—Often buried in preceding T-wave
- P-R interval—Depends on site of supraventricular pacemaker
- Impulses stimulating the heart are not being generated by the sinus node, but instead are coming from a collection of tissue around and involving the atrioventricular (AV) node.

12. The correct answer is d.

- Rhythm—Regular
- Rate—More than 100 beats per minute
- QRS duration—Normal
- P-wave—Visible before each QRS complex
- P-R interval—Normal
- The impulse generating the heartbeats are normal, but they are occurring at a faster pace than normal. Seen during exercise.

13. The correct answer is b.

- Rhythm—Regular
- Rate—Less than 60 beats per minute
- QRS duration—Normal
- P-wave—Visible before each QRS complex
- P-R interval—Normal
- Usually benign

14. The correct answer is a.

- Rhythm—Regular
- Rate—60–100 bpm
- QRS duration—Normal
- P-wave—Visible before each QRS complex
- P-R interval—Normal (<5 small squares. Anything above and this would be first degree block.)
- Indicates that the electrical signal is generated by the sinus node, and is traveling in a normal fashion within the heart.

15. The correct answer is b.

- Rhythm—Regular
- Rate—180–190 beats per minute
- QRS duration—Prolonged
- P-wave—Not seen

- Results from abnormal tissues in the ventricles generating a rapid and irregular heart rhythm. Poor cardiac output is usually associated with this rhythm causing the patient to go into cardiac arrest. Defibrillate this rhythm if the patient is unconscious and without a pulse.

16. The correct answer is a.
- Rhythm—Regular
- Rate—40–60 beats per minute
- QRS duration—Normal
- P-wave—Ratio 1:1 if visible; Inverted in lead II
- P-wave rate—Same as QRS rate
- P-R interval—Variable

17. The correct answer is c.
- Rhythm—Irregular
- Rate—300+, disorganized
- QRS duration—Not recognizable
- P-wave—Not seen
- This patient needs to be defibrillated!!

18. The correct answer is d.
- Rhythm—Flat
- Rate—0 beats per minute
- QRS duration—None
- P-wave—None

19. The correct answer is d.
- Rhythm–Regular
- Rate—Normal
- QRS duration—Normal
- P-wave—Ratio 1:1
- P-wave rate—Normal and same as QRS rate
- P-R Interval—Normal
- Also you'll see two odd waveforms, these are the ventricles depolarizing prematurely in response to a signal within the ventricles. (Unifocal PVCs look alike; if they differed in appearance they would be called multifocal PVCs, as seen above.)

20. The correct answer is c.
- Rhythm—Regular
- Rate—Slow
- QRS duration—Prolonged
- P-wave—Unrelated
- P-wave rate—Normal but faster than QRS rate
- P-R interval—Variation
- Complete AV block. No atrial impulses pass through the atrioventricular node, and the ventricles generate their own rhythm.

21. The correct answer is d.
- Rhythm—Regular
- Rate—Normal or slow
- QRS duration—Prolonged

- P-wave—Ratio 2:1, 3:1
- P-wave rate—Normal but faster than QRS rate
- P-R Interval—Normal or prolonged but constant

22. **The correct answer is c.** The patient is exhibiting signs of a tension pneumothorax.
23. **The correct answer is d.** Current signs and extensive past smoking history.
24. **The correct answer is c.**
25. **The correct answer is c.**
26. **The correct answer is a.**
27. **The correct answer is d.**
28. **The correct answer is c.**
29. **The correct answer is a.**
30. **The correct answer is c.**
31. **The correct answer is a.**
32. **The correct answer is b.**
33. **The correct answer is d.**
34. **The correct answer is b.**
35. **The correct answer is a.**
36. **The correct answer is a.**
37. **The correct answer is a.**
38. **The correct answer is b.**
39. **The correct answer is a.**
40. **The correct answer is d.**
41. **The correct answer is c.**
42. **The correct answer is a.**
43. **The correct answer is b.**
44. **The correct answer is d.**
45. **The correct answer is b.**
46. **The correct answer is d.**
47. **The correct answer is c.**
48. **The correct answer is a.**
49. **The correct answer is b.**
50. **The correct answer is b.**
51. **The correct answer is a.**

52. The correct answer is c.
53. The correct answer is a.
54. The correct answer is d.
55. The correct answer is d.
56. The correct answer is d.
57. The correct answer is d.
58. The correct answer is a.
59. The correct answer is b.
60. The correct answer is c.
61. The correct answer is d.
62. The correct answer is a.
63. The correct answer is d.
64. The correct answer is a.
65. The correct answer is b.
66. The correct answer is a.
67. The correct answer is c.
68. The correct answer is b.
69. The correct answer is b.
70. The correct answer is d.
71. The correct answer is c.
72. The correct answer is c.
73. The correct answer is b.
74. The correct answer is c.
75. The correct answer is d.
76. The correct answer is d.
77. The correct answer is a.
78. The correct answer is d.
79. The correct answer is c.
80. The correct answer is b.
81. The correct answer is c.
82. The correct answer is d.
83. The correct answer is d.
84. The correct answer is d.

85. **The correct answer is b.**

86. **The correct answer is a.** Coronary sinus carries deoxygenated blood from the walls of the heart to the right atrium.

87. **The correct answer is c.**

88. **The correct answer is c.**

89. **The correct answer is a.**

90. **The correct answer is d.**

91. **The correct answer is b.**

92. **The correct answer is c.**

93. **The correct answer is a.**

94. **The correct answer is a.**

95. **The correct answer is b.**

96. **The correct answer is c.**

97. **The correct answer is a.**

98. **The correct answer is c.**

99. **The correct answer is f.**

100. **The correct answer is d.**

101. **The correct answer is e.**

102. **The correct answer is a.**

103. **The correct answer is b.**

104. **The correct answer is d.**

105. **The correct answer is a.**

106. **The correct answer is c.**

107. **The correct answer is a.**

108. **The correct answer is c.**

109. **The correct answer is a.**

110. **The correct answer is c.**

111. **The correct answer is d.**

112. **The correct answer is c.**

113. **The correct answer is a.**

114. **The correct answer is c.**

115. **The correct answer is d.**

116. **The correct answer is d.**

117. **The correct answer is c.**

118. The correct answer is e.

119. The correct answer is d.

120. The correct answer is b.

121. The correct answer is a.

122. The correct answer is c.

123. The correct answer is c.

124. The correct answer is b.

125. The correct answer is b.

126. The correct answer is c.

127. The correct answer is c.

128. The correct answer is a.

129. The correct answer is c.

130. The correct answer is d.

131. The correct answer is c.

132. The correct answer is c.

133. The correct answer is c.

134. The correct answer is b.

135. The correct answer is c.

136. The correct answer is d.

137. The correct answer is c. SLUDGE stands for salivation, lacrimation, urination, defecation, GI upset, and emesis.

138. The correct answer is b.

139. The correct answer is c.

140. The correct answer is c.

141. The correct answer is a.

142. The correct answer is b.

143. The correct answer is a.

144. The correct answer is a.

145. The correct answer is a.

146. The correct answer is b.

147. The correct answer is d.

148. The correct answer is a.

149. The correct answer is a.

150. The correct answer is a.

151. The correct answer is a.

152. The correct answer is a.

153. The correct answer is a.

154. The correct answer is c.

155. The correct answer is a.

156. The correct answer is b.

157. The correct answer is d.

158. The correct answer is a.

159. The correct answer is b.

160. The correct answer is c.

161. The correct answer is a.

162. The correct answer is b.

163. The correct answer is c.

164. The correct answer is a.

165. The correct answer is d.

166. The correct answer is a.

167. The correct answer is c.

168. The correct answer is d.

169. The correct answer is d.

170. The correct answer is b.

171. The correct answer is c.

172. The correct answer is b.

173. The correct answer is d.

174. The correct answer is a.

175. The correct answer is a.

176. The correct answer is a. The crystalloid of choice is normal saline or lactated Ringer's solution because its osmolality is similar to that of the intravascular volume.

177. The correct answer is c.

178. The correct answer is d.

179. The correct answer is a.

180. The correct answer is d.

INDEX

Page numbers followed by *f* or *t* indicate figures or tables, respectively.

E

H

I

J

K

L

M